Atlas of CLINICAL OPHTHALMOLOGY

A **Slide Atlas of Ophthalmology** based on material in this book is available. In the slide atlas format, each of the twenty chapters in the book is presented in a vinyl binder together with labelled and numbered 35mm colour transparencies of each illustration. Each volume contains a list of abbreviated slide captions for easy reference when using the slides. The complete set of slide atlas volumes is contained in a durable presentation slip case. The complete Slide Atlas of Ophthalmology contains a total of 1175 slides, many of which are composite mounts of multiple photographs.

Volume 1	Methods of Ocular Examination	60 slides
Volume 2	The Eyelids	59 slides
Volume 3	The Conjunctiva: Diseases and Tumours	60 slides
Volume 4	Infections of the Outer Eye	56 slides
Volume 5	Allergic Eye Diseases: Episcleritis and Scleritis	60 slides
Volume 6	The Cornea	60 slides
Volume 7	Primary Glaucoma	59 slides
Volume 8	Secondary Glaucoma	57 slides
Volume 9	The Uveal Tract	54 slides
Volume 10	Intraocular Inflammation	59 slides
Volume 11	The Lens	56 slides
Volume 12	Vitreous and Vitreo-Retinal Disorders	60 slides
Volume 13	The Retina: Normal Anatomy and Physical Signs	60 slides
Volume 14	The Retina: Vascular Disease I	58 slides
Volume 15	The Retina: Vascular Disease II	60 slides
Volume 16	The Retina: Macular Diseases and Retinal Dystrophies	60 slides
Volume 17	The Optic Disc	60 slides
Volume 18	Strabismus	59 slides
Volume 19	Neuro-Ophthalmology	60 slides
Volume 20	The Orbit and Lacrimal System	58 slides

Further information may be obtained from:

Gower Medical Publishing Ltd.,
34-42 Cleveland Street,
London W1P 5FB, England

Editors

D. J. Spalton F.R.C.S., M.R.C.P.

Consultant Ophthalmic Surgeon
Consultant Ophthalmologist
Medical Eye Unit
St. Thomas's Hospital
London, U.K.

R. A. Hitchings F.R.C.S.

Consultant Ophthalmic Surgeon
Director Glaucoma Unit
Moorfields Eye Hospital
London, U.K.

P. A. Hunter F.R.C.S.

Consultant Ophthalmic Surgeon
King's College Hospital
London, U.K.

Atlas of CLINICAL OPHTHALMOLOGY

Churchill Livingstone · Edinburgh · London · New York

Gower Medical Publishing · London · New York

Distributed in all countries except USA, Canada and Japan by:
Churchill Livingstone,
Robert Stevenson House,
1–3 Baxter's Place
Leith Walk,
Edinburgh EH1 3AF, UK

Distributed in the USA and Canada by:
J.B. Lippincott Company,
East Washington Square,
Philadelphia, PA. 19105, USA

Distributed in Japan by:
Nishimura Co. Ltd.,
1–754–39, Asahimachi-dori,
Niigata-Shi 951, Japan

ISBN 0-443-03115-0 (Churchill Livingstone)
      0-906923-23-9 (Gower)

Library of Congress Catalog Card Number – 83-080646

British Library Cataloguing in Publication Data

Atlas of Clinical Ophthalmology

1. Eye—Diseases and defects—Atlases
I. Spalton, David J.   II. Hitchings, R.A.
III. Hunter, P.A.
617.7'0022'2   RE71

ISBN 0-906923-23-9

        Project Editors: Marinella Nicolson
                         Steven Cameron

Design and Artwork: Mick Brennan
                    Pam Corfield
                    Julian Dorr
                    Madeleine Hall
                    Lydia Malim
                    Lynda Payne
                    Jeremy Rose
                    Karen Stafford

Re-printed with minor corrections in Italy by Imago Publishing Ltd, 1986

Foreword

Most of us regard the eye and visual system as the paramount sensory system of the body. Not only does the ocular system act as the main receptor connecting us to the outer world, but study of the eye provides numerous clues to the functioning of the entire body. No other organ is as accessible to study, nor is there another site where such precise subjective and objective measurements can be made. Assuming these statements are essentially correct, why is ophthalmology, which deals with the eye and its parameters in both health and disease, so poorly understood by non-ophthalmologists? Perhaps it is because medical school curricula now tend to concentrate on the burgeoning basic sciences, leaving little or no time for students to immerse themselves into the world of the so-called clinical specialities. Could anything be more relevant to all physicians than a solid understanding of vision and the organ system responsible for capturing the speedy, weightless light beam and converting it into the seeing world? The basic medical training of today does not provide medical practitioners with sufficient knowledge to do more than a cursory examination at best and, at worst, leads doctors to fear the eye as some ultra delicate organ they will not properly view or treat. Furthermore, the instrumentation used by eye doctors seems quite foreign and the terminology seems to stump all but the most erudite generalist. Thus, it is no wonder that misconceptions and barriers have arisen which tend to isolate ophthalmology and its practitioners from "mainstream" medical practice.

With this in mind, I commend you to this atlas. Mr. Spalton, his colleagues and the publishers have spared neither expense nor intelligence in producing this volume. It will go a long way to correct the inadvertent mystery that has grown up around a field which, after all, depends upon illumination and openness. The book seems to have been conceived to lay open to every student the "hidden" empire of ophthalmology. Here, in beauteous color, one can see a panoply of the field; instruments, terms, diseases and concepts fully illustrated and accompanied by succinct word capsules. The combination is an awesome one guaranteed to enchant and educate.

This is a big book, but ophthalmology is a vast field. This volume should be required reading for those who know little of ophthalmology and also for those who think they know everything. For the former it will be a foundation stone of inestimable value and for the latter, a touchstone useful for teaching colleagues and patients the nuances of the eye in health and disease.

P. Henkind, New York, 1984

Preface

We hope that this atlas will be used as an introduction to clinical ophthalmology and that for this purpose it will establish itself as an illustrated reference work. Its aim is to provide a high quality and carefully selected collection of colour illustrations to show the type of clinical material which is encountered in general ophthalmological practice. The interpretation of clinical signs and their clinical implications has been emphasised by reference to the relevant embryology, anatomy, physiology and pathology. More rare and esoteric material is included where this is necessary to illustrate a particular point of interest. We have also tried to stress the need to look on the eye as a complete organ and, as so often is the case, as a reflection of disease elsewhere.

We do not intend this book to be used as a textbook in isolation but hope that it will prove useful in conjunction with the standard textbooks on each subspeciality, which generally contain so few illustrations. Detailed references are inappropriate in an atlas of this sort as we feel that the reader is better served by consulting the recognized textbooks for further reading, or details of therapy, and, therefore, a broad bibliography is given at the end of the book.

The gathering of such a diverse collection of photographic material has been a major undertaking which has only been made possible by the help and generosity of numerous friends and colleagues for which we must express our sincere thanks.

D.J. Spalton
R.A. Hitchings
P.A. Hunter

London 1984

Contents

P. A. J. Moriarty F.R.C.S.
Royal Victoria Eye and Ear Hospital
Dublin, Ireland
R. A. Hitchings F.R.C.S.
Moorfields Eye Hospital
London, U.K.

J. R. O. Collin F.R.C.S.
Moorfields Eye Hospital
London, U.K.

P. A. Hunter F.R.C.S.
King's College Hospital
London, U.K.

P. A. Hunter F.R.C.S.
King's College Hospital
London, U.K.

P. A. Hunter F.R.C.S.
King's College Hospital
London, U.K.
P. G. Watson F.R.C.S.
Addenbrookes Hospital, Cambridge, U.K.,
and Moorfields Eye Hospital,
London, U.K.

R. J. Buckley F.R.C.S.
Moorfields Eye Hospital
London, U.K.

R. A. Hitchings F.R.C.S.
Moorfields Eye Hospital
London, U.K.

R. A. Hitchings F.R.C.S.
Moorfields Eye Hospital
London, U.K.

D. J. Spalton F.R.C.S., M.R.C.P.
St. Thomas's Hospital
London, U.K.

10. Intraocular Inflammation   10.1

D. J. Spalton F.R.C.S., M.R.C.P.
St. Thomas's Hospital
London, U.K.

11. The Lens   11.1

N. A. Phelps Brown F.R.C.S.
Nuffield Laboratory of Ophthalmology
Oxford, U.K., and
Radcliffe Hospital
Oxford, U.K.

12. Vitreous and Vitreo-Retinal Disorders   12.1

D. McLeod F.R.C.S.
Moorfields Eye Hospital
London, U.K.

13. The Retina: Normal Anatomy and Physical Signs   13.1

D. J. Spalton F.R.C.S., M.R.C.P.
St. Thomas's Hospital
London, U.K.
J. Marshall, Ph.D
Institute of Ophthalmology
London, U.K.

14. The Retina: Vascular Diseases I   14.1

D. J. Spalton F.R.C.S., M.R.C.P.
St. Thomas's Hospital
London, U.K.
J. S. Shilling F.R.C.S.
St. Thomas's Hospital
London, U.K.
T. J. ffytche F.R.C.S.
Moorfields Eye Hospital, London, U.K. and
St. Thomas's Hospital, London, U.K.

15. The Retina: Vascular Diseases II   15.1

J. S. Shilling F.R.C.S.
St. Thomas's Hospital
London, U.K.
D. J. Spalton F.R.C.S., M.R.C.P.
St. Thomas's Hospital
London, U.K.
T. J. ffytche F.R.C.S.
Moorfields Eye Hospital, London, U.K. and
St. Thomas's Hospital, London, U.K.

16. The Retina: Macular Diseases and Retinal Dystrophies   16.1

T. J. ffytche F.R.C.S.
Moorfields Eye Hospital, London, U.K. and
St. Thomas's Hospital, London, U.K.
D. J. Spalton F.R.C.S., M.R.C.P.
St. Thomas's Hospital
London, U.K.
J. S. Shilling F.R.C.S.
St. Thomas's Hospital
London, U.K.

17. The Optic Disc 17.1

D. J. Spalton F.R.C.S., M.R.C.P.
St. Thomas's Hospital
London, U.K.
M. D. Sanders F.R.C.S., M.R.C.P.
St. Thomas's Hospital
London, U.K., and
National Hospital for Nervous Diseases,
London, U.K.

18. Strabismus 18.1

P. Fells F.R.C.S.
Moorfields Eye Hospital
London U.K.
J. P. Lee F.R.C.S., M.R.C.P.
Institute of Ophthalmology
London, U.K.

19. Neuro-Ophthalmology 19.1

D. J. Spalton F.R.C.S., M.R.C.P.
St. Thomas's Hospital
London, U.K.

20. The Orbit and Lacrimal System 20.1

D. J. Spalton F.R.C.S., M.R.C.P.
St. Thomas's Hospital
London, U.K.
J. E. Wright F.R.C.S., M.D.
Moorfields Eye Hospital
London, U.K.

1. Methods of Ocular Examination

P. A. J. Moriarty

R. A. Hitchings

Introduction

The different methods of assessing ocular structure and function are discussed in this chapter. The first section deals with different aspects of vision: acuity, colour and fields. The second section will illustrate the optical and non-optical means of examining the ocular structures.

The methods illustrated are by no means comprehensive but have been selected to illustrate points of principle or the essentials of basic ocular examination. More specialised techniques will be described in subsequent chapters dealing with the relevant topics.

THE PHYSIOLOGY OF VISUAL ACUITY

The measurement of visual acuity is the essential first part of any ocular examination and although the examination technique is simple, the process being measured is complex and requires the interaction of many factors, both physiological and psychological. During the test a target must be detected by the visual apparatus and resolved into its component parts. This information is then transmitted to the cerebral cortex where it is matched against existing memory shapes and the patient must then signal recognition of the target to the examiner.

Visual acuity is a measure of the capability of the visual system to resolve a target and this resolution is dependent upon three main factors; the background illumination, the target illumination and the visual angle the target subtends at the nodal point of the eye.

Background Illumination

Background illumination alters the level of retinal adaptation. Low light levels stimulate the rod system; the receptor density and level of retinal integration of this system are less than that of the cones, and consequently acuity is also low. At high levels of illumination the cone system is stimulated and acuity is maximal.

To obtain the best visual acuity, illumination should be kept in the optimal photopic range. Due to the effect of reduction of retinal illumination by lens opacities, cataract patients may be seeing in the mesopic to low photopic range where the acuity is proportional to background illumination. In these patients an increase in the ambient lighting will give them better vision provided light scatter by the cataract does not counter this.

Fig. 1.1 This graph shows visual acuity plotted against background illumination. The best acuity in the scotopic (rod sensitive) area of the curve is 20/200, whereas under photopic (cone sensitive) conditions this increases to 20/13. The curve flattens once optimal conditions are reached and then reduces (not shown) due to the effects of dazzle.

In clinical work the best visual acuity is sought with illumination kept at the upper photopic levels, and under these conditions visual acuity is a measure of cone function. This can be shown by comparing the graphs which show cone density and the visual acuity relative to the foveal centre. The curves show a direct relationship between high visual acuity and cone density proving that the anatomical area responsible for maximum visual acuity is the cone bearing part of the retina, the fovea.

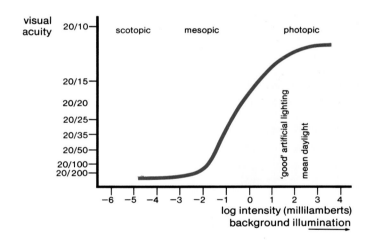

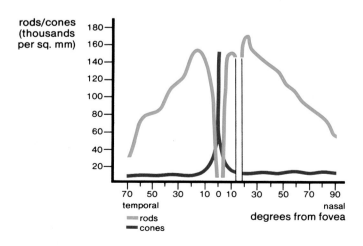

Fig. 1.2 Cone and rod density plotted against degrees from the foveal centre (after Osterberg).

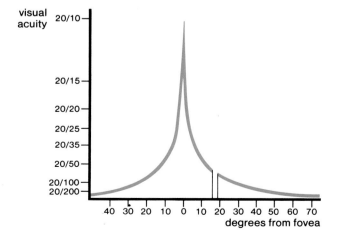

Fig. 1.3 Visual acuity plotted against degrees from the fovea.

Contrast

The eye detects objects by responding to the differing levels of illumination at the target edges, or contrast:

$$\text{contrast} = \frac{\text{background illumination} - \text{target illumination}}{\text{background illumination}}$$

Fig. 1.4 The graph of visual acuity plotted against contrast shows the rapid improvement in acuity as contrast increases, and the difference that background illumination makes to the acuity under the same conditions of contrast. The upper curve is plotted at a higher background illumination than the lower curve. As contrast increases the two merge and the illumination difference becomes irrelevant. Marked above the curves are the contrast ranges of clinical test material and normal printed materials such as newsprint. From this, one can see that patients may see more clearly under test conditions using high contrast typeface than they do at home, where ambient lighting may also be reduced.

In clinical acuity tests black letters are displayed on a white background giving a contrast value of approximately 80%. In the normal eye under photopic conditions the threshold contrast is about 1%.

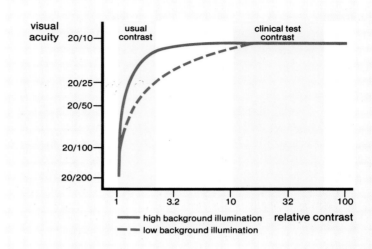

Visual Angle

Fig. 1.5 All objects in the visual field subtend an angle at the nodal point of the eye called the visual angle. Visual resolution can be expressed as the visual angle at which the components of an object can be resolved. Experimentally, the smallest detectable line subtends 0.5″ of arc, or x 0.033 the diameter of a retinal cone, and the contrast is 1% between the stimulated and adjacent receptors. Detection of this target is a function of "just noticeable contrast" rather than visual resolution.

Clinical tests to determine visual resolution use Snellen letters, as seen here, in which the visual angle subtended by the component parts is 1′ of arc.

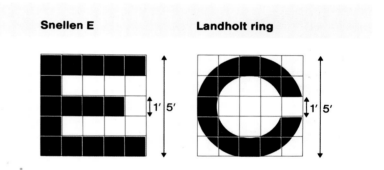

Image Distortion by Optical Aberrations

Fig. 1.6 Light rays passing through the eye are degraded by the inbuilt aberrations of the system, increasing the blur at the margins of images; the loss in edge contrast reduces the resolving power of the visual system. The three main causes of optical degradation are chromatic (top) and spherical aberration (centre) and diffraction (bottom).

The refraction of light varies according to its wavelength (top). It is increased for short wavelengths (blue) and decreased for long wavelengths (red) so that white light tends to be focussed as a coloured blur, and the contrast at the image edge becomes degraded by coloured fringes.

The refractive surfaces of the eye tend to have more effective power at the periphery than at the central paraxial zones. This causes the edge of an image to be blurred by the resulting "line spread" (centre). Spherical aberration increases if the pupil size is larger than 3 mm.

Light projected through an aperture passes through the centre but is absorbed and retransmitted at the edges. The wave fronts of retransmitted light then cause interference patterns which increase the line spread of the image focussed beyond the slit (bottom). Experiments show that diffraction line spread increases if the pupillary aperture is less than 3 mm. Since larger pupillary apertures increase chromatic and spherical aberration the best compromise is achieved with a 2.4 mm diameter pupil; this correlates well with visual acuity plotted against pupil diameter.

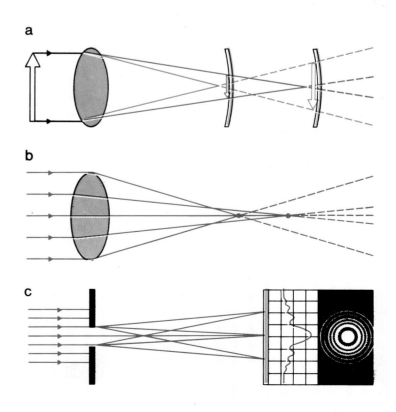

MEASUREMENT OF VISUAL ACUITY
Laser Interference Fringes
Measurement of best retinal acuity has been tried using laser interferometry. This avoids the normal focussing mechanisms of the eye and clinically may give an indication of potential post operative vision in selected cataract patients. It does not work well in very dense opacities and is a difficult technique to explain to older patients. Its best use is in patients with moderate lens opacities, and some retinal disease, in determining whether a reduction in visual acuity is due to retinal or lens changes.

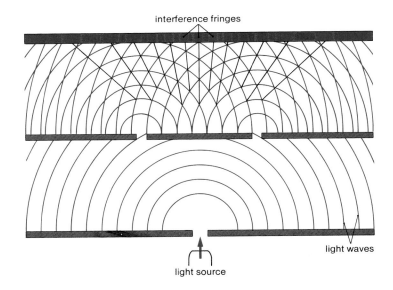

Fig. 1.7 A helium neon laser, of low output, is collimated and split into two beams which are projected into the eye to focus at a point just behind the lens. The wave fronts from the two beams of light produce interference fringes on the retinal surface visible to the patient. The spatial frequency of the fringes and their orientation may be altered to test the patient's response and visual acuity.

Fig. 1.8 This picture shows the appearance of these fringes of dark and bright red light as seen by the patient. The lower half of the picture shows the images after · distortion with tissue paper (simulating lens opacity). Although the image is degraded the fringe pattern is still visible.

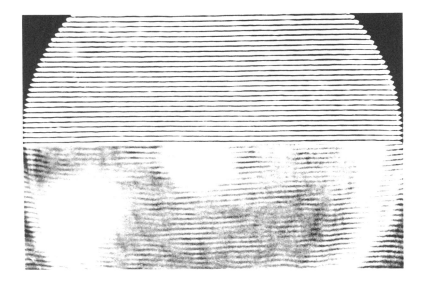

Grating Acuity
In order to resolve the component parts of an object, differences in contrast have to be detected, and clinical tests have been designed to measure this contrast sensitivity. These take the form of light and dark stripes, or gratings, which reflect light in a sine wave pattern and are displayed at variable spatial frequency and contrast values. These patterns can be generated electronically on a T.V. screen or graphically as on a clinical test card. The spatial frequency of the stripes increases along the horizontal axis from left to right and their contrast value decreases in moving up the vertical axis. As the frequency of the stripes increases towards the minimum resolvable

acuity (30−40 cycles/s, or 1−0.7′ of arc), contrast between the stripes decreases. The highest resolvable frequency can only be seen with high contrast; above this the grating appears grey because the contrast is no longer sufficient to resolve the stripes. As the grating frequency reduces there is insufficient contrast to distinguish the stripes from the background illumination.

Patients who have had optic neuritis may retain good Snellen acuity but may have a low threshold on the grating tests due to a low contrast sensitivity. This may be apparent to the patient, when acuity in the affected eye is reduced under conditions of low contrast, such as in a fog.

Fig. 1.9 The lines of this clinical test card (left) are most visible near the centre of the chart but disappear on either side.

If grating visibility is plotted on a graph whose axes are contrast and spatial frequency, a bell shaped curve is formed called the "spatial frequency contrast sensitivity function" or, more commonly, the "spatial modulation transfer function". This curve corresponds to the line of grating visibility shown on the clinical test card.

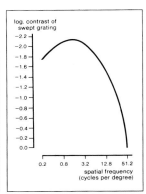

Test Types

Gratings give results close to the best attainable visual acuity, but they are difficult to use clinically and are reserved for research purposes. More commonly, tests of minimum legible acuity are used to measure the resolvable gap between elements of high-contrast type letters. The letters are arranged so that gaps of different visual angles are shown on a decreasing scale. The standard letter, designed by Snellen, when viewed from 20 ft (6 m) subtends an angle of 5′ at the eye and each of the gaps within the letter an angle of 1′ (Fig. 1.5).

Fig. 1.10 Letters were constructed so that they would subtend the same visual angle when viewed at distances up to 200 ft. These letters were then mounted on a card and viewed at 20 ft (6 m). The smallest line of letters which can be resolved by the patient is noted. The test distance is then divided by this line to give a fraction. If the patient sees at 20 ft as far as the 40 ft line, the visual acuity is expressed as:

$$\frac{20 \text{ ft}}{40 \text{ ft}} = \text{visual acuity of } 20/40$$

This can also be measured in metres 6/12, as a fraction 0.5, or as the angle subtended by the smallest gap of the letter, 2′. Normal visual acuity is 20/20, and 20/15 for young adults.

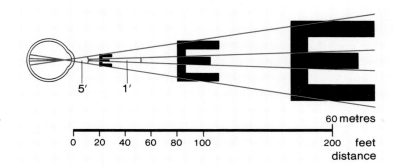

Fig. 1.11 Snellen test types, however, also rely on factors such as literacy and legibility. For example, an L is easier to read than an A. To prevent aberration in the acuity score, individual letters are matched for difficulty against a Landholt broken ring test (Fig. 1.5.), in which the orientation of the gap varies. The score can be compared to that using Snellen letters; any psychological bias can then be eliminated by only using letters of the same Landholt score. Landholt rings can also be used with illiterate patients; alternatively, the patient can be asked to match a cut out letter 'E' with the same letter at different orientations.

Distance visual acuity is tested at 20 ft (6 m) to eliminate complications from presbyopia or accommodation. Near vision is tested by reading test types with appropriate spectacle correction but whilst this is a useful index of visual function, particularly in elderly patients, the correlation with distance acuity is poor. Thus, most patients with an acuity of 20/60 can still manage to read N5 size print.

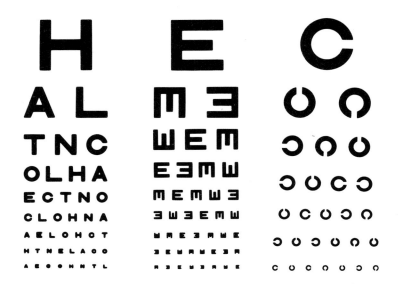

COLOUR VISION

Objects reflect different wavelengths of light and give rise to the sensation of colour. Colour appreciation is a function of cone receptors which respond to light in the visible spectrum; each of the three populations of cones has its own spectral sensitivity range. Different spectral frequencies stimulate each of the cone populations to a different degree so that all colour within the visible spectrum can be matched by differential stimulation.

Colour perception is maximal in the centre of the retina but extends out to 25 or 30 degrees of the visual field. Beyond this, red/green perception disappears and then, in the periphery, all colour perception is absent.

Fig. 1.12 Investigation of the spectral sensitivity curves of the human retina shows peaks at 440-450 nm (blue), 535-555 nm (green) and 570-590 nm (red or yellow). This figure illustrates the way in which the wavelength ranges of the cone sensitivities overlap; the curves have a gentle slope on the high frequency side and a rapid fall off on the lower frequency side, i.e. towards red.

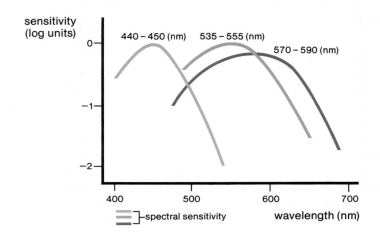

Fig. 1.13 Any colour in the visible range can be matched by a mixture of three reference wavelengths; the intensity of the colour is balanced by the algebraic sums of the intensities of the reference wavelengths. So that:

$$A4\lambda_4 = A1\lambda_1 \text{red} + A2_2\text{green} + A3\lambda_3\text{blue} \quad (A4 = \text{required colour}).$$

A universally accepted reference system for the matching of colours is that set out by the Commission Internationale de l'Éclairage or CIE. This system may be represented by a chromaticity diagram. The three reference wavelengths are 450 nm, 520 nm and 650 nm, and any colour can be matched by varying the luminosity of each wavelength or by the addition of white light.

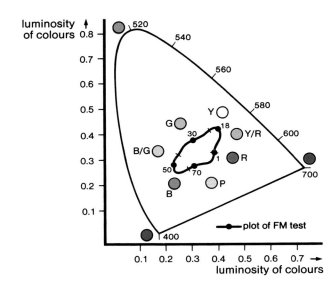

Clinical testing of colour vision

In clinical testing of colour vision there are many types of equipment available. The Farnsworth Munsell "100" hue test and the Ishihara pseudo-isochromatic test plates are most commonly used and will be discussed here.

There are three major groups of colour anomalies, protan deficiency (red), deutan (green), tritan (blue and yellow). Total absence of one population is called anopia, e.g.

protanopia. A relative deficiency is termed an anomaly, e.g. protanomaly. The classification is more complex than this but beyond the scope of the chapter. Patients who have abnormal cone populations will not be able to match some colours visible to a normal patient, but within certain spectral areas they may have normal colour matching.

Fig. 1.14 By plotting colour matches on a CIE chart the anomalous results will show in great detail as can be seen in this diagram where the colour confusion loci are shown for protanomaly. These are lines along which separation of colours is not possible by a patient with red deficiency, but the time taken for this test precludes its use as a clinical method. (This diagram has been overlaid by an FM score sheet from the same patient, see Fig. 1.16. Note the axis of orientation has been rotated so that the colour system of the CIE system and FM test are congruent.)

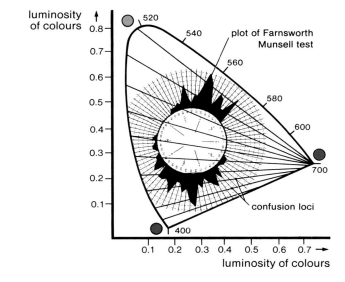

Fig. 1.15 A more useful clinical arrangement is the Farnsworth Munsell test in which a series of coloured tiles, 84 in number, are arranged in 4 separate trays. As one can see in Fig. 1.13, the colour match for each of these tiles can be plotted within the CIE area. In the test the difference between the tiles is graded so that there is one unit of "just noticeable difference" between them and each of the 4 trays covers a different range of the colour spectrum. Trays of tiles are taken one at a time and jumbled; the patient views these under a standard white light and rearranges the tiles in chromatic order between two reference tiles placed at each end of the tray. The misalignment of the tiles from their correct position in the chromatic series is then scored and marked on a standard chart, and the greater the displacement the higher the score.

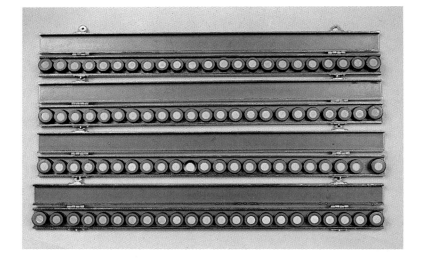

Fig. 1.16 In the normal person there would be only one or two tiles misplaced and the scoresheet would have the appearance of a small circle. In the different colour anomalies, however, the chart becomes distorted along a particular axis. The axis of distortion is typical for a particular colour deficiency, and examples of the axis for protanomaly, deuteranomaly and tritanomaly are shown.

The Farnsworth Munsell scoresheet can be superimposed upon the CIE confusion loci diagram in Fig. 1.14. Here we see that the axis of the scoresheet is tangential to the confusion loci of the CIE diagram. One should note that the Farnsworth Munsell test does not pick up the confusion between colours opposite each other in the circle since these tiles are in different trays and the opportunity for confusion does not arise.

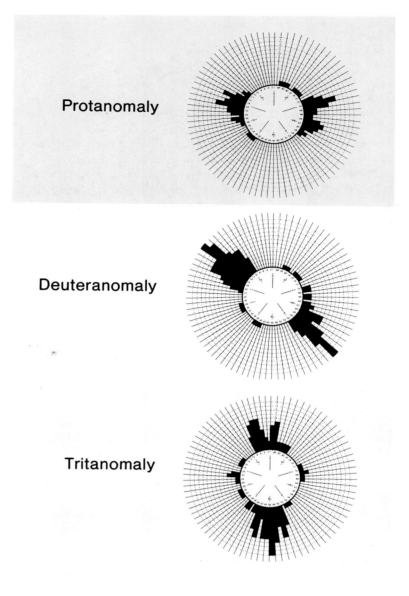

Protanomaly

Deuteranomaly

Tritanomaly

Fig. 1.17 A more rapid test for red/green confusion (which is the commonest colour defect) is the Ishihara pseudo-isochromatic test plates. These are a series of test plates where a matrix of dots are arranged to show a number in the centre. The dots making up the numbers are visible to people of normal colour vision but are confused with adjacent colours by those who are red/green deficient. The colour dots are designed to be isochromatic so that dots making the letters cannot be perceived by contrast difference. A trial and test plate are displayed with and without a green filter. The green filter makes the test number almost disappear but the trial plate number is still easily visible. Apart from congenital colour defects, acquired macula disease tends to produce blue/yellow defects whilst in optic nerve lesions red/green defects appear as an early and important clinical sign, readily elicited with the Ishihara plates (cf. Neuro-Ophthalmology, Chapter 19).

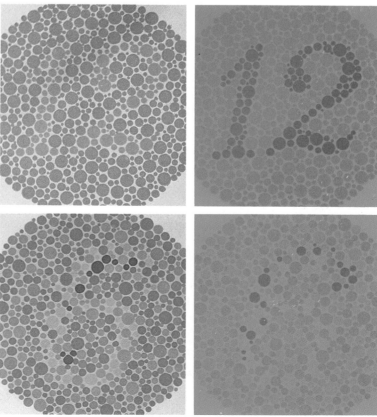

VISUAL FIELDS

The area in space perceived by the eye is called the visual field. The retina has a variable sensitivity and the visual fields are usually plotted to show this. Lines of equal sensitivity, isopters, connect points where a target of the same size and brightness is first perceived.

The area of the visual field depends on the size, brightness and colour of the target and its contrast to background illumination. Psychological factors will influence the patients concentration and good fixation is essential for accuracy. Refractive errors must be corrected when testing the central field, but have little influence on the peripheral fields (outside the central 30° of field). Small pupil sizes (less than 2mm) will simulate constriction of the field area. The visual fields can be tested by many pieces of apparatus, all of either a static or kinetic type, although some instruments have been designed to use both forms of testing. Kinetic perimetry involves the detection of a moving target whilst static perimetry involves the detection of a stationary target of increasing brightness. Sometimes a stationary target cannot be perceived whereas an equivalent moving one can. This is known as the Riddoch phenomenon.

Fig. 1.18 This figure shows a typical visual field as plotted on a Bjerrum tangent screen. The visual field, which is marked off in degrees from the fovea, is not circular but displaced laterally and downwards. The upper and medial limits are approximately 60°, the temporal 100° and the inferior 75°. In the temporal field, the exit of the optic nerve is marked by a blind spot 7.5° in height and 5.5° wide whose centre is 15° from the centre of foveal fixation. Due to the prominence of the brow and nose, there may be artefacts projected onto the field nasally and superiorly which the examiner must be able to correct.

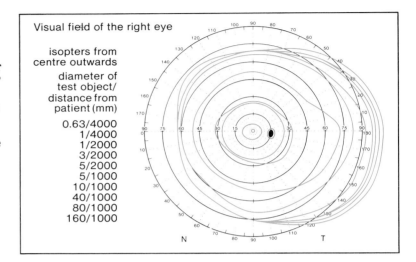

Fig. 1.19 The plot of the visual field isopters can be represented in a three dimensional form called Traquair's Island, in which the isopters appear as contour lines on the island. The visual field and the slope of the field contour is not static but varies with the background illumination. Under mesopic conditions the gradient of sensitivity away from the central area is much more gentle than under photopic conditions where the peripheral retina is desensitized. For this reason it is important that visual field comparisons are made under similar conditions of retinal adaptation.

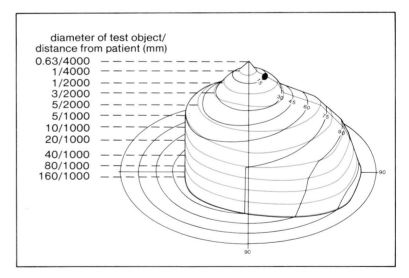

Clinical Visual Field Testing

Fig. 1.20 The fields can be tested by many means. The simplest is by confrontation. The technique involves the examiner sitting opposite the patient with approximately 1 metre distance between them. They cover opposite eyes so that the uncovered eyes have mutually congruent fields. The examiner then introduces a test target into the field (fingers, hatpin, bottlecap) until the target is perceived by the patient. The patient and examiner's fields are congruent, so the presence of a defect is noted by an absence of patient response when the object is visible in the examiner's field. A red target is especially useful for detecting neurological defects in the central field, since the retrobulbar pathways are mainly concerned with macular vision (central 30° of field). With practice a confrontation field can be obtained from almost any patient.

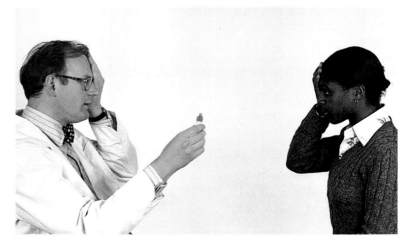

Fig. 1.21 The Goldmann Perimeter (left) is usually used to produce a kinetic field but can be adapted for some basic static perimetry. It is made up of a hemispherical bowl which is uniformly illuminated and onto which are projected target lights of varying size and brightness. Target size, brightness, colour, background illumination and fixation are all controlled.

The patient sits at the machine with the eye to be tested fixed on the centre of the hemisphere (right). Fixation is checked by an observation telescope mounted at the central fixation point. The target lights are then introduced by the projector into the patient's visual field while a pantograph arm moves across a standard recording chart. As the patient signals perception of the spots of light, the examiner marks the chart and eventually builds up an isopter to this particular target. The test is usually undertaken at several isopters of target size and brightness producing a kinetic field which demonstrates the area and density of field loss. A static assessment can be made by flashing the target light within the appropriate isopter.

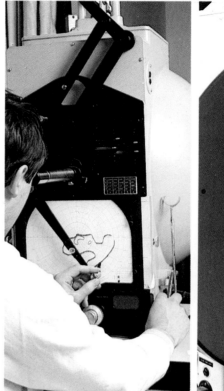
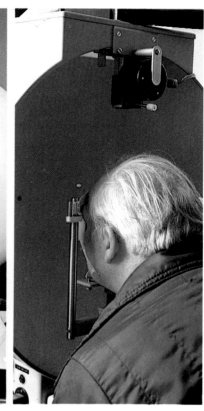

Fig. 1.22 A more rapid assessment of the central 30° field can be obtained by the Friedman Analyser. This is a static perimeter, and consists of a screen with a series of spot targets set in a black background. These spots deliver a flash of light which is of constant size but variable intensity. The screen is illuminated by a standard light source and the patient placed at a 330 mm distance. At the beginning of the test the central macular threshold is established by varying the illumination of a flash seen at fixation. The field test is then run 0.2 log units of light above this and flashes are displayed in set patterns on the field; the threshold illumination, at which each flash is seen, is recorded. On the scoresheet the target dots are left unmarked if the flashes are seen at threshold. If seen at a higher intensity this is recorded, and if not seen at all the particular site is blacked in.

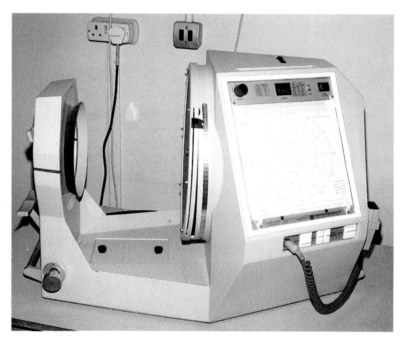

Fig. 1.23 This shows a Friedman field of a patient compared to that obtained on a Goldmann Perimeter. Target size and illumination is recorded on the table at the bottom right hand corner of the Goldmann field. Both tests require good concentration from the patient and a skilled operator, but produce standardized fields for long term follow up. Static perimetry allows itself to be adapted for automated field testing but this does not overcome the need for comprehension and concentration on the part of the patient.

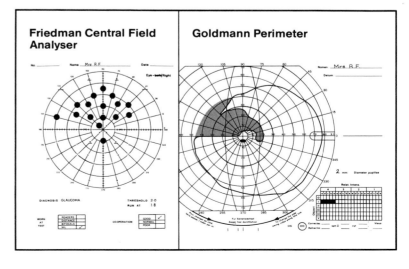

Friedman Central Field Analyser | Goldmann Perimeter

EXAMINATION OF THE EYE
Slit Lamp (Biomicroscope)

The slit lamp consists of a moveable light source and binocular microscope with which to illuminate and view the eye. In its basic form it is used to examine the anterior segment but is easily adapted for the posterior segment.

Fig. 1.24 A slit lamp is seen here (left) together with its optics (right). Light arising from a tungsten filament lamp in the lamp house passes through a condensor to a variable slit mechanism which allows the length and width of the slit to be altered at will. Below this is a tray for various filters to be inserted in the light path. The beam is directed into the eye by a mirror and focussed so that the focal plane is the same as that for the viewing microscope. The microscope incorporates a two stage magnification changer which alters the objective lenses without moving the focal plane. Height and focussing is altered by the use of a joy-stick control. The different ways in which ocular features can be viewed using the slit lamp are illustrated in the following figures.

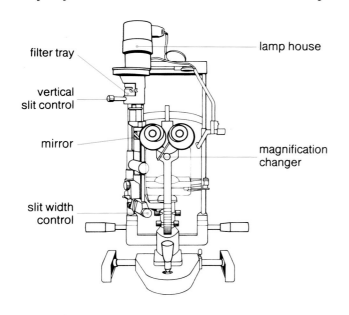

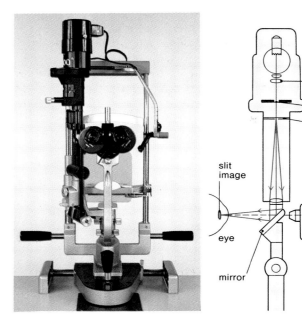

Fig. 1.25 The differences in detail obtained by using full aperture illumination (left) as apposed to that of the slit beam (right) are shown. The slit beam produces a narrow optical section of the anterior segment which throws the various anatomical components into relief. From the slit beam painting one can also see that the anterior vitreous gel is clearly visible using this form of examination.

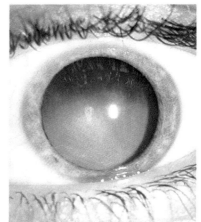
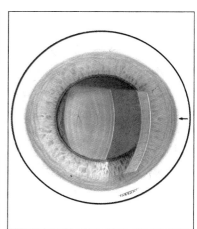

Fig. 1.26 Some features on the eye do not show up well with direct or slit beam illumination and in these cases it is often better to offset the beam of light so that the feature is illuminated by scattered light from the surface of the eye (scleral scatter). This is illustrated here; on the left the blood vessel is illuminated directly by the slit beam (only a narrow portion of it can be seen corresponding to the width of the slit), as compared to the offset beam picture on the right where the vessel is thrown into relief.

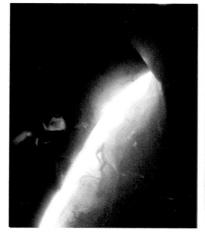
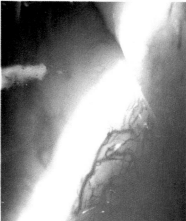

Fig. 1.27 Another form of illumination which highlights special features within the eye is that of retro illumination. On the left, light which has been reflected from the retina and shows as a diffuse red glow highlights a cataract which has formed after the introduction of silicone oil into the vitreous cavity. In the picture on the right, light reflected from the iris surface illuminates a dendritic ulcer in the corneal epithelium. The swollen epithelial cells which are involved in the infection are shown particularly well by the retro illuminated cornea.

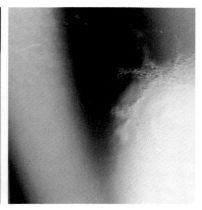

Specular Reflection
Fig. 1.28 When a beam of light traverses a heterogeneous optical medium, most of the light is transmitted but at each optical interface a proportion of light is reflected (specular reflection). This phenomenon is employed in a particularly useful technique for examining the corneal endothelium and, although this can be performed on routine slit lamp biomicroscopy, it has been used to advantage by specialised specular microscopes.

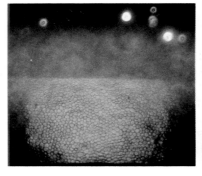

Fig. 1.29 The angle of illumination is adjusted, when viewing the endothelial cells, to reduce the relatively intense reflection from the epithelial surface. The typical endothelial pattern seen by this method is shown on the left; on the right is a photograph taken with a specular microscope producing extra magnification.

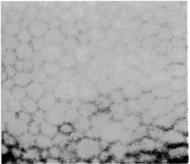

Examination of the Corneal Curvature
Measurement of the corneal curvature is essential in the fitting of contact lenses and also in the follow up of patients with diseases of the cornea such as keratoconus. More recently, measurement of the corneal curvature has become important with the use of intra-ocular lenses where selection of the correct lens power is dependent upon knowing the axial length of the eye and the radius of curvature of the cornea. A simple piece of apparatus for qualitative examination of corneal curvature and distortion was the Placido's disc; a more modern derivation of this instrument is the photokeratoscope.

Fig. 1.30 The photokeratoscope (left) projects a series of illuminated rings onto the corneal surface. These are reflected and then viewed through the instrument. A permanent record can be made with a polaroid camera, a picture of which can be seen on the right. Computer analysis reveals any distortion of the rings, giving information on the corneal curvature and meridians of astigmatism. This technique is especially useful in assessment of irregular astigmatism such as that seen in keratoconus or corneal scarring (cf Fig. 6.60).

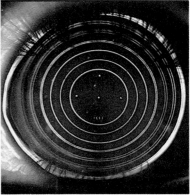

Fig. 1.31   A more simple piece of equipment for measuring the corneal curvature is the Schiøtz type of keratometer. Essentially, this is a microscope with a fixed working distance so that when the cornea is in focus the apparatus is a fixed distance from it. There are two illuminated objectives (bottom picture), green and red; these are mounted on a curved track (to keep them equidistant from the cornea) on either side of the central telescope. When the images of the two coloured objectives (mires) are seen on the cornea in apposition, the end point has been reached and the corneal curvature can be read directly from a scale on the arms supporting the objectives, either in millimetres of radius or dioptres. Alignment of the horizontal bars in the images allows the axis of astigmatism to be measured. These are aligned by rotating the objectives around the axis of the telescope. To prevent any relative movement of the images when viewing the cornea the instrument incorporates a doubling device so that both images move together.

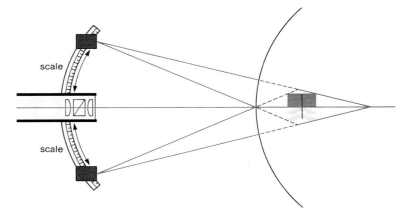

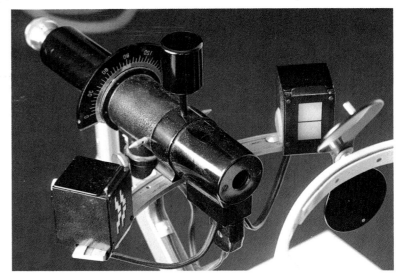

Pachymetry

Fig. 1.32   The thickness of the cornea and depth of the anterior chamber can be measured by similarly designed instruments which differ only in their calibration. A narrow vertical slit beam of light is projected axially on the cornea and viewed at an angle of 40°. The image is viewed through a glass block which has been split horizontally; one half is fixed and the other allowed to rotate on a vertical axis. This produces a horizontally split slit image of the anterior segment with the lower image fixed and the upper moveable by rotating the upper glass block.

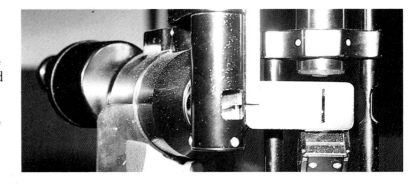

Fig. 1.33   The optics, as seen on the left, are complicated but give a split image view of the anterior segment of the eye. In the case of anterior chamber depth measurement, the posterior surface of the cornea in one half image can be aligned with the anterior lens surface in the other half image (right). This is achieved by revolving the moveable half of the glass block and the movement is read on the scale at the top of the instrument.

Measurement of corneal thickness is undertaken in a similar way except the posterior edge of the cornea in one split image is aligned with the anterior edge of the cornea in the other image. In calibrating the instrument, assumptions have to be made for the refractive index of the corneal tissue. In disease where the cornea has become swollen, the refractive index changes and some authorities believe that pachometer units are a more accurate expression of corneal thickness than millimetres. Anterior chamber dimensions can also be measured ultrasonically but this is less convenient.

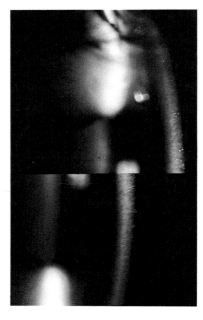

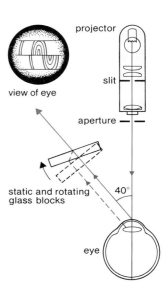

Examination of the Angle of the Eye

Due to the curvature of the cornea, reflected light from the angle of the eye hits the cornea at an angle greater than the critical angle and so is reflected rather than transmitted. In order to see structures in this area, various optical devices have been constructed, the commonest of these being the gonioscopic mirror.

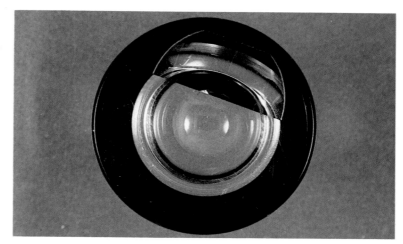

Fig. 1.34   The gonioscope is a solid perspex contact lens within which is mounted a small mirror so that the structures of the angle of the eye can be easily viewed.

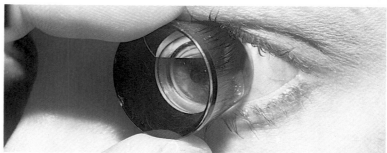

Fig. 1.35   This figure shows a Goldmann gonioscope lens *in situ* on the patient's eye; the structures which are visible by this technique are reviewed in Glaucoma, Chapter 7. The full circumference of the angle can be inspected by rotating the contact lens on the surface of the eye to give a 360° view.

Measurement of Intraocular Pressure

The pressure within the globe can be measured by the use of a tonometer. There are various models of this but applanation tonometry is used most commonly in clinical practice. This works on the principle that a force required to flatten a given area of corneal apex will be proportional to the intra-ocular pressure that maintains the corneal curvature.

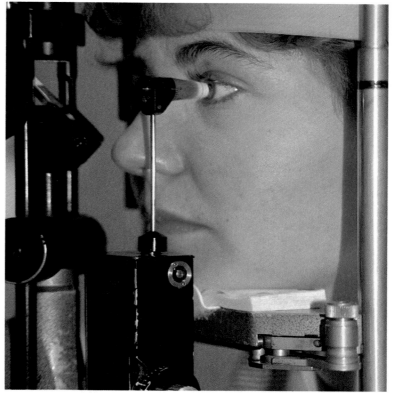

Fig. 1.36   The area of the tonometer head is such that the surface tension force of the tear film and the elastic tension within the cornea are equal and cancel each other out. The applanation head has a clear centre which incorporates a prismatic doubling device. The cornea is illuminated with cobalt blue light and viewed co-axially through the applanation head (top), the tear film having been stained by fluorescein to identify the meniscus around the applanating head. The applanation head is gently brought to rest on the surface of the anaesthetized cornea; its force is increased by revolving a graduated wheel at the base of the instrument which is calibrated in millimetres of mercury. The bottom figure shows the end point at which the intraocular pressure is measured. One can see the split image of the tear film meniscus around the tonometer head outlined by the semicircular fluorescein rings whose edges are just overlapping. If the pressure on the tonometer head is too low the split rings do not touch; if it is too high, they overlap. Corneal depression is minimal so that the amount of aqueous humour or choroidal blood displaced does not produce a change in intra-ocular pressure.

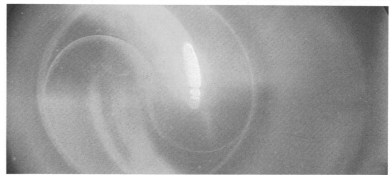

OPHTHALMOSCOPY

There are two types of instrument, the direct and indirect.

The Direct Ophthalmoscope

This instrument incorporates a light source focussed directly onto the retina through a small angled mirror which either fills half or the whole of the aperture. The mirror centre is unsilvered so that the illuminated retina can be seen through it. Between the returning light rays and the examiner's eye there is a revolving magazine of lenses which usually range from +30 to −30 dioptres which correct any inherent refractive error of either the patient or the examiner. Changing the depth of focus in the eye allows the ophthalmoscope to be used to view not only the posterior segment but also opacities in the media, especially in the lens, when retro-illuminated.

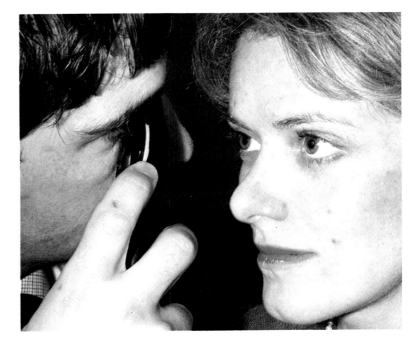

Fig. 1.37 This photograph shows the instrument in use with the examiner viewing the patient's right eye with his right eye, which would be reversed when viewing the left. Pupillary dilatation is essential for the best retinal view.

Fig. 1.38 The field of view with the direct ophthalmoscope is quite small, approximately 6½° with a magnification of ×15; the image is erect and real. A green or "red-free" filter is particularly useful in observing nerve fibre and small vessel detail.

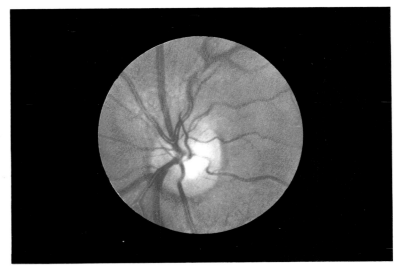

The Indirect Ophthalmoscope

Indirect ophthalmoscopy can be performed with a uniocular method but is normally undertaken with a binocular stereoscopic instrument. A light source is directed into the patient's eye by an adjustable mirror and the reflected light is then gathered by a condensing lens (normally of the power of either +20 or +28 dioptres) to form a virtual inverted image of the retina. The size of the image varies according to the power of the indirect lens; the greater the power of the lens, the smaller the image. A +13 lens magnifies the retina by aproximately 2½ times.

Indirect ophthalmoscopy has the advantages of providing high intensity illumination, stereopsis and a wide field of view as well as allowing a dynamic assessment of vitreoretinal pathology. Its disadvantages are that the image is inverted and considerable skill is needed to use the instrument.

Fig. 1.39 The examiner can be seen using the instrument holding the condensing lens at an appropriate distance from the patient's eye. He is standing behind the patient so that the inverted image that is seen corresponds to the normal erect appearance.

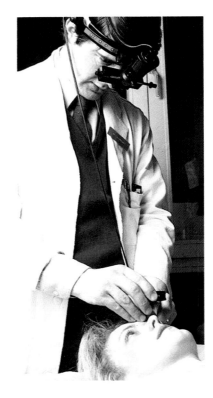

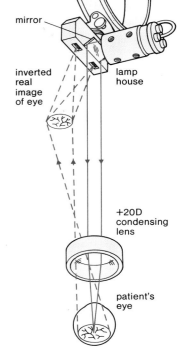

mirror

inverted real image of eye

lamp house

+20D condensing lens

patient's eye

Fig. 1.40 The image size and field of view of the fundus as seen through the indirect ophthalmoscope using a +28 dioptre lens. The additional benefit of using a high dioptric value lens is that a clear view of the fundus may be obtained with a relatively small pupil size, if full dilatation is not possible.

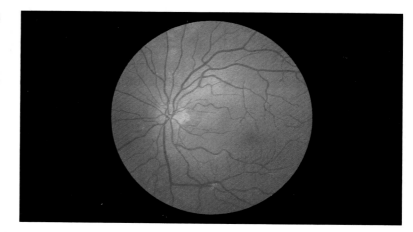

Fig. 1.41 Further detail, especially at the retinal periphery, can be seen by augmenting examination with the use of an indentor which pushes peripheral retinal areas into the field of view of the instrument. Indentation of the retinal structures may also help to highlight any pathology, and movement of the indentor allows dynamic forces to be assessed.

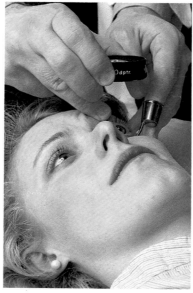
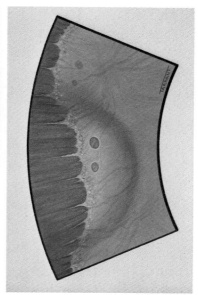

Goldmann 3-mirror Contact Lens

Other techniques involving the slit lamp can be used to examine the posterior segment of the eye, namely by using the Goldmann 3-mirror contact lens, a fundus viewing lens, or a Hruby lens. All three of these devices essentially neutralise the positive lens power of the eye inherent in the corneal curvature and allow stereoscopic examination and laser treatment of the fundus using the slit lamp.

Fig. 1.42 One can see that the Goldmann 3-mirror contact lens is made up of a central viewing area which has a concave surface (left). This allows it to be placed on the cornea of the eye, any curvature disparity being overcome by the use of an optical coupling such as saline or hypromellose. The different areas of the retina that can be viewed through the angled mirrors of this instrument are illustrated on the right.

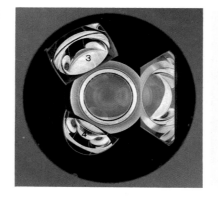
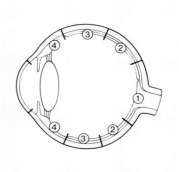

Fig. 1.43 This figure shows the Goldmann 3-mirror lens on a patient's eye.

The peripheral retina may be brought into view by indenting the periphery. The lens is held in a special cup that carries an indentor, analogous to indenting with the indirect ophthalmoscope.

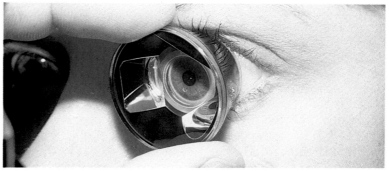

Fig. 1.44 The fundal lens is optically the centre part of the Goldmann 3-mirror lens but is smaller and more convenient to use when viewing the central retina alone (top). A small flange on the lens fits behind the eyelids thus retaining the lens on the patient's eye. As an alternative non-contact method one can use the Hruby lens (bottom). This is a -55 dioptre lens which is placed close to the corneal surface and negates the inherent refraction of the eye. It produces a real erect image in front of the retina which has to be viewed at moderately high magnification to obtain a good image size.

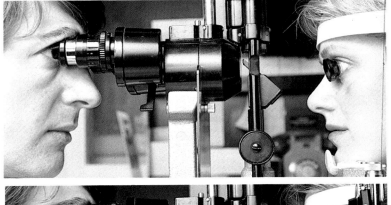

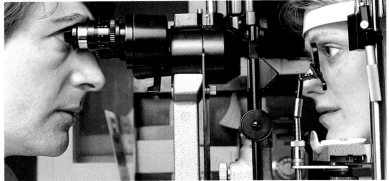

Fig. 1.45 This ray diagram illustrates the optics of the Hruby lens.

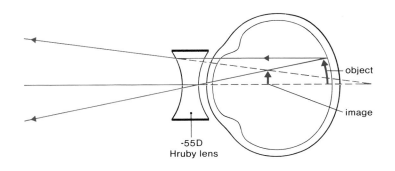

ELECTRICAL TESTS OF RETINAL FUNCTION

The electrical response to light, generated by the eye as a mass potential (i.e. a whole eye response), can be used to assess retinal function both clinically and experimentally. Electrodiagnostic tests are particularly useful in differential diagnosis of inherited retinal dystrophies. Tests in common clinical practice consist of the electro-oculogram (EOG), the electroretinogram (ERG) and the visual evoked response (VER) which is a test of conduction in the retrobulbar visual pathways.

Dark adaptation is sometimes used in conjunction with these tests and is also considered here. Electrodiagnostic tests have not yet been standardized so that responses and normal values differ between laboratories.

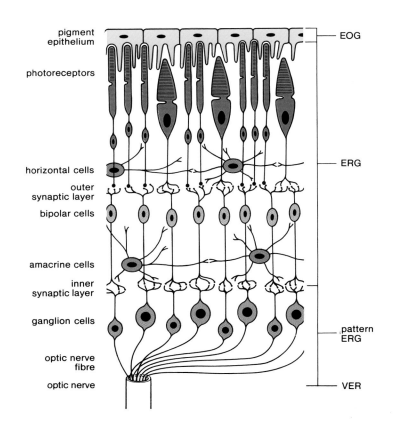

Fig. 1.46 This diagram shows the regions of the retina which are responsible for generating the various potentials. The EOG is generated by the retinal pigment epithelium and photoreceptors. The ERG is generated in the bipolar layer, probably by Müller cells, but is dependent on impulses from the photoreceptors. The ERG is usually normal in the presence of retinal ganglion cell disease but the newly introduced pattern ERG may represent function further along the visual pathway, possibly in the ganglion cells themselves. The VER is an index of conduction in the retrobulbar pathways.

Dark Adaptation

Fig. 1.47 This test measures the increase in retinal sensitivity with time due to photoreceptor pigment regeneration. The visual threshold to a flash of light is plotted against time after preadaptation to a standard amount of light. Normally after about 7 minutes of adaptation, the sensitivity of the scotopic system (rods) overtakes that of the photopic system (cones). After 25 to 30 minutes, rhodopsin should have fully regenerated and retinal sensitivity reached its peak. Defects in rod metabolism such as retinitis pigmentosa will produce abnormally high thresholds at this time. In practice, the same information can be gained more easily by ERG and EOG.

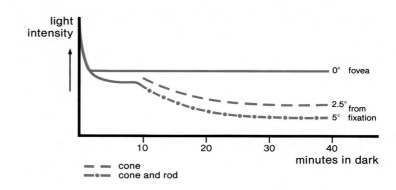

Electro-oculogram

Fig. 1.48 Within the eye itself there is a standing potential between the retina and cornea of about 6 millivolts, with the cornea positive to the retina. This arises from the interactions in the retinal pigment epithelial layer. This potential can be measured by electrodes placed on the skin at the medial and lateral canthi.

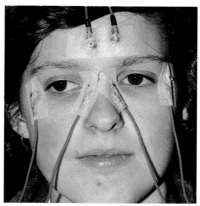

Fig. 1.49 The patient is asked to fixate on target lights which alternate from left to right causing a 30° excursion of the horizontal eye movements. Movements of the potential between the electrodes induces a current which is then amplified and displayed on recording equipment. The potential which can be measured in this way varies according to the level of background illumination.

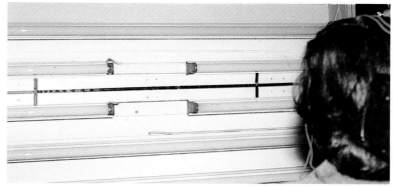

Fig. 1.50 Clinically the pupils are fully dilated and the induced potential is measured first in the dark for 12 to 15 minutes, during which time the potential falls to a minimum. The patient is then exposed to intense light and the rise in potential is measured at its peak. The ratio of the potentials measured in the light and the dark is converted to an algebraic fraction and the light rise should be in excess of 180% to be within the normal range. Measurements lower than this usually represent retinal disease at the level of the pigment epithelium.

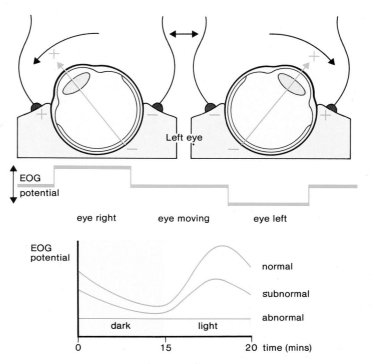

Fig. 1.51 Typical tracings of a normal patient compared to a sufferer of retinitis pigmentosa are illustrated. Measurement of the EOG requires active co-operation of the patient. Although readings are not affected by opacities in the ocular media, low responses can be found normally in myopes and in the elderly, and also after ocular surgery or injury.

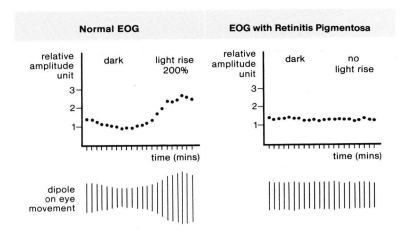

Electro-Retinogram

The electro-retinogram measures the mass retinal response to a flash of light using a corneal electrode and neutral electrodes placed on the skin around the orbital margin.

Fig. 1.52 A patient can be seen wired up, prior to the examination, with neutral electrodes taped to the forehead and orbital rim. The corneal electrode itself is a thin foil of gold leaf place gently behind the lower eyelid so that it contacts the cornea. In infants the ERG can be recorded under general anaesthesia.

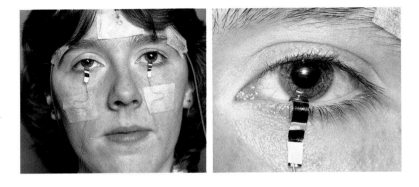

Due to many different methods and techniques used to record the ERG there is no typical response. However, there is usually a biphasic wave with an initial negative trough (A wave) followed by a larger positive peak (B wave). The latency (from stimulus to onset of the A wave), the implicit times (stimulus to peak of A or B wave) and the amplitude of the A or B waves can be measured. The ERG varies with the stimulus duration, intensity, colour and the state of retinal adaptation.

The great value of the ERG lies in its ability to differentiate rod and cone responses. This can be achieved either by measuring the responses under photopic or scotopic conditions, using red or blue light or the phenomenon of flicker fusion. The latter measures the ERG to a flashing light which increases in frequency until the photoreceptors can no longer differentiate the individual flashes and the electrical signal is no longer recordable.

More sophisticated analysis of the ERG shows that if a really intense stimulus is used a deflection occurs preceding the A wave. This is known as the early receptor potential (ERP) and probably correlates with photochemical changes in the photoreceptors. Intense stimuli give rise to oscillatory potentials on the ascending limb of the B wave and are probably derived from the amacrine cells in the inner nuclear layer. Finally, experimental techniques of focal and pattern ERG's are being used as research tools.

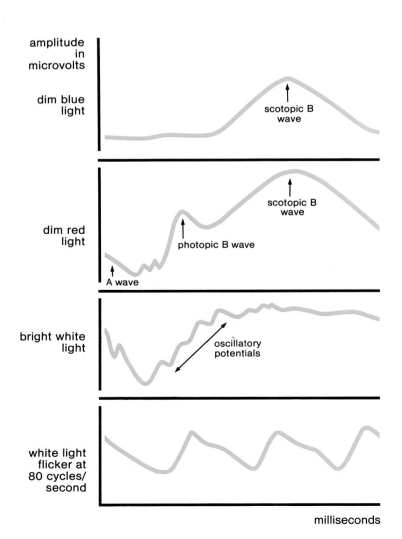

Fig. 1.53 This diagram shows the different wave forms obtained by altering the stimulus. Under dim blue light only the scotopic B wave is recorded. With dim red light an A wave is seen as well as photopic and scotopic peaks in the B wave. An intense bright white light produces oscillatory potentials on the ascending limb of the B wave. In a normal patient discrete responses are seen in response to a flashing light of up to 80 cycles/second.

Fig. 1.54 Comparison of ERG responses in a patient with cone dystrophy and a patient with retinitis pigmentosa. In cone dystrophy (left) the amplitude of the scotopic B wave is normal, but the photopic B wave is abolished (dim red). Response to bright light is present but reduced and delayed, and discrete flicker responses are not elicited. In retinitis pigmentosa (right) the converse is seen; the scotopic B wave is absent, the photopic responses are present but reduced in amplitude, and flicker fusion is preserved.

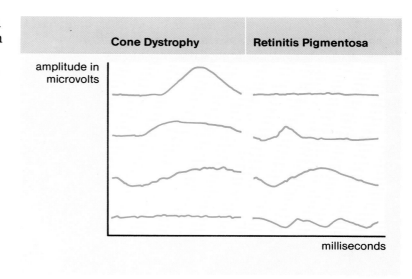

Visual Evoked Response

The conduction of visual signals from the eye to the occipital cortex can be measured by adapting the EEG response to a visual stimulus. The eye is stimulated by a bright flash of light (flash VER) or by observing an alternating chequer board pattern of white and black squares (pattern VER). The latter has the advantage that total retinal luminance remains constant and a wave form is generated that is consistent and largely derived from macular photoreceptors. The pattern VER response varies with the stimulus characteristics, pupillary size, retinal adaptation and visual acuity as well as psychological factors and recording techniques.

Fig. 1.55 The response is recorded by placing occipital and reference electrodes on the scalp and repeated responses are analysed by computer averaging. The amplitude and latency of the first deflection (PI peak) from the stimulus can be measured and the wave form studied. In this recording from a normal patient the PI peak has a latency of 118 msecs. and a high amplitude. A tracing from a patient with acute retrobulbar neuritis shows a low amplitude peak which is delayed to 170 msecs. With clinical improvement the amplitude increases but the delay in the response remains.

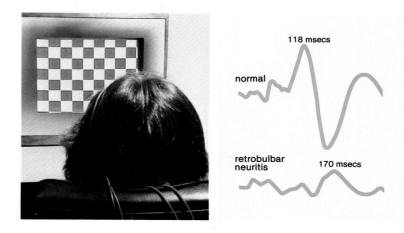

ULTRASOUND EXAMINATION OF THE EYE

The ocular anatomy can be investigated using a beam of ultrasonic sound, usually in excess of 18,000 hertz, directed at the eye. The sound beam is reflected at interfaces of changing tissue density and the reflected beam can be analysed to give information about the internal ocular structure.

Fig. 1.56 With the A-scan mode of investigation a transducer is coupled to the eye (with a water bath or gel) and the reflected sound beams measured by a receiver, the display being shown in the lower part of the diagram. The echo peaks match a section across the eye and their amplitude corresponds to the ultrasonic interfaces.

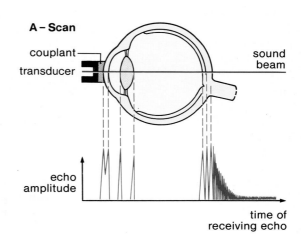

Fig. 1.57 An experienced operator can discern changes of the ocular anatomy and in this diagram the different patterns of ultrasonic sound can be seen to show a mass within the globe of the eye. In some cases analysis of the echo pattern will correlate with the histological appearance of the lesion, allowing a diagnosis to be made (eg. choroidal haemangioma, Chapter 10). The A-scan is now used more routinely for measurement of the axial length of the eye in the preoperative assessment before intraocular lens implantation, to ensure that the correct lens power is chosen after cataract extraction.

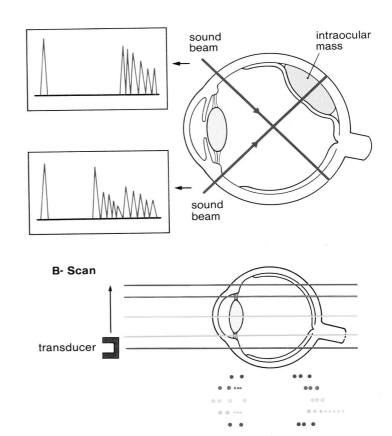

Fig. 1.58 If the A-scan linear echoes are displayed as points of light whose intensity is proportional to the echo amplitude and the eye is scanned across several planes, a cross-sectional image is formed known as B-scan. This method allows both static and dynamic examination of the ocular contents and is very useful in the assessment of retinal and vitreous pathology (see Chapter 12).

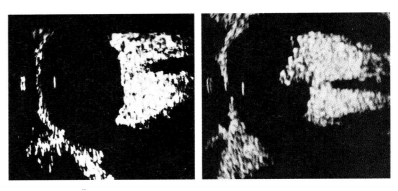

Fig. 1.59 A normal B-scan compared to an abnormal one showing the same intra-ocular mass as that of the A-scan picture in Fig. 1.57.

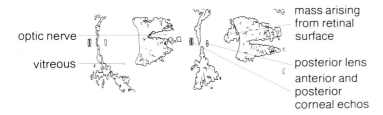

NUCLEAR MAGNETIC RESONANCE (NMR)
Computerized tomography has become well established over the last 10 years in the investigation of orbital and neuro-ophthalmological problems (ref. Ch. 19 and Ch. 20). More recently NMR has been developed but is still experimental. It measures hydrogen atom density within tissue using large electro-magnets to produce a magnetic

flux. This aligns the axis of spin of electrons about the hydrogen atom. A radio signal is pulsed through the tissue at right angles to the magnetic field and this gives a secondary misalignment of spin axis. When the signal is switched off, the spin axis realigns with the magnetic field and causes the emission of a weak radio signal which is then analysed to form the image.

Fig. 1.60 This shows an NMR scan through the brain, orbit and cranial fossa. This does not, as yet, produce the resolution of a CT scan but in the future has the possibility of giving more useful biological information; for example, the viability of tumours following treatment, or better definition in areas when CT scanning is poor, such as the posterior cranial fossa or optic canals.

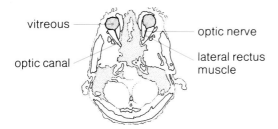

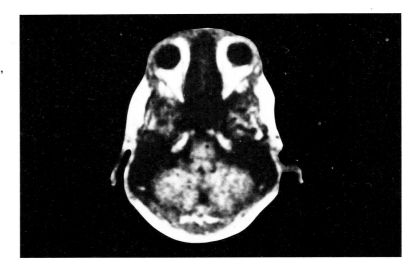

2. The Eyelids

J. R. O. Collin

NORMAL ANATOMY

The structure of both the upper and lower eyelids is similar. It consists of an anterior lamella or layer of skin and orbicularis muscle, and a posterior lamella of tarsal plate and conjunctiva. The orbital septum extends from the orbital rim and separates the pre-septal orbicularis muscle from the pre-aponeurotic fat pad. The lid retractors lie between this pre-aponeurotic fat pad and the globe. The upper lid retractors consist of the levator palpebrae superioris muscle, the aponeurosis, and the superior tarsal muscle (Müller's muscle). The lower lid retractors arise from the sheath of the inferior rectus muscle and are similarly composed of an aponeurosis and smooth muscle layer (the inferior tarsal muscle).

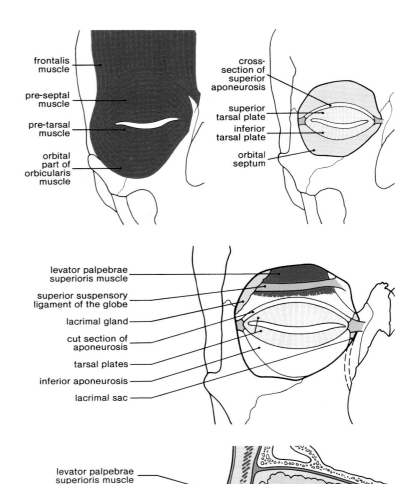

Fig. 2.1 Diagrammatic view of the structures of the normal eyelid. The orbicularis muscle can be divided into three parts but these are not separate anatomically. These are the pre-tarsal, the pre-septal, and orbital parts of the orbicularis muscle. The pre-tarsal and pre-septal parts together form the palpebral section of the orbicularis muscle, which is responsible for blinking, while the orbital part is responsible for forced lid closure. Removal of the orbicularis muscle shows the underlying tarsal plates and orbital septum. The superior aponeurosis is the tendon of the levator muscle which inserts between the orbicularis muscle bundles and is responsible for the skin crease.

Fig. 2.2 The pre-aponeurotic fat pad lies behind the orbital septum. If it is elevated, the levator palpebrae superioris muscle with its aponeurosis is seen. Whitnall's ligament (the superior suspensory ligament of the globe) is a thickening in the aponeurosis which helps to support the aponeurosis and the upper lid retractors. It runs from the periostium of the lacrimal gland fossa to the trochlea of the superior oblique muscle. The inferior aponeurosis is the anterior extension of the connective tissue from Lockwood's ligament (the inferior suspensory ligament of the globe) and is continuous posteriorly with the sheath around the inferior rectus muscle.

Fig. 2.3 The upper lid structures can be compared in diagrammatic and histological vertical sections. The levator palpebrae superioris muscle divides into an anterior lamella (the aponeurosis) and a posterior lamella (Müller's muscle), both of which are responsible for lifting the eyelid. The connective tissue between the levator muscle and the superior rectus muscle (the common sheath) extends forward to support the upper conjunctival fornix (superior suspensory ligament of the fornix).

Fig. 2.4 Histological section of the upper lid corresponding to the cross-sectional diagram of Fig. 2.3.

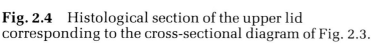

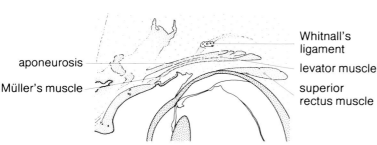

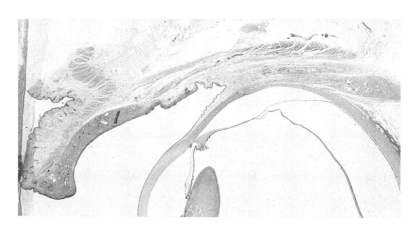

Fig. 2.5 Sections of the lower lid show the arrangement of the lower lid retractors. A condensation of fascia around the inferior oblique muscle forms the inferior suspensory ligament of the globe (Lockwood's ligament). This is analogous to Whitnall's ligament in the upper eyelid. It is attached medially and laterally in the region of the canthal tendons and can support the globe if the orbital floor is removed. The inferior aponeurosis extends forwards from Lockwood's ligament with the inferior tarsal muscle (analogous to Müller's muscle in the upper lid). These are the lower lid retractors, which are responsible for depressing the lower eyelid on down-gaze because of their connection with the inferior rectus muscle. A forward extension of the connective tissue associated with the lower lid retractors forms the inferior suspensory ligament of the fornix and anterior part of Tenon's capsule.

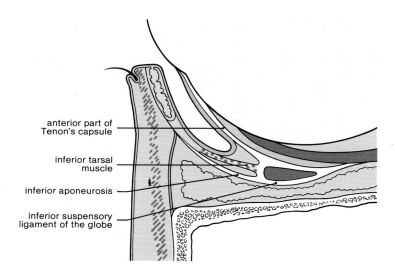

Fig. 2.6 Histological section of the lower lid corresponding to the cross-sectional diagram of Fig. 2.5.

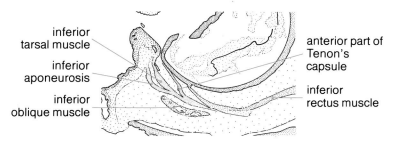

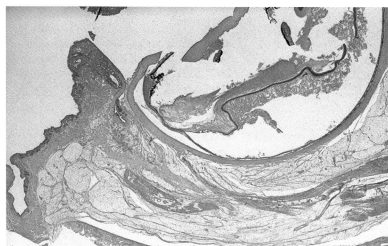

ENTROPION
Entropion, or inversion of the lid margin, may be congenital or acquired. The acquired variety can be the result of ageing changes (involutional entropion) or cicatricial changes affecting the posterior lamella of the eyelid (cicatricial entropion).

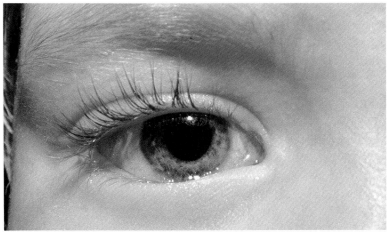

Fig. 2.7 Congenital lower lid entropion is caused by hypertrophy of the skin and underlying orbicularis muscle. A mild degree of this hypertrophy is common in young children (epiblepharon) and rarely, the eyelid margin itself inverts (congenital entropion). Should this fail to improve with age and cause irritation of the eye, it should be corrected by the excision of the hypertrophied skin and underlying orbicularis muscle.

Fig. 2.8 Involution (senile) entropion is a common condition caused by a combination of ageing changes affecting the orbicularis muscle, the lower lid retractors, the tarsal plate, the medial and lateral canthal tendons, and the orbital fat. A variety of operations have been described to correct various combinations of these defects. These include sutures or incisions designed to prevent the upward movement of the pre-septal muscle, tightening the lower lid retractors, eversion of the upper border of the tarsal plate, horizontal lid and canthal tendon shortening procedures.

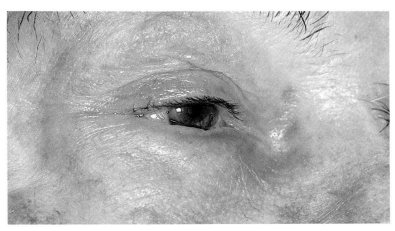

Fig. 2.9 Cicatricial changes can affect either the upper or lower lid and lead to entropion. This patient has scarring and shrinkage of the tarsal plate and conjunctiva. Common causes include trauma, acid and alkali burns, trachoma, and other chronic conjunctival inflammations such as ocular pemphigoid, Stevens-Johnson syndrome, etc. It may be possible to correct a cicatricial entropion with an everting procedure and rotation of the tarsal plate, but if there is a marked degree of lid retraction a posterior lamella graft will be required.

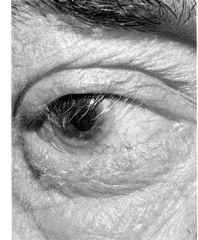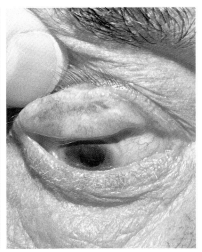

ECTROPION

Ectropion, or eversion of the lid margin, may be congenital or acquired. The acquired forms are the result of ageing changes (involutional), lumps (mechanical), scarring of the anterior lamella of the lid (cicatricial), or weakness of the orbicularis muscle (paralytic).

Fig. 2.10 Congenital ectropion may affect all four lids. In neonates and very young children it can be caused by crying and spasm of the orbicularis muscle. This does not usually require any treatment. If there is a shortage of skin, as in the case illustrated here, skin-replacement is necessary with a graft or flap.

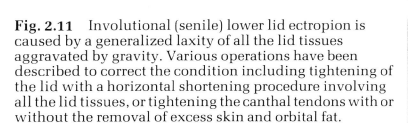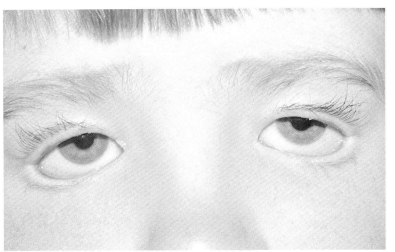

Fig. 2.11 Involutional (senile) lower lid ectropion is caused by a generalized laxity of all the lid tissues aggravated by gravity. Various operations have been described to correct the condition including tightening of the lid with a horizontal shortening procedure involving all the lid tissues, or tightening the canthal tendons with or without the removal of excess skin and orbital fat.

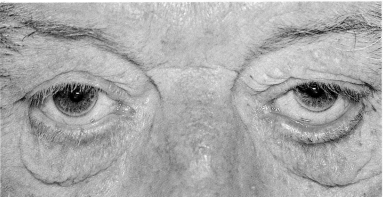

Fig. 2.12 Any form of lump on the lower lid can lead to a mechanical ectropion. The patient illustrated here has a localized neurofibroma of the lower lid and treatment involves the removal of the tumour.

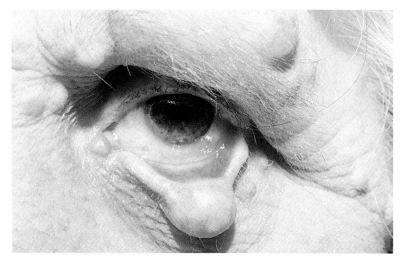

Fig. 2.13 Cicatricial lower lid ectropion can be caused by any condition which leads to a shortage of skin. This patient fell off his bicycle and lost skin: the resultant scarring caused a cicatricial ectropion. Surgical correction involves excision of the scar tissue, and replacement of the skin. The lid must be shortened at the same operation if it has been excessively stretched by the scarring.

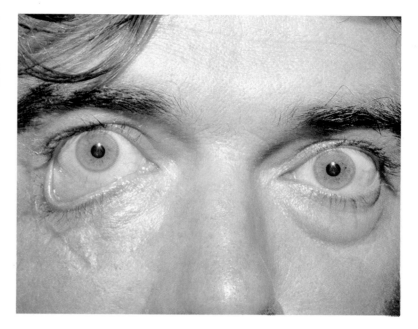

Fig. 2.14 Paralytic ectropion is caused by weakness of the orbicularis muscle (seventh nerve palsy) and subsequent lid laxity. Surgical treatment tends to be unsatisfactory and involves tightening of the lower eyelid, usually with a medial and lateral canthoplasty. If the cornea is at risk from exposure due to defective closure of the eyelid, this can be treated in the acute stage with a temporary tarsorrhaphy. Should the defective closure persist, however, further procedures may be required to reduce the size of the palpebral aperture permanently and so improve eyelid closure.

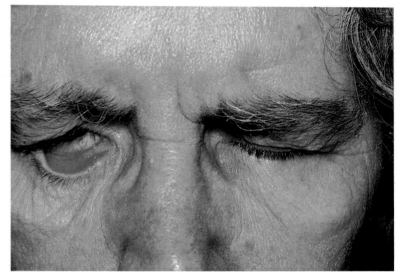

EYELID RETRACTION

The most common cause of upper and lower lid retraction is dysthyroid eye disease but any condition which involves the eyelid retractors can cause lid retraction, e.g., trauma, tumour infiltration, etc., as well as neurological conditions affecting the mid-brain. Eyelid retraction must be differentiated from conditions such as proptosis and high myopia, as well as from contra-lateral ptosis, etc. Treatment depends on the cause, but it is possible to reduce the vertical height of the palpebral aperture by recessing the lid retractors with or without the insertion of a graft, e.g., of sclera.

Fig. 2.15 This patient has unilateral upper lid retraction due to dysthyroid disease.

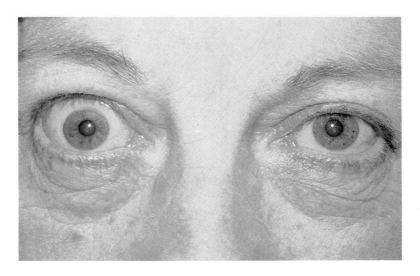

PTOSIS

Conditions which cause ptosis can be divided into those which are congenital and those which are acquired. The most common cause of congenital ptosis is an isolated dystrophy of the levator palpebrae superioris muscle which may be either unilateral or bilateral. Some patients are born with a non-dystrophic type of ptosis, e.g., due to a neurogenic or aponeurotic defect, but these may also occur after birth and can therefore be considered under acquired causes of ptosis. Any aponeurotic weakness can lead to ptosis, and an acquired defect associated with involutional changes is the probable cause of the common involutional (senile) ptosis. Neurogenic causes of ptosis include conditions leading to IIIrd nerve palsy, the various aberrant regeneration syndromes, and involvement of the sympathetic nervous system (Horner's syndrome). Myogenic ptosis is caused by a myopathy involving the levator muscle and is usually due to a progressive external ophthalmoplegia. Myasthenic ptosis is the result of a conduction defect at the neuromuscular junction, while a mechanical ptosis can be caused by any lump on the upper lid (cf. Figs. 2.38 and 2.40). Cicatrizing conditions which involve the upper conjunctival fornix may also lead to a mechanical ptosis. Trauma may produce a mechanical ptosis by direct involvement of the lid retractors (cf. Fig. 2.59): trauma can also cause ptosis by involvement of the aponeurosis or by affecting the nerve supply to the upper lid retractors.

Pseudoptosis can result from a volume deficit (such as is associated with microphthalmia or post-enucleation), or from various other conditions such as excess upper lid skin or a hypotropia.

A useful classification of the causes of ptosis can be given by considering them under the headings of congenital, acquired, or pseudoptosis.

Congenital: – Dystrophic
                – Non-dystrophic

Acquired: – Aponeurotic defects
                – Neurogenic – third nerve and aberrant regeneration syndromes, Horner's syndrome
                – Myogenic
                – Myasthenia
                – Mechanical

Pseudoptosis: – Volume deficit, hypotropia, etc.

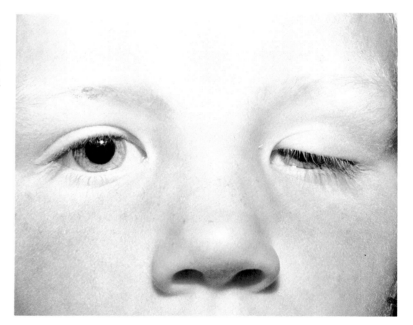

Fig. 2.16 This boy has unilateral congenital dystrophic ptosis in which the lid margin occludes the pupillary access and therefore interferes with the development of normal vision. Under these circumstances, an urgent effort should be made to lift the eyelid to expose the visual axis in an attempt to prevent amblyopia and stimulate normal visual development.

If the visual axis is not occluded by the eyelid, it is reasonable to delay correction of a congenital ptosis until the child is old enough for a more accurate assessment when definitive ptosis surgery may be performed. This usually occurs around the age of four years.

The type of surgery is governed primarily by the levator muscle function which is assessed by the extent of upper lid movement between full up- and down-gaze with the frontalis muscle prevented from acting by pressure over the brow. If the levator function is good, the lid retractors can be shortened: if it is poor, however, an alternative source of lift must be found and a frontalis muscle brow suspension procedure is often indicated.

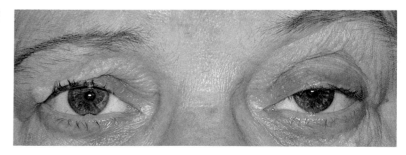

Fig. 2.17 Involutional (senile) ptosis may be the result of an aponeurotic defect. This patient has an elevated skin crease on the ptotic side due to the aponeurotic defect, and the brow is elevated because of frontalis muscle overaction which attempts to raise the lid by raising the eyebrow.

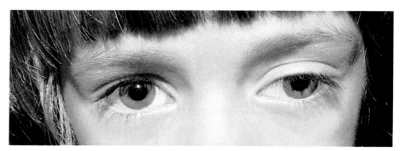

Fig. 2.18 In this example of a partial third nerve palsy, the ptosis is associated with a divergent eye and large pupil on the same side.

Fig. 2.19 Horner's syndrome is caused by damage to the sympathetic nerve supply to the orbit. This results in a mild degree of ptosis and a small pupil. In this case, the iris is less pigmented on the involved side which suggests a congenital lesion of the sympathetic system.

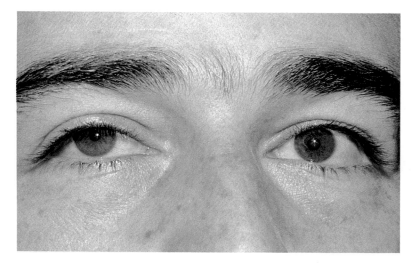

Fig. 2.20 Marcus Gunn (jaw-winking) ptosis is characterized by elevation of the ptotic lid when the mouth is opened or when the jaw is moved laterally, usually to the side opposite the ptosis. The eyelid may even become retracted as in the case illustrated here. The condition is caused by an exaggerated synkinesis between the pterygoid muscles and the levator muscle which probably results from a congenital brain stem abnormality.

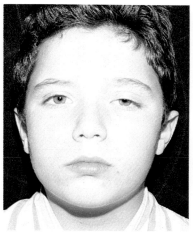
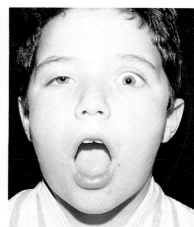

Fig. 2.21 An ocular myopathy usually presents with a bilateral progressive ptosis and involvement of all the extraocular muscles, with limitation of all movements of the globe and eyelids. It covers a group of syndromes which may be associated with other abnormalities such as a pigmentary retinopathy, cataracts, a shoulder girdle myopathy, dysphagia, and short stature. If the orbicularis muscle is involved, eyelid closure will be defective. A cardiac conduction block may be present and makes general anaesthesia hazardous. The biochemical defects are thought to occur in mitochondrial metabolism. Surgical correction of the ptosis should be approached cautiously since the condition is progressive and may involve eyelid closure as well as opening. Various forms of ptosis prop may be tried.

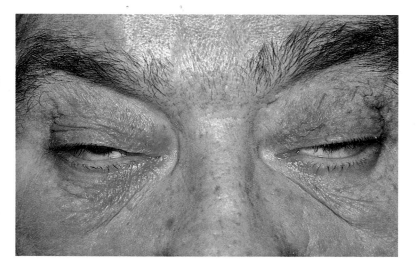

Fig. 2.22 Excessive upper lid skin (dermatochalasis) is usually the result of involutional changes involving the skin and may present as a pseudoptosis. The excess skin can be removed with a blepharoplasty.

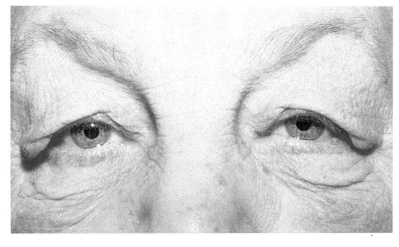

EYELID TUMOURS

Eyelid tumours may be benign or malignant. Although an attempt can be made to diagnose them clinically on their appearance and the histology, a biopsy is often required to ensure the correct treatment.

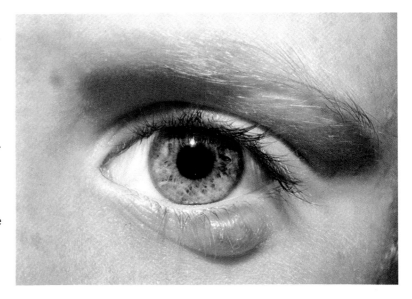

Fig. 2.23 A meibomian cyst (chalazion) is formed by a blockage of one of the meibomian glands in the tarsal plate. Clinically, it presents in the acute stage as a red tender swelling within the tarsal plate of the upper or lower eyelid. This either resolves completely or leaves a firm nodule. Treatment is initially conservative, with heat and local antibiotics, but if resolution does not occur it may be treated surgically by incision and curettage.

Fig. 2.24 Histology shows the centre of a chalazion to have spaces that contained liberated sebaceous secretions. There is a surrounding inflammatory cell infiltrate with phagocytic cells, some of which are multinucleate.

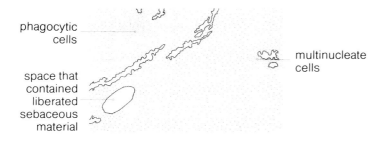

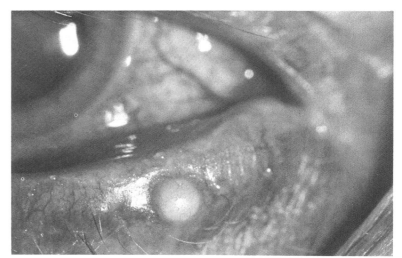

Fig. 2.25 Cysts of Moll are translucent and filled with clear fluid from retained watery secretions of a sweat gland. The condition is treated either by excision or by marsupialization of the cyst.

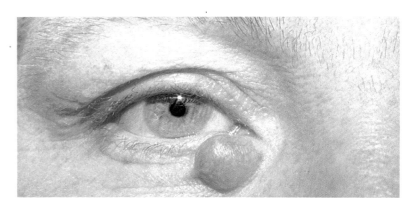

Fig. 2.26 A cyst of Zeis is filled with oily secretions from blockage of one of the specialized sudorific glands associated with the cilia. It can be either incised or marsupialized if it does not resolve spontaneously.

Fig. 2.27 Sebaceous cysts appear as yellowish-white lumps in the skin and have a central punctum. They are caused by retained cheesy secretions from ordinary skin sweat glands and can be treated by simple excision.

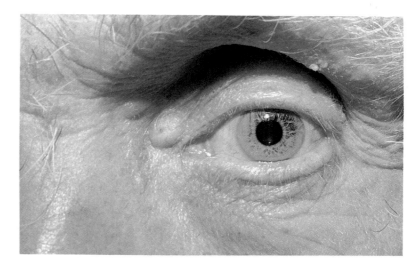

Fig. 2.28 Skin deposits of cholesterol, which classically occur around the inner canthus, are known as xanthelasma. They may be either idiopathic or associated with a hypercholesterolaemic state. Local treatment consists of excision or cautery if necessary. Patients, especially young patients, may need further investigation for a hyperlipidaemia.

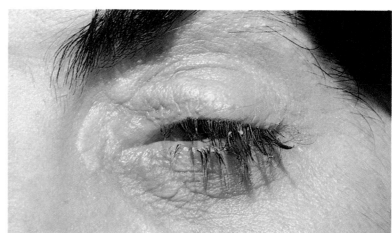

Fig. 2.29 Histology of a xanthelasma shows large histiocytic cells filled with foamy cytoplasm which represents engulfed lipids. The cells have small round nuclei.

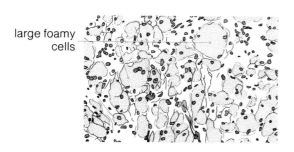

large foamy cells

Fig. 2.30 A squamous papilloma is a benign overgrowth of squamous epithelium. Keratin may build up on the surface of a squamous papilloma to form a cutaneous horn. The lesion can usually be simply excised.

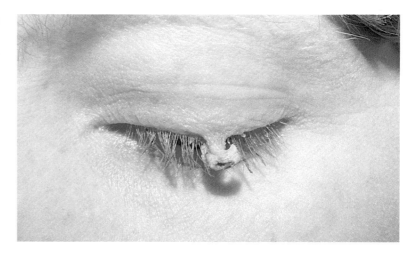

Fig. 2.31 The histology of a squamous papilloma shows that excessive epithelium forms fronds about a central fibrovascular core.

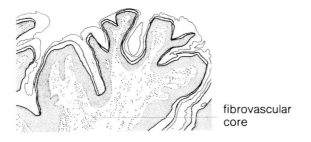

fibrovascular core

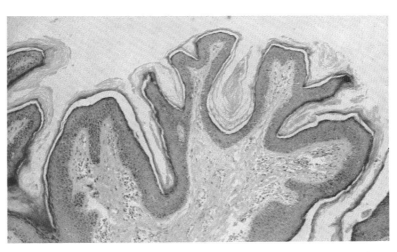

Fig. 2.32 Basal cell papilloma (seborrhoeic keratosis) is a benign overgrowth of the basal cells in the epithelium. It presents in the elderly as a thickened pigmented area of skin with papillary changes and can be simply excised.

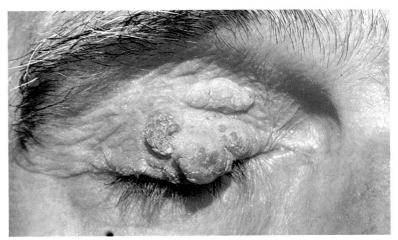

Fig. 2.33 Histology of a basal cell papilloma shows proliferation of the basal cells in the epithelium with the formation of keratin nests. The lesion is entirely benign and has no potential for malignant change. Patients usually have similar lesions elsewhere.

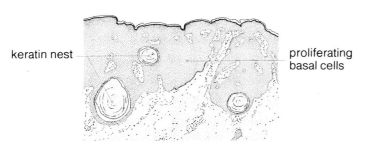

keratin nest

proliferating basal cells

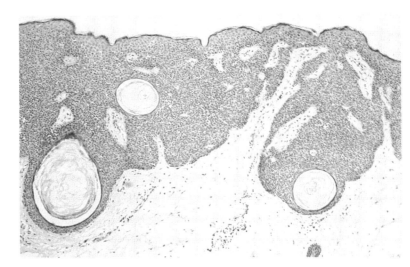

Fig. 2.34 Senile keratosis (actinic or solar keratosis) presents as a dry, scaly, minimally raised lesion with excess keratin. There is an underlying squamous dysplasia which may occasionally proceed to frank malignancy and form a squamous cell carcinoma. The lesion is best excised. It occurs mainly in elderly people with fair skins who have been exposed to excessive sunlight.

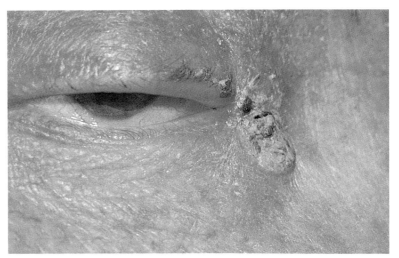

Fig. 2.35 The essential histological features of senile keratosis are stromal changes (comparable to those in a pingueculum) with pronounced keratosis and atypical cells in the epithelium.

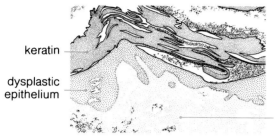

keratin

dysplastic epithelium

stromal degeneration

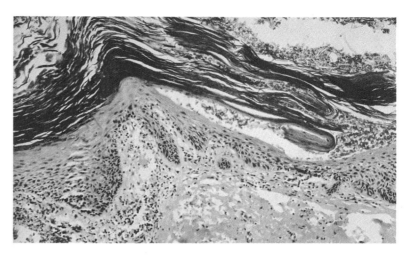

Fig. 2.36 A kerato-acanthoma is a rapidly growing epithelial lesion with a central core of keratin. It usually grows vigorously over a three-month period and then involutes spontaneously. Should involution not occur, however, the lesion should be excised since a small proportion may develop into a squamous cell carcinoma.

Fig. 2.37 Histology of a kerato-acanthoma shows a central plug of keratin surrounded by hyperplastic epithelium which does not extend further than the superficial layers of the dermis. The dermis itself shows chronic inflammatory cellular infiltration.

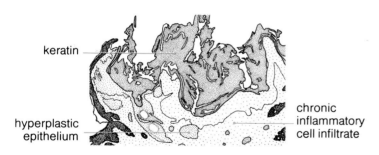

keratin

hyperplastic epithelium

chronic inflammatory cell infiltrate

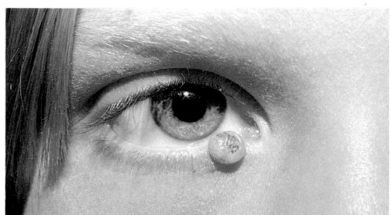

Fig. 2.38 A haemangioma can present either as a local (left) or generalized (right) eyelid mass with vascular changes which are more or less prominent. They are benign but, if they are large enough and affect the upper lid, they may induce amblyopia in children. Many involute spontaneously but if necessary surgery, steroids, radiotherapy, lasers, corrosive injections, or carbon dioxide snow can be tried.

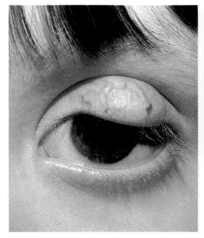

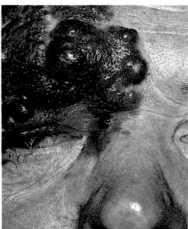

2.11

Fig. 2.39 The pathology of a lid haemangioma shows a mass of proliferated capillaries, some of which are canalized whereas others remain as a solid core of endothelial cells. The lesion is a hamartoma.

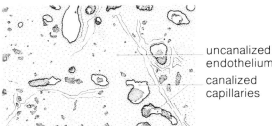

uncanalized endothelium

canalized capillaries

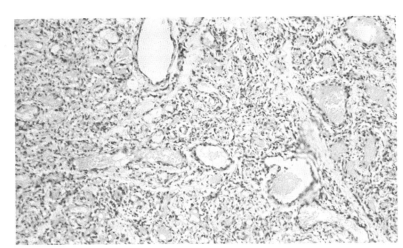

Fig. 2.40 An eyelid neurofibroma can be either diffuse, as in this example of a plexiform neuroma, or localized (cf. Fig. 2.12). A local lesion may be excised but large lesions can only be debulked. They are hamartomas and occur as part of von Recklinghausen's disease. This child also has partial hemihypertrophy of the face and orbital dysplasia as well as an optic nerve glioma.

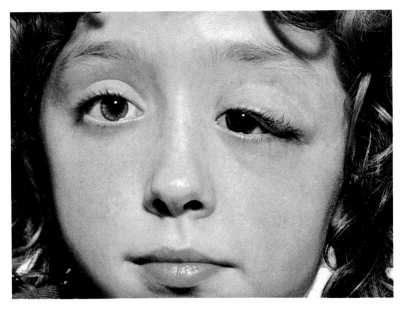

Fig. 2.41 Histology of a local neurofibroma shows a nodular proliferation of both Schwann cells and fibroblasts beneath the epidermis. Silver stains commonly demonstrate neuronal axons in the lesion.

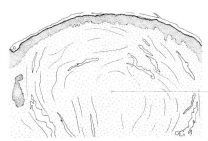

proliferating Schwann cells and fibroblasts

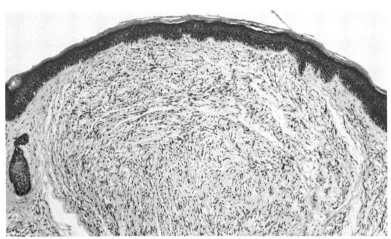

Fig. 2.42 Basal cell carcinoma is the most common malignant eyelid tumour and usually occurs on either the lower eyelid or at the medial canthus. It can present in many different forms and treatment is by either surgery, radiotherapy, or cryotherapy. All of these procedures are effective and the choice depends on the site of the lesion and the physician's preference. Surprisingly, of the tumours that are incompletely excised, only about twenty-five percent will recur clinically. This is an example of a relatively benign type of basal cell carcinoma with a classical pearly margin laced with blood vessels and a central shallow ulcerated base.

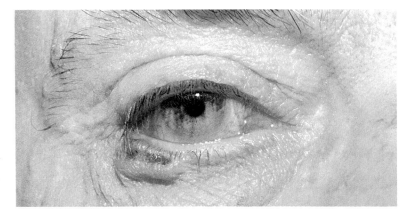

Fig. 2.43 This pathology slide of a basal cell carcinoma shows a proliferation of basal cells around a central ulcer with a rolled margin. The adenoid differentiation is not uncommon in basal cell carcinomas.

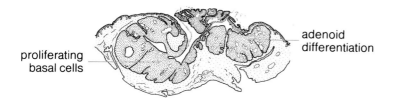

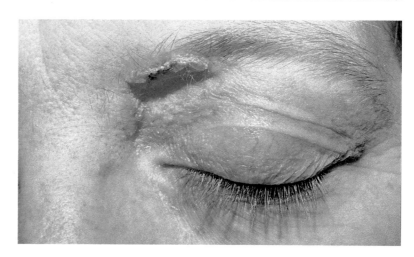

Fig. 2.44 This example of basal cell carcinoma shows a more malignant type (morpheic or sclerosing variety), with a less clearly defined margin. This requires a wide surgical excision to prevent recurrence.

Fig. 2.45 The pathology of a morpheic or sclerosing type of basal cell carcinoma shows islands of proliferating basal cells which have extensively infiltrated the underlying stroma. The surface epithelium is relatively normal in this slide, which explains the clinical difficulty in defining the margins of such lesions.

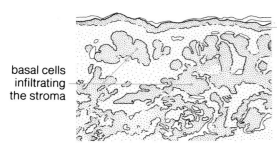

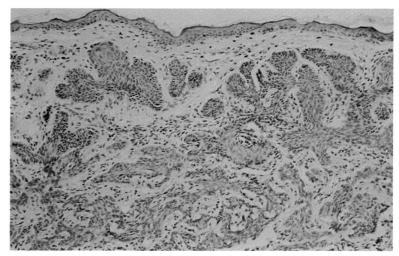

Fig. 2.46 Basal cell carcinomas spread by direct extension and may be highly invasive although they do not metastasize. In this example, an extensive basal cell carcinoma has spread to involve surrounding structures.

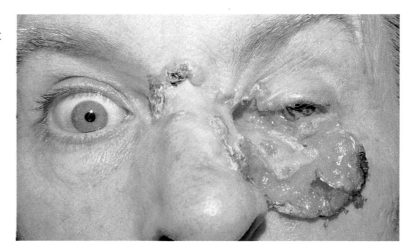

Fig. 2.47 Squamous cell carcinoma may arise de novo or from a pre-existing senile keratosis or kerato-acanthoma. They are especially common in the rare syndrome of xeroderma pigmentosa. The lesion has an everted edge and is relatively more common on the upper eyelid. They may metastase to the regional lymph nodes. Treatment is usually surgical excision.

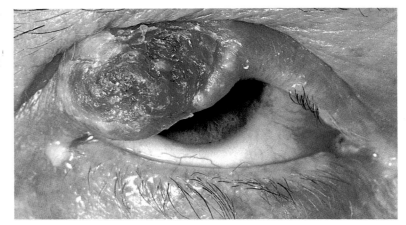

Fig. 2.48 The pathology of squamous cell carcinoma shows proliferating squamous cell epithelium which is extensively infiltrating the underlying stroma. The keratin pearls and extensive inflammatory changes in the underlying stroma are common.

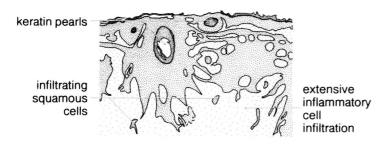

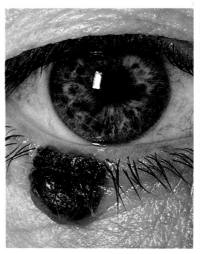

Fig. 2.49 A malignant melanoma can arise de novo or from a pre-existing naevus. Any pigmented eyelid lesion which is growing should be excised in order to prevent local invasion and metastasis. Warning signs of malignant change in a naevus are a rapid increase in size of the lesion, satellite lesions, ulceration, or haemorrhage. These examples show early malignant change in a pre-existing naevus (left) and an advanced malignant melanoma (right).

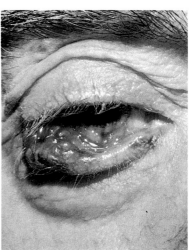

Fig. 2.50 Pathology of a malignant melanoma shows proliferation of atypical melanocytes within the epithelium. There is invasion of the underlying stroma, which shows an inflammatory reaction.

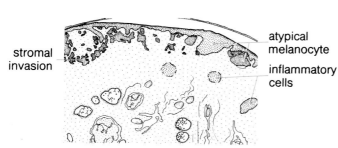

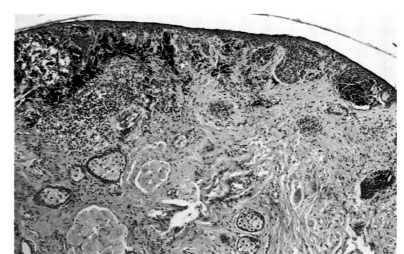

Fig. 2.51   Meibomian gland carcinoma may occur either in a localized or a more generalized form. When the carcinoma is relatively localized, it often presents as a persistent and recurrent meibomian cyst. These localized tumours, as in this example, can be treated surgically.

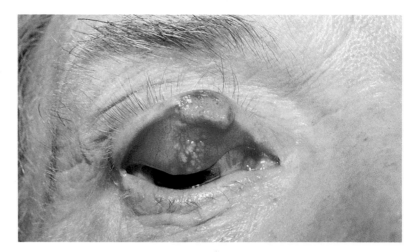

Fig. 2.52   The more generalized form of meibomian gland carcinoma often presents as a severe unilateral and persistent chronic blepharitis, as in this case. Diffuse disease normally carries a poor prognosis and may be treated by a combination of radiotherapy and surgery including exenteration.

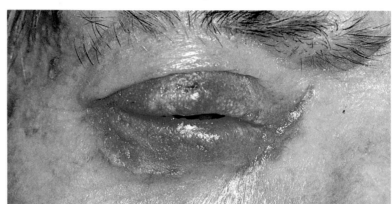

Fig. 2.53   The pathology of meibomian gland carcinoma shows cells with foamy vacuolated cytoplasm and large hyperchromatic nuclei. Mitotic figures are also seen.

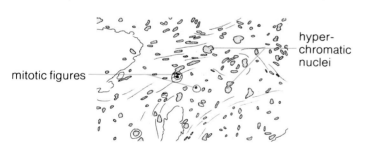

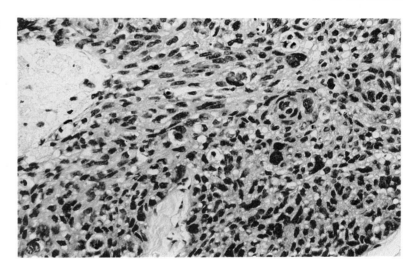

TISSUE DEFICIENCY AND TRAUMA

Patients may be born with eyelid tissue defects or, defects may be acquired subsequently from either accidental or iatrogenic trauma.

Fig. 2.54   Epicanthic folds are abnormal folds of skin at the medial canthus which result from a relative shortage of tissue. They are common in childhood, especially in children of oriental origin, but they may also be acquired as a result of tissue loss from trauma (Fig. 2.58). Congenital epicanthic folds are important because the child may present with pseudostrabismus. They usually become less obvious with age but if they persist, both congenital and acquired folds can be treated by a variety of plastic surgery procedures.

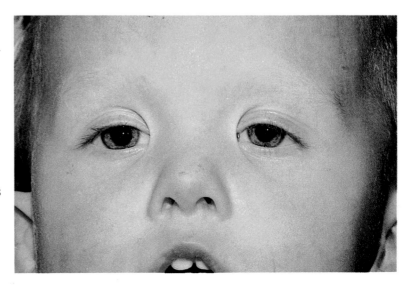

Fig. 2.55 Congenital lid colobomas are the result of a failure of normal development of the eyelid and closure of the facial clefts. Urgent repair is only required if the defect is so severe that the cornea is likely to suffer permanent damage from exposure.

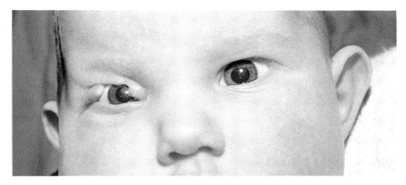

Fig. 2.56 Full-thickness loss of eyelid tissue, as in this case following a caustic burn, may result in corneal exposure and requires sophisticated techniques of lid reconstructive surgery. Conjunctival damage is often present, creating problems of symblepharon and loss of ocular motility, a dry eye, or damage to the lacrimal drainage system.

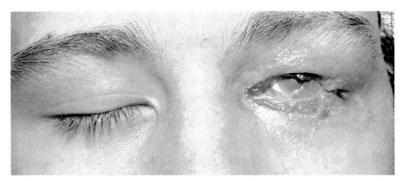

Fig. 2.57 A lateral traction injury to the eyelid can avulse it from the medial canthal tendon, lacerating the lacrimal drainage apparatus without loss of lid tissue. Many cases of avulsion follow assault.

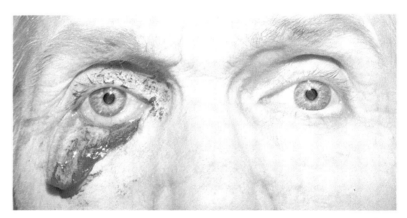

Fig. 2.58 Pigment and dirt, which is not adequately removed at the time of the original injury, can become ingrained into the tissues and lead to the tattooing shown in this patient who had been involved in an explosion.

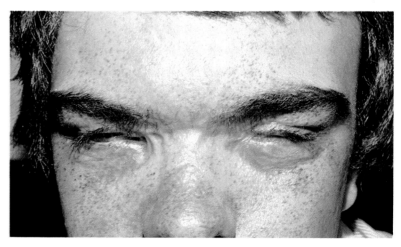

Fig. 2.59 In this patient, severe injuries around the orbit as in this case, have caused orbital wall fractures and avulsion of the medial canthal tendon, resulting in a traumatic telecanthus. Such a severe injury may also cause ptosis as in this case, from either direct injury to the levator complex, injury to the nerve supply, or by causing enophthalmus following a blow-out fracture.

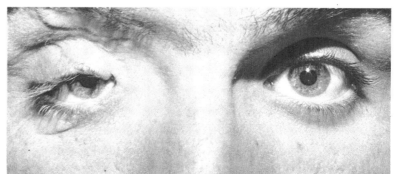

3. Conjunctival Disease and Tumours

P. A. Hunter

THE NORMAL CONJUNCTIVA

The conjunctiva is the transparent mucous membrane which lines the inner surfaces of the eyelids and is reflected over the anterior sclera before terminating at the limbus. In the embryo, it is developed from the ectoderm covering those structures and is formed during the third month of intrauterine life as the eyelids grow together.

A healthy conjunctiva is essential for normal ocular function. Its chief purpose is the maintenance of a suitable corneal environment, through its contribution towards the stability of the tear film, its secretion of some nutrients in the tears, and in its role in defence against exogenous disease.

Fig. 3.1 The conjunctiva consists of a bulbar portion investing the anterior part of the globe (except for the cornea), and two palpebral portions which cover the posterior aspects of the upper and lower eyelids. The palpebral and bulbar conjunctiva are continuous via the upper and lower fornices.

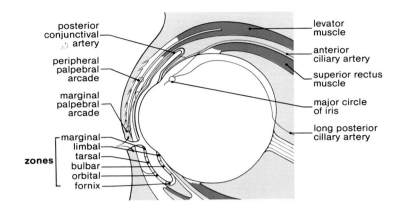

Fig. 3.2 The bulbar conjunctiva is normally transparent making the subconjunctival and episcleral blood vessels easily visible. Its anterior limit is the limbus where the epithelium becomes continuous with that of the cornea. The normal limbal arcade of blood vessels (formed by the anastomosis of the terminal branches of the posterior conjunctival and anterior ciliary vessels) may extend a short distance into the cornea, but in so doing terminates in an even border with the clear cornea.

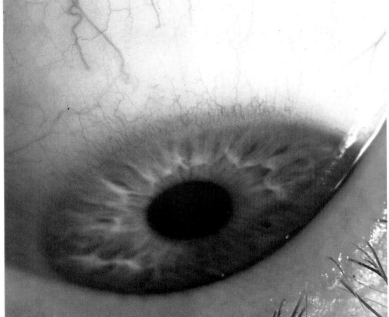

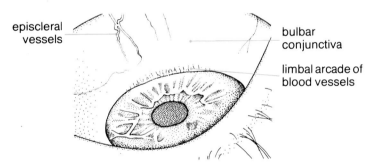

Fig. 3.3 The lower palpebral conjunctiva may be readily inspected by gentle downward traction on the lower eyelid. It is slightly thicker than the bulbar conjunctiva and is highly vascular, especially in its tarsal portion where it derives its blood supply from the tarsal arcades. The lower fornix itself has fewer blood vessels but a greater amount of lymphoid tissue and mucus-secreting glands.

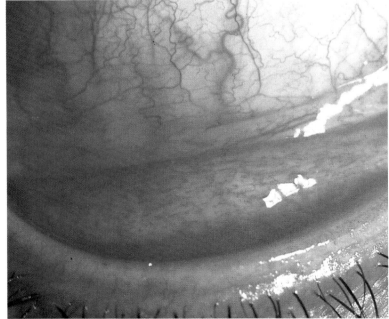

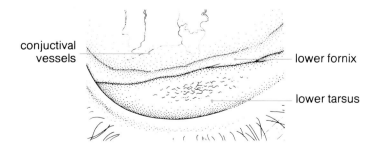

Fig. 3.4 The upper tarsal conjunctiva is inspected by everting the upper eyelid. As in the lower lid, it is firmly adherent to the underlying tarsal plate. The blood supply is derived from the palpebral arcades whose branches are readily visible. A small number of lymphoid follicles can often be seen at the medial and lateral aspects of its upper border.

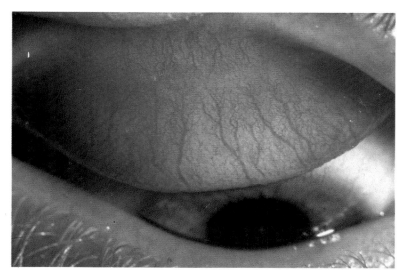

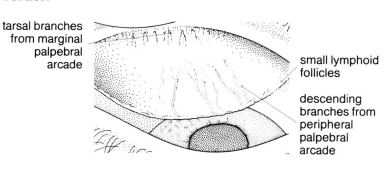

Fig. 3.5 The upper fornix is only visible on double eversion of the upper eyelid using a retractor. Here the posterior conjunctival vessels are visible and interspersed with yellowish patches of inactive lymphoid tissue.

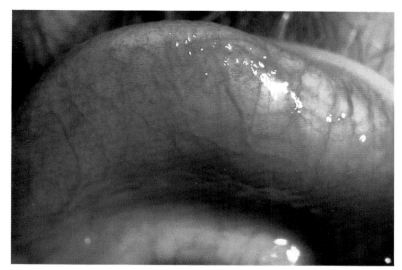

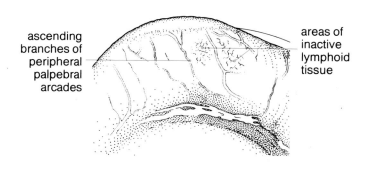

Fig. 3.6 The microscopic anatomy of the conjunctiva shows it to consist of non-keratinizing squamous epithelium overlying a substantia propria. In its tarsal portion, the connective tissue elements of the latter form a fine network creating a papillary structure, but towards the fornices it is looser and contains elastic fibres, blood vessels and lymphoid tissue. In addition, the conjunctiva contains numerous goblet (mucus-secreting) cells, especially in the fornices, and the accessory (lacrimal) glands of Krause and Wolfring.

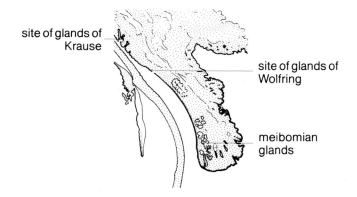

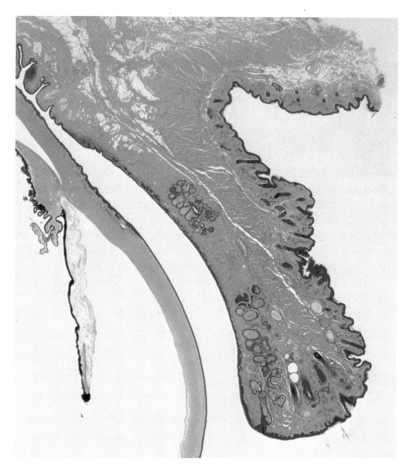

PATHOLOGICAL CHANGES OF THE CONJUNCTIVA

The conjunctiva may undergo a variety of changes either during the course or as a result of disease processes. Recognition of the types of change may give valuable information as to the aetiology of the disease. These principal pathological changes are demonstrated in this section.

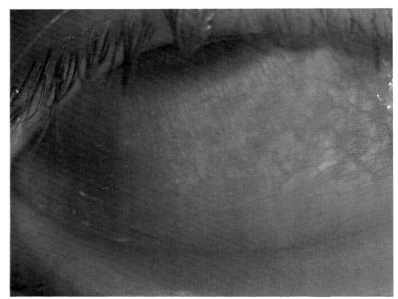

Fig. 3.7 Hyperaemia of the conjunctiva may occur as part of an acute inflammatory process or in response to chronic irritative factors. There is an increase in the number, calibre, and tortuosity of the vessels producing a characteristic bright red appearance. Hyperaemia is often associated with an increase of vascular permeability giving rise to oedema, infiltrate or, as in this case, small subconjunctival haemorrhages.

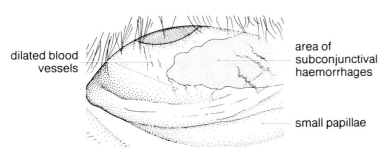

Fig. 3.8 Congestion of the conjunctival vessels arises as a result of impaired venous drainage which if severe may additionally produce oedema of the conjunctiva (chemosis). The characteristic dusky red coloration results from a prolonged circulation time within the conjunctiva.

Chemosis may, of course, arise without venous congestion. This occurs most commonly in association with acute allergic states when the pale swollen conjunctiva takes on a jelly-like appearance (cf. Diseases of the Cornea – Chapter 6).

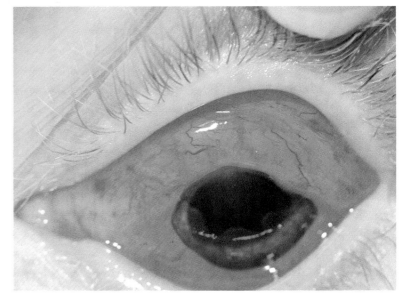

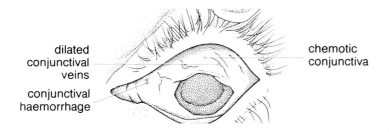

Fig. 3.9 Subconjunctival haemorrhages most frequently arise spontaneously when they appear as bright red patches extending to the limbus. They may result from an episode of raised venous pressure, for example, following coughing, or less commonly from blood dyscrasias, vessel anomalies or trauma. In this last instance, if no posterior limit to the haemorrhage is defined, the blood may have resulted from a middle or anterior cranial fossa fracture and patients should be examined with this in mind.

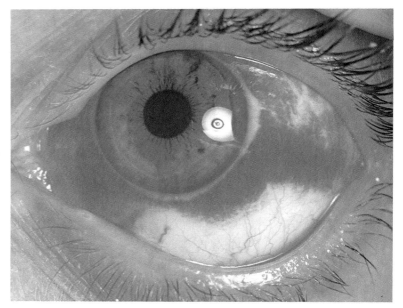

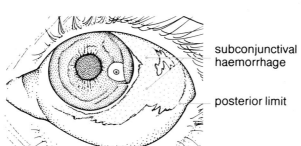

Fig. 3.10 Papillae are seen in the palpebral conjunctiva during acute inflammatory states and represent an exaggeration of some aspects of the normal conjunctival anatomy. Clinically, they can be recognized as small elevations of the conjunctiva which together give the tissues a velvety appearance. Each papilla contains a central dilated arteriole with a surrounding clear or slightly infiltrated zone of swollen conjunctiva. Usually, they can only be seen on biomicroscopic examination, but in some chronic conditions giant papillae may form which can be seen with the naked eye. (cf. Diseases of the Cornea — Chapter 6).

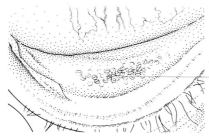

small papillae showing central arteriole

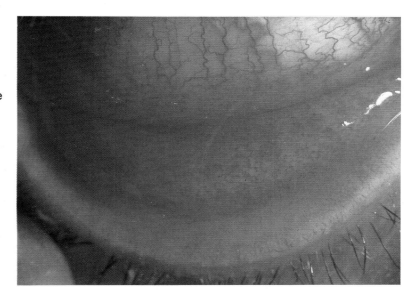

Fig. 3.11 Histologically, the conjunctiva between individual papillae can be seen to be connected to the underlying tarsal plate by the fibrous network normally present in the substantia propria. A dilated central blood vessel can be seen in some papillae in this section: many chronic inflammatory cells are also present.

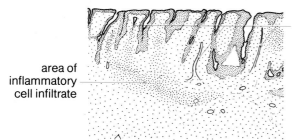

dilated arterioles

area of inflammatory cell infiltrate

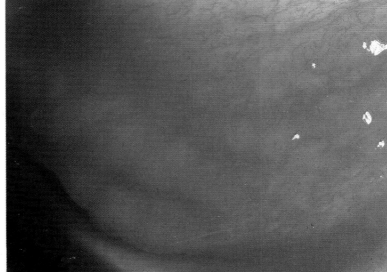

Fig. 3.12 The clinical appearance of follicles is of large pinkish or pale grey elevations lying beneath the conjunctival epithelium with small blood vessels frequently visible on their surface. In the early stages, they are present only in the fornices but may extend onto the tarsi if the disease becomes chronic. They are especially associated with those conditions in which cell-mediated immune mechanisms are involved, such as viral disorders and drug hypersensitivity.

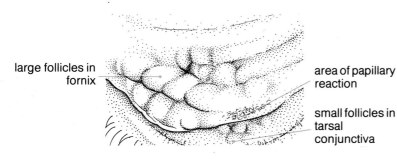

large follicles in fornix

area of papillary reaction

small follicles in tarsal conjunctiva

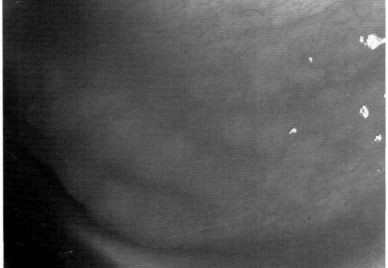

Fig. 3.13 Follicles consist of aggregations of lymphocytes. In chronic states, they may begin to resemble a germinal follicle with a paler staining area surrounded by darker lymphocytes when stained with haematoxylin and eosin.

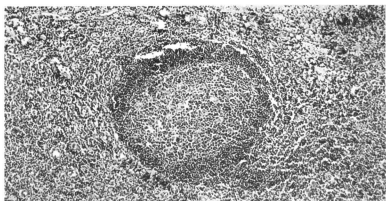

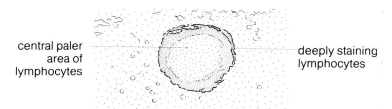

central paler area of lymphocytes

deeply staining lymphocytes

Fig. 3.14 Pseudomembrane formation on the surface of the conjunctiva is seen in cases of severe acute conjunctivitis. A fibrinous exudate forms which is initially loosely adherent to the underlying tissues. At this stage, it may be wiped from the surface with a cotton swab, often revealing a bleeding conjunctival surface. It may later become more firmly attached and organize as scar tissue.

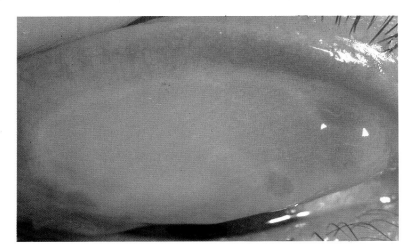

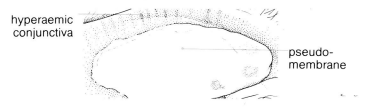

hyperaemic conjunctiva

pseudo-membrane

Fig. 3.15 Conjunctival scarring may be the end result of a wide variety of inflammatory processes and its effects on the eye vary from insignificant to devastating depending on its effects on the tear film and lid architecture. Localized superficial linear scarring may have little clinical significance, as in this example which followed a severe viral conjunctivitis.

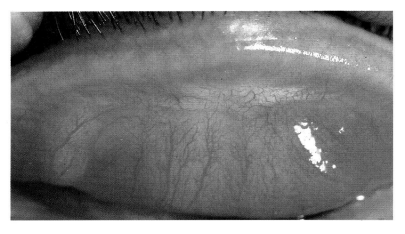

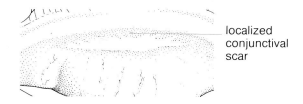

localized conjunctival scar

Fig. 3.16 Extensive diffuse scarring resulting from trachoma may have serious effects on the eye by diminishing the protective functions of the lids and conjunctiva. Contraction of the scar may result in entropion, trichiasis, and lid shortening. Obliteration of

the normal mucus-secreting cells may affect the stability of the tear film. This example also shows some fibrovascular proliferation in the surface of the scar tissue which may subsequently add to the already extensive scar by further fibrosis.

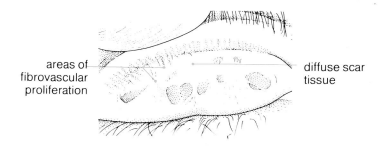

areas of fibrovascular proliferation

diffuse scar tissue

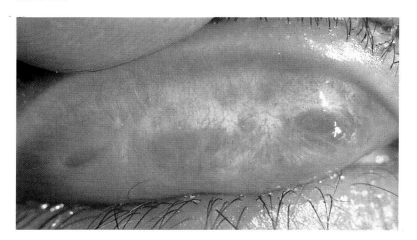

Fig. 3.17 Symblepharon is an adhesion between the conjunctiva covering the lids and the globe. In this example, severe conjunctival adhesions developed following a lime burn. Disorders of ocular motility and poor lid closure with corneal exposure or instability of the tear film may result.

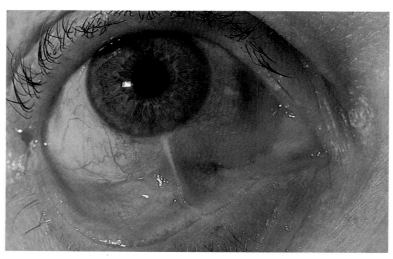

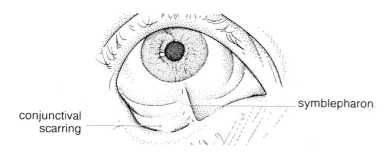
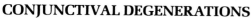

conjunctival scarring — symblepharon

CONJUNCTIVAL DEGENERATIONS

Degenerative changes in the conjunctiva rarely produce serious effects on ocular function and, in many instances, their recognition serves mainly to exclude progressive disease. Degenerative changes may occur either as a result of age, or may be related to exposure of the eye to sun, wind or weather over long periods. This later group of disorders can be distinguished by their distribution in the interpalpebral area of the globe.

Fig. 3.18 Pingueculae may be formed in the conjunctiva adjacent to the limbus on the nasal side, or later on the temporal side. They are raised yellowish patches which gradually enlarge until they abut the cornea but do not encroach upon it. Histologically, they are formed by elastotic degeneration of collagen within the substantia propria.

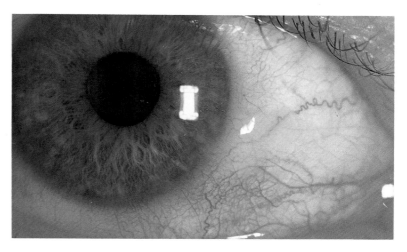

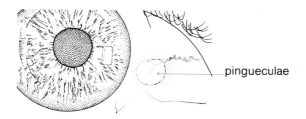

pingueculae

Fig. 3.19 A pterygium is a raised triangular area of bulbar conjunctiva which actively invades the cornea to produce visual symptoms if the pupillary area is involved. In temperate climates the condition progresses only very slowly, but in sunny, hot dusty regions of the world it can represent a serious threat to vision. It is usually bilateral with the nasal side of the interpalpebral area being affected most commonly. Examination of the leading edge and body of the lesion shows whether the pterygium is active by the degree of vascular dilatation in the bulk of the lesion. Surgical removal is indicated if visual impairment is threatened or if the lesion causes discomfort, but the recurrence rate may be as high as thirty to fifty percent in those countries with a high degree of solar exposure and successful removal presents a considerable surgical challenge.

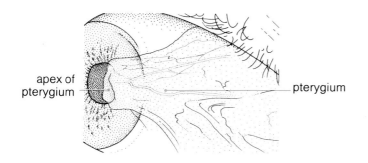

apex of pterygium — pterygium

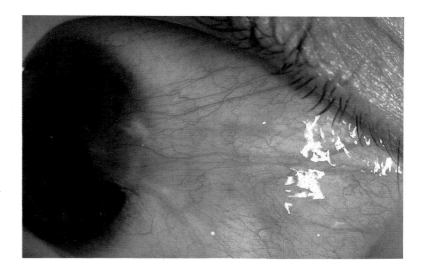

Fig. 3.20 The histology shows marked fibroblastic activity under the apex of the pterygium where Bowman's membrane has been destroyed. Elsewhere, the pterygium consists of acellular hyaline material covered by thinner conjunctival epithelium and pseudoelastic degeneration, similar to that observed in a pinguecula (which probably represents the initial stage of the disease). This initial irregularity is thought to disturb the uniformity of the tear film causing a localized alteration in the tear meniscus and a focal area of drying (a dellen), which stimulates corneal inversion.

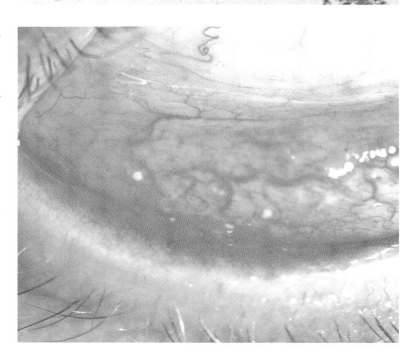

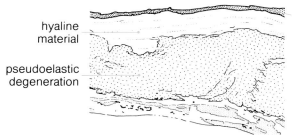

Fig. 3.21 Concretions are minute hard yellow spots seen in the palpebral conjunctiva of elderly people, although they may also be the result of chronic inflammatory disease. They rarely cause symptoms but, if large, they occasionally project through the surface of the conjunctiva to produce a foreign body sensation and will stain with bengal rose or fluorescein. If necessary, they may be removed using a needle point under topical anaesthesia. They are formed by cellular degeneration when the products remain trapped in small recesses of the conjunctiva and become calcified.

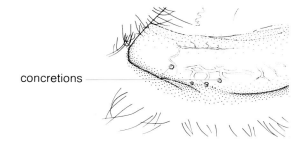

CYSTS

Conjunctival cysts may be congenital (a dermoid cyst) or acquired during life (as a result of trauma; implantation cysts; or in the form of retention cysts).

Fig. 3.22 Conjunctival retention cysts are common and usually develop in the accessory lacrimal gland of Krause. These are thin-walled cysts filled with clear watery fluid and usually do not cause any symptoms. If large, they may be excised or marsupialized.

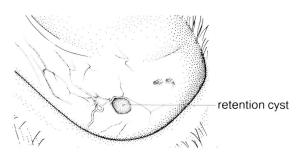

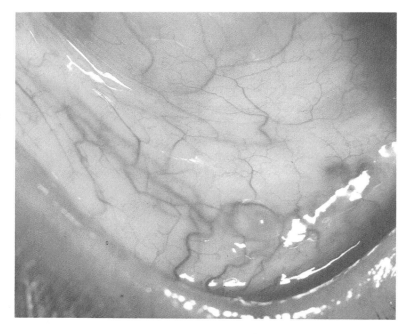

Fig. 3.23 Dermoid cysts are congenital tumours involving tissue of mesodermal and ectodermal origin. They appear as raised circumscribed pale yellowish growths and are generally situated at the lower temporal limbus where they involve the cornea, conjunctiva and sclera. They are normally present at birth and, although

enlargement is unusual, removal may be justified on cosmetic grounds when the child is nearing school age. If the deeper layers of the cornea are involved, a lamellar keratoplasty may be required to restore corneal thickness and reduce astigmatism.

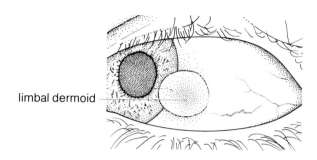

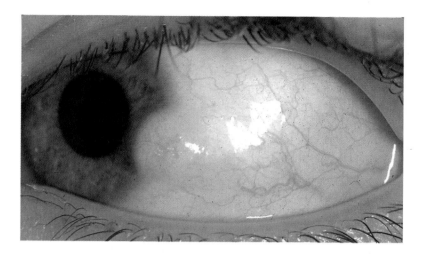

Fig. 3.24 Children with dermoid cysts should be examined for other signs of Goldenhar's syndrome, (first branchial arch syndrome) – accessory auricles, limbal and orbital dermoids, sometimes with maldevelopment of the jaw.

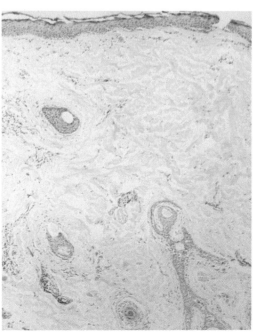

Fig. 3.25 The histology of a limbal dermoid shows it to consist of abundant collagen with a surface covering of stratified squamous epithelium. A variety of tissues may be present within the collagen matrix, as in this example where islands of sweat gland ducts and a hair follicle are visible.

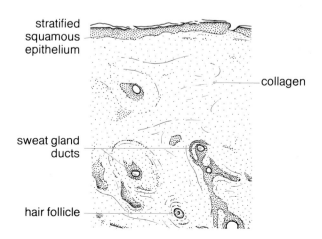

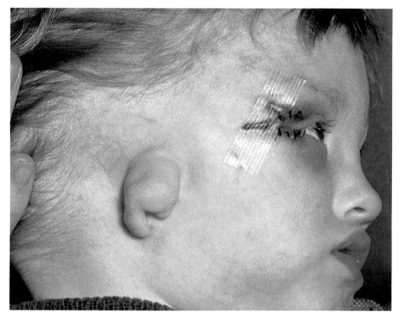

NON-PIGMENTED TUMOURS OF THE CONJUNCTIVA

The clinical differentiation between conjunctival and corneal tumours, hypertrophic and neoplastic processes and benign and malignant conditions may prove immensely difficult on the basis of a single examination.

Where doubt exists, several examinations over a period of time (with the aid of serial photographs) may be required to observe the evolution of a lesion and, in some cases, biopsy will be required to establish a diagnosis.

Fig. 3.26 Tumours may be classified, according to their tissue of origin, into those arising from the surface epithelium (or its associated glandular elements), connective tissue, vascular, lymphoid tissue or peripheral nerves. Pigmented lesions of the conjunctiva are an important group of conditions which will be considered in detail in a separate section.

A Classification of the Origins of Conjunctival Tumours

Tissue of Origin	Benign	Malignant
Epithelium		
a – surface epithelium	kerato-acanthoma dyskeratoses papilloma	Bowen's disease squamous carcinoma
b – glandular origin	adenoma	pleomorphic adenoma
Connective Tissue	fibroma myxoma osteoma	sarcoma
Vascular	haemangioma	angiosarcoma
Reticulososis	lymphoid hyperplasia	lymphoma lymphosarcoma
Peripheral nerve	neurofibroma neurilemmoma	malignant schwannoma
Pigmented	naevus	melanoma

Fig. 3.27 Dyskeratosis is a term that encompasses a variety of pathological changes taking place within the corneal and conjunctival epithelium and which may present clinically as a dry white plaque on the surface of the globe (leucoplakia). The disease may arise as a result of a variety of chronic irritative factors such as radiation and topical drug therapy. In this unusual example, dyskeratosis followed prolonged miotic therapy in a case of aphakic glaucoma. The dry, keratinized white plaque shows clearly against the chronically inflamed conjunctiva, which has taken up fluorescein stain.

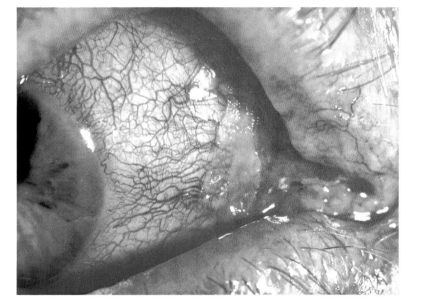

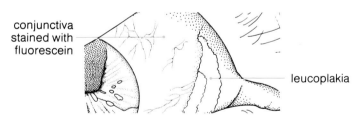

Fig. 3.28 Some of the histological features of dyskeratosis are shown in this example where epithelial hyperplasia is associated with excessive keratin formation. There is underlying pseudoelastic degeneration and, in this case, a chronic inflammatory reaction is present as indicated by the lymphocytes in the subepithelial layers.

It is not uncommon for dyskeratotic lesions to undergo malignant change and produce an invasive carcinoma. Such lesions should therefore be excised if there is any suspicion of malignancy.

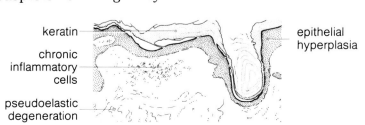

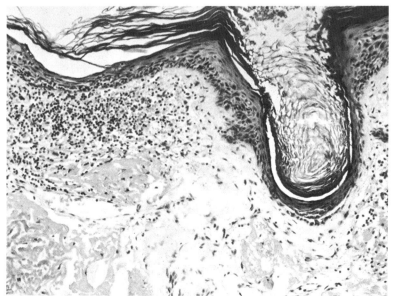

Fig. 3.29 Papillomata arising in the conjunctiva are usually soft pink pedunculated lesions with a slightly irregular surface. They occur most commonly in patients over forty years of age either at the caruncle or in the fornices. They may occasionally be multiple. When a papilloma occurs at the limbus, it may invade the cornea to which it becomes firmly adherent. Treatment is by excision, and should where possible, include, an area of healthy conjunctiva around the base.

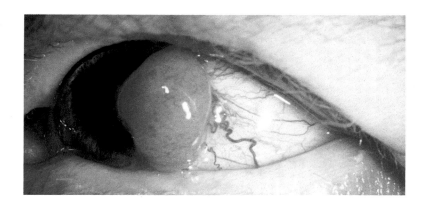

Fig. 3.30 Histologically, a conjunctival papilloma contains a fibrovascular stalk with processes extending towards the surface of the lesion which consists of greatly thickened stratified squamous epithelium.

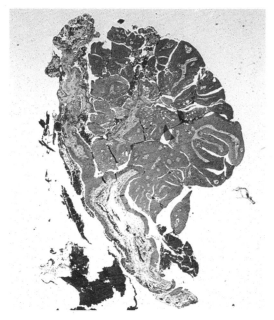

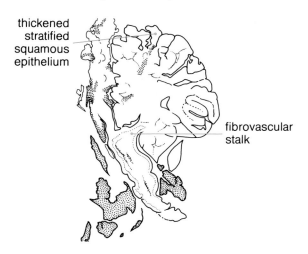

thickened stratified squamous epithelium

fibrovascular stalk

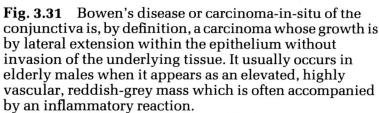

Fig. 3.31 Bowen's disease or carcinoma-in-situ of the conjunctiva is, by definition, a carcinoma whose growth is by lateral extension within the epithelium without invasion of the underlying tissue. It usually occurs in elderly males when it appears as an elevated, highly vascular, reddish-grey mass which is often accompanied by an inflammatory reaction.

Bowen's disease should be treated by local excision and a striking feature of corneal involvement is the ease with which the lesion is stripped from the Bowman's membrane.

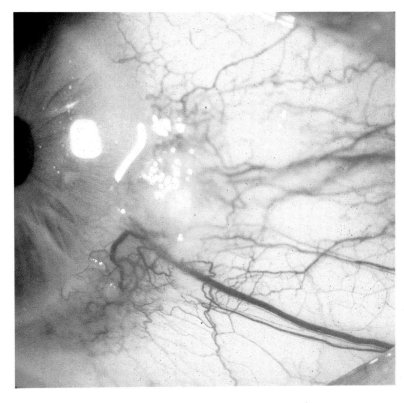

Fig. 3.32   The histological features of Bowen's disease are a proliferation of the basal cells of the epithelium, with partial loss of their normal polarity and hence their regular palisades. The nuclei are hyperchromatic and mitotic figures are common. The basement membrane is intact and, as indicated previously, spread is by lateral growth.

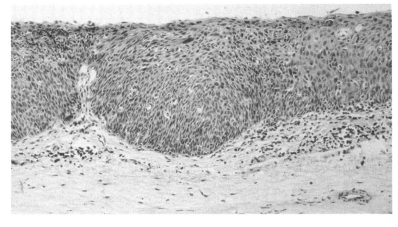

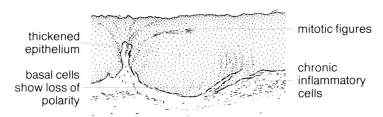

Fig. 3.33   Squamous cell carcinoma (epithelioma) of the conjunctiva is a relatively rare condition which develops most commonly at the limbus in the interpalpebral zone. It starts as a small grey nodule which, as in this example, becomes almond-shaped as it extends around the limbus.

Large feeder vessels have developed which, when associated with tumours of the eye, should always give rise to the suspicion of malignancy. In its early stages, such a lesion may be treated by wide local excision but recurrences are common.

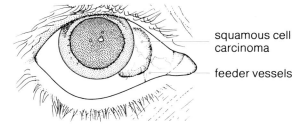

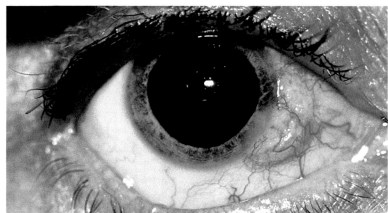

Fig. 3.34   A more advanced case of squamous cell carcinoma with extensive progression around the limbus and invasion onto the cornea. Note the prominent feeding vessel.

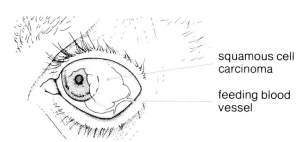

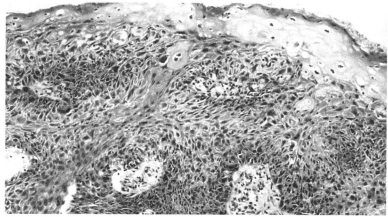

Fig. 3.35   Histology of a moderately well differentiated carcinoma with keratin formation on its surface. In contrast to papilloma, there is marked pleomorphism of the basal cells which have broken through the basement membrane into the underlying tissues.

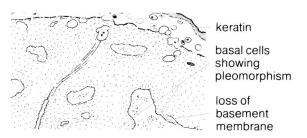

Fig. 3.36 This example of a small haemangioma of the conjunctiva had been present for many years with no alteration in size. The feeding vessels reflect the vascular nature of the lesion rather than its malignancy.

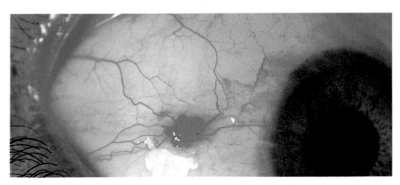

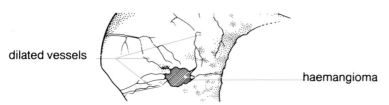

Fig. 3.37 The histology of a similar capillary angioma is shown in this illustration. There is focal proliferation of blood vessels lined by normal endothelial cells. The overlying conjunctival epithelium is thinned.

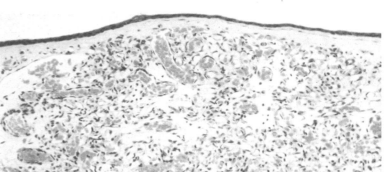

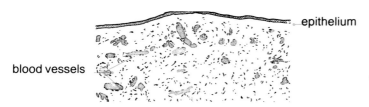

Fig. 3.38 This is an example of benign lymphoid hyperplasia in the conjunctiva. The lesion presents as a slowly growing diffuse tumour involving the bulbar conjunctiva and the fornices. The unaffected conjunctiva appears normal and thereby distinguishes the condition from the lymphoid follicles seen in cases of inflammatory conjunctivitis.

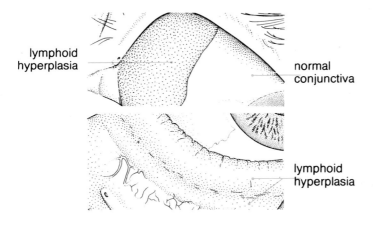

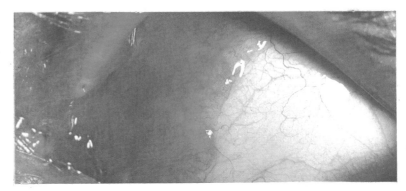

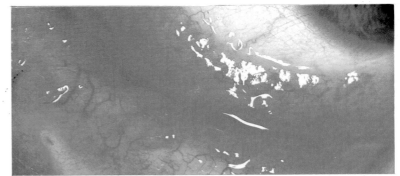

Fig. 3.39 In histological section, a mixture of lymphoblasts (with paler staining nuclei) and lymphocytes (with darker nuclei) can be seen. No mitotic figures are visible and the surface of the lesion is covered by a thinner epithelium. The histological differentiation of benign or malignant conjunctival lymphomas can be extremely difficult, and the clinical picture and follow-up for lymphoma elsewhere is most important. Recent studies with cell markers for T and B lymphocytes are likely to lead to a reclassification of these tumours.

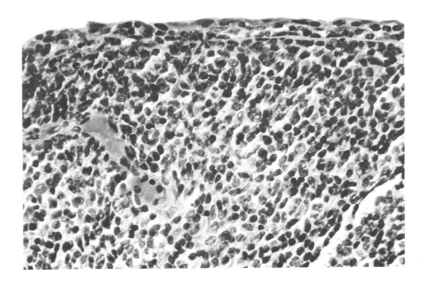

PIGMENTED LESIONS OF THE THE CONJUNCTIVA

The melanocytes of the conjunctiva are derived from the neural crest in the same way as those of the skin or uveal tract. A wide variety of pigmented conjunctival lesions is seen clinically, which are frequently difficult to diagnose and have varying degrees of malignant potential. Freckles and naevi are usually thought of as congenital lesions, although they may not be apparent at birth. They tend to become more pigmented and larger with age, and especially at puberty. Junctional and compound naevi have a low malignant potential.

Excess melanin in the conjunctiva is known as melanosis and may be either a congenital or acquired disease.

Fig. 3.40 A classification of pigmented lesions of the conjunctiva.

A Classification of Pigmented Lesions of the Conjunctiva

Freckles

Naevi –
  junctional
  subepithelial
  compound
  blue naevi

Congenital Melanosis Oculi
  (± naevus of Ota)

Acquired Melanosis –
  primary precancerous
  secondary to drugs etc.

Malignant Melanoma

Melanosis

Congenital melanosis oculi is seen as an isolated condition or as part of a naevus of Ota where there is a unilateral blue naevus of the skin of the face and eyelid: these patients have an increased risk of choroidal malignant melanoma but do not carry any extra risk of developing conjunctival malignancy.

Acquired melanosis may be due to a variety of causes such as exposure, drugs, or Nelson's syndrome, but primary acquired melanosis of the conjunctiva carries a high risk of the patient developing multiple malignant melanomas. Although malignant melanomas of the conjunctiva will invade locally and metastasize to the regional lymph glands, their growth tends to be slow and small lesions do well with local treatment, especially cryotherapy.

Congenital melanosis may be either epithelial (when it appears as localized pigment flecks in the bulbar conjunctiva) or subepithelial (when it is diffuse and may be associated with the cutaneous naevus of Ota). This is a diffuse unilateral slate-grey discoloration seen on the lids and face which has the histological features of a blue naevus. Neither form has been shown to have any tendency towards malignant change in the conjunctiva.

Fig. 3.41 This example of congenital subepithelial melanosis shows a large bluish-grey area of pigmentation extending back to the limbus. The edge of the lesion is slightly mottled and the very dark iris indicates associated melanosis bulbi which may sometimes accompany the condition and carries a higher than normal risk of developing choroidal malignant melanoma. For this reason, patients should be observed at yearly intervals but otherwise require no treatment. Diffuse slate-grey pigmentation of the eyelids from the naevus of Ota can also be seen in this patient.

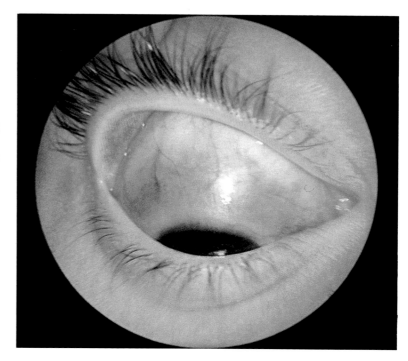

Fig. 3.42 One form of acquired melanosis associated with long-standing conjunctival disease is shown in this case of ectropion in a black patient. Similar pronounced pigmentary changes may be seen in the conjunctiva of patients with trachoma or onchocerciasis and probably reflect a high rate of conjunctival epithelial turnover associated with chronic disease. Acquired melanosis in Caucasian individuals is of far greater significance where it may represent a pre-malignant condition (see Fig. 3.44).

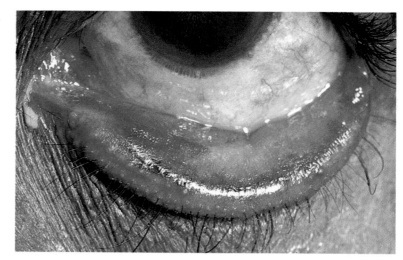

Fig. 3.43 Benign naevi, although embryonic in origin, are not always present at birth and in many cases they may not become apparent until adulthood. They are common lesions and their usual site is at the limbus, as this example where the pigmented area contrasts markedly with the white sclera. They tend to grow slowly but, providing they do not undergo rapid change or develop feeder vessels, no treatment is required. A simple excision is easy to perform, however, and removes any worry of potential malignant change.

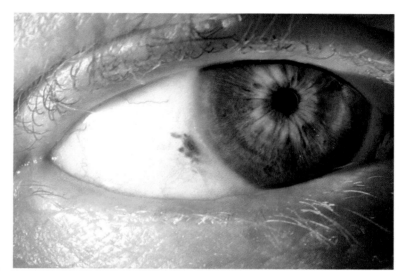

Fig. 3.44 Compound naevi tend to be elevated lesions which, histologically, contain both epithelial and subepithelial elements. In this example, a densely pigmented raised naevus is situated on the caruncle. Treatment is by simple excision.

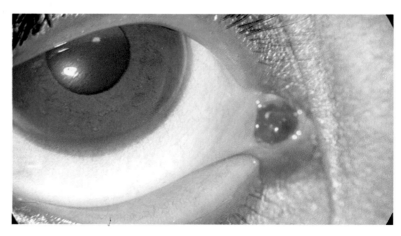

Fig. 3.45 A predominant feature in the histology of many benign naevi is a cystic component which is not always obvious clinically. These appear when epithelial downgrowths become nipped off by naevus cells and lead to mucus accumulation. Naevus cells are the small cells with a deeply staining nucleus and little cytoplasm.

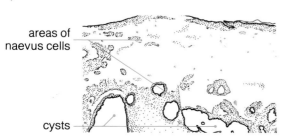

areas of
naevus cells

cysts

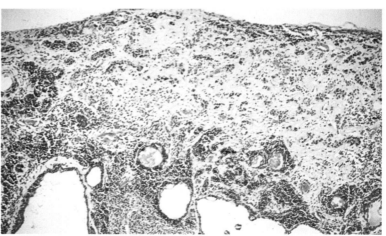

Fig. 3.46 Malignant melanomas of the conjunctiva may arise spontaneously, from a pre-existing naevus, or an area of precancerous melanosis. They occur with equal frequency in males and females, most commonly between the ages of forty and sixty years. This is an example of a malignant melanoma arising at the limbus and spreading into the cornea. Many feeding blood vessels are visible. Localized lesions may be treated by excision of the affected conjunctiva with a wide margin of tissue.

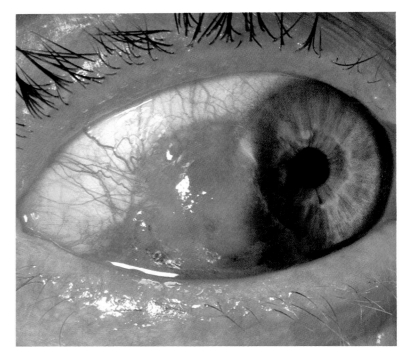

Fig. 3.47 This slide shows mutiple malignant melanomas of the conjunctiva arising in areas of acquired precancerous melanosis. All patients with acquired melanosis should be followed at regular intervals with serial photography. Pigmented areas which increase in size or develop feeding vessels should be excised and examined histologically for evidence of malignancy.

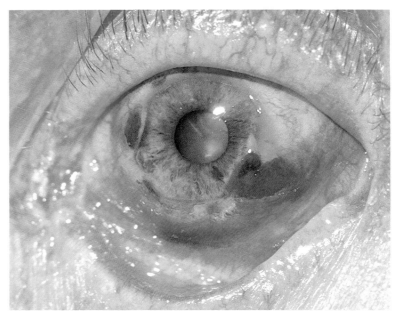

Fig. 3.48 Malignant melanomas may spread by direct means or by seeding to other parts of the conjunctival sac. In this example, a melanoma on the upper tarsus has given rise to lesions at the lid margin, elsewhere in the conjunctiva, and at the upper limbus. In this instance exenteration of the orbit, including the eyelids, offers the only surgical way of removing all potential tumour-bearing tissue.

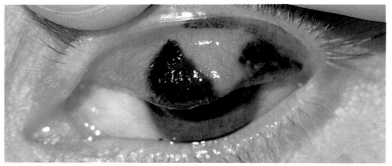

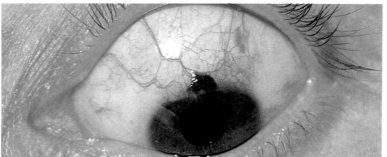

Fig. 3.49 This gross example of a neglected malignant melanoma shows a fungating tumour which has arisen from the anterior part of the globe and spread onto the cheek. In spite of its size, there was no direct invasion of neighbouring orbital or facial structures and no evidence of distance metastases.

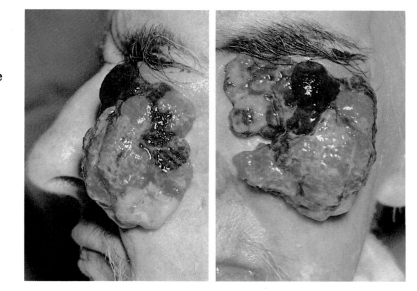

Fig. 3.50 This specimen, removed by limited exenteration, shows the position and extent of a malignant melanoma in macroscopic section. A large conjunctival melanoma is visible occupying over one-third of the anterior surface of the globe in the section shown. No invasion of the globe has taken place.

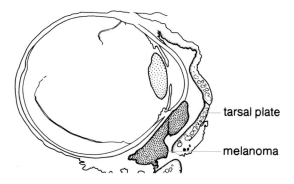

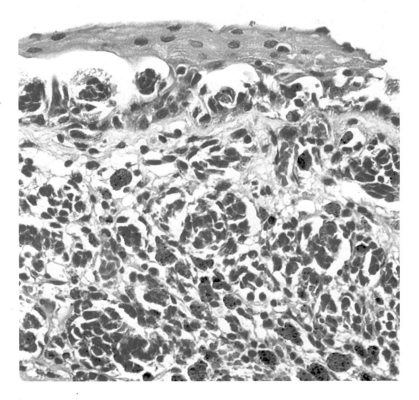

Fig. 3.51 A high-powered histological section of a malignant melanoma of the conjunctiva shows large numbers of tumour cells with densely-staining nuclei, some of which can be seen invading the necrotic epithelium. Many mitotic figures are present. Macrophages, containing abundant melanin pigment granules are prominent, together with many blood vessels.

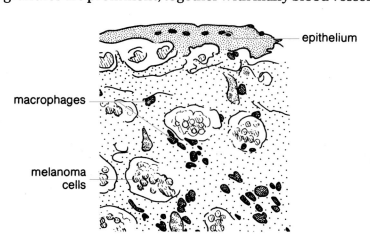

Drug-Induced Pigmentation

Pigmentation of the conjunctiva may be the result of an adverse reaction to long-term drug administration.

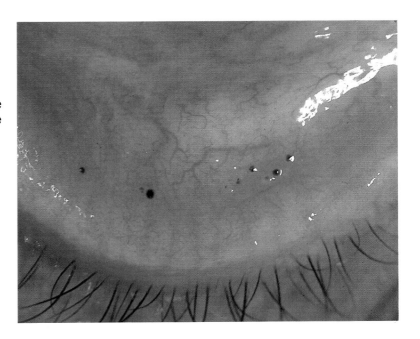

Fig. 3.52 Melanin pigment may be present in the conjunctiva as a result of the long-term use of epinephrine drops used in the treatment of glaucoma. The epinephrine undergoes oxidation when trapped in pre-existing conjunctival pockets, concretions, or cysts resulting in discrete "granules" which usually cause no symptoms.

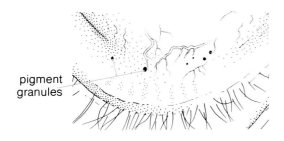

Fig. 3.53 Argyrosis of the conjunctiva and cornea is due to the deposition of silver which used to result from the long-term topical use of silver-containing therapeutic preparations. The conjunctiva develops slate-grey areas of pigmentation which is seen here most clearly as the caruncle. A pinguecula is also present on the bulbar conjunctiva. Silver deposition in the cornea appears as a broad greyish band affecting Descemet's membrane in the periphery.

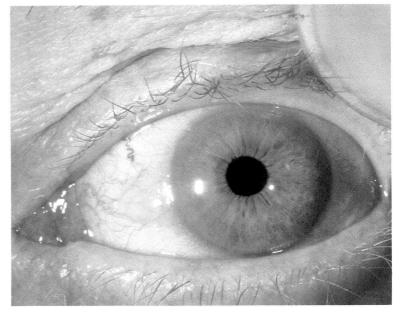

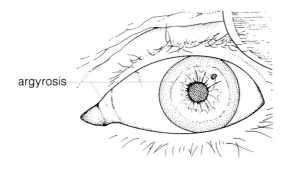

Fig. 3.54 At greater magnification, under slit illumination, refractile deposits are seen at the level of Descemet's membrane and the deeper parts of the stroma. The epithelium is unaffected. Similar conjunctival and corneal pigmentation is a feature of chronic mercury deposition either from mercurials which used to be incorporated in drops as a preservative, or in industrial workers exposed to the metal over many years. Copper is deposited similarly in the cornea as the Kayser-Fleischer ring of Wilson's disease. (cf. Diseases of the Cornea – Chapter 6).

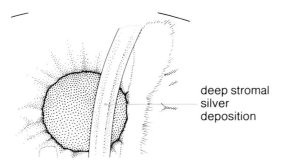

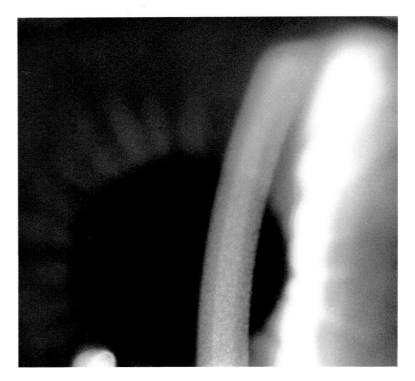

MISCELLANEOUS CONJUNCTIVAL CONDITIONS

The majority of conditions which present with inflammation of the outer eye may be ascribed to broad disease categories which are, for example, infective, allergic or traumatic in origin. There remains, however, a small number of conditions where the pathogenesis is still uncertain and some of these are considered below.

Superior Limbic Keratoconjunctivitis

Fig. 3.55 Superior limbic keratoconjunctivitis is an uncommon form of conjunctivitis in which changes appear in the upper limbus and tarsal conjunctiva. The extent of the conjunctival changes can be demonstrated by the installation of rose bengal drops which reveal a punctate staining of the conjunctiva over the upper limbus from the ten o'clock to the two o'clock positions. Most cases are associated with a history of dysthyroid eye disease, as in this case, when there is also puffiness of both eyelids and lid retraction. The disease may be related to abnormalities in the conjunctival mucus together with the physiological abrasion of the upper eyelid. Symptoms of ocular discomfort can be relieved by wetting agents.

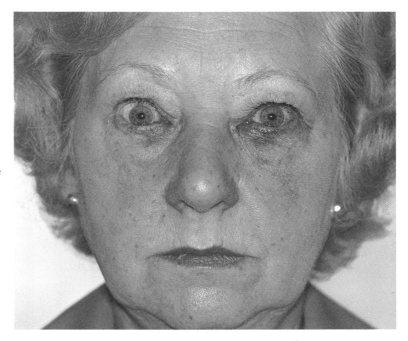

Fig. 3.56 Typically, there is bilateral involvement which is best seen in the position of down gaze. The changes are more marked in the left eye where a diffuse limbal infiltration extends on to the cornea and upwards on to the bulbar conjunctiva.

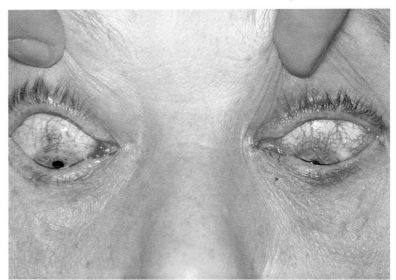

Fig. 3.57 This patient demonstrates a less marked example of superior limbic keratoconjunctivitis in which the changes are limited to scattered punctate staining of the limbus, associated with mild hyperaemia.

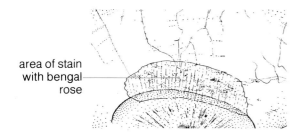

area of stain with bengal rose

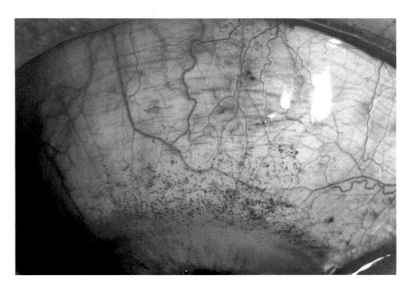

Ligneous Conjunctivitis

Fig. 3.58 Ligneous conjunctivitis is a rare condition of unknown aetiology which is associated with the massive development of granulation tissue on the conjunctiva. It usually involves the upper tarsus, but may include the lower tarsal or bulbar conjunctiva, and is more common in young children. Ligneous conjunctivitis has an acute onset, which may be related to acute infection or minor surgical trauma, and thereafter runs a chronic course.

Initially, a yellowish-white fibrinous pseudo-membrane is formed, which is thicker than in pseudo-membranous conjunctivitis, and then becomes compacted and invaded by granulation tissue, making its removal difficult. The aetiology of the disease seems to be related to excessive production of an abnormal mucus and some success has been achieved in its treatment with intensive topical mucolytic therapy.

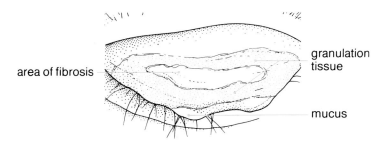

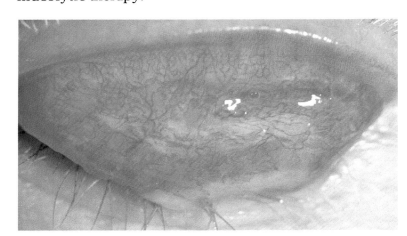

Fig. 3.59 The pathological features of ligneous conjunctivitis include a loss of the conjunctival epithelium which is replaced by an eosinophilic amorphous material that exhibits the staining characteristics of fibrin. Haemorrhage is interspersed in this amorphous material and there is a chronic inflammatory infiltrate in the underlying stroma.

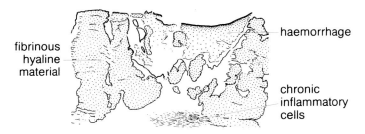

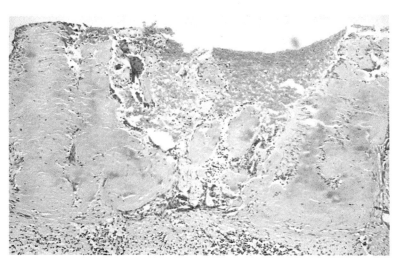

Giant Papillary Conjunctivitis

Fig. 3.60 Giant papillary conjunctivitis is a chronic condition affecting the upper tarsal conjunctiva. It has been described in patients wearing soft contact lenses and in association with protruberant suture ends at the upper limbus, following cataract removal. In this example, a hard contact lens has produced giant papillae at the medial end of the upper border of the tarsus with a fine papillary

reaction elsewhere. The presence of eosinophils and mast cells in the papillae have led some authors to suggest an allergic basis for the reaction, although the condition can be distinguished from vernal conjunctivitis by the lack of changes elsewhere in the conjunctiva, the lack of an atopic background history and the presence of an associated foreign body in the eye.

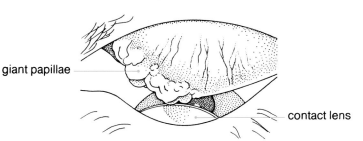

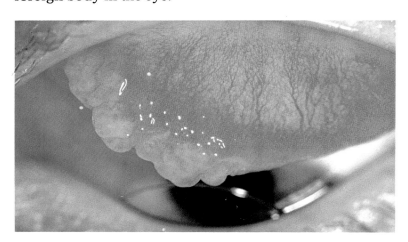

4. Infections of the Outer Eye

P. A. Hunter

VIRAL INFECTIONS

Viruses and related organisms are probably responsible for the major proportion of infections of the outer eye. They produce a wide variety of disease ranging from transient forms of conjunctivitis to the devastating blindness of trachoma, which results from repeated infection by chlamydia. The spread of infection may occur by direct inoculation from an infected source, from indirect transmission by fomites, or, occasionally, by droplet transmission. Where no specific therapy exists, symptomatic treatment is usually all that is required until resolution takes place but, in the case of herpes and chlamydial infections, accurate diagnosis is essential if the appropriate treatment is to be given. Where the diseases exist in epidemic or hyperendemic forms, public health measures may prove to be the only methods of controlling the spread of infection.

Adenovirus

Adenovirus infection may be due to a variety of different serotypes which can vary in their clinical presentation and epidemiology, although many features are common to all.

A typical case presents with acute bilateral, but unequal swelling and erythema of the eyelids. There may be associated pre-auricular lymph node enlargement, a history of contact with other similar cases, or a previous illness of the upper respiratory tract.

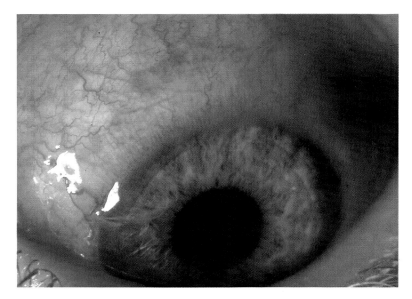

Fig. 4.1 The early stages of the disease are often accompanied by a profuse watery discharge with marked hyperaemia of the bulbar conjunctiva. This patient also has small conjunctival haemorrhages which sometimes present in the acute phase.

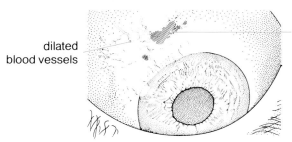

Fig. 4.2 During the first few days, the palpebral conjunctiva is hyperaemic with a fine papillary reaction. Small amounts of mucopurulent discharge are often produced (bottom).

Similar changes are visible over the upper tarsus where, in severe cases, exudation of fibrin may combine with mucus and lead to pseudomembrane formation. This photograph also shows typical hyperaemia and small subconjunctival haemorrhages (top).

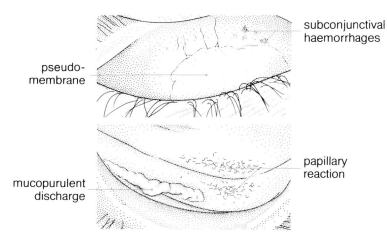

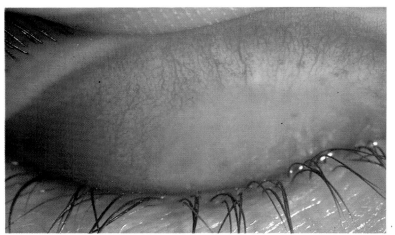

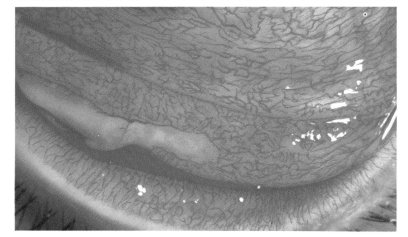

Fig. 4.3 During the first weeks, small follicles appear in the lower fornix which may later involve the tarsal surface. In the early stages, as in this example, the follicles are greyish-white with slightly raised areas appearing in the subepithelial layers of the inflamed conjunctiva (top).

During the second week of the illness, the follicles usually persist although they become more discrete with resolution of the acute inflammatory changes found elsewhere in the conjunctiva. The lower photograph is the same eye taken three days later. By the second or third week, the conjunctival disease has usually resolved. The condition is self-limiting although symptomatic relief may be obtained by the use of topical antibiotics.

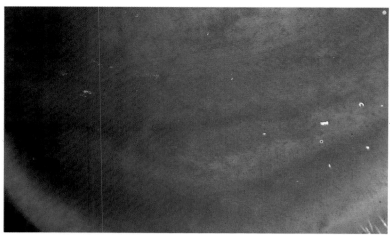

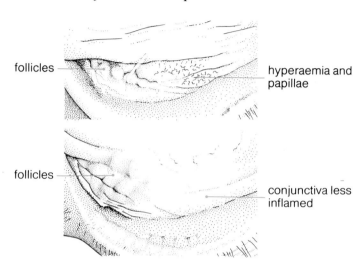

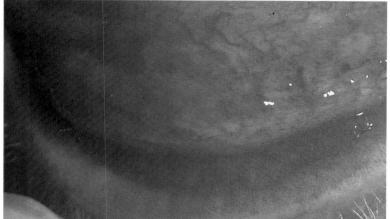

Fig. 4.4 Adenoviral keratitis is seen in the more severe forms of the disease and is particularly associated with serotypes 8, 11 and 19. It starts in the first weeks as a fine punctate epithelial keratitis which later becomes associated with subepithelial infiltrates (left). The associated oedema then resolves gradually and the edges harden to produce discrete circular opacities (right).

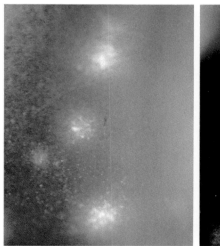

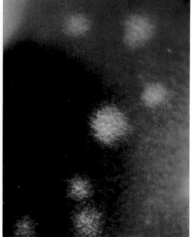

Fig. 4.5 The small circular subepithelial opacities, which are typically placed centrally in adenovirus infections, may persist for many weeks, months, or, rarely, even years. This patient was photographed two years after the initial infection. Although symptomatic relief in persistent adenoviral keratitis may be obtained by the use of topical steroid preparations, the opacities tend to recur following withdrawal of steroids.

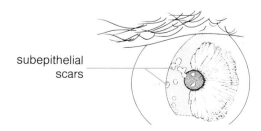

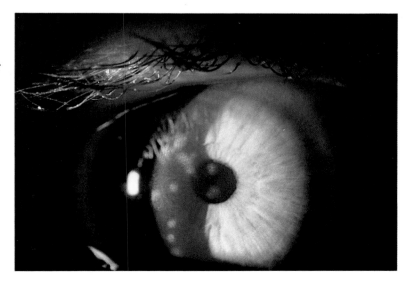

4.3

Herpes Simplex

In the past, ocular disease has usually been associated with herpes simplex virus (HSV) type I, but this pattern may be changing with the increasing isolation frequency of herpes simplex virus type II.

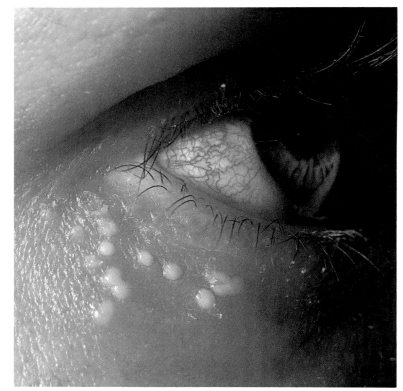

Fig. 4.6 Primary herpetic blepharoconjunctivitis affects non-immune individuals following inoculation from an infectious source. The infection begins as a vesicular and then a pustular eruption on the skin near the lids and is frequently associated with conjunctival inflammation. In this patient, the conjunctival inflammation is associated with hyperaemia of the bulbar conjunctiva.

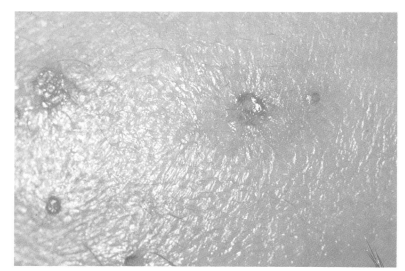

Fig. 4.7 The skin lesions evolve during the first week to form crusts. These fall off to reveal characteristic ulcers which usually heal during the course of the second week.

Fig. 4.8 Ulceration of the mucocutaneous junction of the lid margin is common and may be a feature of recurrent attacks at a later date.

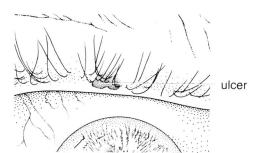

ulcer

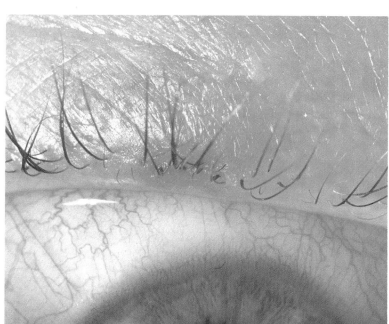

Fig. 4.9 Herpes simplex conjunctivitis is often present in the primary disease when it is invariably associated with a tender, enlarged, pre-auricular lymph node. It is frequently accompanied by purulent discharge, and the lower fornix and tarsus show a mixed papillary and follicular reaction (bottom).

This photograph of the upper tarsus shows small areas of conjunctival ulceration which may be present near the lid margin in the acute stages (top). These may be easily overlooked in the presence of marked hyperaemia. Herpetic conjunctivitis may be satisfactorily treated by the use of a topical antiviral preparation such as idoxuridine ointment.

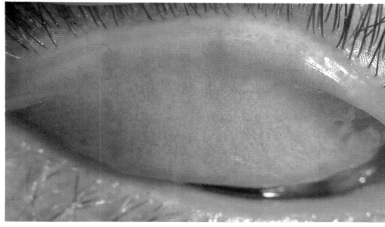

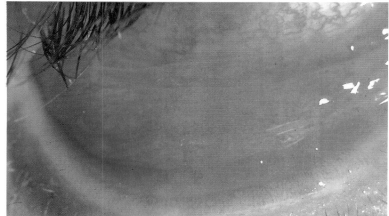

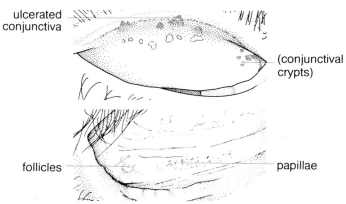

ulcerated conjunctiva

(conjunctival crypts)

follicles

papillae

Fig. 4.10 Herpes simplex keratitis is usually unilateral. Small single or multiple dendritic ulcers are rarely seen in the primary disease, but, as in this case, are a common manifestation of recurrent herpes simplex infection in an already immunized host. Following a primary infection, herpes simplex virus lies latent within the trigeminal ganglion and is transmitted to the eye by the Vth nerve, producing recurrent disease which is often associated with stress or systemic illness.

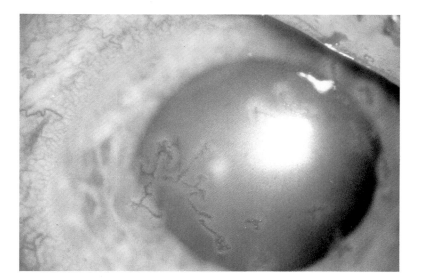

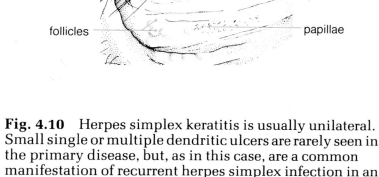

dendritic ulcers

Fig. 4.11 This higher powered photograph shows a classical dendritic ulcer stained with bengal rose with no visible stromal involvement. Treatment usually consists of a topical antiviral preparation with or without initial débridement of the affected area.

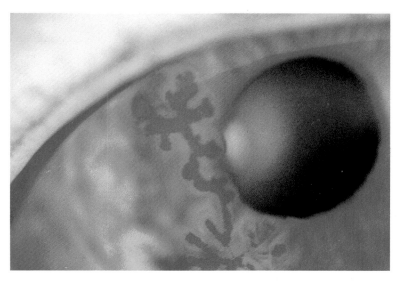

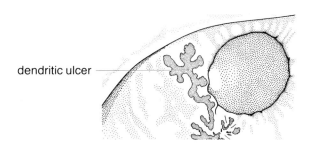

dendritic ulcer

Fig. 4.12 More severe ulceration due to herpes simplex is characterized by either 'amoeboid' or 'geographical' configurations and almost invariably results from the inadvertent use of topical steroids in keratoconjunctivitis caused by herpes simplex. Persistent treatment with steroids will lead to corneal destruction and perforation.

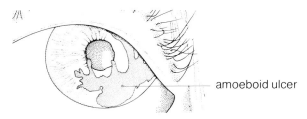

amoeboid ulcer

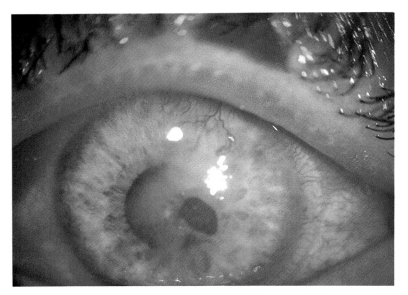

Fig. 4.13 Chronic active stromal herpes simplex keratitis usually involves some reactivation of virus replication and associated immune responses. This patient has an area of ulceration surrounded by stromal oedema and infiltrate in an old herpetic scar. Previous vascularization had occurred and blood vessels can be seen invading the superficial cornea. Topical weak steroid preparations with antiviral cover are usually indicated to suppress the inflammatory reaction and minimize subsequent scarring.

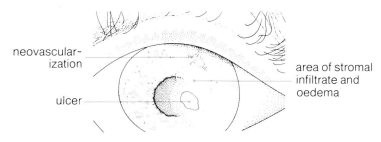

neovascular-
ization

area of stromal
infiltrate and
oedema

ulcer

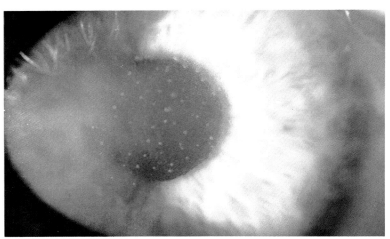

Fig. 4.14 Disciform keratitis can arise with or without previous corneal ulceration and presents as an area of stromal oedema associated with uveitis. This patient presented with a diffuse stromal haze and central multiple keratic precipitates indicating an active anterior uveitis.

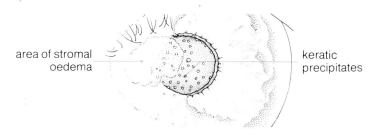

area of stromal
oedema

keratic
precipitates

Fig. 4.15 This photograph shows an end-stage of chronic herpes simplex keratitis with vascularization and lipid deposition in an old stromal scar. A well pronounced arcus senilis is also present.

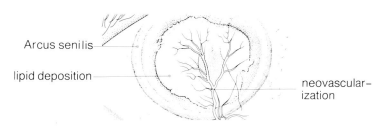

Arcus senilis

lipid deposition

neovascular-
ization

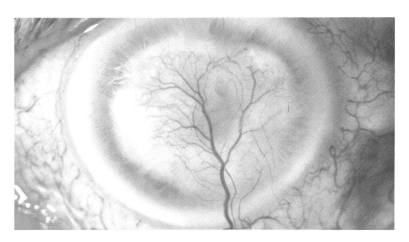

Fig. 4.16 The histological features of active herpes simplex stromal keratitis show an intact corneal epithelium with destruction of parts of Bowman's membrane, beneath which there are collections of lymphocytes and plasma cells. Vascularization of the corneal stroma is also evident with oedema and destruction of the normal pattern of corneal lamellae.

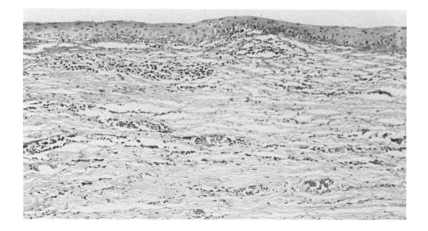

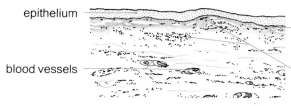

Herpes Zoster

Herpes zoster ophthalmicus results from activation of latent varicella zoster virus in the trigeminal ganglion. It involves the first division of the trigeminal nerve whose distribution it follows exactly.

Fig. 4.17 Involvement of the external nasal branch of the trigeminal nerve is often associated with ocular infection by herpes zoster ophthalmicus. This patient illustrates the healing phase of the rash during the second week when crusts have started to form and the erythema is subsiding.

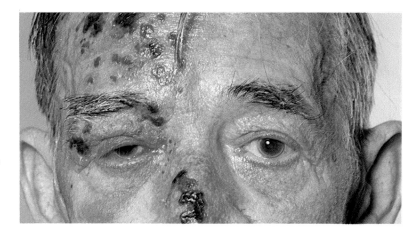

Fig. 4.18 The late stigmata zoster infection include marked atrophy and depigmentation of the skin, sometimes associated with more extensive tissue destruction from arteritis and inflammation. In this case, there is full thickness loss of part of the upper eyelid on the affected side.

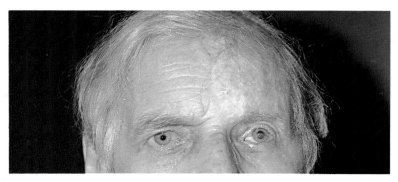

Fig. 4.19 This is an unusual example of a rash in the early stages with erythema, oedema of the lower lid and vesicle, and pustule formation following the distribution of the second division of the trigeminal nerve. Ocular involvement is much less common in this instance.

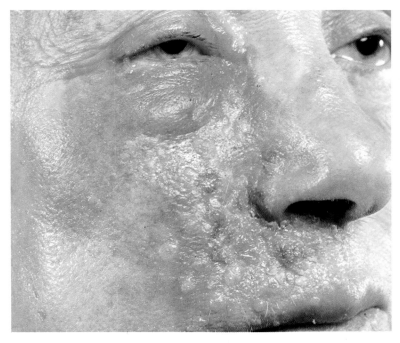

Fig. 4.20 Conjunctivitis and keratitis are features of ocular involvement during the early stages of the disease. Corneal 'pseudodendrites' from mucus deposition may form, but these can be distinguished from the dendrites of herpes simplex infection by their elevated appearance, peripheral location, poor staining with fluorescein compared with rose bengal, and their ability to be wiped easily from the corneal surface. Disciform keratitis may also be a feature of corneal disease in herpes zoster when changes are seen which are identical to those of herpes simplex infection (cf. Fig. 4.17).

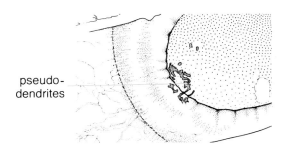

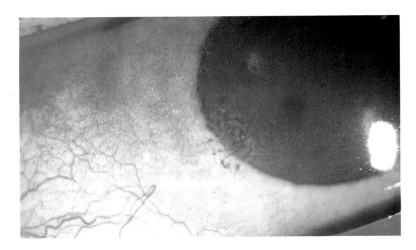

Fig. 4.21 Uveitis is present in approximately fifty percent of cases with ocular involvement and is frequently accompanied by iris vasculitis. Secondary glaucoma is common. The uveitis starts during the third or fourth week of the illness and usually requires treatment with topical steroids for many months. Sector iris atrophy is a characteristic late finding in such patients. Examination of the pupil margin on direct illumination may show loss of the pigmented border in a section that reacts poorly to light (top).

The loss of the pigmented layers can be seen more dramatically on retroillumination where it has a sectorial distribution corresponding to a portion of the iris vascular supply (bottom).

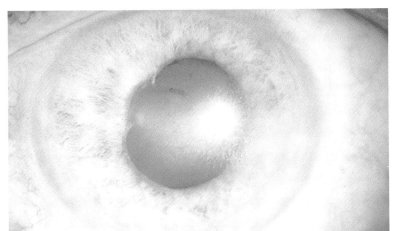

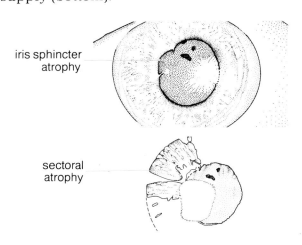

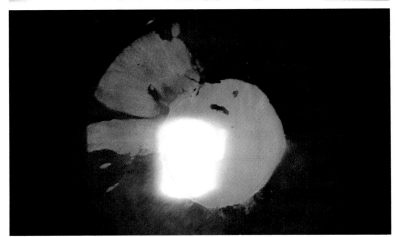

Vaccinia

Ocular vaccinia is caused by the accidental secondary inoculation of the eye with infected material from a vaccination site. It may be expected to occur with decreasing frequency as the practice of mass smallpox vaccination gradually disappears.

Fig. 4.22 Vaccinia may produce a widespread indolent lid ulceration, follicular conjunctivitis, and keratitis. The reaction was more severe in this subject owing to the presence of facial eczema

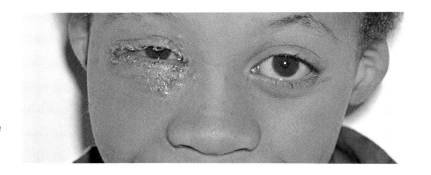

Fig. 4.23 This example of ocular vaccinia shows the disease at a pustular stage associated with conjunctival hyperaemia. It may progress to produce an ulcerative blepharitis associated with a follicular conjunctivitis.

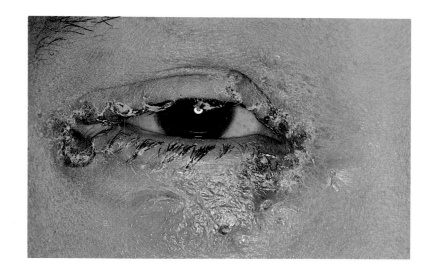

Molluscum Contagiosum

The virus of molluscum contagiosum commonly affects the skin of the face and eyelids. Ocular involvement occurs only when a lesion is present at or near the lid margin.

Fig. 4.24 Molluscum contagiosum produces characteristic raised skin lesions with umbilicated centres which may be either single or, as in this case, multiple.

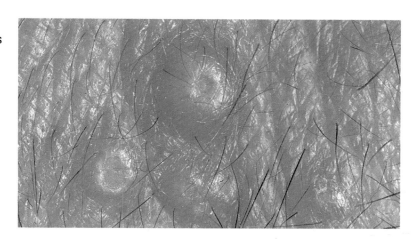

Fig. 4.25 If a molluscum lesion occurs on the lid margin (top), virus particles may be shed into the lower conjunctival sac where they may produce a secondary follicular conjunctivitis (bottom). This is thought to be due to an immune reaction without direct conjunctival invasion by the organisms. The conjunctivitis thus produced is readily cured by removing the offending lid lesion, which in this case (top) is somewhat unusual in that it lacks the typical umbilicated centre.

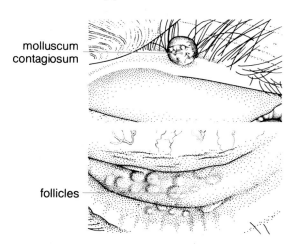

molluscum contagiosum

follicles

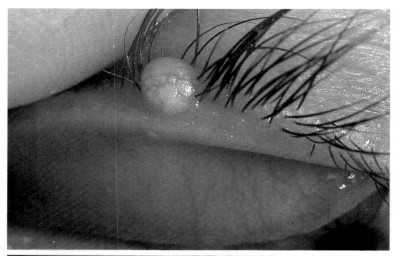

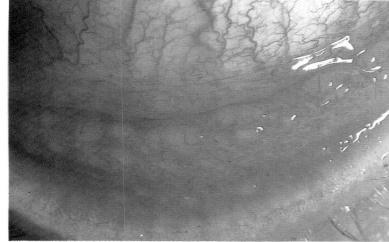

Fig. 4.26 The characteristic histological feature of a molluscum lesion is the presence of large numbers of eosinophilic inclusion bodies. These appear in the cytoplasm of the hyperplastic epithelium which forms lobules, and the enlarging bodies are discharged centrally on to the umbilicated surface of the lesion. There is a fibrous capsule and, except in the central portion, the surface is covered by normal epithelium.

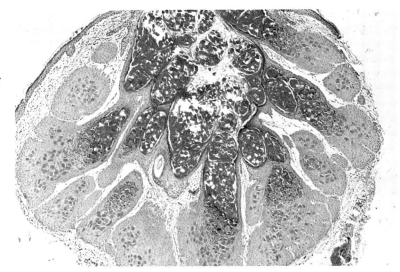

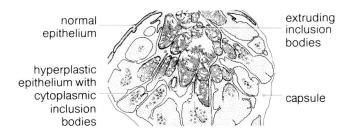

CHLAMYDIAL INFECTIONS
Inclusion Conjunctivitis

Inclusion conjunctivitis (TRIC conjunctivitis) is a form of follicular conjunctivitis caused by sub-group A chlamydia of the serotypes D-K. It is a sexually transmitted disease which follows direct or indirect oculo-genital contact.

Fig. 4.27 The onset of inclusion conjunctivitis is usually gradual in that it develops over a period of several weeks. A typical case shows the formation of large follicles in the lower (bottom) and upper (top) fornices.

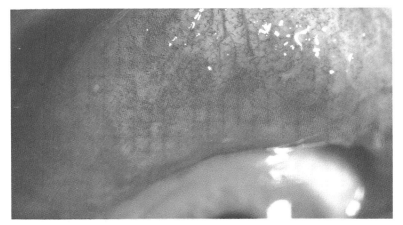

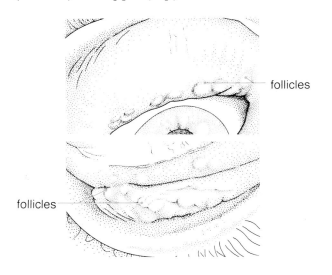

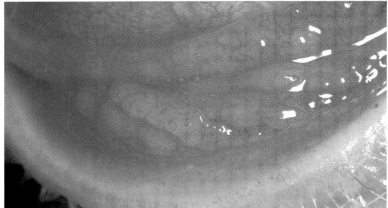

Fig. 4.28 The follicular response later spreads on to the tarsal conjunctiva where the follicles tend to be smaller and are associated with other inflammatory signs including a papillary reaction.

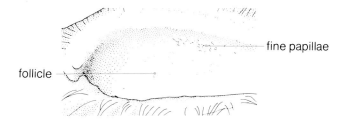

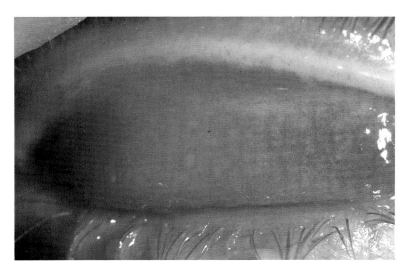

Fig. 4.29 Superficial keratitis may develop in the form of small greyish-white epithelial and subepithelial infiltrates. These infiltrates may be distinguished from those seen in adenovirus by their tendency towards a peripheral distribution and their association with early pannus formation.

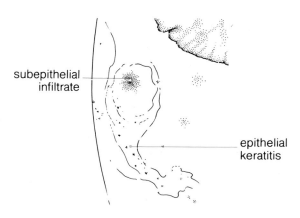

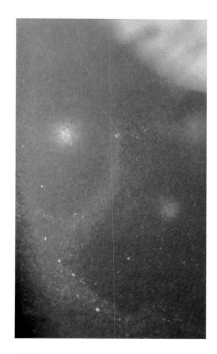

Fig. 4.30 Inclusion conjunctivitis is transmitted sexually and is associated with cervicitis in women and urethritis in men. Procitis may also be present. This patient has well developed follicles on the cervix and these are a characteristic feature of chlamydial genito-urinary infections. Ocular disease may be treated with local tetracycline ointment but all cases should be screened for both chlamydial-genital infection and other sexually transmitted diseases which may be associated.

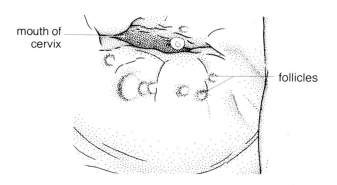

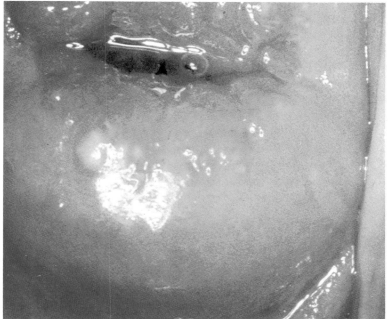

Fig. 4.31 In the newborn, where infection may be acquired via the birth canal, chlamydia are an important cause of ophthalmia neonatorum. Progression of the disease in neonates is different from that in the adult in that an oedematous, papillary conjunctivitis is produced in neonates in which the palpebral conjunctivae readily invert themselves with gentle pressure on the lids from the examiner's fingers. Pseudo-membrane formation is present on the lower tarsus.

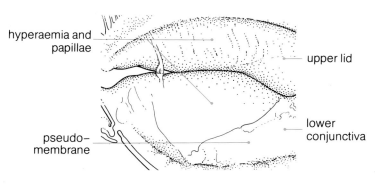

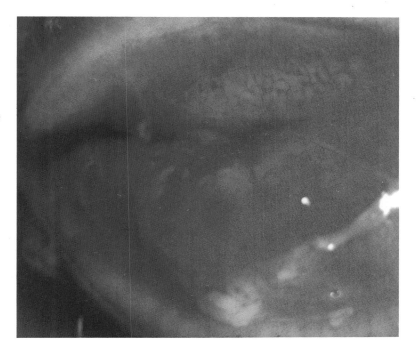

4.11

Fig. 4.32 Chlamydia are obligatory intracellular parasites and are therefore usually classified with other viruses. They differ from the latter, however, in having organelles and also in their sensitivity to some antibiotics.

The diagnosis of chlamydial infection is made by either direct culture, serological methods, or the demonstration of inclusion bodies (Halberstaedter-Prowazek bodies) in the conjunctival scrapings. Subgroup A chlamydia can be stained with iodine or Giemsa stains (left) and in the latter instance, are more readily seen when viewed with polarized light (right).

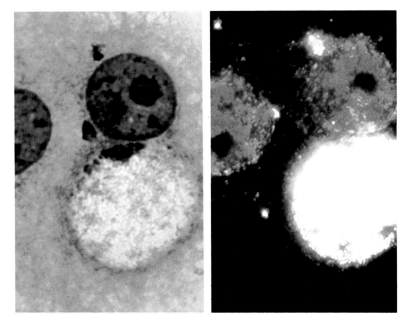

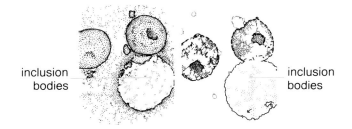

Trachoma

Trachoma is the result of repeated infection by subgroup A chlamydia of serotypes A-C, often with superimposed bacterial infection. Transmission usually occurs from eye to eye and, in its classical description, stages I and II would appear to be clinically indistinguishable from TRIC conjunctivitis.

Fig. 4.33 Stage III trachoma is defined as active disease with scar formation. The limbal changes consist of active pannus formation, i.e., a palisade of dilated limbal blood vessels and diffuse infiltrate invading the upper cornea. Large limbal follicles can also be seen.

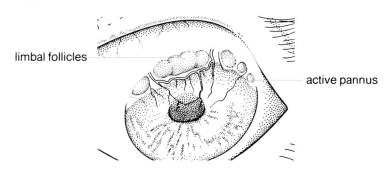

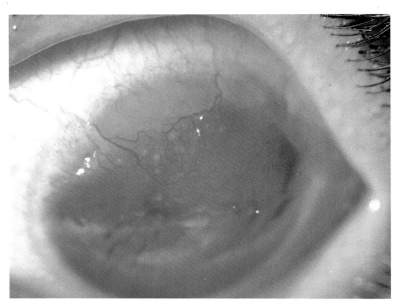

Fig. 4.34 The palpebral conjunctiva shows a combination of diffuse and reticular scar formation in addition to a follicular and papillary reaction.

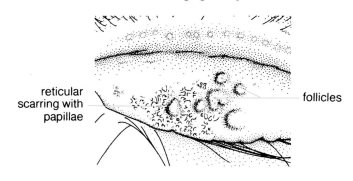

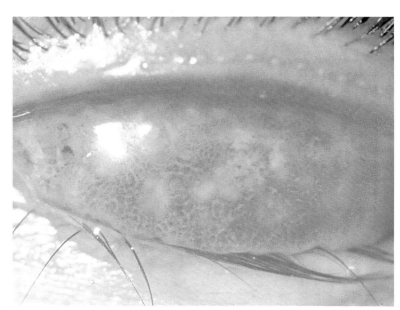

Fig. 4.35 Stage IV disease is characterized by superficial and deep scarring of the conjunctiva with no follicular or papillary changes. Dense scar tissue near the upper lid margin may contract leading to the formation of Arlt's line.

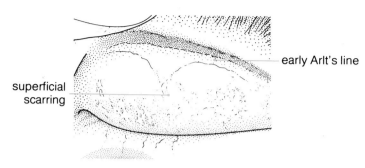

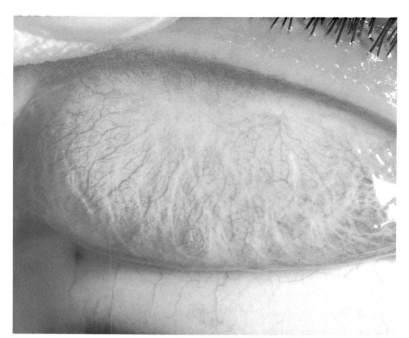

Fig. 4.36 The limbal changes in stage IV trachoma are characteristic, with inactive pannus (down-growth of vessels and scarring without infiltration) in which shallow depressions, known as Herbert's pits, can be seen.

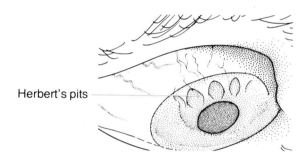

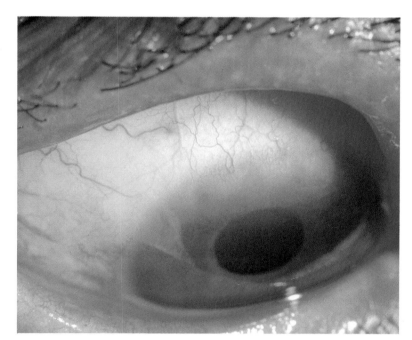

Fig. 4.37 The complications of severe trachoma result from the contraction of conjunctival and deep scar tissue which lead to cicatricial entropion, trichiasis, and lid shortening (which may in turn lead to further corneal damage). There is marked corneal scarring associated with drying, also as a result of old conjunctival disease.

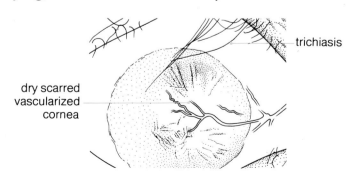

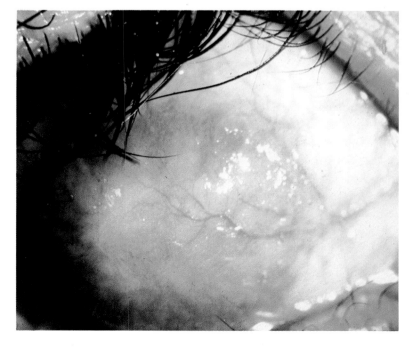

BACTERIAL INFECTIONS

Bacterial infections of the outer eye usually respond rapidly to treatment with antibiotics although, under certain circumstances, serious complication may follow. Superficial infections of the lids and conjunctivae may be treated with topical broad spectrum antibiotic preparations while deeper infections such as dacryocystitis and orbital cellulitis require systemic administration. The most serious bacterial infections are those involving the cornea and these require urgent intensive therapy if loss of the eye through an endophthalmitis is to be avoided.

Blepharitis

Fig. 4.38   Acute bacterial infections of the eyelid usually take the form of a stye (external hordeolum) in which a lash follicle becomes infected, or acute chalazion (internal hordeolum), in which one of the meibomian glands of the eyelid is involved as in this patient. In a stye, the abscess 'points' and subsequently discharges around the base of an eyelash, whereas a chalazion remains as a localized tender swelling. This swelling may persist as a chronic granuloma.

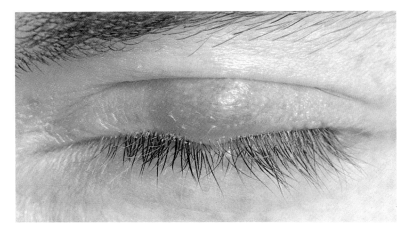

Fig. 4.39   Histology of chalazion shows lipid globules associated with multinucleated giant cells and pale epitheloid cells. There is also round cell infiltration.

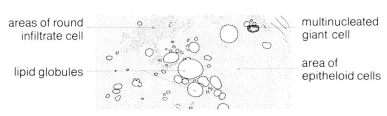

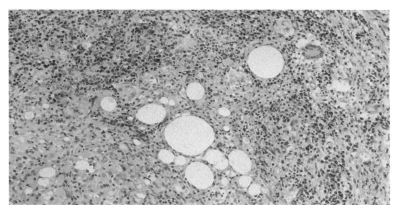

Fig. 4.40   Chronic infective blepharitis is a common condition, frequently bilateral, which is usually of staphylococcal origin. It is characterized by the presence of crusts and scales on the lid margins which may be erythematous and slightly swollen. The eyelashes are irregular and fewer in number than normal.

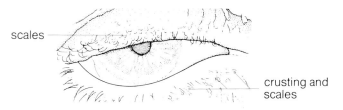

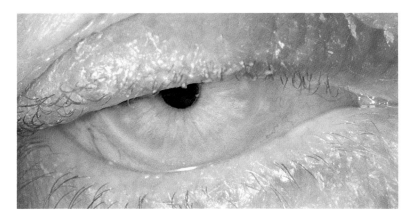

Fig. 4.41   Excessive meibomian secretion may also be a feature of chronic blepharitis, especially in the presence of acne rosacea. This photograph shows the characteristic facial appearance of the condition (left) together with the rhinophyma associated with sebaceous hypertrophy (right).

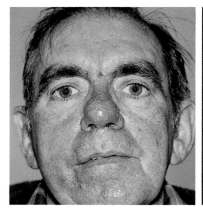
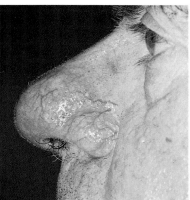

Fig. 4.42 Acute marginal infiltrates are yellowish-white in colour and may appear at the periphery of the cornea either singly or with involvement of more than one quadrant. Localized injection of the conjunctiva is present. This is thought to be the result of a localized hypersensitivity reaction.

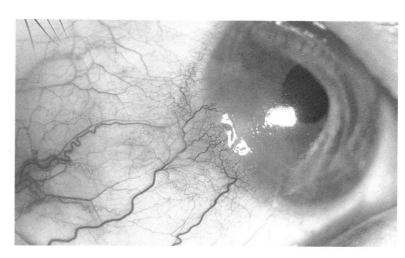

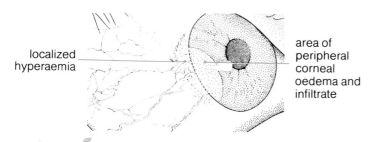

localized hyperaemia

area of peripheral corneal oedema and infiltrate

Fig. 4.43 Superficial punctate keratitis, superficial scarring, and peripheral corneal vascularization are also seen in both chronic blepharitis and rosacea which occasionally involve some thinning of the peripheral cornea, although perforation is rare.

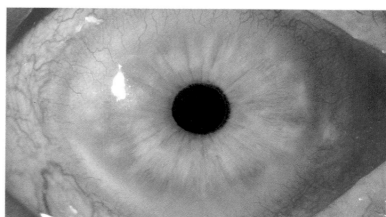

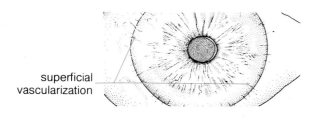

superficial vascularization

Conjunctivitis

Fig. 4.44 Bacterial conjunctivitis is characterized by its acute onset, profuse thick discharge, and its rapid response to topical antibiotic therapy. Diagnosis depends on the demonstration of causative organisms by standard bacteriological techniques. Important causes include Staphylococcus, pneumococcus, Moraxella, Haemophilus, and gonococcus. The conjunctivitis may be secondary in origin, as in this case where it is associated with an acute dacryocystitis.

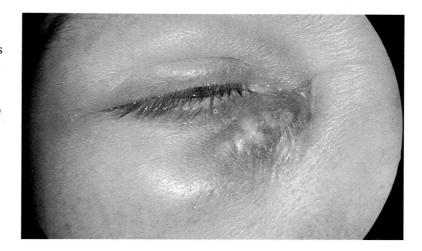

Keratitis

Fig. 4.45 Bacterial suppurative keratitis usually results from the breakdown of the corneal epithelium allowing organisms to gain access to the corneal stroma. In this case, due to Pseudomonas aeruginosa, a diffuse grey infiltrate is present over approximately half the cornea and is associated with a central area of corneal melting (seen here as thinning) and epithelial loss.

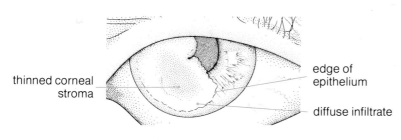

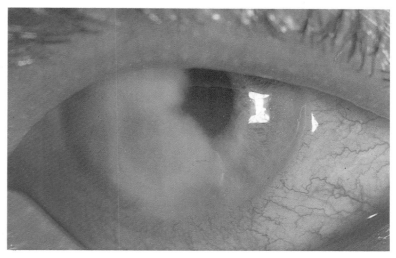

thinned corneal stroma

edge of epithelium

diffuse infiltrate

4.15

Fig. 4.46 This second case, due to pneumococcal infection of a vernal ulcer, shows a dense white infiltrate associated with inflammatory exudate within the anterior chamber. If loss of the eye is to be prevented, such patients require immediate admission to hospital with appropriate specimens taken from Gram stain and bacterial culture from the conjunctiva, the cornea, and sometimes from the anterior chamber.

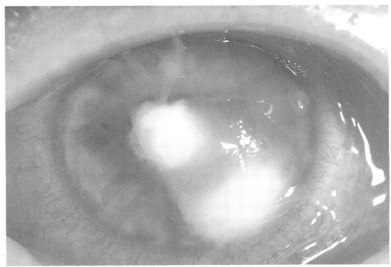

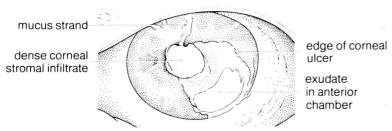

Fig. 4.47 Although various causative organisms may present differing clinical pictures, the diagnosis should be based only on the precise bacteriological methods outlined above. Two corneal scrapings are shown here: the presence of gram negative rods gives a presumptive diagnosis of Pseudomonas species (left): streptococci morphological identification of the causative organisms (right) enables the appropriate antibiotic therapy to be chosen and intensive local treatment to commence before definitive cultures are available. Useful diagnostic information will be found by Gram stains in approximately seventy percent of bacterially infected eyes whereas the causative organism will be grown in only about fifty percent of patients.

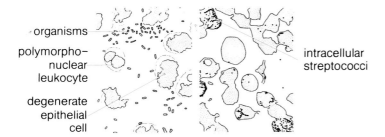

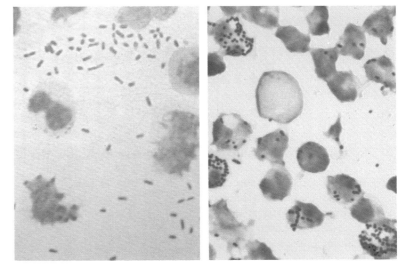

FUNGAL INFECTION
Fungi are relatively uncommon ocular pathogens, especially when considered in the context of their widespread distribution in the environment. Patients who are immuno-compromised or have a history of exposure to contaminated soil, such as agricultural workers, are two groups who may be considered to be at risk.

Keratitis
Fig. 4.48 It may be clinically impossible to distinguish fungal keratitis from bacterial keratitis. Fungal keratitis should be suspected, however, in those cases which fail to respond to adequate antibiotic therapy. This photograph shows a large corneal ulcer with secondary hypopyon occupying half the anterior chamber.

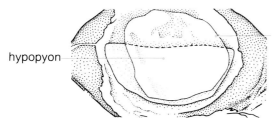

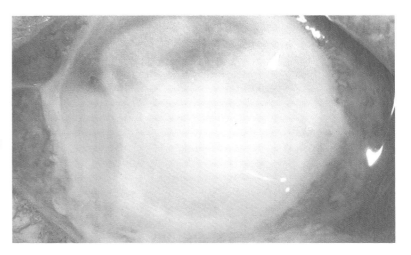

Fig. 4.49 Fungal hyphae may indicate the diagnosis when seen on corneal scraping. Culture methods for the isolation and identification of fungi take two-to-three weeks; all cases of suppurative keratitis should therefore be cultured for fungi at the time of their presentation if there is any possibility of fungal infection. Valuable time is not therefore lost should a bacterial cause be excluded at a later date.

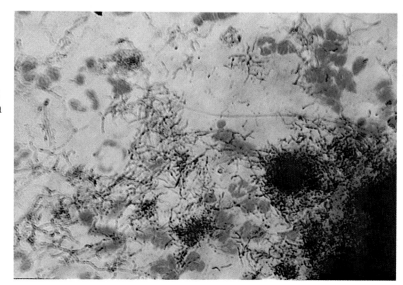

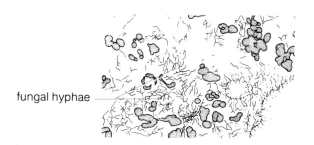

fungal hyphae

PARASITIC DISEASE AND INFESTATIONS
Ocular infestation by parasites is an important cause of ocular disease in tropical and subtropical regions of the world. Among the many forms of helminthic infestation, onchocerciasis is one of the leading causes of blindness in the world.

Onchocerciasis
Fig. 4.50 Onchocerciasis is caused by a threadworm, onchocerca volvulus. The adult worm lives in fibrous subcutaneous nodules into which the females discharge large numbers of microfilariae. These microfilariae migrate in the subcutaneous tissues and, when ingested by the simulium fly, can be transmitted to other individuals.

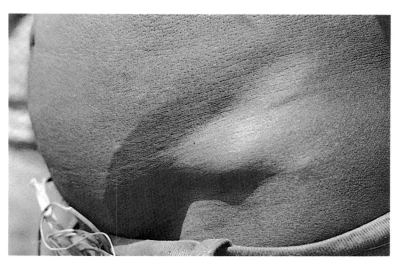

Fig. 4.51 In addition to the nodules, the skin changes of onchocerciasis include a painful and intensely itchy rash which is probably of an allergic nature and is frequently seen during treatment when the microfilariae are being killed in large numbers.

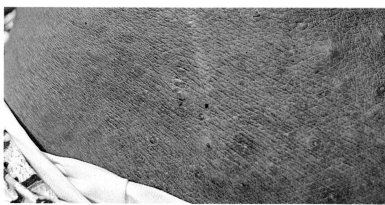

Fig. 4.52 Ocular involvement by the microfilariae has been demonstrated in the conjunctiva and cornea. The microfilariae can be seen as curved or spiral shapes when they are present in their mobile state.

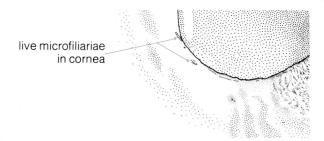

live microfiliariae in cornea

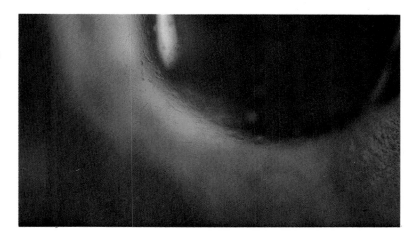

Fig. 4.53 In advanced cases of corneal disease, parasitic infestation results in a sclerosing keratitis with marked pigment migration.

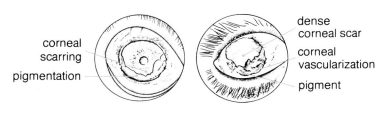

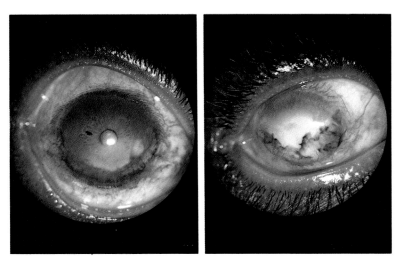

Fig. 4.54 The posterior segment involvement takes the form of focal choroido-retinitis associated with diffuse pigment epithelial changes over a large area. Optic nerve involvement may occur producing atrophy and associated field changes. Both new pigment epithelial changes and an increase in pre-existing field defects have been reported following treatment with diethyl carbamazine.

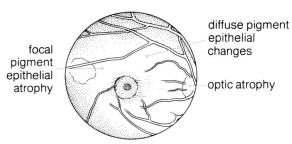

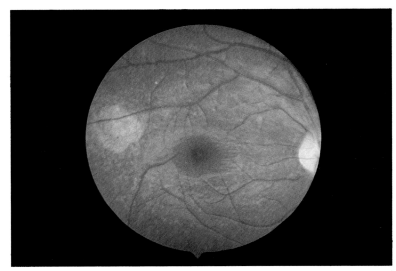

Pediculosis

Fig. 4.55 This photograph illustrates the empty egg cases (nits) on the eyelashes in a case of pediculosis pubis infestation causing a chronic blepharitis. Eyelash infestation is from the pubic louse. Treatment with eserine ointment paralyses the lice on the lashes and all patients require additional treatment for the deinfestation of their pubic hair.

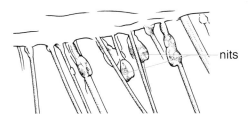

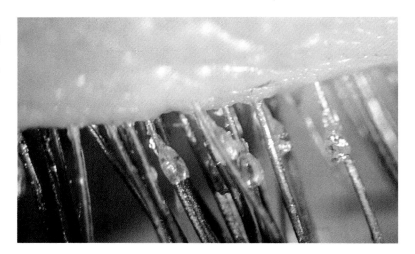

Fig. 4.56 A pubic louse clinging to a pubic hair to which is attached an egg case.

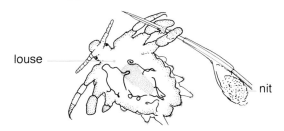

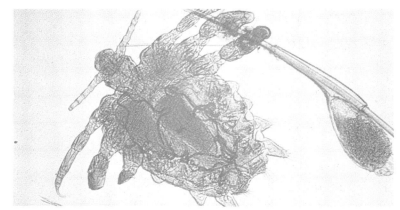

5. Allergic Eye Diseases: Episcleritis and Scleritis

P. A. Hunter

P. G. Watson

ALLERGIC REACTIONS
Immediate Hypersensitivity
The external eye is under constant immunological challenge from a wide variety of substances, which may lead to the development of one of many conditions that can be loosely grouped together as allergic eye disease. The chief factors which determine the outcome of such challenges are the size and duration of the antigenic load and the immunological status of the individual. Local or systemic immune mechanisms may be involved, to produce immediate hypersensitivity, complement-mediated, or delayed hypersensitivity reactions.

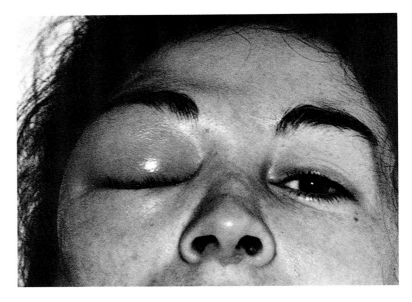

Fig. 5.1   Acute periorbital oedema is a common manifestation of immediate hypersensitivity and it may follow the systemic administration of antigen in a sensitized individual, such as in the ingestion of certain foods or drugs. The reaction is frequently associated with high titres of circulating IgE antibody, being mediated via the release of histamine and other pharmacologically active substances from mast cells in the skin and mucosal tissues. It usually produces symmetrical bilateral lid oedema, which may also be accompanied by conjunctival chemosis and urticarial skin rashes. Acute unilateral signs may result from local inoculation and histamine release in the skin, as in this example where the reaction followed an insect bite.

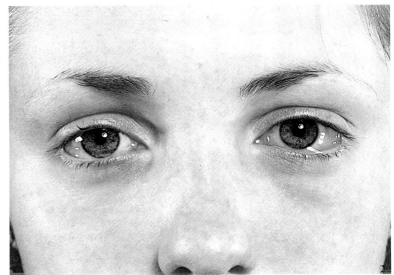

Fig. 5.2   Acute conjunctival chemosis may occur in the absence of lid swelling as an immediate hypersensitivity response to local inoculation of antigenic substances (frequently pollens) directly into the conjunctival sacs of a sensitized individual. The level of response depends on the degree of previous sensitization and the dose of antigen. In this patient, although both conjunctivae are chemotic and slightly hyperaemic, the signs are more pronounced in the left eye, reflecting a higher antigenic load in that eye.

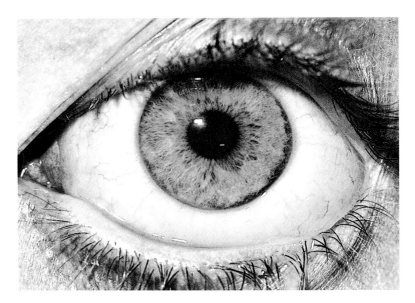

Fig. 5.3   This illustration shows the left eye from Fig. 5.2 in greater detail. There is a swelling of the bulbar conjunctiva giving the typical gelatinous appearance associated with mild hyperaemia of the blood vessels. Although the symptoms may be alarming, they usually resolve spontaneously over a few hours. Antihistamine drops may provide symptomatic relief.

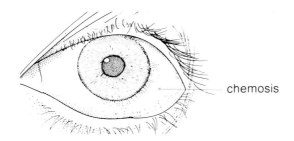

chemosis

Vernal Disease

Vernal conjunctivitis is an IgE-mediated disorder which is an ocular manifestation of atopy. This condition often includes severe forms of eczema, hay fever and asthma, which characteristically start early in life. The disease is chronic, with seasonal exacerbations and remissions, and predominates in young males. Treatment is aimed at controlling the conjunctival disease during the acute attacks by intensive steroid drops. It is important to reduce such treatment as soon as possible to avoid steroid glaucoma, and this may be facilitated by the additional use of cromoglycate drops. These may be successful in controlling the disease when used alone in less severe forms of the disease.

Fig. 5.4 This boy, who suffers from vernal conjunctivitis, shows a typical eczematous rash on his forehead and cheeks. There is an associated slight bilateral ptosis reflecting the chronic inflammatory upper conjunctival disease.

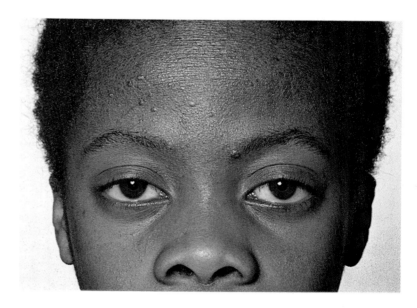

Fig. 5.5 The conjunctival changes found over the upper tarsus consist of giant papillae, typically described as having a 'cobblestone' appearance. Although these papillae persist during quiescent phases of the disease, they become swollen when the disease becomes active (as in this example), and are infiltrated by oedema and inflammatory cells, with abundant abnormal mucus situated both on the surface and in the crevices between the papillae.

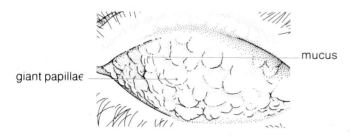

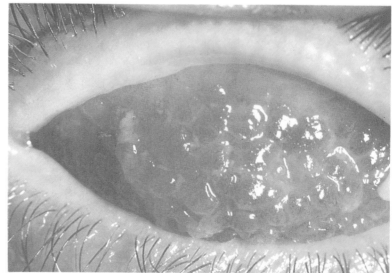

Fig. 5.6 The changes in the lower tarsal conjunctiva and fornix are less striking but equally typical. The superficial conjunctiva is heavily infiltrated by cells and oedema, thus obscuring most of the normal vascular pattern. There is also mucus accumulation in the lower fornix.

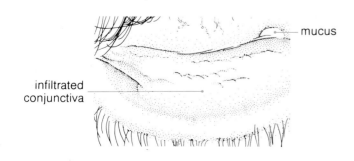

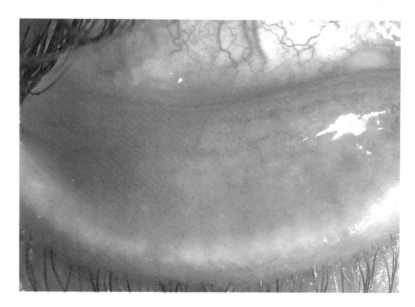

Fig. 5.7 Limbal changes may occur in vernal conjunctivitis in the absence of marked tarsal papillae. These 'vegetations' are heavily infiltrated with inflammatory cells and appear as greyish, gelatinous swellings at the upper limbus in this patient. The blood vessels are not unduly prominent and there is no mucus visible.

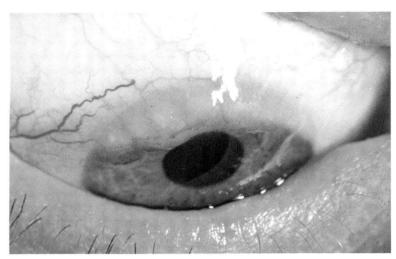

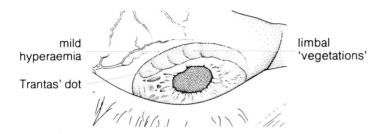

Fig. 5.8 Trantas' dots are also a feature of vernal conjunctivitis. They are small white, elevated epithelial lesions seen at the upper corneal limbus. In this example, they are associated with a greyish corneal infiltrate and superficial vascularization.

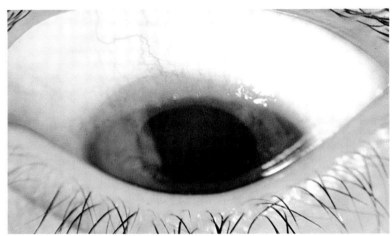

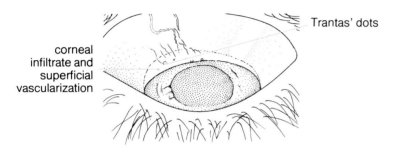

Fig. 5.9 This low-powered histological section of vernal conjunctivitis shows the flat-topped contour of the giant papillae with the conjunctiva heavily infiltrated by round cells. The section also includes part of the normal underlying tarsal plate and meibomian glands.

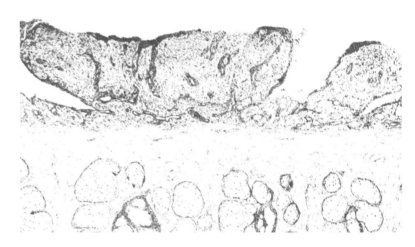

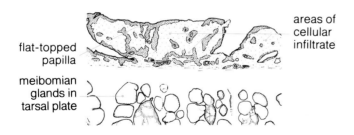

Fig. 5.10 A high-powered section of vernal conjunctivitis shows typical papillae with epithelial downgrowth to form crypts, at the base of which lie the mucus-producing goblet cells. The papillae have a loose stroma in which collections of lymphocytes and plasma cells can be seen. Eosinophils, which are present in great numbers during the active phase of the disease, are not seen in this section.

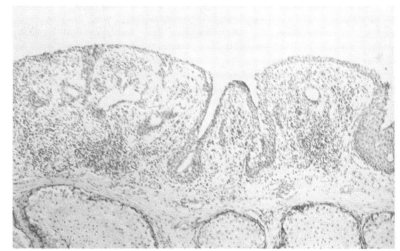

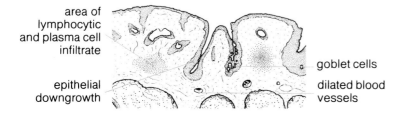

Fig. 5.11 This patient illustrates the early corneal changes seen in vernal disease. There is an early fine punctate epithelial keratopathy consisting of fine grey dots which may, in more severe forms of the disease, become confluent.

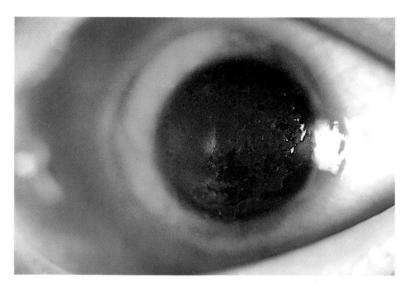

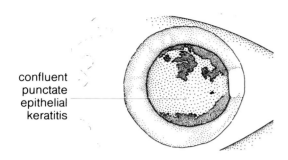

Fig. 5.12 A vernal ulcer can characteristically develop in the upper half of the cornea during active phases of the disease. The edge of the ulcer is surrounded by whitish, heaped-up epithelium. The base is composed of abnormal mucus which is deposited with fibrin and other serum constituents as a grey plaque. When established, this plaque prevents healing occurring. Superficial vessels can be seen extending into the cornea from the adjacent limbal arcades. An area of superficial corneal infiltration can be seen nearer the limbus on the nasal side of the cornea.

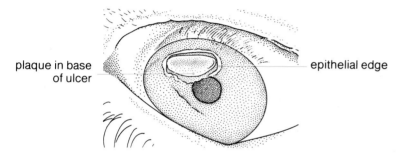

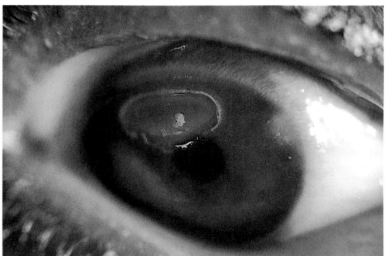

Fig. 5.13 This is a more severe example of a vernal ulcer showing a large area of central ulceration with established plaque formation. This example helps to illustrate the non-wetting properties of the plaque and the heaped-up epithelial edge, which is indicative of poor healing in the presence of plaque. Peripheral to the ulcer the cornea is relatively clear, although limbal vessels are starting to grow centrally. The conjunctiva is hyperaemic and a strand of typically 'stringy' mucus lies on the surface of the eye.

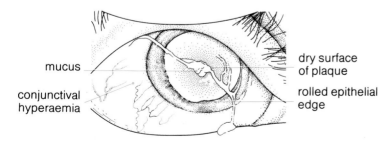

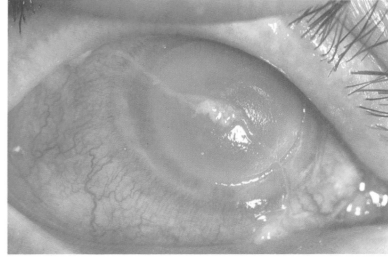

Fig. 5.14 Following treatment with intensive local steroids and acetylcysteine drops, this cornea has become re-epithelized, leaving a typical ring scar at the site of the ulcer. In established cases, it is necessary to remove the mucous plaque by superficial keratectomy and prevent the production of additional mucus in order to allow healing to take place.

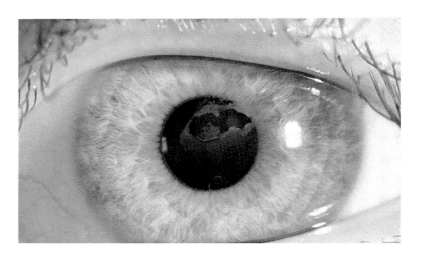

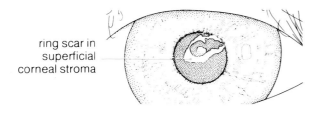

ring scar in superficial corneal stroma

Mucous Membrane Pemphigoid

This autoimmune disorder is believed to be caused by the cytotoxic effect of antibody and complement acting against autologous tissue components. The conjunctivae become chronically inflamed with typical areas of epithelial ulceration associated with thick mucus discharge. Conjunctival vesicles are rare. As the disease progresses, there is conjunctival scarring leading to symblepharon and entropion formation and tear film instability. Cutaneous involvement is minimal and usually limited to the mucosal junction at the mouth and anus. Topical steroids are needed to suppress the conjunctival inflammation.

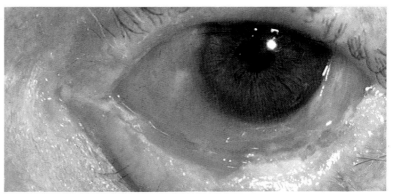

Fig. 5.15 Early disease usually obliterates the caruncle and causes progressive loss of the fornices with broad symblepharon.

This example (top) shows the early changes in mucous membrane pemphigoid. There is a broad symblepharon and a foamy keratin plaque.

The slow inexorable progression of the disease is illustrated by this picture (bottom) of the same patient one year later. The inflammation diminishes as more scarring occurs, as do the conjunctival plaques. The scarring, which has progressed to involve the inferior half of the cornea, will eventually cover it completely.

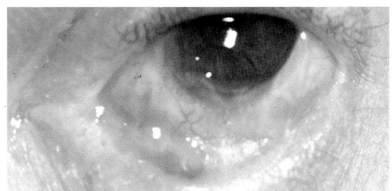

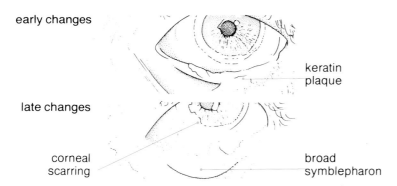

early changes

late changes

keratin plaque

corneal scarring

broad symblepharon

Fig. 5.16 This example illustrates a late stage of mucous membrane pemphigoid with symblepharon formation, corneal scarring, and vascularization resulting from corneal drying: this is associated with loss of mucus-producing cells in the conjunctiva. The lashes have been removed during the course of the disease to prevent further corneal trauma from trichiasis and cicatricial entropion.

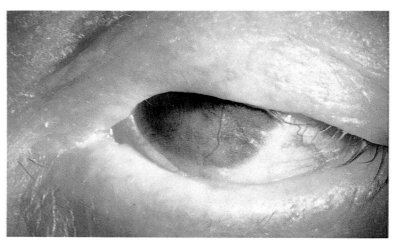

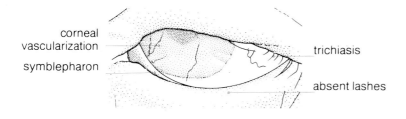

corneal vascularization

symblepharon

trichiasis

absent lashes

Fig. 5.17 A high-powered section of the conjunctiva in mucous membrane pemphigoid (stained with haematoxylin and eosin) shows a thickened conjunctival epithelium with epidermalization and total absence of goblet cells. The epithelium has a 'prickle cell' layer and is covered by a thin layer of keratin. The underlying stroma shows a chronic inflammatory cellular infiltration and oedema.

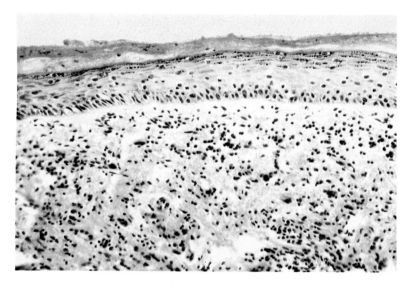

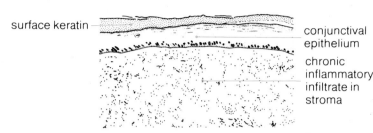

Fig. 5.18 Specific staining methods may be used to demonstrate the presence of autoimmune antibodies in a variety of mucous membrane disorders. A conjunctival biopsy has been treated with peroxidase-labelled anti-human IgG to show deposits of immunoglobulin (stained brown) around individual epithelial cells, which have been counterstained with malachite green. In pemphigus, the antibodies are found in the intercellular zone (as in this slide), while in pemphigoid, the staining lies along the basement membrane. The brown staining of the epithelial surface is a washing artifact incurred during the preparation of the section.

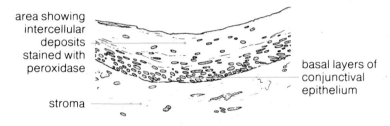

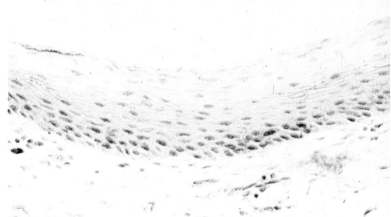

Erythema Multiforme

Erythema multiforme is an acute hypersensitivity reaction in which an immune vasculitis is precipitated by the deposition of circulating antigen complexed with complement-fixing antibody. It frequently follows the administration of drugs, such as sulphonamides or phenobarbitone, bacterial infection, or viral infections such as herpes simplex. The disease is characterized by its acute onset and lasts two to three weeks, during which time complete resolution occurs. In some cases, serious complications, such as renal failure, may develop.

Fig. 5.19 The rash of erythema multiforme starts on the extensor surfaces of the arms and legs and spreads to involve the trunk. The skin lesions consist of an area of erythema surrounding a paler centre, which may ulcerate to give a 'target' appearance. The lesions heal without scarring.

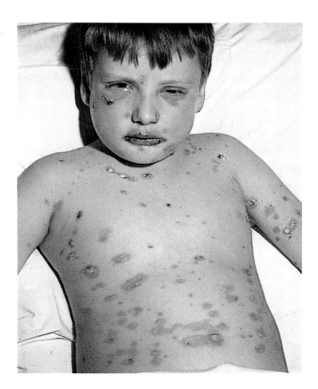

Fig. 5.20 In its more severe form, with mucous membrane involvement, erythema multiforme is known as the Stevens-Johnson syndrome. This patient shows extensive oral ulceration involving the upper and lower lips. Patients are acutely ill, losing serum and protein through their skin, unable to eat and at grave risk of secondary infection. Systemic steroids, fluid replacement and prophylactic antibiotics are the basis of treatment.

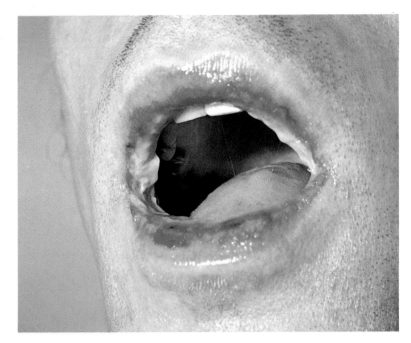

Fig. 5.21 Stevens-Johnson syndrome produces similar ulcerative changes in the conjunctiva where a severe pseudomembranous conjunctivitis may ensue. In the resolving phase, healing is accompanied by scar formation, seen here on the lower tarsus, which may eventually give rise to a dry eye.

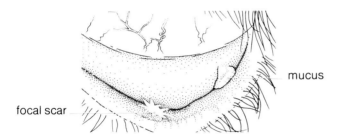

focal scar   mucus

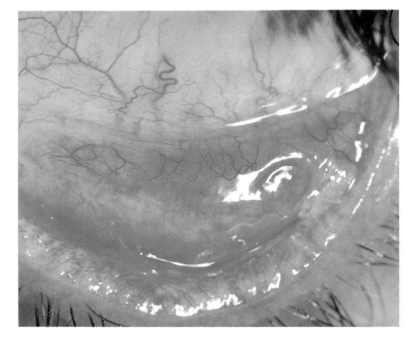

Fig. 5.22 Symblepharon formation is a frequent result of ocular involvement in erythema multiforme. In this example, a fibrous band is seen at the medial canthus stretching from the lower punctum across to the bulbar conjunctiva. These symblephara are narrow, in contrast to the broad bands of ocular pemphigoid.

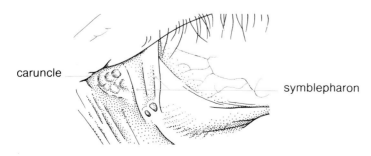

caruncle   symblepharon

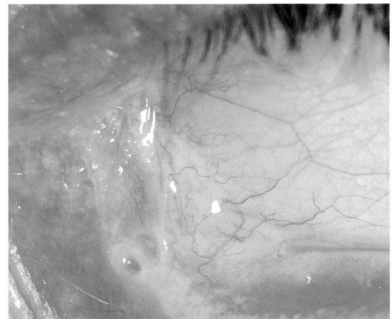

Fig. 5.23 Histological changes in end-stage erythema multiforme may be similar to those seen in mucous membrane pemphigoid. Patchy epidermalization of the conjunctiva has taken place, as evidenced by rete peg formation, thickened epithelium with a prickle cell layer, and keratin formation, giving the histological appearance of skin without hair follicles or other appendages. The underlying stroma shows marked fibrous tissue formation.

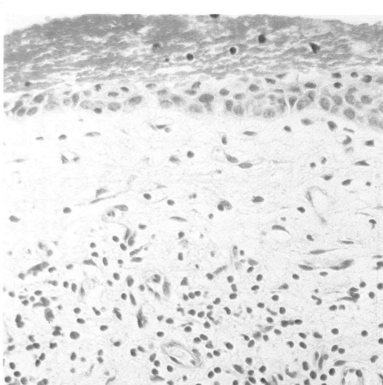

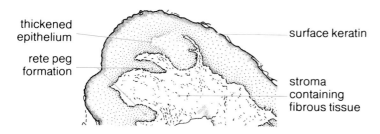

Fig. 5.24 A high-power view of a section of conjunctiva in the acute phase of Stevens-Johnson syndrome shows a thinned conjunctival epithelium with fibrinous exudate on the surface. The stroma has been heavily infiltrated by lymphocytes and eosinophils: the occasional polymorphonuclear leucocyte is also present.

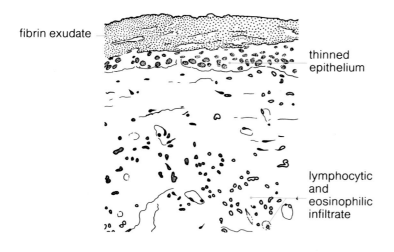

Drug Hypersensitivity Reactions

Contact hypersensitivity reactions are a common problem which frequently arise from the use of cosmetic preparations, contact lens solutions, topical drops and ointments. Such responses are produced by delayed (cell-mediated) hypersensitivity. The skin changes on the lids are those of a contact dermatitis while the conjunctiva shows a primarily follicular response. Patients complain of irritation of the eye, discharge, and, especially, of itchiness.

Fig. 5.25 This patient illustrates the typical dermatitis following three weeks of treatment to the right eye with topical neomycin drops. The right lower eyelid is erythematous and slightly swollen, while the skin of the upper eyelid and around the left eye is entirely normal. Lower down the face, the appearance of the skin of both cheeks is rosacea-like and is unrelated to the hypersensitivity reaction.

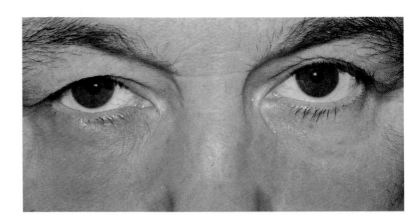

Fig. 5.26 In a more severe reaction, such as in this case where the patient had received atropine ointment, the swelling and erythema are more marked, the area of involvement is more extensive, and the skin may take on a weeping eczematous appearance.

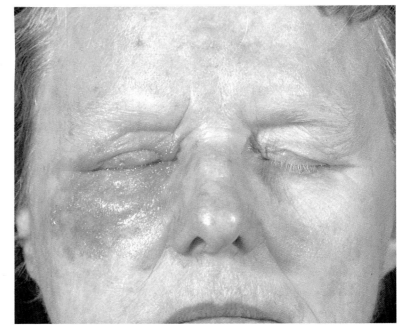

Fig. 5.27 The conjunctival changes shown in this slide are the result of hypersensitivity to trifluorothymidine drops, but similar changes may be seen with a variety of other drops, including pilocarpine, eserine, idoxuridine and many of the topically applied antibiotics. The whole lower tarsus and fornix are covered by follicles which also extend on to the bulbar conjunctiva. There is also an associated conjunctival oedema and hyperaemia.

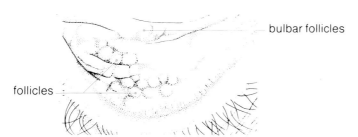

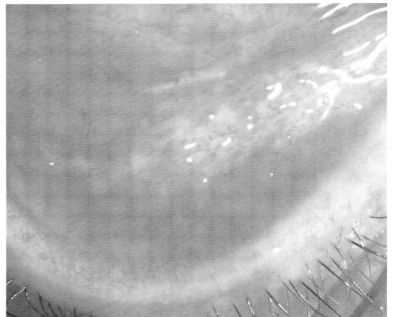

Fig. 5.28 The upper tarsus of the same patient as in Fig. 5.27 shows hyperaemic vessels and follicles extending from the medial side along the upper edge of the tarsus.

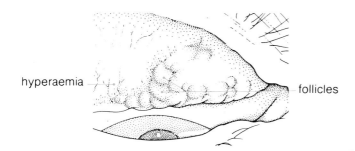

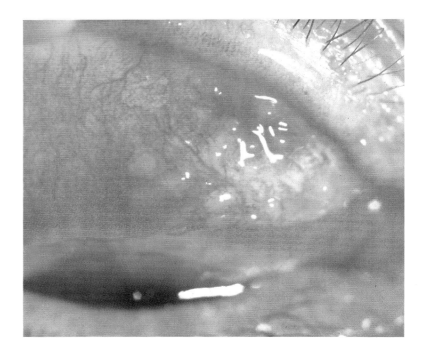

Fig. 5.29 Bulbar follicles are frequently seen in drug hypersensitivity reactions. This illustration shows a typical grouping of bulbar follicles at the limbus of a sensitized patient who has recommenced treatment with trifluorothymidine drops.

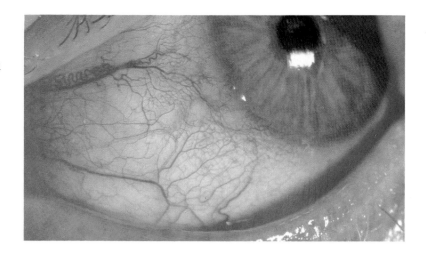

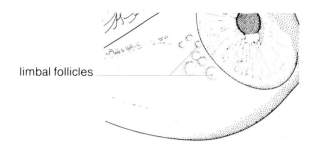

limbal follicles

TOXIC REACTIONS OF THE CONJUNCTIVA
Drug-Induced Reactions

Normal conjunctiva and cornea may undergo changes in response to drugs and other chemicals without evidence of an immunological reaction. Antiviral preparations may interfere with normal cellular metabolism leading to defective epithelial turnover. In the cornea, this may be apparent by the presence of a punctate epithelial keratopathy or poor epithelial healing.

Antibiotics or preservatives in drops may produce changes in the surface microanatomy which may severely affect function if continued for long periods. These toxic changes usually disappear once the stimulus has been recognized and removed.

Fig. 5.30 Topical preparations may produce a non-specific response, as in this case of a thiomersal-induced conjunctival reaction. Such preservatives, which are common to many preparations, especially solutions for soft contact lens use, may produce a marked hyperaemia of the vessels associated with a fine papillary reaction. Reversal of changes over a period of several weeks occurred when the patient changed to treatment with a preservative-free solution.

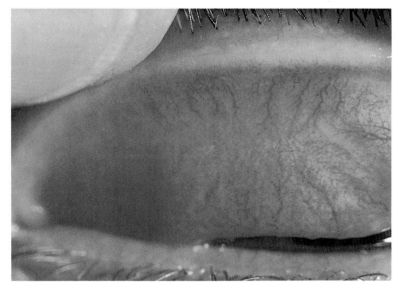

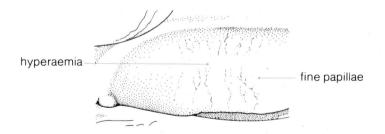

hyperaemia

fine papillae

Fig. 5.31 Chronic drug toxicity reactions in the conjunctiva may be produced by prolonged drop administration, as in this unusual example where pilocarpine and neutral epinephrine drops had been used over many years. Dyskeratotic changes are seen over the whole of the lower fornix and tarsus with extension on to the bulbar conjunctiva on the medial side. Keratin sheet formation is visible as a whitish, non-wetting surface in those areas of conjunctiva which might be expected to have most contact with the drug. The lower punctum appears to have been completely obliterated and the remaining visible conjunctiva is hyperaemic.

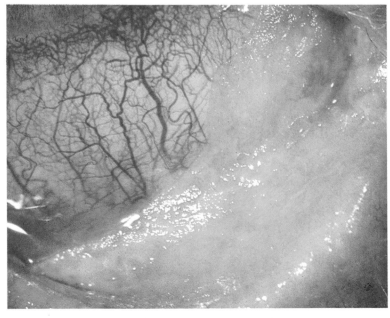

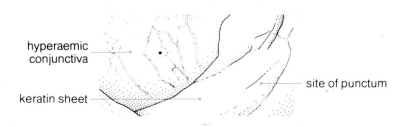

hyperaemic conjunctiva

keratin sheet

site of punctum

Fig. 5.32 This patient has developed squamous metaplasia involving the conjunctival surface near the lid margin, following prolonged idoxuridine therapy. A thick, white, keratin plaque is present with the normal conjunctival mucous membrane replaced by stratified squamous epithelium, which has obliterated the meibomian orifices along the lower lid margin.

The diagnosis of drug-induced hypersensitivity and toxic reactions is usually established by a combination of the history and the reversal of changes following withdrawal of the drug.

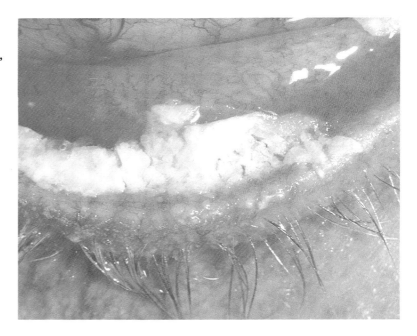

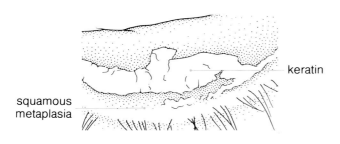

Chemical Burns

Chemical injuries account for the most severe toxic reactions of the eye. Those involving alterations in pH may produce permanent damage as a result of changes that develop immediately on contact. First aid measures, especially prompt immersion of the eye in cold water, to dilute the chemical, are therefore vital in determining the outcome of such an injury. Burns due to ammonia and other alkaline chemicals are undoubtedly the most serious, in view of their rapid ocular penetration (often within minutes of contact), causing severe intraocular damage.

Fig. 5.33 This patient illustrates the acute changes occurring in the skin and outer eye immediately following an ammonia burn. There are large ulcerated areas associated with erythema involving the skin of the upper and lower eyelids. The conjunctiva is chemotic and haemorrhagic and there is loss of corneal epithelium over the lower half of the cornea.

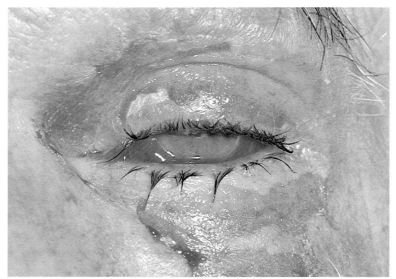

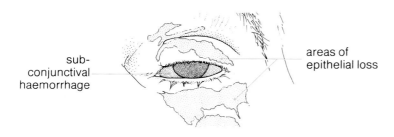

Fig. 5.34 This is the appearance of the bulbar conjunctiva immediately following a severe alkali burn, and shows the typical appearance with a complete absence of the normal conjunctival vascular markings in a dense white, slightly chemotic conjunctiva. There is complete loss of the whole of the corneal epithelium and early sloughing of necrotic conjunctiva beneath the upper tarsus.

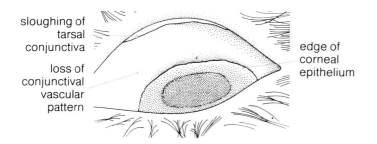

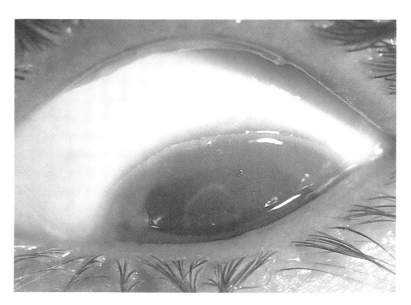

Fig. 5.35 In the same patient as Fig. 5.33, conjunctival necrosis occurred some weeks after the ammonia burn. The whole upper tarsal conjunctiva is pale, yellowish and swollen, with poorly defined vessels. The upper edge is starting to slough away from the underlying tissues.

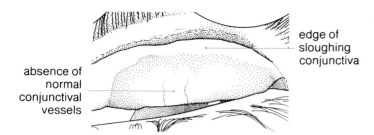

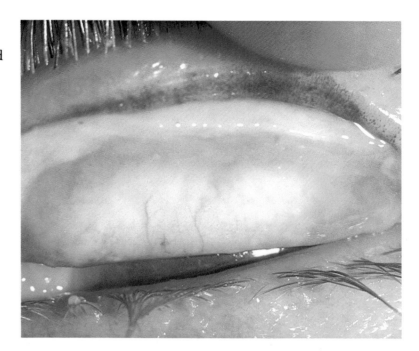

Fig. 5.36 The late corneal changes of the same patient are shown six weeks later. The corneal stroma has become oedematous and is undergoing melting, as evidenced by the ectatic shape. There is failure of epithelization over the central part of the cornea.

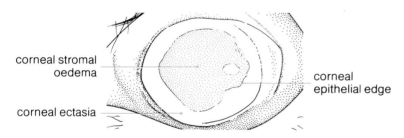

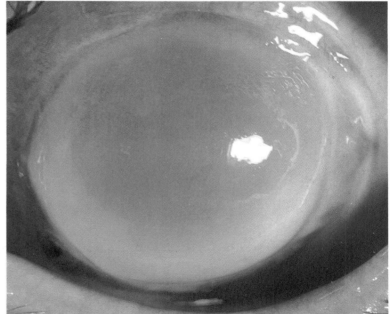

Fig. 5.37 Healing of the corneal tissues may eventually take place in the presence of massive neovascularization of the cornea. There is diffuse stromal scarring associated with thinning and facetting of the cornea. The corneal problems are usually compounded by abnormalities in the tear film from the conjunctival damage; this, together with the neovascularization, produces a poor prognosis for corneal grafting.

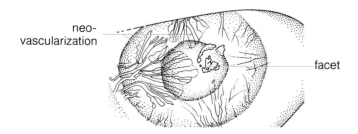

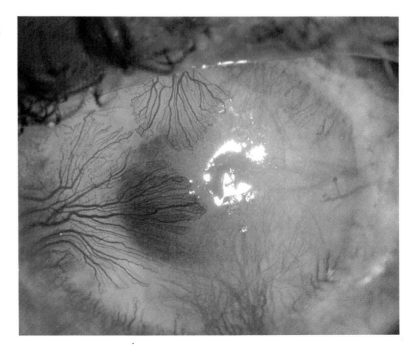

5.13

DRY EYES (Keratoconjunctivitis Sicca)

Keratoconjunctivitis sicca is a common cause of chronically irritable sore eyes which usually occurs in the late middle-aged and elderly female due to a gradual reduction in the lacrimal secretions. Similar symptomatology and findings may be present in other conditions where other components of the normal tear film, such as mucus and meibomian secretions, are reduced or absent. Dry eyes have a deficient or unstable tear film, which contains mucus and debris and has a poor or absent meniscus at the lid margins. In severe cases, mucus filaments can be seen attached to the cornea and these exacerbate the symptoms.

Apart from idiopathic keratoconjunctivitis sicca, similar changes are seen with rheumatoid arthritis, Sjögren's syndrome, Mikulicz's syndrome, and local conjunctival conditions caused by trauma, infection, or drugs.

Fig. 5.38 The clinical picture of keratoconjunctivitis sicca shows diffuse punctate epithelial erosions over the lower one-third of the corneal epithelium which stain as red spots with bengal rose: the staining usually extends on to the lower bulbar conjunctiva in the exposure area. There is some associated conjunctival hyperaemia.

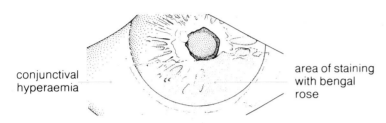

conjunctival hyperaemia

area of staining with bengal rose

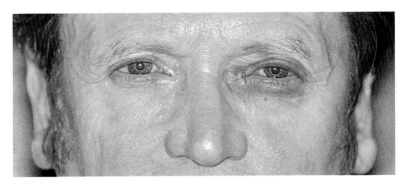

Mikulicz's Syndrome

Fig. 5.39 Mikulicz's syndrome is usually caused by sarcoidosis. As well as keratoconjunctivitis sicca resulting from dacryoadenitis, there is bilateral parotitis. This is the same patient as shown in Fig. 5.37. There is characteristic bilateral parotid swelling from glandular infiltration.

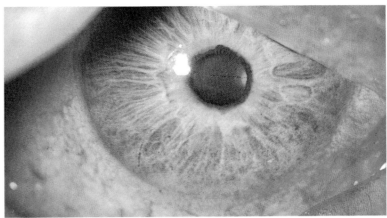

Fig. 5.40 A more common association of keratoconjunctivitis sicca is rheumatoid arthritis. Among sufferers of the disease, fifteen percent may be expected to develop dry eyes, although usually not severe. This example shows the changes associated with advanced rheumatoid arthritis of the hands, including the swollen metacarpal phalangeal joints, ulnar deviation, swan-neck deformities of the fingers, and the skin changes associated with vasculitis.

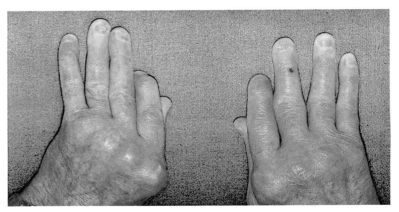

Sjögren's Syndrome

Sjögren's syndrome is typically seen in elderly women and is characterized by a combination of dry eyes, a dry mouth and rheumatoid arthritis.

Fig. 5.41 This patient illustrates the typical changes associated with Sjögren's syndrome. Patients also have a small but statistically significant risk of developing a lymphoma. Mild cases respond to treatment with wetting agents. Occlusion of the lacrimal puncta by cautery is a useful way of alleviating symptoms in the more severe cases.

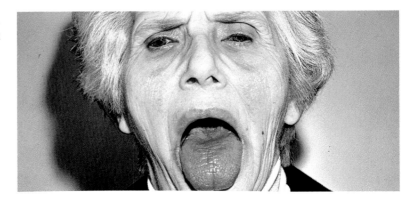

Nutritional Xerophthalmia

Nutritional xerophthalmia is one of the two main clinical manifestations of vitamin A deficiency – the other being night blindness. It occurs primarily in children under the age of ten in conditions of malnutrition, and may also affect the skin and mucous membranes of the alimentary tract. It is a leading cause of world blindness with an estimated 20,000 children becoming blind annually as a result of the disease.

Treatment of the eye condition is readily effected in the early stages of the disease by oral administration of a single dose of 100,000 I.U. of vitamin A. Prevention through large scale programmes of dietary education should eliminate the worst effects.

Fig. 5.42 In the vitamin A-deficient eye there is a drying and wrinkling of the conjunctiva associated with the development of 'Bitot's spots.' These spots are small, white, cheese-like patches which may have a foamy appearance and do not wet easily. At this stage, a punctate keratopathy may also appear.

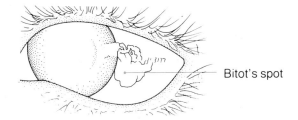

Bitot's spot

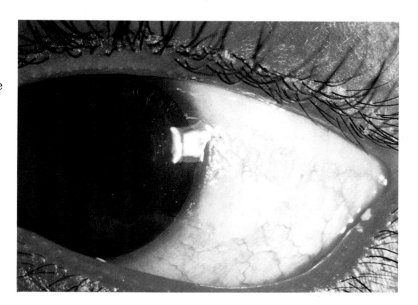

Fig.5.43 This photograph demonstrates a late stage in the development of vitamin A deficiency in which the corneal epithelium is lost over the lower nasal part of the exposed eye. Note the dry, wrinkled conjunctiva.

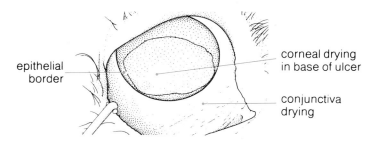

epithelial border

corneal drying in base of ulcer

conjunctiva drying

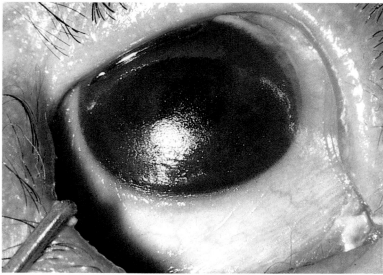

Fig. 5.44 In advanced keratomalacia, the whole cornea becomes softened and opaque. At this stage, the clinical picture is often complicated by secondary infection: in this case, secondary infection has resulted in perforation of the globe and endophthalmitis.

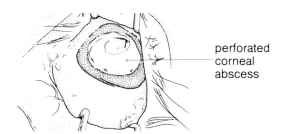

perforated corneal abscess

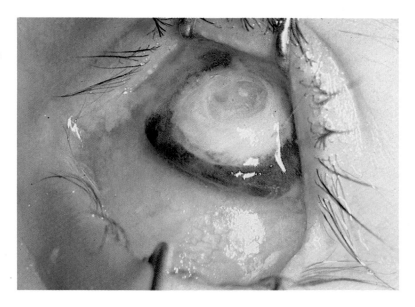

5.15

Fig. 5.45 The histological appearance of the conjunctiva in advanced keratomalacia shows a thickened epithelium with keratin formation, which stains red with a Masson stain. There is loss of goblet cells and the appearance of a prickle cell layer immediately above the basal layer.

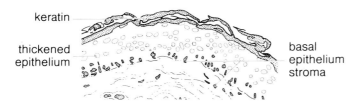

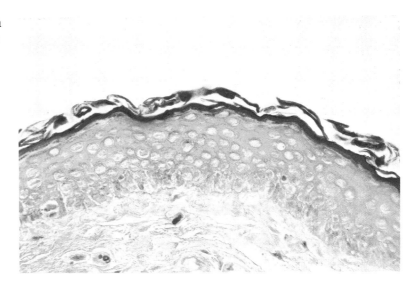

DISEASES OF THE SCLERA AND EPISCLERA

Although the sclera and episclera may be affected by a wide range of diseases including degenerations, congenital anomalies, and neoplastic processes, the most common and most important forms of disease in clinical practice are the inflammatory disorders. These are broadly classified as scleritis and episcleritis. The sclera is composed of collagen and elastic fibres, and is subject to a range of disease processes which affect connective tissue elsewhere in the body – hence its association with chronic inflammatory joint disease and conditions such as systemic lupus erythematosus and rheumatoid arthritis. The episclera, likewise, consists of connective tissue but, unlike the sclera, is vascularized and is responsible, in part, for the nutrition of the sclera and for providing the cellular response to inflammation. Scleritis is, therefore, always accompanied by overlying episcleritis.

The sclera is the protective coat of the eye and consists of bundles of collagen and elastic tissue which are approximately 10μ–15μ in width and 100μ–150μ in length, and are arranged in a criss-cross manner. Such a structure is well adapted to the functions of the sclera,

which are to provide a firm protective coat for the intraocular contents, and to resist distortions of the globe by the extraocular muscles.

Anteriorly, the sclera is pierced by the anterior ciliary vessels to join the major circle of the iris and is continuous with the corneal stroma, which differs in structure from the sclera both in its regular arrangement of the collagen bundles, and in its state of partial dehydration. Posteriorly, the sclera is pierced by the optic nerve and by canals which carry the posterior ciliary nerves and vessels, and the vortex veins. A knowledge of the thickness of the sclera is important in ocular surgery – it varies from 0.3mm (immediately behind the insertion of the recti muscles) to 1–1.35mm at the posterior pole. Anteriorly at the limbus, the thickness is 0.6mm, and at the equator it varies between 0.4 and 0.6mm.

The episclera (Tenon's capsule) acts as a synovial membrane for smooth movement of the eye. It is a fibroelastic structure covering the sclera and carries a vascular network which consists of a deeper visceral layer and a superficial parietal layer.

Fig. 5.46 The vascular supply of the anterior episclera and sclera are best examined using a slit lamp. The importance of understanding the vascular anatomy lies in the clues that it provides in differentiating clinical patterns of inflammation.

Three layers of vessels are visible. The conjunctival plexus is the most superficial layer and can be distinguished clinically by its ability to be moved over the underlying structures. The superficial episcleral plexus is a radially arranged series of vessels within Tenon's capsule. These superficial vessels anastomose at the limbus with the conjunctival vessels, and the underlying deep plexus. The deep episcleral plexus lies in the visceral layer and is closely applied to the sclera. The vessels in this layer are arranged in an irregular (non-radial) fashion and, unlike the conjunctival and superficial layers, will not be blanched by a drop of 1 in 1,000 epinephrine.

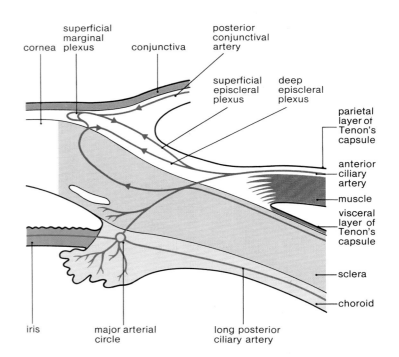

Fig. 5.47 Normal fluorescein angiogram of the anterior segment. The first vessels to fill are the perforating arterioles adjacent to the limbus. These vessels arise from the anterior ciliary vessels whose branches surround Schlemm's canal (left). From these vessels, the limbal and both the deep ducts and superficial episcleral vessels are filled (right).

Simultaneously, the posterior conjunctival vessels fill from the tarsal arcade.

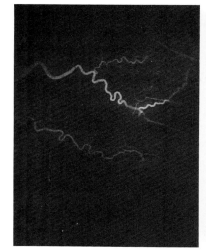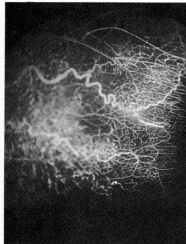

Episcleritis

Episcleritis is a benign self-limiting inflammation which occurs in young adults and may be bilateral. The presenting features include redness and mild discomfort with occasional watering. Severe pain and photophobia are not characteristic features and may help to differentiate the condition from a scleritis or keratitis. No associated systemic condition is found in the majority of patients, but up to thirty percent may have an associated general finding such as herpes zoster, collagen disease, or evidence of allergy.

Treatment in the form of steroid drops or systemic non-steroidal anti-inflammatory drugs will be effective shortening the course of the condition. Episcleritis may be divided into simple (diffuse) inflammation and that associated with episcleral nodules

Fig. 5.48 Diffuse episcleritis may affect a sector or the whole anterior segment of the globe. In this example, the radial superficial episcleral vessels are dilated and, although there is some associated engorgement of the conjunctival and deep episcleral plexus, there is no scleral swelling. Treatment with topical steroids produced resolution within a few days. Episcleritis may recur, but no ocular damage results.

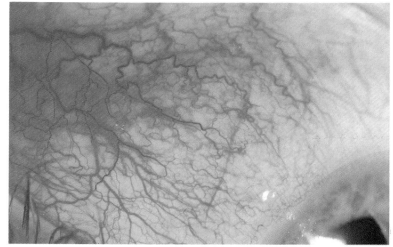

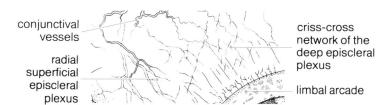

conjunctival vessels

radial superficial episcleral plexus

criss-cross network of the deep episcleral plexus

limbal arcade

Fig. 5.49 In nodular episcleritis, the oedema and infiltration of the episclera are localized to one or more sites, with engorgement of episcleral vessels around a central pale nodule. The nodules are mobile on the underlying sclera and, unlike scleral nodules, do not undergo necrosis. Resolution of nodular episcleritis tends to occur more slowly than in simple episcleritis, and topical steroids or flurbiprofen applied either locally or given systemically, may be used. Steroid therapy may be associated with a rebound phenomenon and treatment should be reduced gradually after the signs have disappeared.

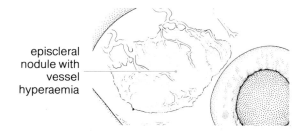

episcleral nodule with vessel hyperaemia

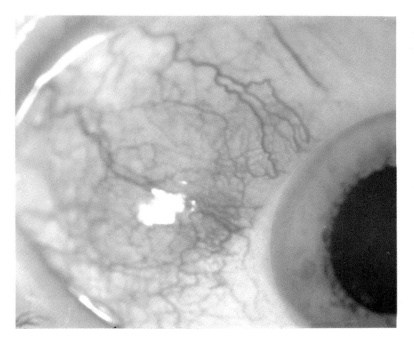

Fig. 5.50 Early and late films of anterior segment angiography from another patient with episcleritis show rapid filling of normal capillaries without distortion of the normal vascular pattern.

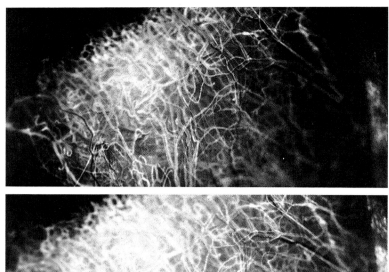
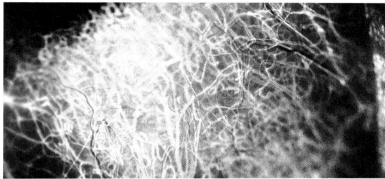

Scleritis

Scleritis, unlike episcleritis in which resolution takes place without damage, is a destructive disease. Four clinical types of scleritis are recognized: nodular anterior, diffuse anterior, necrotizing anterior, (termed scleromalacia perforans when it occurs without inflammation), and posterior scleritis. The majority of patients with necrotizing scleritis have an underlying causative systemic factor, as do a third of patients with the diffuse form of the disease. Necrotizing scleritis is caused through a vasculitis of the vessels of the anterior segment of the eye and is therefore associated with the vasculitis which accompanies rheumatoid arthritis, systemic lupus erythematosus, Wegener's granuloma, polyarteritis nodosa, and Crohn's disease.

'Severe pain is the dominant feature, which may be associated with photophobia and visual disturbance. The inflammation of the eye, which is also a prominent feature,

has a deeper red colouration, and an overlying episcleritis is invariably present as well. If the superficial episcleral vessels are blanched with ten percent phenylphrine or epinephrine 1 in 1,000, the congestion of the deeper vessels and swelling of the sclera are more readily visible.

Venulitis is a characteristic of this condition which leads to vaso-occlusion and later vaso-obliteration. These changes can be detected with fluorescein angiography.

Nodular and diffuse anterior scleritis will usually respond to systemic therapy with non-steroidal anti-flammatory agents such as flurbiprofen, if the vascular tree remains patent on fluorescein angiography. Local steroids may provide symptomatic relief but do not, of course, affect the underlying disease process. Following resolution, increased transparency of the sclera can be seen.

Fig. 5.51 Diffuse anterior scleritis usually shows widespread changes, although it may occasionally be confined to a segment. The injection is a deeper red than in simple episcleritis and all levels of blood vessels are involved (left).

Nodular anterior scleritis may appear similar to nodular

episcleritis on superficial examination, but the nodules are tender, associated with scleral swelling, and cannot be moved over the tissues (right). There are inflammatory changes around the nodule, but the remaining sclera appears normal. Necrosis is a rare sequela.

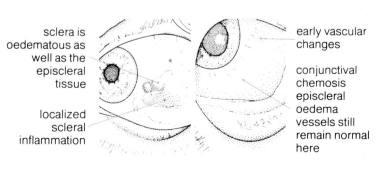

sclera is oedematous as well as the episcleral tissue

localized scleral inflammation

early vascular changes

conjunctival chemosis episcleral oedema vessels still remain normal here

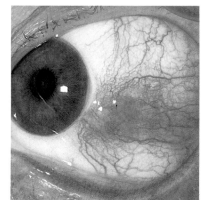
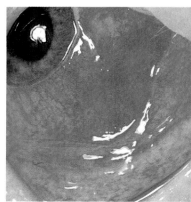

Fig. 5.52 Necrotizing anterior scleritis is the most serious variety of these conditions. If this is found and not treated immediately, the condition will be progressive and may extend to involve the whole anterior segment. The first indication of necrotizing change is vaso-occlusion or venular shutdown of areas of episcleral and scleral vessels. The eye still appears congested in these areas.

A first attack in which there is no vascular shutdown should be treated with flurbiprofen or indomethacin in high doses, which are gradually reduced when the disease is controlled. Severe attacks or recurrences and evidence of vaso-occlusion require large doses or systemic anti-inflammatory drugs or steroids (prednisolone 80-120 mg daily) in order to control the disease. Perforation of the globe is very rare. Scleral grafting is required only if there is evidence that the affected sclera is the source of auto-antigen.

Although there may be acute congestion of vessels in the affected area, fluorescein angiography reveals that there is a shutdown of the venous circulation in this area.

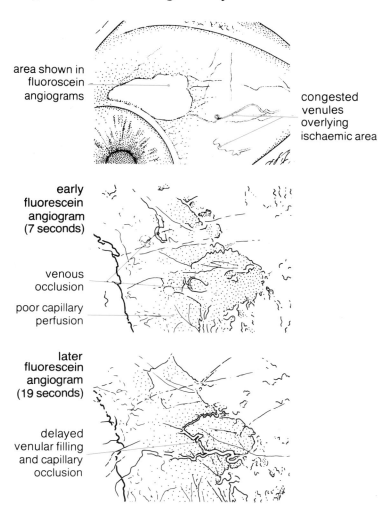

area shown in fluoroscein angiograms

congested venules overlying ischaemic area

early fluorescein angiogram (7 seconds)

venous occlusion

poor capillary perfusion

later fluorescein angiogram (19 seconds)

delayed venular filling and capillary occlusion

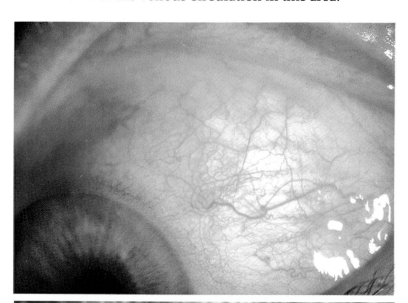

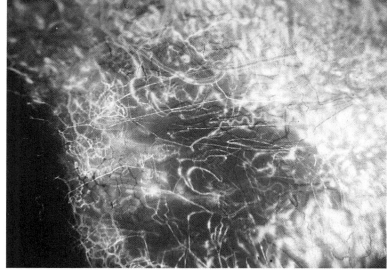

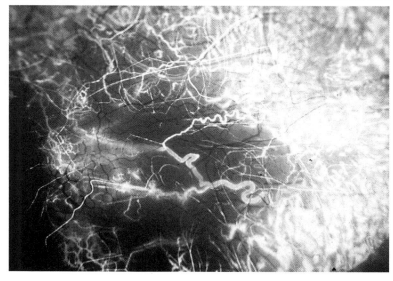

Fig. 5.53 A change in colour of the underlying sclera indicating infarction of the deep tissues. In this case, there is no perfusion of the overlying vessels in spite of these being congested.

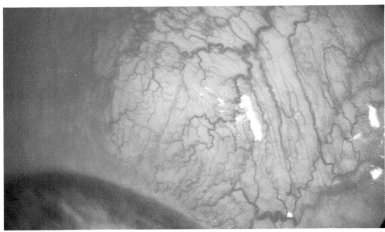

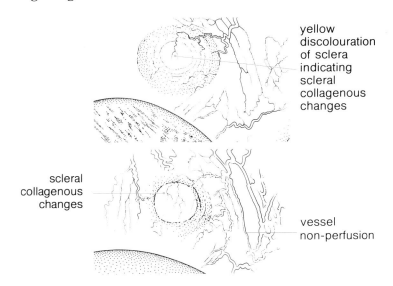

yellow discolouration of sclera indicating scleral collagenous changes

scleral collagenous changes

vessel non-perfusion

Fig. 5.54 Ten days later, breakdown and ulceration of the affected area are apparent.

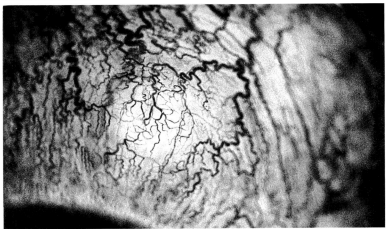

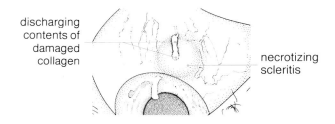

discharging contents of damaged collagen

necrotizing scleritis

Fig. 5.55 Localized progressive necrotizing scleritis or sclerokeratitis can be precipitated by surgical procedures (in this case a peripheral iridectomy) in susceptible individuals.

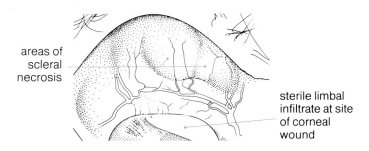

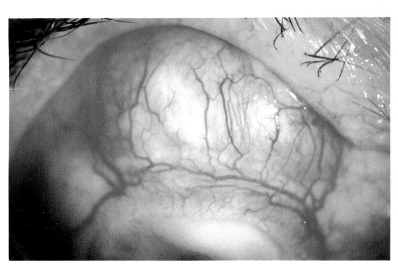

areas of scleral necrosis

sterile limbal infiltrate at site of corneal wound

Fig. 5.56 Scleromalacia perforans is characterized by progressive thinning of the sclera in the absence of symptoms and without inflammatory signs, as a result of arteriolar occlusion of the deep vascular network. It is nearly always associated with severe long-standing rheumatoid arthritis. In this example, scleral thinning has resulted in conjunctival ulceration and guttering of the adjacent cornea. Treatment is ineffective unless undertaken in the very earliest stages of the process. However, no active measures need be taken to replace the damaged sclera.

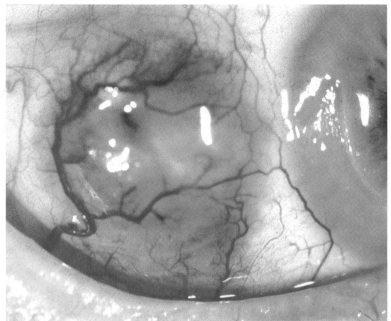

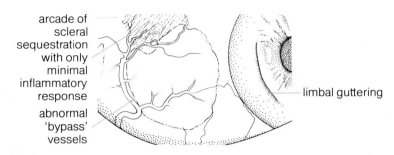

Fig. 5.57 Posterior scleritis is a seriously under-diagnosed condition. The patient may present with ocular pain, a severe exudative retinal detachment, macular oedema, or disc swelling. With severe inflammation, there may also be proptosis and extraocular muscle involvement. The diagnosis may be easily overlooked unless careful inspection of the anterior sclera is performed; inflammatory signs are often only apparent in the more posterior aspects. Fundus examination of a relatively mild case shows slight optic disc swelling and subretinal fluid producing macular folds.

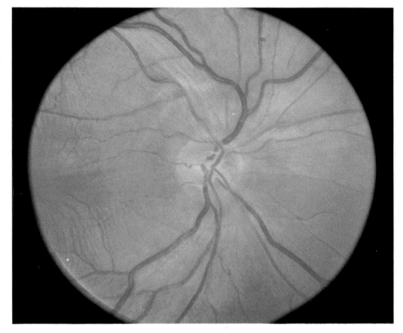

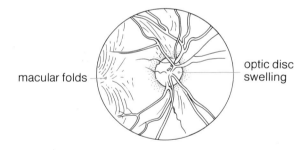

Fig. 5.58 An ultrasonic B-scan or orbital C.T. scan is helpful in confirming the diagnosis of posterior scleritis by demonstrating the scleral thickening with secondary choroidal and periocular inflammation.

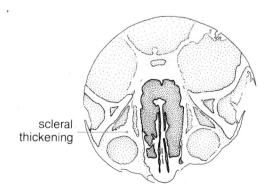

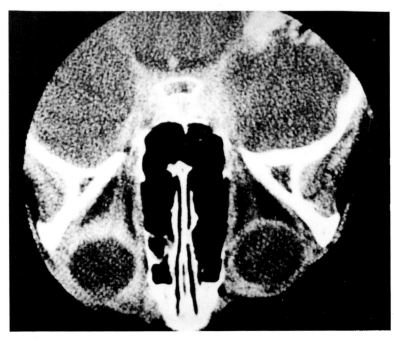

5.21

Fig. 5.59 Sclerokeratitis may complicate an anterior scleritis when a diffuse peripheral opacity may develop in the adjoining corneal stroma. In active disease, the whole thickness of the stroma adjacent to a patch of scleritis may become oedematous and may vascularize later. With resolution of activity, a dense white opacity persists and lipid deposition in the cornea is common. This type of active limbitis is often accompanied by an acute rise is intraocular pressure.

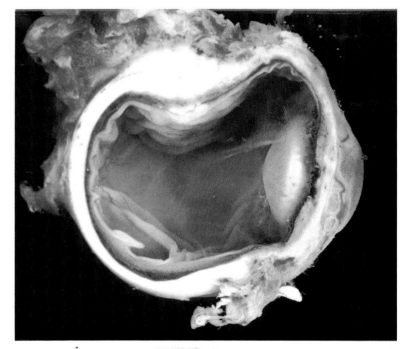

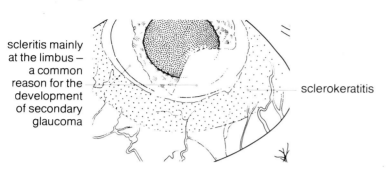

scleritis mainly at the limbus — a common reason for the development of secondary glaucoma

sclerokeratitis

Fig. 5.60 In severe scleritis, the granulomatous process not only involves the anterior segment but extends, as here, to involve the posterior sclera and adjacent orbital tissue, giving rise to retinal detachment, disc oedema, and limitation of ocular movement.

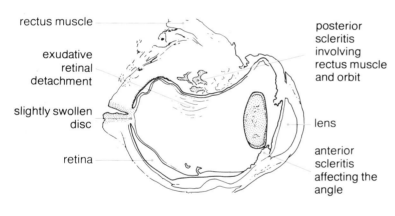

rectus muscle

exudative retinal detachment

slightly swollen disc

retina

posterior scleritis involving rectus muscle and orbit

lens

anterior scleritis affecting the angle

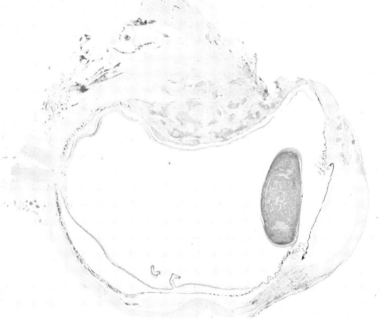

6. The Cornea

R. J. Buckley

THE NORMAL CORNEA

The normal cornea is an almost perfectly transparent, nearly circular window in the scleral envelope of the eye. The diameter of the posterior surface is 11.7 mm; its anterior surface constitutes an ellipse whose horizontal diameter is 11.7 mm (normal range: 10.5 to 13.0 mm) and whose vertical diameter is 0.9 mm less. The central zone of the cornea has a radius of curvature of 7.8 mm anteriorly (normal range: 6.75 to 9.25 mm) and 6.6 mm posteriorly. More peripherally the anterior curvature is flattened, more nasally than temporally and more above than below. The thickness of the cornea is 0.52 mm centrally (normal range: 0.50 to 0.54 mm) increasing to around 0.65 mm in the periphery.

The cornea consists of the epithelium, the stroma and the endothelium; both the stroma and the endothelium are derived from embryonic mesoderm. 90% of the corneal substance is made up by the stroma, which is composed of parallel lamellae of collagen fibrils in a glycosamino-glycan ground substance.

Anteriorly, the stroma is specialized into Bowman's membrane (layer), which is 10-13μ thick and appears amorphous under the light microscope. The basement membrane of the epithelium lies on this layer. The epithelium is 50-100μ thick and comprises a basal layer, two or three layers of wing cells and two layers of surface cells. The anterior surface of the epithelium appears smooth by light microscopy, but the electron microscope reveals microvilli whose function it is to interact with the mucus layer of the tear film. It is the tear film which gives the cornea its smooth and brilliant surface and which forms the major refractive interface of the eye.

Posteriorly, the stroma is bounded by Descemet's membrane and the endothelium. The endothelium, which is actually a mesothelium, is a monolayer of non-dividing cells 5μ thick which secrete Descemet's membrane. The process continues throughout life; at birth the membrane is 2-3μ thick but in old age it reaches 20-30μ. Descemet's membrane is composed of fine collagen fibrils and is particularly resistant to inflammatory processes. It inserts peripherally into Schwalbe's line at the filtration angle. The endothelium has a smooth posterior surface.

The oxygen and nutritional requirements of the cornea are met by the atmosphere and tear film anteriorly and the aqueous posteriorly; the limbal circulation contributes only at the periphery. When the eyes are shut, oxygen is derived from the conjunctival capillaries, but the partial pressure beneath closed lids (55 mm Hg) is only one third of the atmospheric partial pressure (160 mm Hg). Water is removed from the stromal ground substance by the active 'pumping' of the endothelium, which is thus fundamental in maintaining the cornea at its normal hydration, thickness and clarity.

Fig. 6.1 The histological preparation (left) demonstrates the layers of a normal cornea, stained with haematoxylin and eosin. The slit lamp view (right) shows, in the specular zone, the bright featureless gleam of the air/tear film interface, and the dimmer endothelial/aqueous interface in which details of the endothelial cells are seen.

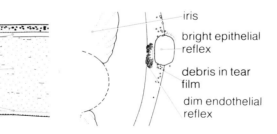

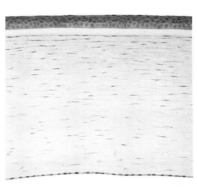

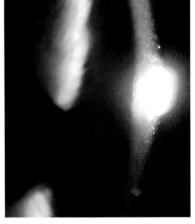

Fig. 6.2 This figure shows the appearance of the normal corneal endothelium as seen with the clinical contact specular microscope. The cells are roughly equal in size and shape; most of them are hexagons in this two-dimensional view. (The specular micrographs in this volume are presented at the same linear magnification, approximately ×100; the single exception is figure 6.4.)

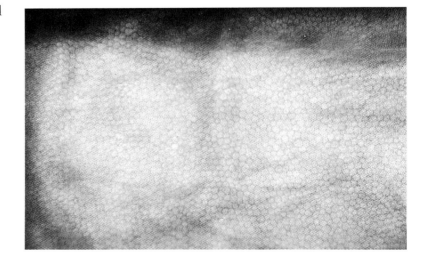

Fig. 6.3 Scanning electron micrographs of the epithelial surface (left) and the endothelial surface (right) at the same magnification. The surface epithelial cells are irregular in size and shape and possess microvilli. The endothelial cells are mostly hexagonal; cilia are occasionally seen on their posterior faces. Magnification of both frames is ×750.

Fig. 6.4 This is a montage of specular micrographs of a normal cornea, with the applanation artefacts which are known as posterior corneal rings. These concentric irregular elliptical rings form in predetermined positions for each individual. They may represent the locations of ties between the corneal lamellae which limit tangential slip and which maintain its normal non-spherical profile. These rings can be used clinically to relocate, and therefore follow sequentially, specific areas of endothelium.

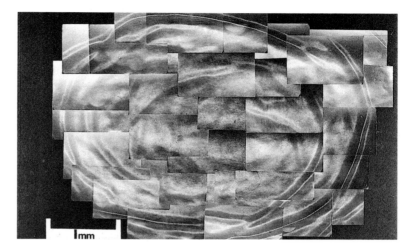

CONGENITAL ABNORMALITIES

Congenital abnormalities of the cornea are rare. Anomalies of size and shape may be found in an otherwise healthy eye. However, corneal disorders are more often present in association with other ocular defects as in, for example, buphthalmos or the anterior chamber cleavage syndromes.

Fig. 6.5 Megalocornea may be present from birth and need not be associated with raised intraocular tension. The most usual cause of a large corneal diameter is, however, congenital or infantile glaucoma, which can stretch the coats of the eye from late foetal life to three years of age. This condition, which is not uncommon, is termed buphthalmos (ox-eye). Three fifths of patients are male; two thirds of cases are bilateral, but the corneas are often unequally affected; seven eighths of cases are sporadic, the remainder showing autosomal recessive transmission.

Buphthalmos may also occur in association with neurofibromatosis, or the Sturge-Weber syndrome, as in this example. Here the naevus flammeus affects the right side of the face, and the right eye is buphthalmic.

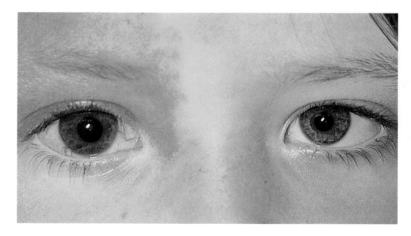

Fig. 6.6 When the corneal diameter increases, as a part of the enlargement of the whole eye in buphthalmos, splits in Descemet's membrane appear. These are known as Haab's striae, and are very similar in appearance to, but histologically different from, the curvilinear lesions of posterior polymorphous corneal dystrophy (Fig. 6.57).

The figure shows examples from the same patient in ordinary diffuse illumination (left) and in microscopic specular reflection (right). The endothelial cells are enlarged as is frequently seen in buphthalmos, even in cases which have not had surgical treatment.

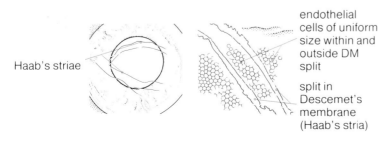

Haab's striae

endothelial cells of uniform size within and outside DM split

split in Descemet's membrane (Haab's stria)

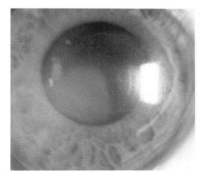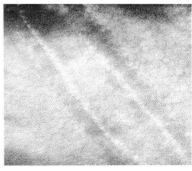

6.3

Fig. 6.7 In keratoglobus, a rare bilateral condition, the corneal diameter is within normal limits but the cornea becomes ectatic throughout with consequent production of myopic irregular astigmatism. Neither in this condition nor in megalocornea, in which the corneal diameter is abnormally large, is there an association with glaucoma. The stroma is thin; sometimes Descemet's membrane ruptures, producing acute hydrops corneae as in keratoconus (Fig. 6.11).

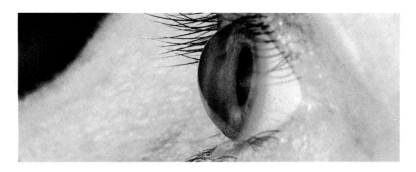

Fig. 6.8 Localized posterior keratoconus is a rare condition of uncertain aetiology. It is probably part of the spectrum of mesenchymal dysgenesis of the anterior segment which also includes posterior embryotoxon, Axenfeld's anomaly, Rieger's anomaly, iridogoniodysgenesis and Peter's anomaly (Chapter 7).

In this example localized posterior keratoconus is seen

in flat illumination on the left and slit illumination on the right. There is a small round area of smooth excavation of the posterior cornea; the endothelium appeared normal throughout. The anterior profile of the cornea is normal, as is usual in this condition. Only if the area of posterior excavation is large enough to cause secondary ectasia is vision likely to be much affected.

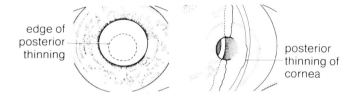

edge of posterior thinning

posterior thinning of cornea

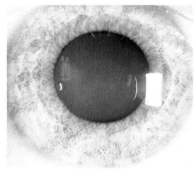
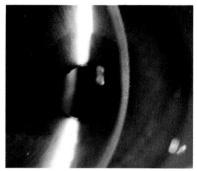

CORNEAL OPACIFICATION

The cornea can lose its transparency by several means, including oedema, drying, deposition, cellular infiltration, vascularization and scarring. In cases other than the deposition of non-transparent materials, the basic mechanism involves the disorganization of the normal regular arrangement of collagen fibres in the stroma. They may separate in oedema, approximate in cases of drying, and in the case of scarring randomly-arranged fibres may be added. Examples of these mechanisms are described below. Degenerations and dystrophies are discussed in subsequent sections.

Oedema

The cornea becomes oedematous if the barrier and pumping functions of the endothelium (and, to a much lesser extent, of the epithelium) are upset. There are many possible causes but endothelial cell malfunction is virtually always the common factor. In the open eye, some dehydration occurs through exposure.

Patients with minimal corneal oedema see rainbow haloes around polychromatic lights; further oedema blurs acuity. Fluid in the epithelium forms cystic spaces (bullous keratopathy) which can rupture causing painful epithelial defects.

Fig. 6.9 Corneal oedema, indistinguishable from that which occurs clinically, is seen as a post mortem change in fresh donor eyes. The accumulation of metabolites in the stagnant aqueous humour is the primary cause and this is frequently augmented by cooling, which slows the endothelial pump. The first visible sign of oedema is the appearance of fine, straight, branching dark lines in the posterior stroma, seen here in an eye photographed 4½ hours post mortem (left). Greater oedema and hence greater thickening produces folding of Descemet's membrane (DM), seen in this example 22½ hours post mortem (right).

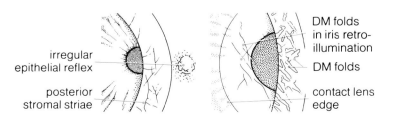

irregular epithelial reflex

posterior stromal striae

DM folds in iris retro-illumination

DM folds

contact lens edge

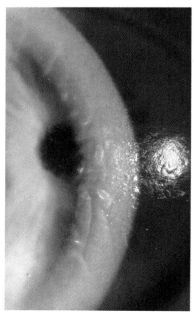
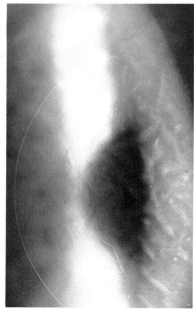

Fig. 6.10 Folds in Descemet's membrane seen clinically are termed striate keratitis. This frequently occurs following endothelial insult, whether hypoxic, traumatic or toxic, and is transient unless there is substantial permanent damage. This example, photographed on the day after cataract extraction, shows striate keratitis and also epithelial bullae, which are secondary to stromal oedema. Such bullae are often seen adjacent to surgical wounds, and are caused by local endothelial cell damage.

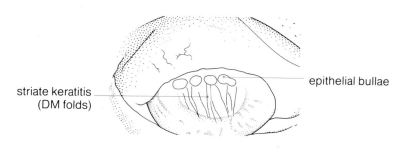

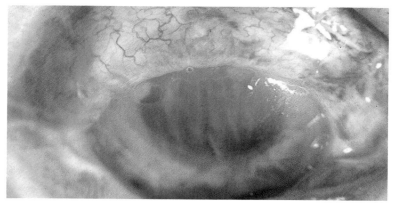

Fig. 6.11 If Descemet's membrane is ruptured, either spontaneously in conditions such as keratoconus and buphthalmos or as the result of trauma, a patch of gross stromal oedema, usually very clearly demarcated, results. This resolves over a matter of weeks: the endothelial cells around the rupture migrate over the bare area, re-establish a continuous monolayer, and secrete a basement membrane. This example of acute hydrops occurred in a case of keratoconus.

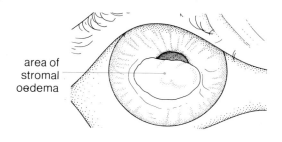

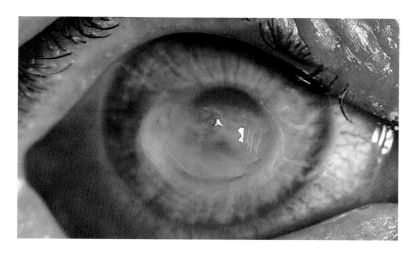

Fig. 6.12 The most serious type of corneal graft rejection is that directed at the corneal endothelium by cytotoxic T-lymphocytes. An early stage of graft rejection is seen in this example. Careful examination of the endothelial surface might show a 'rejection line' of cellular constituents, rather like a continuous line of keratic precipitates, preceding the area of stromal oedema in its steady advance across the cornea. The initial graft oedema may clear either spontaneously or with the aid of intensive steroid therapy, but if endothelial damage is too severe the oedema will persist indefinitely. An early stage of graft rejection is seen in this example. The effect of steroid therapy in this patient was subsequently monitored by corneal thickness measurements.

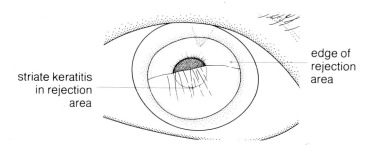

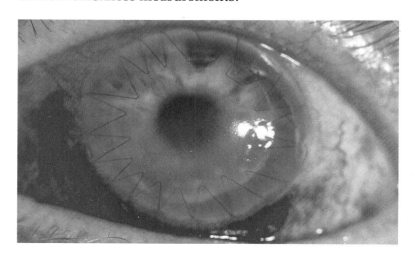

Drying

Drying of the cornea results first in damage to the epithelium, with consequent risk of infection and scarring. Dryness may result from tear film instability or lid or conjunctival disease. The corneal sensory innervation appears to be important in maintaining a healthy epithelium.

Fig. 6.13 A saucer-shaped excavation of the cornea, known as a dellen, can form adjacent to an elevation (usually at the limbus) which either prevents normal apposition of the lid to the corneal surface or disturbs the pre-ocular tear film. The epithelium within the dellen may be somewhat eroded, but there is essentially no loss of tissue, and the condition responds to rehydration by padding the eye. This example, stained with Rose Bengal, was associated with local conjunctival elevation following squint surgery to an aphakic eye.

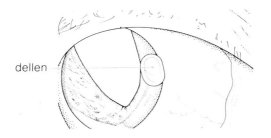

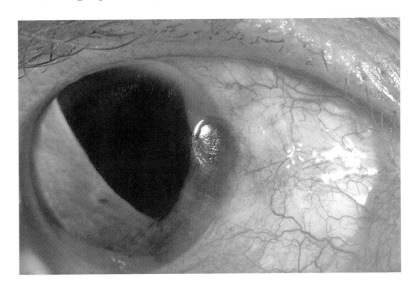

Fig. 6.14 In severe keratoconjunctivitis sicca, threads of dried mucus and epithelial cell debris become attached to particularly dry locations on the corneal epithelium. This condition is known as filamentary keratitis. Rose Bengal stains mucus and devitalized cells; in this example it is seen staining the filaments more avidly than is the fluorescein which has also been instilled. Filamentary keratitis produces severe discomfort and photophobia; treatment lies in tear film augmentation and topical mucolytic agents.

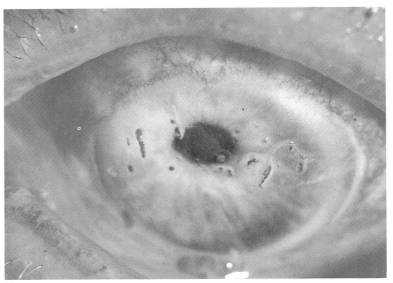

Fig. 6.15 Severe drying of the cornea occurs in exposure keratitis, where the lids are deficient in anatomy or function; the situation is worsened if Bell's phenomenon is not present. In cases of leprosy, as shown here, infiltration of the lids and denervation of the orbicularis oculi muscle result in permanently open eyes. Chronic drying of the cornea (left) has resulted in neovascularization and scarring. On the right is a leprous face with its characteristic fixed stare.

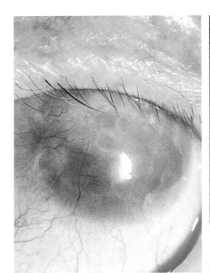 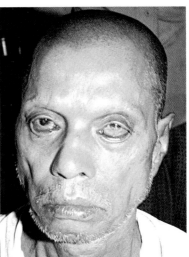

Fig. 6.16 Neurotrophic keratitis results from partial or complete corneal denervation. The extreme condition, which results from complete loss of function of the ophthalmic division of the trigeminal nerve, is known as neuroparalytic keratitis. Very soon after denervation the surface epithelial cells of cornea and conjunctiva lose their microscopic projections which hold the mucin layer of the tear film. The tear film becomes unstable due to the non-wetting surface and the eye is very vulnerable to infection and minor trauma. In the example shown, there is a shallow ulcer due to loss of epithelium, and the surrounding epithelium is grey and unstable. A permanent tarsorrhaphy may prove necessary for corneal protection.

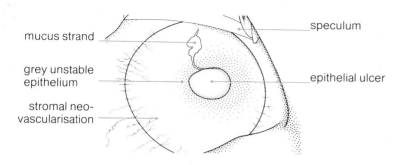

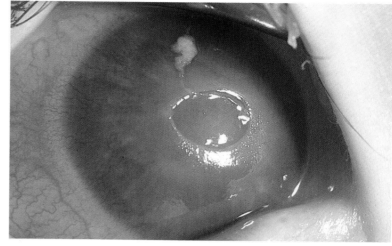

- mucus strand
- grey unstable epithelium
- stromal neo-vascularisation
- speculum
- epithelial ulcer

Deposition

A variety of substances, both organic and inorganic, can be deposited in the corneal tissues with resulting loss of corneal transparency.

Fig. 6.17 Calcium is frequently deposited in the superficial layers of inflamed corneas, often a considerable time after the inflammation has apparently ceased. Such corneas are almost invariably neovascularized. The example on the left shows calcium deposition in the lower half of the corneal periphery in a case of chronic exposure keratitis. The more severe example on the right shows calcium plaques at the level of Bowman's layer following an ammonia injury.

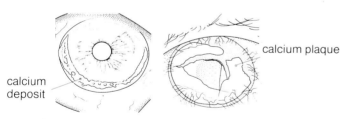

- calcium deposit
- calcium plaque

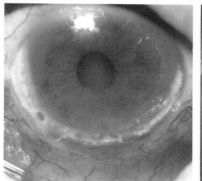

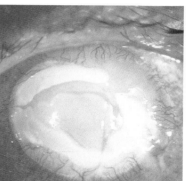

Fig. 6.18 Silver, if topically applied to the eye, is deposited in the deepest layers of the corneal stroma, as well as in the conjunctiva (argyrosis; ref. Chapter 3). It is now less frequently used as a medication, but it may still present a hazard for certain industrial workers. The slit lamp view shows bluish-grey discoloration of the posterior corneal layers. The specular micrograph shows finely divided silver deposits apparently outlining some endothelial cells. Patients are usually asymptomatic.

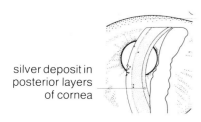

- silver deposit in posterior layers of cornea

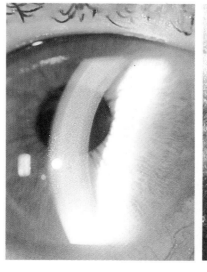

Fig. 6.19 Haemosiderin is deposited in the normal cornea as the Hudson-Stähli line; it is commoner in older than in younger subjects and in injured corneas of any age. The roughly horizontal brown line, situated at the level of the basal epithelial cells, usually occurs at the junction of the lower and middle thirds of the cornea. It does not extend to the limbus. A Hudson-Stähli line is shown on the left.

A precisely similar deposition occurs in most cases of keratoconus, but here the deposit apparently surrounds the base of the cone. The ring, named after Fleischer, is frequently incomplete. The example shown is illuminated by blue light, which makes the ring darker and more visible. As is so often the case, the ring is not concentric with the geometrical axis of the cornea; nor is it circular, but rather a horizontal oval.

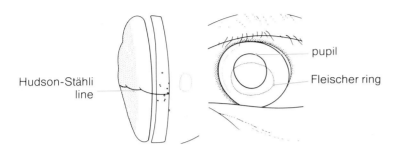

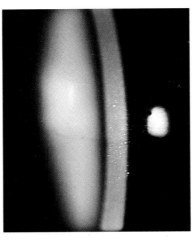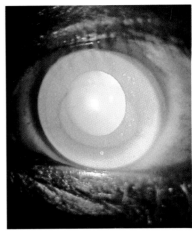

Fig. 6.20 Hepatolenticular degeneration (Wilson's Disease) has as its ocular sign the deposition of a copper compound at the corneal periphery at the level of Descemet's membrane: the Kayser-Fleischer ring. It is

usually a brownish colour, and is only seen in longstanding untreated cases. It fades away with treatment of the general disease.

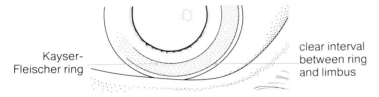

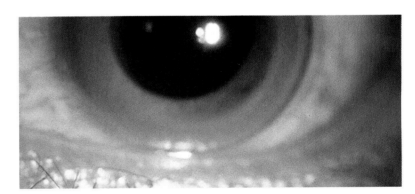

Fig. 6.21 A ferrous foreign body impacted on the surface of the cornea is a very common minor injury. Within minutes or hours the particle stains the epithelial layers (and the superficial stroma, if Bowman's layer is breached) with the formation of a rust ring. A ferrous foreign body is seen here with a surrounding rust ring (top).

If the cornea is subjected to repeated bombardment by small ferrous particles, the endothelium may show toxic features. The bottom illustration is a specular micrograph from a man whose occupation involved grinding iron and steel on a wheel and who declined to wear protective goggles. The corneas showed areas of endothelial cell enlargement (i.e. local depletion) such as the one seen in the lower half of the illustration.

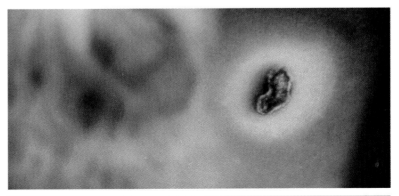

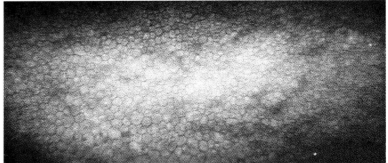

Fig. 6.22 The normal negro eye shows melanin pigmentation of the limbus, and pigmented cells often extend a little distance on to the corneal periphery. In the variety of vernal disease seen in parts of Africa, this pigmentation becomes much more marked; exceptionally, the whole of the cornea may be covered by pigmented epithelium. This condition is associated with limbal inflammation and corneal epithelial erosion. The characteristic limbal hyperplasia is seen in this example in which the view of the iris and pupil is obscured by uniform corneal epithelial pigmentation.

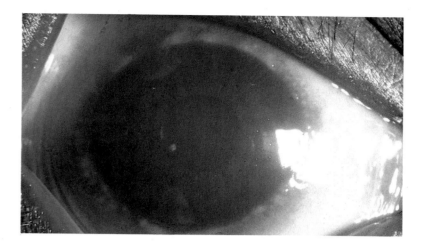

Fig. 6.23 Keratic precipitates (KP) are discussed in other chapters. Pigmented granules on the endothelial surface, or perhaps melanocytes, are shown here and these can simulate KP. The slit lamp view shows quite large particulate brown deposits on the central posterior corneal surface. The specular micrograph shows another example in which very small, brightly-reflecting pigmented granules are superimposed on the endothelial mosaic. In both cases the pigment derived from the iris following intra-ocular surgery, but similar appearances are seen with Krukenberg spindles of the pigment dispersion syndrome (Chapter 7).

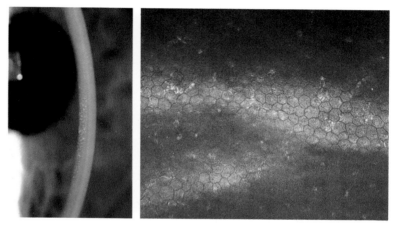

Fig. 6.24 Blood staining of the cornea occurs either as a result of a long-standing hyphaema or, rarely, as a direct extension of subconjunctival haemorrhage. Occasionally, abnormal vessels present in the cornea may bleed, producing an intrastromal haematoma. These examples show the results of a severe traumatic hyphaema (top) and an acute subconjunctival haemorrhage (bottom) in which the associated pathology has resolved.

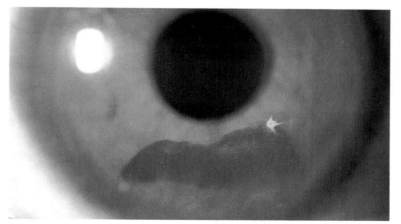

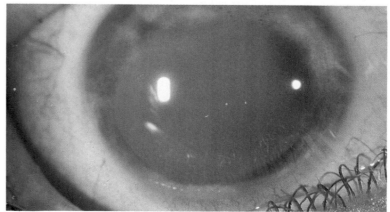

Fig. 6.25 The Wessely ring is an immune phenomenon seen in the cornea for two reasons: the cornea is avascular, so that some immune reactions are greatly slowed; and it is transparent, so that such reactions can be seen. The Wessely ring consists of neutrophils attracted to the site of antigen-antibody complex deposition. The antigen is derived from the more central region (for example, bacterial products) and the antibody diffuses inwards from the limbus. In this example a Wessely ring surrounds a small area of corneal infection by *Staphylococcus aureus*.

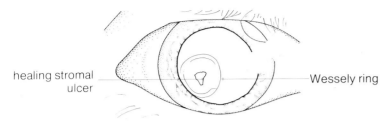

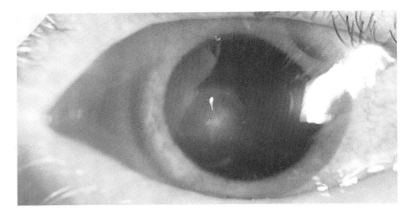

Fig. 6.26 The accumulation of lipid in the cornea is usually associated with corneal neovascularization rather than with a disorder of fat metabolism. This example of peripheral lipid infiltration occurred in a patient who had worn scleral contact lenses for many years with subsequent peripheral corneal neovascularization. Such gross changes are uncommon.

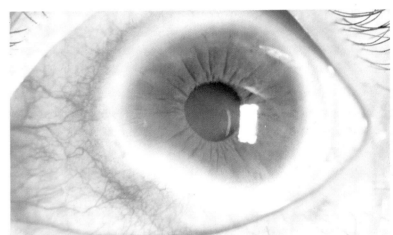

Fig. 6.27 Arcus occurring in youth is usually due to chronic inflammation, though it may be seen in hyperlipidaemias. Patients under thirty years of age should be referred for vascular assessment in the absence of local ocular disease. The example of arcus juvenalis shown here occurred in a case of vernal disease. In this condition, arcus is not uncommonly seen deposited beyond the vascular pannus at the upper corneal pole. It slowly waxes and wanes according to the degree of limbal inflammation.

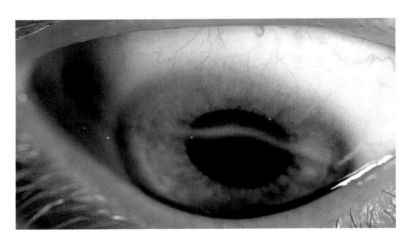

Fig. 6.28 Another deposition occurring in vernal disease is superficial corneal plaque, which complicates chronic epithelial loss and whose constituents are altered mucus, cellular debris and fibrin (Chapter 5). Other diseases in which corneal plaque is seen include herpes simplex, herpes zoster and dry eye syndromes. This example is a case of long-standing herpes simplex keratitis. The plaques, in band distribution, were intraepithelial and contained calcium and fibrin. They were easily removed by superficial keratectomy.

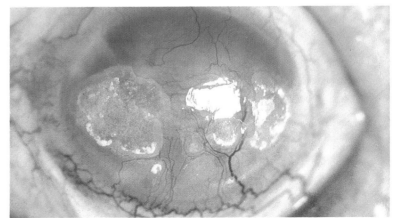

Fig. 6.29 Cornea verticillata (also known as vortex dystrophy) is a whorl-like deposition in the epithelium, usually centred in the lower third of the cornea. It occurs as a rare congenital condition unassociated with systemic disease. However, it is seen much more commonly in Fabry's disease or associated with treatment with phenothiazines, chloroquin, indomethacin and amiodarone. All patients receiving amiodarone in normal doses show cornea verticillata, which persists for many weeks or even months after the drug is discontinued; it does not usually cause symptoms or ocular damage. The example shown is of one such case.

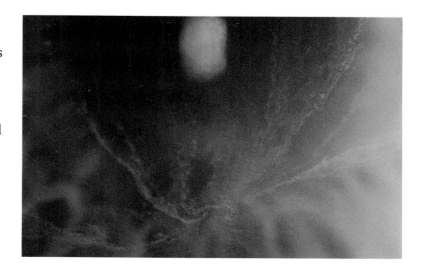

Cellular Infiltration

Fig. 6.30 Corneal ulceration is discussed in Chapter 4. A punctate keratitis is a common sign of a variety of insults to the corneal surface, including bacterial and viral infections, the products of allergic reactions, ultraviolet light and drug toxicity. The example here is of punctate epithelial erosion (the lesions becoming coalescent superiorly) in active vernal keratitis. The lesions are stained with rose bengal.

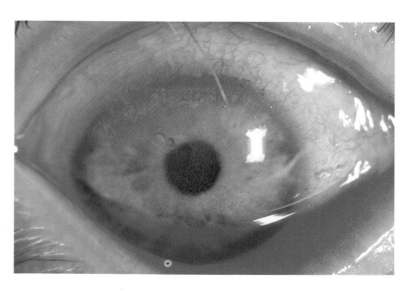

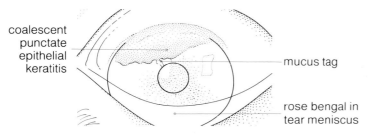

coalescent punctate epithelial keratitis

mucus tag

rose bengal in tear meniscus

Fig. 6.31 Thygeson's superficial punctate keratitis is a specific bilateral keratitis in which there is minimal conjunctival inflammation and minimal stromal involvement. The lesions are characteristically coarse and sparse. The condition, first described in 1950, runs a relapsing course over several years, occurs at any age, and has no systemic disease association. A viral aetiology has been postulated but no infective agent has been conclusively demonstrated. In this fairly severe example (left), the lesions, which are intraepithelial and frequently slightly raised, are stained with rose bengal. This photograph (right) of a group of Thygeson's keratitis lesions shows their typical appearance at high magnification.

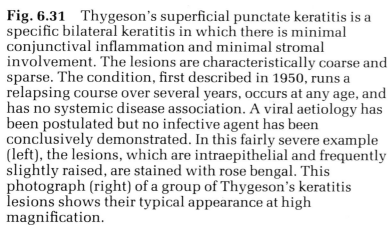

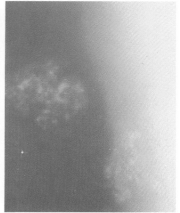

Fig. 6.32 This example of punctate subepithelial keratitis was photographed in a case of resolving adenovirus keratoconjunctivitis. The epithelial surface over the lesions was completely smooth. (Examples of corneal ulceration due to infection will be found in Chapter 4.)

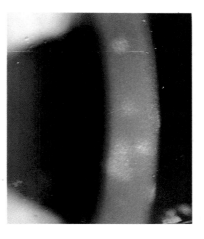

Fig. 6.33 Marginal ulceration of the corneal epithelium and stroma is typical of staphylococcal sensitivity and is usually accompanied by signs of blepharoconjunctivitis.

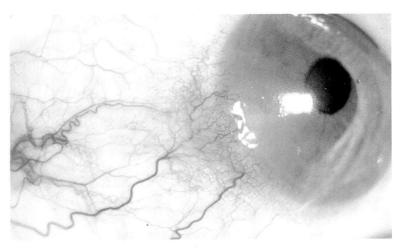

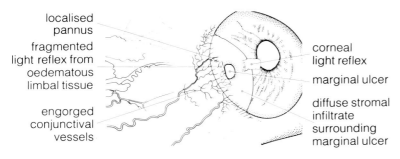

localised pannus
fragmented light reflex from oedematous limbal tissue
engorged conjunctival vessels
corneal light reflex
marginal ulcer
diffuse stromal infiltrate surrounding marginal ulcer

Fig. 6.34 Inflammation of the corneal stroma is known as interstitial keratitis. The majority of cases are due to congenital syphilis, and may be associated with other stigmata such as Hutchinson's teeth, deafness and depressed nasal bridge. The keratitis is seen in children and adolescents and is considered to be an immune reaction. It starts with corneal clouding which progresses to neovascularization ('salmon patch'). After some months the haze and the vessels resolve, leaving only light stromal scarring and 'ghost' vessels. The endothelium is damaged by the inflammation, so that corneal decompensation may supervene, usually many years later. This example of resolved interstitial keratitis shows stromal opacities and 'ghost' vessels. The patient shown on the right had interstitial keratitis, deafness and abnormal teeth. Other ocular signs of congenital syphilis are an iritis and a chorioretinitis in the active stages, and later cataract.

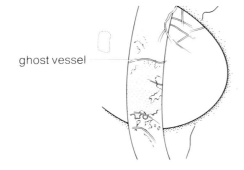

ghost vessel

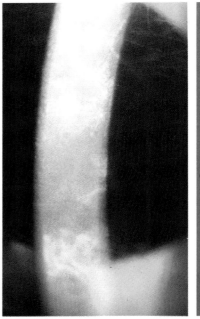

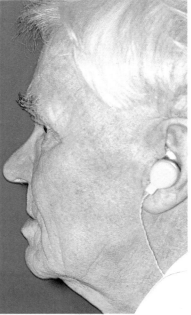

Vascularization

Fig. 6.35 Pannus, the extension of limbal blood vessels into the previously avascular corneal stroma, is always preceded by inflammation, whether infective, toxic, hypoxic or of another aetiology. Common examples are seen in trachoma and in contact lens-related corneal hypoxia or irritation. The example on the left occurred in a severe case of molluscum contagiosum keratoconjunctivitis. Another example is seen in the fluorescein angiograph on the right, which shows leakage of dye from the abnormal new vessels.

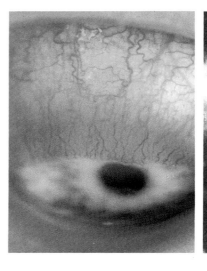

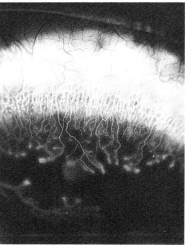

Fig. 6.36 Staphylococcal blepharokeratoconjunctivitis sometimes results in extensive neovascularization of the corneal stroma. This example occurred in a young girl who also had a chronic papillary conjunctivitis. The condition, which was bilateral, was at first wrongly diagnosed as vernal disease.

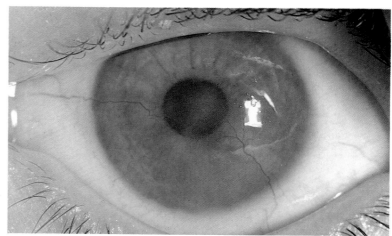

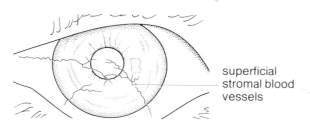

superficial
stromal blood
vessels

Fig. 6.37 Neovascularization following exposure to mustard gas is characterized by ampulliform dilations. This example shows, in addition, stromal scarring and plaque formation.

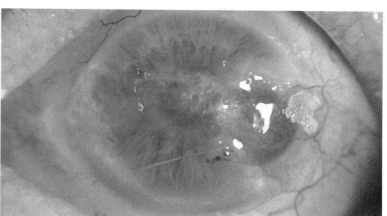

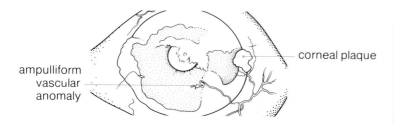

ampulliform
vascular
anomaly

corneal plaque

Fig. 6.38 The sequel of corneal neovascularization, as in this example following penetrating corneal injury, is often opacification due to fibrous tissue and lipid deposition. Uveal vessels have contributed to the picture.

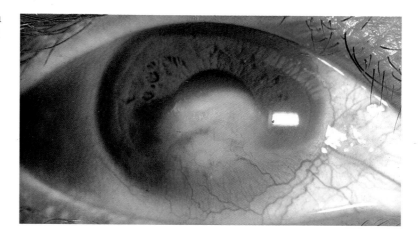

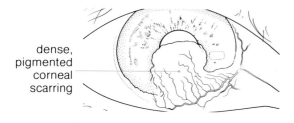

dense,
pigmented
corneal
scarring

Scarring

The cornea when injured can heal by avascular scarring, a process unique to this tissue. Immediately after injury, polymorphs appear in the stroma; the keratocytes surrounding the wound proliferate, come to resemble fibroblasts and migrate towards it. Macrophages reach the area a little later, scavenge cellular debris and transform into fibroblasts. Mast cells are also found in the healing corneal stroma.

The injured epithelium quickly regenerates and slides over the wound surfaces; no regeneration of the damaged endothelium is possible, but these cells also have some power to slide over denuded corneal stroma.

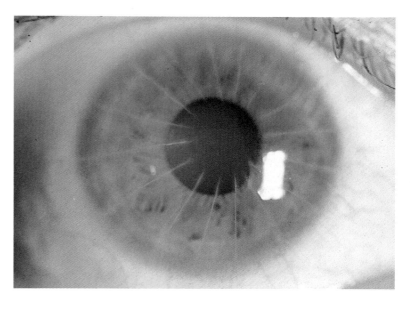

Fig. 6.39 Examples of avascular corneal healing are seen in simple sterile wounds, corneal grafts in avascular beds, and, in recent times, following refractive keratoplasty. The example shows avascular healing following radial keratotomy for the reduction of myopia.

DEGENERATIONS

Minor degenerative changes occurring in the cornea are so common that in many instances their presence provokes no comment. Such changes are always benign and offer no threat to vision. Rarely, either as a result of longstanding ocular disease or for reasons not understood, degenerative changes occur which may progress and cause blindness.

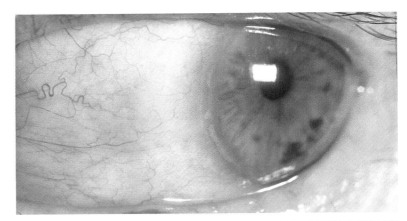

Fig. 6.40 Vogt's limbus girdle (top), is frequently seen in middle-aged and elderly people and occurs in the interpalpebral zone both nasally and temporally. There may or may not be a clear interval between it and the limbus. The opacity is at the level of Bowman's layer and is of no clinical significance, but must be differentiated from early deposits due to hypercalcaemia.

Arcus senilis (bottom) is seen in nearly all middle-aged and elderly people. There is a clear zone between it and the limbus. The deposition, which occurs at all levels of the stroma, is of lipid. This patient has had a cataract extraction, and has silk sutures in a corneo-scleral section.

These two conditions are considered to be age-related degenerations.

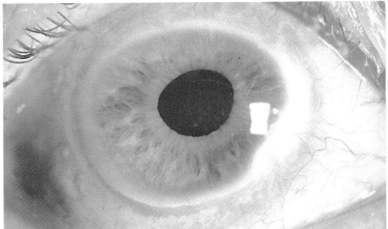

Fig. 6.41 Band keratopathy is seen in hypercalcaemia and as a sequel to almost any severe ocular disease. It is also frequently seen in phthisical eyes. Calcium is deposited in the superficial stroma, in Bowman's layer and in the deep epithelium. The distribution in the interpalpebral zone, in which a clear interval is found between the ends of the band and the limbus, is characteristic.

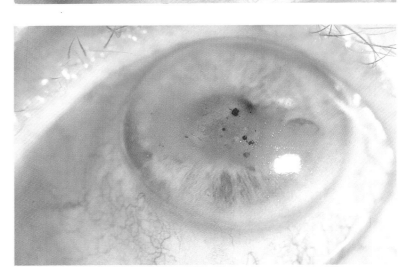

Fig. 6.42 Salzmann's nodular degeneration is rare but can follow a variety of corneal inflammations, especially phlyctenular disease and trachoma. The example shown followed vernal disease of many years' standing. The deposits, which form elevations of the corneal surface, are of hyaline material. They are associated with areas of destruction of Bowman's layer and of the subjacent stroma.

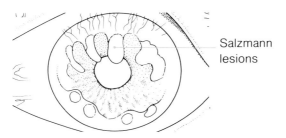

Salzmann lesions

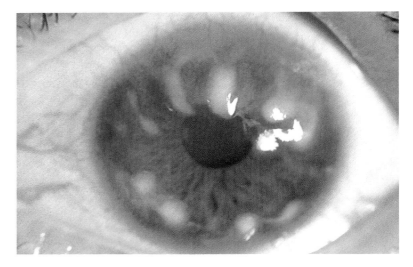

Fig. 6.43 Terrien's marginal degeneration is a rare bilateral condition which chiefly affects males in early middle age. Vascularizing peripheral infiltration is followed by stromal thinning and the appearance of a gutter just within the limbus. Before this is clinically obvious, keratometry may show a marked corneal astigmatism, which is responsible for the visual deterioration characteristic of this condition.

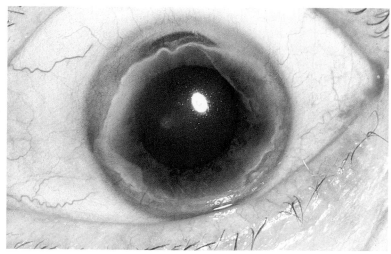

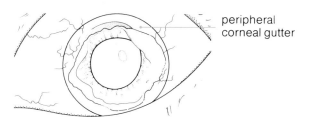

peripheral corneal gutter

Fig. 6.44 Mooren's ulcer has some of the hallmarks of an immunopathological disease. Immunoglobulin has been found bound to corneal epithelium, and autoantibodies to epithelium are sometimes present in the serum.

Peripheral infiltration proceeds to stromal melting which usually progresses around the entire cornea, typically leaving an overhanging corneal edge. The central zone is often spared, though frequently it is oedematous. The condition usually resolves when it has encompassed the corneal periphery, but in some cases it proceeds centrally destroying the entire cornea. Perforation is a frequent complication and may lead to loss of vision and of the eye.

An early progressive example (left) and a late quiescent one extending through 360° (right) are shown.

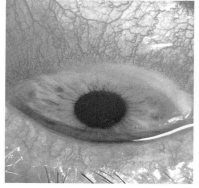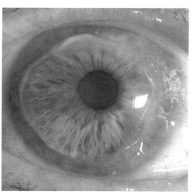

Fig. 6.45 Ichthyosis of the skin is sometimes accompanied by a degeneration of the deep corneal stroma. It is said that this is more likely to be seen in the X-linked condition. Dry scaly skin covers the whole body (the 'dirty neck syndrome') (bottom). Grey punctate and linear opacities are seen at the level of Descemet's membrane. These are seen in the slit-lamp photograph (top) and, in the same case, by specular microscopy (top right). The depth of the peculiar reflective layer is such that endothelial cells are seen in focus at the same time.

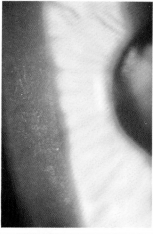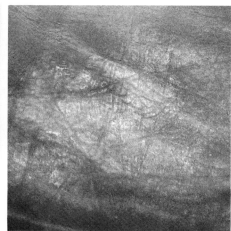

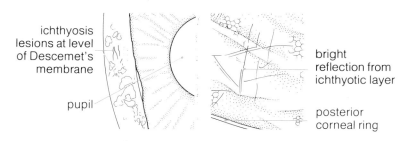

ichthyosis lesions at level of Descemet's membrane

pupil

bright reflection from ichthyotic layer

posterior corneal ring

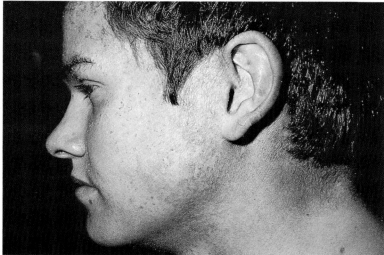

Fig. 6.46 The three conditions (essential iris atrophy, Chandler's syndrome, Cogan-Reese/iris naevus syndrome) known collectively as the iridocorneal endothelial (ICE) syndrome are described in Chapter 8. Only the specular microscopic appearances will be described here.

This example of Chandler's syndrome shows the different appearance of the endothelium in the normal and the affected eye. The abnormal cells are seen on the left. They are markedly enlarged and show dark, light, or dark and light inclusions. This appearance is similar to that sometimes seen in animal eyes in experimental adverse conditions. Histologically, the endothelial cells take on an epithelial appearance, and an abnormal collagenous layer is interposed between the cells and Descemet's membrane. The appearance of the unaffected endothelium of the fellow eye is seen on the right.

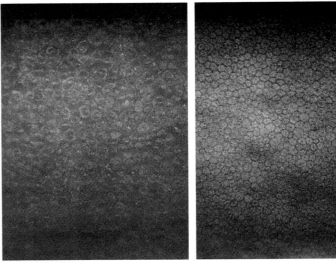

Fig. 6.47 In another case of Chandler's syndrome, geographical endothelial dysplasia is seen (left). The abnormal cells to the right appear to be compressing the normal cells to the left. There is a sharp border between the two cell populations. In the zone of retroillumination ('relief mode') in the upper part of the illustration, no features separate the two cell groups. This indicates that their posterior profiles are smooth and similar; in fact, normal.

Another example of Chandler's syndrome (right), shows relief mode only. The specular mode, which should appear in the lower half of the image, was obscured by stromal oedema. The relief mode shows a fine guttata-like irregularity of the posterior corneal profile, such as that described by Chandler himself.

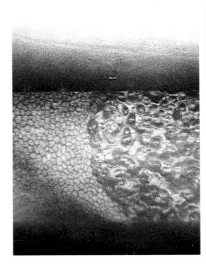

DYSTROPHIES
Corneal dystrophies can be classified by their anatomical site within the cornea and their mode of inheritance. Many dystrophies are extremely rare and only the more common examples seen in clinical practice are illustrated.

Dystrophies involving the epithelium and anterior stroma tend to present with recurrent epithelial erosions, while those involving the deeper cornea usually present with bilateral loss of visual acuity.

Anterior Membrane
Fig. 6.48 Non-traumatic recurrent corneal epithelial erosion is one manifestation of the map-dot-fingerprint epithelial dystrophy which is frequently referred to as Cogan's dystrophy. The condition may, in fact, be asymptomatic, and an autosomal dominant transmission can be demonstrated. Histologically the

epithelial basement membrane is found to be abnormal. The epithelial lesions are best observed by retro-illumination, either from the iris or from the fundus. The three examples here show microcysts (dots) (left), fingerprint lines (centre), and geographical (map) lesions (right).

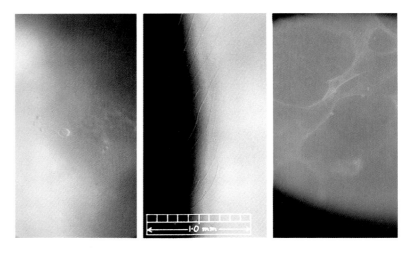

Fig. 6.49 Meesmann's dystrophy is an autosomal dominant hereditary condition in which cysts are present between the epithelial cells. These cysts are areas of cellular degeneration. The example shown is of an advanced case in which patches of subepithelial fibrosis were present in addition to the intraepithelial cysts.

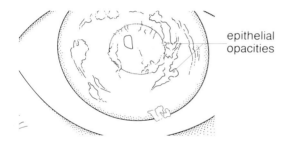

intra-epithelial microcysts

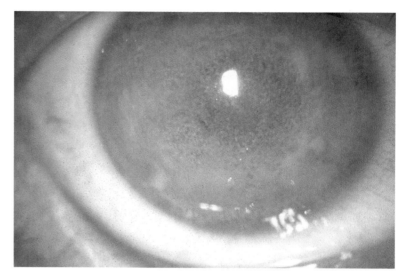

Fig. 6.50 The dystrophy of Reis and Bücklers is an autosomal dominant condition characterized by fragmentation of the collagen of Bowman's layer and recurrent epithelial erosion. Fine thread-like opacities are seen at the level of Bowman's layer. The primary cause of this dystrophy is not known.

epithelial opacities

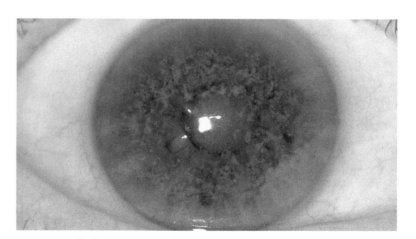

Stroma

Fig. 6.51 Granular dystrophy is an autosomal dominant condition which becomes manifest in the first decade of life, although vision may be unaffected until early middle age. Milky white spots occur in the superficial stroma, with a clear area adjacent to the limbus. The lesions are sharply delineated and may assume a variety of shapes. The deposits, which are seen histologically to occur at all levels in the stroma, consist of amorphous proteinaceous material which may derive from the keratocytes. The histological example is stained with Masson trichrome; the abnormal deposits are stained red.

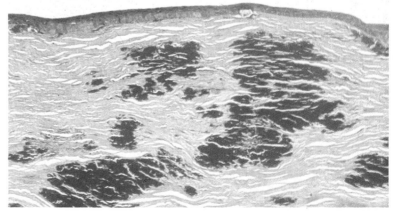

Fig. 6.52 Lattice dystrophy, an autosomal dominant condition, appears in the first decade of life. The cornea has a ground glass appearance owing to surface irregularity, and characteristic branching pipestem lesions are seen at all levels in the stroma. The periphery is spared. The condition has been described as a form of localized amyloidosis of the corneal stroma because of the characteristic histochemical staining features.

In the slit lamp view (left) the lesions are best seen in retro-illumination at the edges of the iris reflex. The two histological examples show the same solitary focus of deposition, corresponding to a cross-section of a lattice line. The specimen is stained with congo red, which when viewed through crossed polarizing filters shows the green dichroism and birefringence characteristic of amyloid.

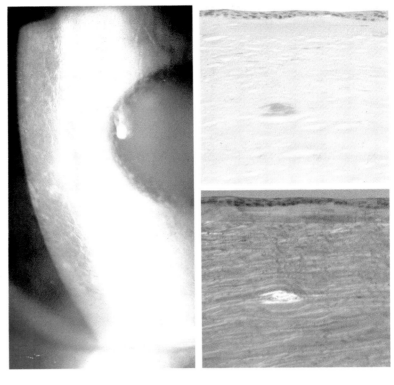

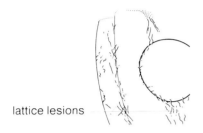

lattice lesions

Fig. 6.53 Macular dystrophy is transmitted as an autosomal recessive trait. It becomes evident in the first decade of life. The greyish-white spots seen in the corneal stroma tend to be superficial centrally and deep peripherally; the extreme periphery is not usually spared. Between the lesions, which are not clear-cut like those of granular dystrophy, the stroma is diffusely cloudy.

Recurrent epithelial erosion is sometimes a feature. The basic histological feature is the accumulation of an abnormal acid glycosaminoglycan in the keratocytes. The histological illustration shows deposits of blue-stained mucoid material beneath the epithelium and between the stromal lamellae (Alcian blue stain).

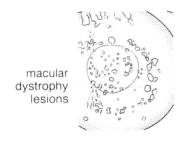

macular dystrophy lesions

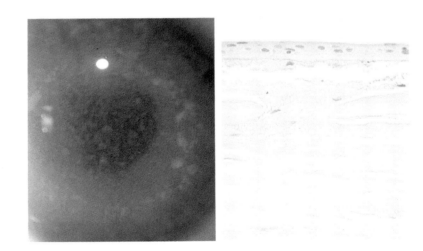

Posterior Membrane

Fig. 6.54 A few guttata (excrescences of Descemet's membrane) may be observed in healthy young corneas. Guttata become more numerous with advancing age. They represent local thickening of Descemet's membrane, caused by the deposition of new collagenous tissue by individual cells or groups of cells. Cornea guttata and Fuchs's dystrophy may represent different parts of the same disease spectrum.

The specular micrograph shows cornea guttata in a symptomless middle-aged woman. The guttata, whose positions are marked by the dark areas interrupting the endothelial mosaic, interrupt specular reflection and for this reason appear dark. Their apparent size is enhanced in the specular microscopical image.

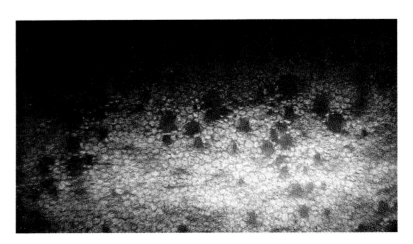

Fig. 6.55 In Fuchs's dystrophy the basic lesion lies in the guttata of the corneal endothelium. The condition is inherited as an autosomal dominant trait with variable expression, and tends to affect women more severely than men. It is bilateral but usually asymmetrical. The guttata are most numerous in the central cornea and spread peripherally as the condition advances. As the guttata increase in number, the density of the endothelial cell population decreases. Stromal oedema, at first only detectable by pachometry but later associated with posterior stromal striae (Fig. 6.9, left), eventually results in epithelial oedema and bullous keratopathy. Patients usually present in later life with poor acuity from corneal oedema.

Fine epithelial bullae are seen in the slit lamp view (top) at the edges of the area of iris retro-illumination. At a histological level (bottom), flat-topped excrescences of Descemet's membrane can be seen of which the endothelial lining is so atrophic as to be barely discernible (periodic acid-Schiff stain, ×100).

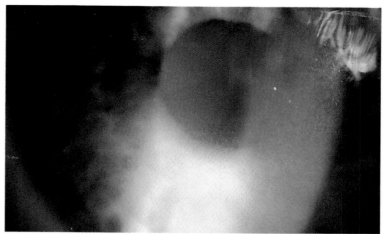

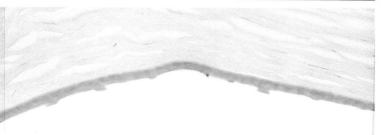

Fig. 6.56 The specular micrograph of a patient with Fuchs's dystrophy shows enlarged endothelial cells and guttata, and, in the relief mode zone in the upper third of the image, the characteristic profile of the guttata is clearly seen. In addition to these excrescences (which are dark above) there are some minute dimples (which are light above). The significance of the dimples is not known.

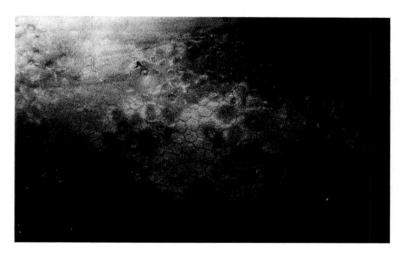

Fig. 6.57 Posterior polymorphous dystrophy is a common abnormality of the endothelium and Descemet's membrane which is usually symptomless. It is inherited as an autosomal dominant trait with variable expression. The basic defect is in the endothelial cells, which take on epithelial characteristics and fail to secrete a normal Descemet's membrane. Three distinct lesions are seen clinically. These are the vesicular, curvilinear and geographical types. The example on the left shows the first two types in fundus retro-illumination. The specular micrograph, from the same case, shows a vesicular lesion and a part of a curvilinear lesion. The endothelial cells are markedly enlarged (i.e. depleted in number) and there are guttata associated with the actual lesions.

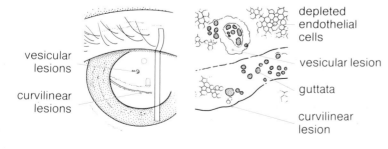

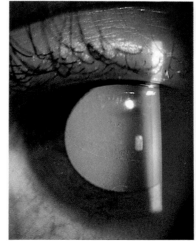

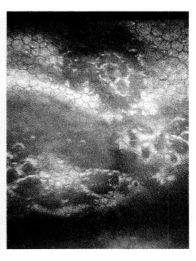

Fig. 6.58   This is an example of a more severe case of posterior polymorphous dystrophy, in its geographical form. A more generalized posterior corneal opacity is seen in the slit-lamp view. The specular micrograph shows profound endothelial cell depletion and a host of abnormal features. At present, it is difficult to relate these to the known histological findings.

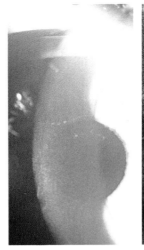
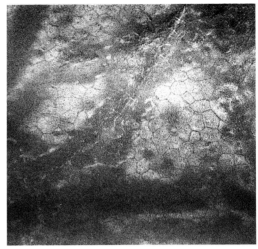

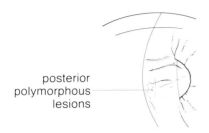

posterior polymorphous lesions

Ectasia

Keratoconus can be considered to be primarily a dystrophic condition because of its occasional hereditary transmission. There is an abnormality of corneal collagen which results in thinning and ectasia of the central cornea (not necessarily centred on the geometrical axis). The condition is associated with atopy, aniridia, mongolism and pigmentary retinopathy, among other conditions. It is always bilateral, though usually asymmetrical, and occurs more frequently in males than in females; it usually becomes manifest in the second decade of life when increasing astigmatism develops. Initially, vision can usually be improved by the use of rigid contact lenses but the later stages of the disease can only be treated by penetrating keratoplasty.

The base of the cone is usually surrounded by an iron-containing ring, named after Fleischer (Fig. 6.19). The clinical course is sometimes marked by episodes of acute stromal oedema (hydrops corneae, Fig. 6.11) when Descemet's membrane ruptures.

Fig. 6.59   This figure illustrates the characteristic conical profile of the cornea of a patient with keratoconus (top). If the condition is well marked, the lower lid margin is distorted when the patient looks down. This gross sign is known as Munson's sign (bottom).

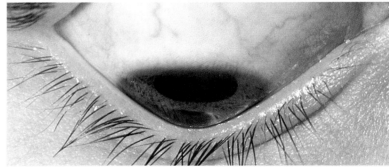

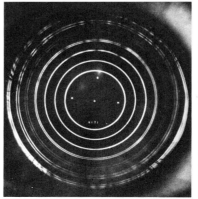

Fig. 6.60   Corneal pachometry, especially performed regionally, is likely to provide the earliest evidence of keratoconus. Apart from thinning, irregular corneal astigmatism is present in the early stages. This is often detectable with the keratometer but is more easily seen by photokeratoscopy. These two examples, reproduced at the same magnification, show a normal cornea (left) and a fairly advanced case of keratoconus (right). The keratoconic cornea is steep and irregular.

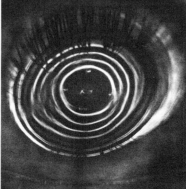

7. Primary Glaucoma

R. A. Hitchings

Introduction

Glaucoma is the name given to a group of ocular conditions which are characterized by a raised intraocular pressure. This is usually associated with typical changes to the optic disc and in the visual field, but identical changes can occasionally be seen in patients whose intraocular pressure has never been raised (low-tension glaucoma). It has been estimated that approximately three hundred people per one hundred thousand suffer from glaucoma: the prevalence increases with age and, in some studies, glaucoma has been shown to affect one percent of the population over forty years of age.

Glaucoma can be classified either as a primary defect or as an abnormality secondary to other ocular conditions such as uveitis or steroid therapy. Approximately ninety-five percent of glaucoma is of the primary form and is the subject of this chapter. Primary glaucoma may itself be divided into three major categories: open angle; closed angle and congenital. The approximate incidence of these three types is sixty-six percent, thirty-three percent and one percent respectively. Whatever the type of glaucoma or its aetiology, four basic facts concerning the eye are necessary in order to assess the disease and the amount of damage to the eye: these are the intraocular pressure, the appearance of the angle of anterior chamber, the state of the optic disc, and the visual field.

PATHOGENESIS OF NERVE DAMAGE

In spite of considerable interest and a great deal of investigation, the precise mechanism whereby raised intraocular pressure inflicts damage on the optic disc is still not fully understood.

Loss of nerve fibres could result either from vascular damage and anoxia due to raised intraocular pressure, or from mechanical factors acting on the axons as they bend through ninety degrees in order to leave the eye at the optic disc. Glaucomatous cupping of the disc reflects neuronal and possibly glial cell loss from the disc substance. It is not known, however, whether vascular damage occurs primary or secondary to these changes. The optic disc is supplied by the posterior ciliary arterioles and perfusion pressure in these vessels is a balance between ophthalmic artery pressure, intraocular pressure and venous pressure. A reduction in ophthalmic artery pressure or an increase in intraocular pressure or venous pressure will consequently lower the perfusion pressure in the disc tissue, but this relationship may not be entirely straightforward because of possible autoregulatory influences. Perfusion pressure can be measured directly in animals but human studies rely on indirect evidence such as fluorescein angiography, which has not provided consistent information in the case of glaucoma. Evidence that vascular mechanisms may be involved in the pathogenesis of glaucoma is supported by the not uncommon finding of splinter haemorrhages at the disc margin in some patients with glaucoma.

Different patients are able to withstand raised intraocular pressures to a greater or lesser degree; some eyes can sustain a pressure in the 20-30mm Hg for many years without signs of neuronal loss (ocular hypertension) whereas others will have rapidly progressive disease at much lower pressures. This anomaly, and the typical arcuate fibre field loss resulting from glaucoma, has drawn attention to the structural anatomy of the optic disc. Retinal glanglion cells seem able to withstand a raised intraocular pressure of the levels seen in chronic open angle glaucoma, but it has been postulated that the stretching of axons as they pass through a cupped optic disc interferes with axoplasmic transport and hence causes neuronal death. The bowing and posterior displacement of the lamina cribrosa in a cupped disc result in a longitudinal stretching and lateral posterior displacement of the retinal axons. The lamina cribrosa has a sieve-like structure of approximately six hundred pores through which pass the retinal nerve fibre bundles. There is some evidence that the lamina cribrosa may be weaker superiorly and interiorly, thereby accounting for the predilection of these regions to early nerve fibre loss (with corresponding visual field loss) in glaucoma.

AQUEOUS HUMOUR FORMATION AND INTRAOCULAR PRESSURE

Aqueous humour forms at a rate of about $2\ \mu$ litres/min, the fluid volume of the anterior chamber being completely changed over a period of approximately one hundred minutes. The aqueous is secreted by the ciliary epithelium in a combination of active and passive processes. About seventy percent of aqueous appears to be actively secreted and, in this respect, sodium transport appears to be crucial. The remaining thirty percent of the aqueous is derived via the mechanisms of ultrafiltration, diffusion, osmotic pressure, and ion gradients. It has been suggested that the outer non-pigmented epithelium of the ciliary body is responsible for the active transport of sodium ions, while the inner pigmented epithelium controls the penetration of substrates to this active site.

The aqueous humour provides oxygen and nutrients to the intraocular structures as well as removing their waste metabolites. When compared with plasma, aqueous humour contains higher concentrations of ascorbic acid and glutathione, and lower levels of proteins.

Normal intraocular pressure is determined by the balance between the production and removal of aqueous: it varies between individuals, and in each individual at different times of the day, such intra-individual variations forming the diurnal curve. Plasma cortisol levels seem to be important in determining the normal diurnal rhythm and it is probable that a number of hormonal influences affect intraocular pressure either directly (by production in the ciliary body), or indirectly (through some elusive central regulation mechanism) to keep both eyes at similar pressures.

While the ciliary epithelium does not have a neuronal supply, blood vessels in the ciliary body are well endowed with sympathetic fibres through which drugs such as neutral epinephrine, guanethidine, and timolol probably exert their influence.

Fig. 7.1 Bulk flow of aqueous through the eye begins in the region of the ciliary epithelium, flows past the equator of the lens through the posterior chamber and the pupil to reach the anterior chamber. Aqueous leaves the anterior chamber and enters the canal of Schlemm via the trabecular meshwork. It then passes into collector channels and aqueous veins, to reach the episcleral veins. Resistance to flow is greatest at the trabecular meshwork.

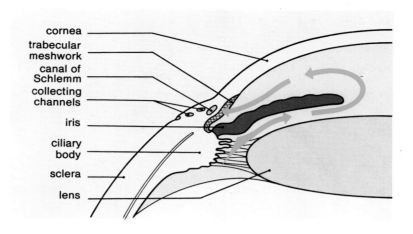

Fig. 7.2 In the normal eye, the average pressure drop between the posterior chamber and the episcleral vessels is about 8mm Hg. The pressure gradient provides the stimulus for aqueous flow and, as can be seen, most resistance to flow occurs in the trabecular meshwork. Whether this resistance is actually within the meshwork plates themselves or at the canal of Schlemm is not known. A small amount of aqueous also leaves the eye by draining into the suprachoroidal space and is known as the uveoscleral outflow.

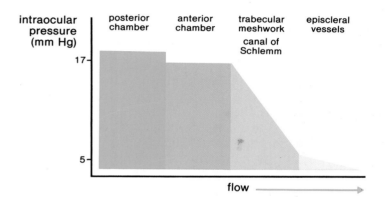

Fig. 7.3 Factors which cause an increase in intraocular pressure include an increase in ciliary epithelium production of aqueous, alterations in the blood-retinal barrier, increased resistance of the conventional outflow channels, formation of anterior synechiae, and an increase in the episcleral venous pressure. (WDT stands for "water drinking test").

Factors Causing Increased Intraocular Pressure

Inflow	Outflow
ciliary epithelium production increase	**"conventional" outflow channels (resistance increased)**
increased fluid load (WDT)	age
increased blood flow to ciliary body?	prostaglandin E1
beta-agonists	silting of trabecular meshwork with debris and pigment cells
altered blood retinal barrier	**other**
with ultrafiltration of fluid into vitreous and anterior chamber (e.g., panretinal photocoagulation for diabetics)	peripheral anterior synechiae
	raised episcleral venous pressure

Fig. 7.4 Factors which may cause a decrease in intraocular pressure include a decrease in aqueous production by the ciliary epithelium, structural alterations in the conventional outflow channels, and an increase in outflow via non-conventional routes. There is probably some sort of central mechanism for the regulation of intraocular pressure which accounts for the fact that pressure remain within a prescribed range and at similar levels in both eyes.

Factors that Lower Intraocular Pressure

Inflow	Outflow
ciliary epithelium production decrease	**"conventional" outflow channels**
reduced blood flow	pilocarpine
dehydration	alpha-agonists
beta-blockers	laser to trabecular meshwork
digitalis	
disease	**other**
age	sclerostomy
surgical destruction	rhegmatogenous retinal detachment
carbonic anhydrase inhibitors	**"non-conventional" outflow increased**
	ciliary effusion
	atropine?
	beta-agonists?

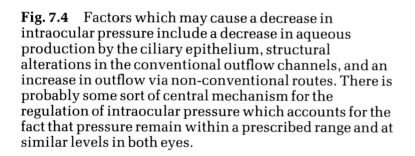

Fig. 7.5 In a population survey of two thousand males aged over forty years, the normal mean intraocular pressure was found to be circa 16.0mm Hg with a standard deviation of 2.5mm Hg. Two standard deviations from the mean are 21mm Hg. This is usually regarded as the (statistical) upper limit fror normal intraocular pressure.

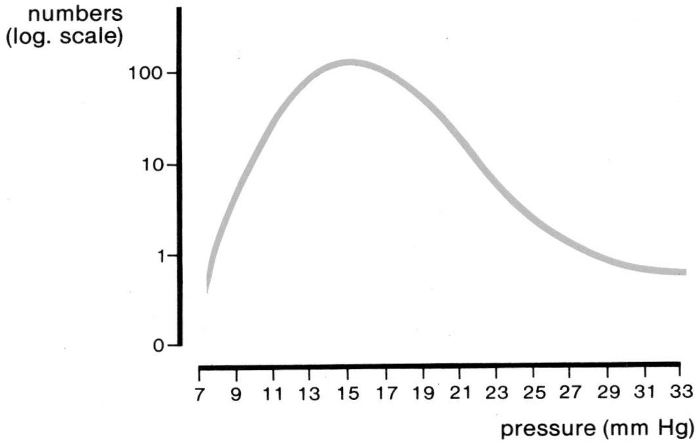

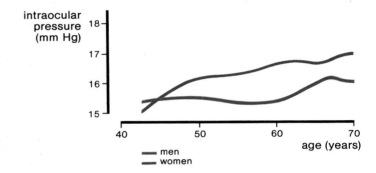

Fig. 7.6 The mean intraocular pressure for both men and women increases with age (and also with increases in systolic blood pressure). Mean pressures for women are consistently higher than those for men, for reasons not fully understood. In the eighth decade of life, two standard deviations above the mean intraocular pressure for women are greater than 24mm Hg, and this has obvious implications for the management of elderly patients.

Fig. 7.7 A diurnal variation in intraocular pressure levels is apparent in both the normal (lower) and glaucomatous (upper) eye and is possibly related to plasma cortisol levels. Peak pressure usually occurs around midday, and the lower pressures result during sleep. There is often a characteristic exaggeration of this diurnal variation in patients with chronic simple glaucoma.

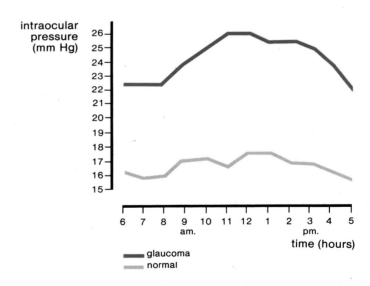

Fig. 7.8 In patients with chronic simple glaucoma, there may be a marked variation in intraocular pressure, well illustrated by the two hourly pressure readings of the right eye of this patient. (Note particularly the rapid pressure rise between 19.00 and 21.00 hours.) There is obviously a need for frequent and repeated intraocular pressure measurements in the management of such patients.

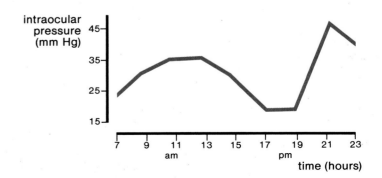

OPEN ANGLE GLAUCOMA

Open angle (chronic simple) glaucoma is insidious in its onset. Central visual acuity is not lost until the late stages of the disease; patients are not usually aware of loss of visual acuity and are normally diagnosed at routine eye examination either by the finding of elevated ocular pressures or by suggestive changes at the optic disc and in the visual field.

There are three situations in which chronic open angle glaucoma has a higher than normal incidence: these are a familial tendency, high myopia, and in association with central retinal vein occlusion.

The inheritance of open angle glaucoma has been investigated extensively and appears to be polygenic. First degree relatives of a patient (parents, siblings, and children) appear to have about a ten-fold increase in the risk of developing the disease. Relatives of a patient should therefore have regular ocular screening examinations, especially after the age of forty. The elevation of intraocular pressure by topical steroids may be mediated by similar mechanisms to those of inherited glaucoma and may enable susceptible individuals to be more easily identified.

The Angle of the Anterior Chamber

The external appearances of an eye with open angle glaucoma do not differ from those of an eye of similar age. Histological changes can be seen within the trabecular meshwork but these do not differ from those of a normal eye when viewed by light microscopy. Gonioscopy is an essential part of the investigation of open angle glaucoma.

Fig. 7.9   In the normal eye, aqueous flow passes through the fenestrated collagenous structure of the trabecular meshwork, which is situated within the angle of the anterior chamber at the junction of the iris and cornea, to reach the episcleral venous plexus. It is then taken up by the endothelium to drain through the canal of Schlemm and into collector channels (in the sclera) which empty into the conjunctival veins. This anastomosis can be seen as 'aqueous' veins in the conjunctiva.

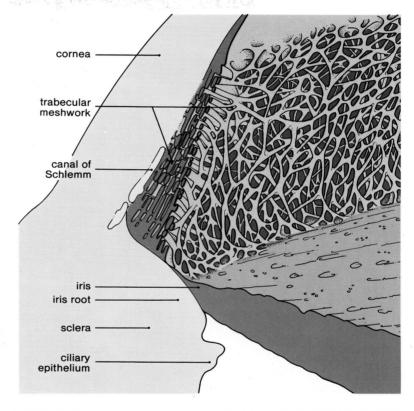

Fig. 7.10   In advanced glaucoma, light microscopy shows a flattening of the trabecular meshwork. There is evidence of both intertrabeculr sclerosis and pigment deposition. These appearances are not pathognomonic for glaucoma alone, however, since they may also be seen in old age.

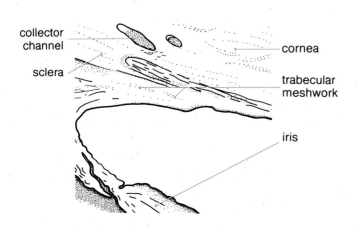

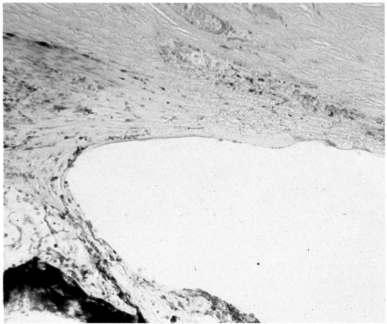

7.5

Fig. 7.11 This composite diagram correlates the gonioscopic and microscopic appearances of the angle of the anterior chamber when both 'open' and 'closed' (see Fig. 7.37) and shows the relationship of the trabecular meshwork to the surrounding cornea, ciliary body and canal of Schlemm.

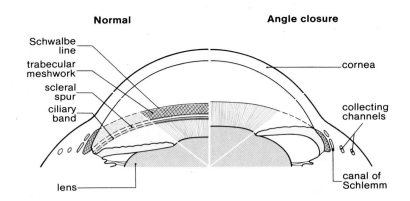

Fig. 7.12 A gonio-photograph of a normal angle shows the featureless appearance of the trabecular meshwork. Its location between the cornea and iris can only be determined by a faint line of pigment (top).

A gonio-photograph of the angle of the anterior chamber in a patient with pigmentary glaucoma shows extensive pigment deposition within the structure of the anterior chamber which is therefore more clearly visible. The trabecular meshwork extends from the anterior pigment deposition (uppermost in this picture) to the ciliary band: there is also a sharply defined mid-trabecular band of pigment (bottom).

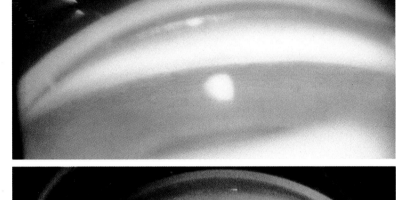

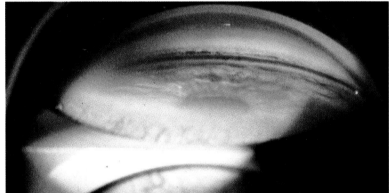

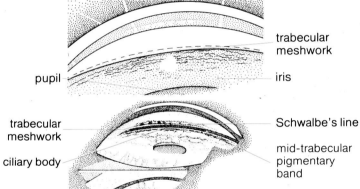

Fig. 7.13 Part of the outflow system from a normal human eye showing Schlemm's canal, the endothelial meshwork, and the corneoscleral meshwork compared with the region from a patient of similar age who was suffering from chronic simple glaucoma and whose intraocular pressure could not be controlled with miotics. It can be seen that Schlemm's canal is open, but the pathways for drainage through the endothelial meshwork and the intertrabecular spaces in the corneoscleral meshwork are obliterated.

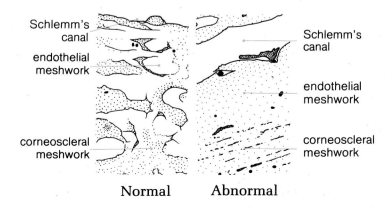

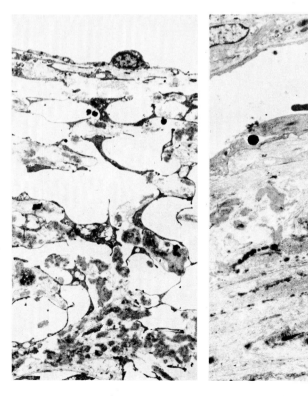

The Optic Disc in Open Angle Glaucoma

Observation of the optic disc is fundamental to the management of any patient with raised intraocular pressure and there is much to be said for serial photography to document disc changes. On examination, it is important to note the size and shape of the disc and particularly, the normal physiological cup. Signs suggestive of glaucoma are asymmetry of the cup size between the eyes, especially when this affects the vertical axis: enlargement of the cup along this axis is a firm indication of neuronal damage in the arcuate fibre areas. Eyes which have a ratio of cup to vertical disc diameter greater than 0.6 have a more significant association with glaucoma. The colour and shape of the neuronal rim should also be observed: notching, sectorial pallor, and grooves in the retinal nerve fibre layer all indicate damage. 'Baring' of the blood vessels results from nerve fibre loss, and the pathological hooking of the vessels under the scleral rim in advanced glaucoma indicates extensive neuronal damage. While these signs are obvious in established glaucoma, their early detection can demand ophthalmoscopy of the highest calibre. These changes can sometimes be seen more easily (and stereoscopically) by routine examination of the disc through the centre of the lens at gonioscopy.

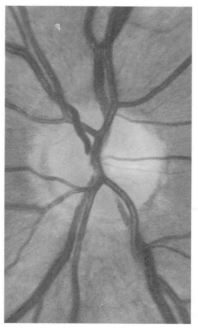
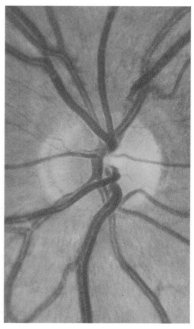

Fig. 7.14 Both optic discs of this patient are normal, being symmetrical in appearance with similar overall dimensions, shape, colour, contour, and having a clearly visible and full retinal nerve fibre layer.

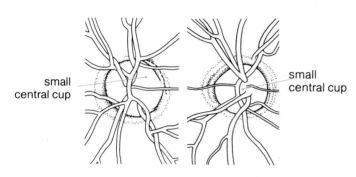

small central cup — small central cup

Fig. 7.15 The central dimple or physiological cup varies in size from patient to patient and is probably dependent on the overall dimensions of the scleral canal; eyes with large scleral canals tend to have larger discs and larger cups. In this patient, the optic discs and cups are large but normal. Signs suggestive of glaucoma are asymmetry of cup size between the eyes, a vertical diameter greater than the horizontal, vertical enlargement or notching of the rim, undermined sharp edges at the nasal and temporal borders, sectorial pallor or loss of the nerve layer, and a cup to disc ratio of greater than 0.6.

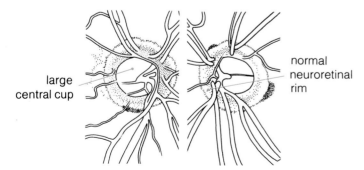

large central cup — normal neuroretinal rim

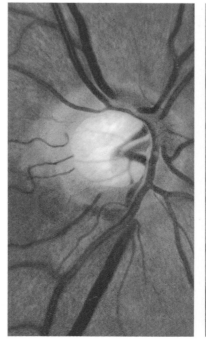
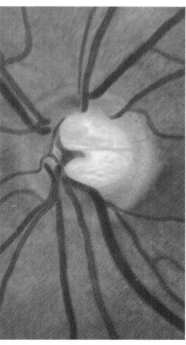

Fig. 7.16 While the right optic disc of this patient is normal, the left shows evidence of chronic simple glaucoma. A comparison of the two discs reveals that the optic cup in the left eye is vertically elongated; there is loss of the neuroretinal rim at the five o'clock position; and pallor of the rim in the inferotemporal quadrant. The retinal nerve fibre layer is less clearly visible adjacent to the deficient neuroretinal rim and the retina is darker in this position. Such a 'groove' in the nerve fibre layer is seen especially in low-tension glaucoma where the usual field defect may be localized and absolute.

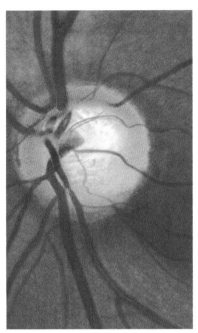
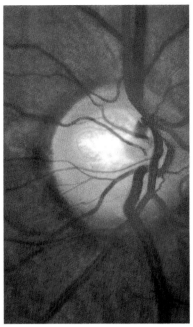

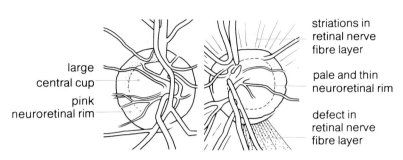

large central cup

pink neuroretinal rim

striations in retinal nerve fibre layer

pale and thin neuroretinal rim

defect in retinal nerve fibre layer

Fig. 7.17 This photograph shows a patient with advanced chronic simple glaucoma in the right eye. There is a marked enlargement of the cup, together with extreme attenuation of the neuroretainal rim and undermining of its margin. The cribriform plate is exposed and bowed posteriorly.

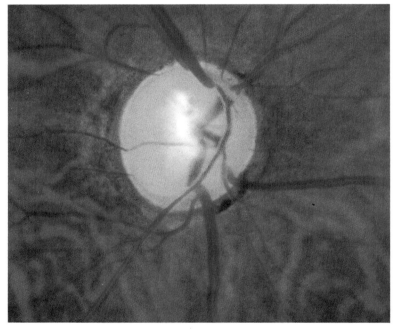

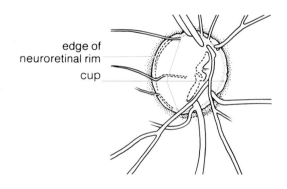

edge of neuroretinal rim

cup

Fig. 7.18 The inferotemporal quadrant of the neuroretinal rim is a typical site for splinter haemorrhages of the optic disc. Many of these occur in patients with low-tension glaucoma. Field defects are not usually associated with the initial haemorrhage but become more likely with recurrent haemorrahges.

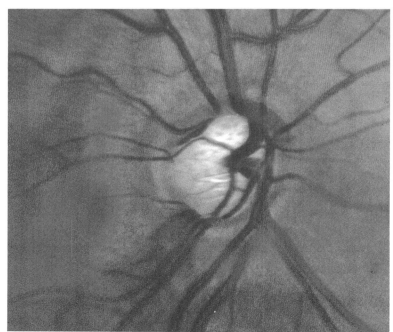

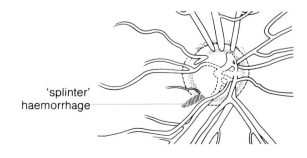

'splinter' haemorrhage

Visual Field Changes in Open Angle Glaucoma

Any visual field test is a subjective assessment of visual function and the results will depend on the patients' attention, mental ability, general health, and enthusiasm as much as the more physiological parameters. Size of visual field varies with the size and brightness of the target, its colour, and the contrast with the background illumination. There are now many sophisticated machines which successfully control these parameters but they all depend on the patients' cooperation and intelligence and their ability to maintain good fixation.

The visual field can be determined either by kinetic perimetry (where the patient sees a moving target) or static perimetry (where the patient detects the illumination of a stationary target in the field). Both of these techniques can be used in the investigation of glaucomatous eye disease where most of the early damage is found within the central twenty-five degrees of field from fixation – this is the area investigated by the Bjerrum screen. With any field technique, best results are obtained by a trained operator with good control of fixation and who ensures that the appropriate refractive correction is applied for the distance at which the test is performed. Pupillary size is important as a pupillary aperture of less than 2mm can constrict the peripheral field and result in test artifacts. A useful visual field can be elicited from virtually any patient and it should always be remembered that good confrontation fields give valuable information with a bed-bound or ill patient.

The normal visual field extends from about fifty degrees from fixation nasally to about ninety degrees on the temporal side. The blind spot lies approximately fifteen degrees from fixation in the temporal field and is about five degrees in diameter.

Fig. 7.19 Size and variation in sensitivity of the normal visual field. The upper chart is graph plotting sensitivity on the vertical axis against distance from the fovea on the horizontal axis. The cut for this horizontal axis has been made at 45° and 225°. It will be noticed that sensitivity is greatest at the fovea and falls of rapidly towards the periphery.

The lower diagram superimposes this graph on the two-dimensional peripheral field obtained with the I-4 target on the Goldmann perimeter. This provides an appreciation of the visual field as a three-dimensional structure (Traquair's 'Island of vision in the sea of darkness').

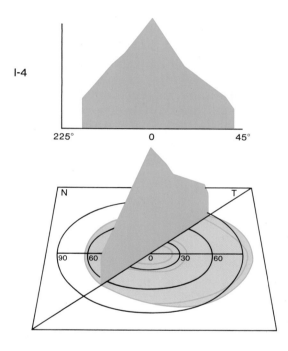

Fig. 7.20 This graph shows a static field cut at 225° and 45° in a patient with a lower arcuate scotoma that abuts onto fixation. Two isopters (I-2, I-4) have been drawn. The smaller target (I-2) is only perceived on one small part of the central field of vision in this patient's eye. The whole of the visual field seen with the I-4 target has also been drawn and it will be noted that the cross-hatched area of greatest sensitivity must therefore be seen at both the I-2 and the I-4 targets.

The lower diagram shows a superimposition of the graph upon the two isopter kinetic Goldmann field. This emphasizes the three-dimensional aspect of the field of vision with severe visual field loss in the lower arcuate system.

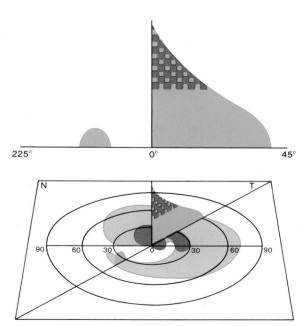

Pathology of the Optic Disc

Fig. 7.21 Low power photomicrograph of a normal optic disc in longitudinal section. There is a considerable increase in the transverse diameter of the optic nerve after it has passed through the scleral canal. This increase is due to myelination of the axons (see Optic Disc, Chapter 17).

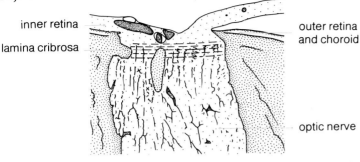

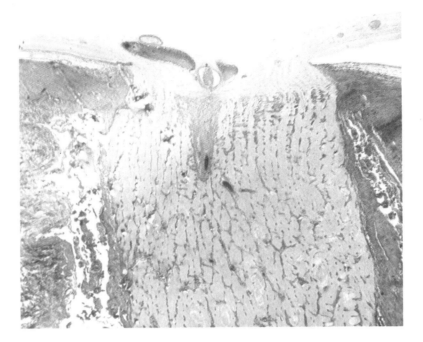

Fig. 7.22 The pathophysiological changes are well demonstrated by these histological sections from an eye with glaucoma secondary to a melanoma of the iris. The patient had an arcuate defect in the upper half of the visual field. The optic disc shows loss of neurons inferiorly (the retina is artifactually detached) (top), and myelin stains show the corresponding degeneration within the optic nerve (bottom).

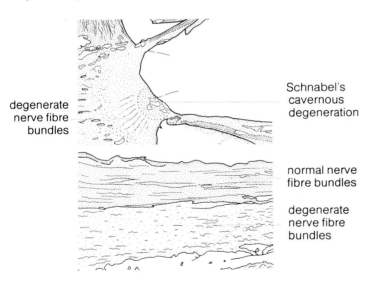

Fig. 7.23 Histological appearance of the optic nerve in an eye with advanced glaucoma. Note the marked backward displacement and stretching of the lamina cribrosa associated with loss and undercutting of the neuroretinal rim.

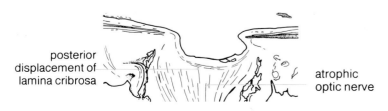

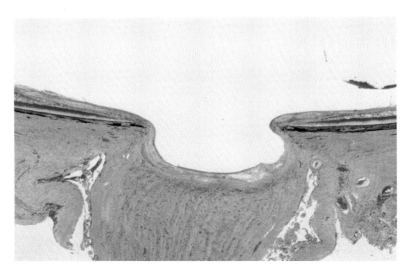

Pigmentary Glaucoma and Pseudoexfoliative Glaucoma

Both pigmentary glaucoma and pseudoexfoliative glaucoma follow obstruction and obliteration of the intra-trabecular spaces by pigment or pseudoexfoliative basement membrane material. They may be considered either as variants of primary open angle glaucoma, or as a specific form of secondary open angle glaucoma.

Pigmentary glaucoma is an uncommon form of primary open angle glaucoma which characteristically affects both eyes of young myopic males. In a typical case, there is loss of pigment epithelium from the posterior iris surface, and corresponding transillumination of the peripheral iris. It

has been suggested that the pigment loss and dispersion is caused by friction between the iris pigment epithelium and the zonular fibres of the lens. Pigment is released and deposited onto the corneal endothelium (Krukenberg's spindle), the trabecular meshwork (usually seen as a dense, dark trabecular band involving the mid-portion of the meshwork (cf. Fig. 7.12)), and the anterior iris surface. Such pigment deposition is known as the pigment dispersion syndrome, not all cases of which develop pigmentary glaucoma.

Fig. 7.24 In this patient, extensive pigment deposition is seen on the anterior surface of the iris, rather like dust particles, lying in the wrinkles formed by iris contraction.

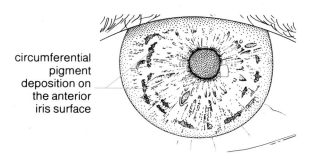

circumferential pigment deposition on the anterior iris surface

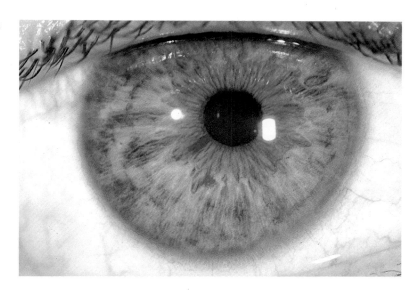

Fig. 7.25 Retro-illumination of the iris of the same patient shows multiple slit-like defects in the pigment epithelium of the peripheral iris.

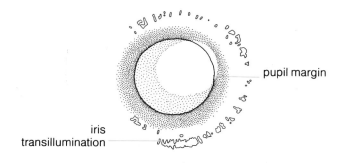

pupil margin

iris transillumination

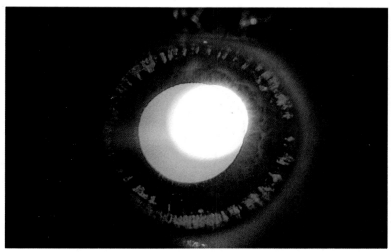

Fig. 7.26 Krukenberg's spindle is the term given to pigment deposition on the posterior corneal surface. The pigment is usually deposited in a vertical band.

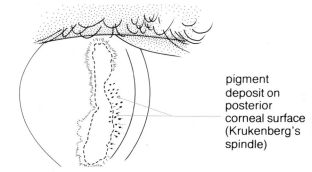

pigment deposit on posterior corneal surface (Krukenberg's spindle)

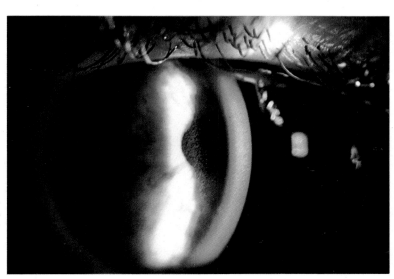

Fig. 7.27 Histological section shows that the angle has extensive pigment accumulation. Pigment granules lie freely between the trabecular plates, or phagocytosed within the endothelium, or in macrophages obliterating the normal pattern and obstructing the outflow. The gonioscopic appearances of the angle in pigmentary glaucoma have been demonstrated earlier (cf. Fig. 7.12).

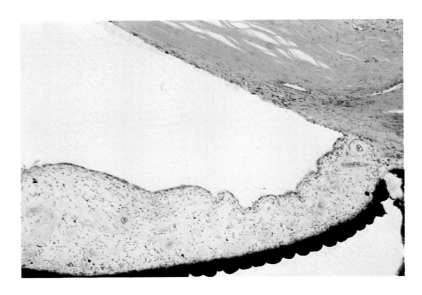

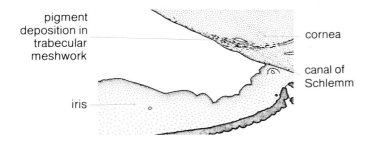

Fig. 7.28 Electron micrograph of the angle demonstrates a characteristic accumulation of the intertrabecular and intracellular pigment granules which is not seen in age-matched normal eyes.

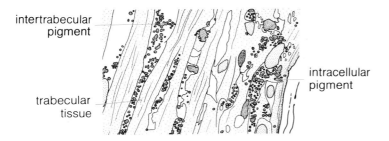

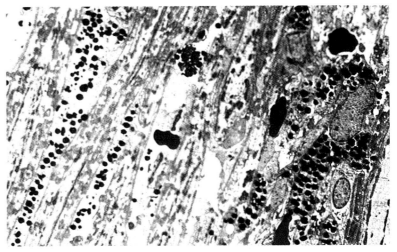

Pseudoexfoliation Glaucoma

Pseudoexfoliation glaucoma is caused by the production of an abnormal fibrillar material which obstructs the trabecular meshwork. It is seen more often in the elderly and appears to be genetically determined, being much more common in people of Scandinavian descent. The source of the abnormal material is unknown but it is supposed to originate from the basement membrane of the ciliary epithelium, the zonule, and possibly the lens capsule, and is seen as dandruff-like flakes on the pupillary margin following pupillary dilatation. It may also be evident on the anterior lens surface in the periphery and pupillary area, but the midzone is often swept free by physiological alteration in pupil size. This material becomes detached and deposited in the trabecular meshwork where it obstructs outflow. Characteristically, pseudoexfoliation glaucoma is relatively resistant to medical therapy. The condition is usually bilateral although one eye may be more severely affected. Gonioscopy shows an open angle with more pigmentation in the meshwork than would normally be expected.

Fig. 7.29 The clinical diagnosis of pseudoexfoliation glaucoma is made by observing the dandruff-like apperance of the fibrillar material on the pupillary margin.

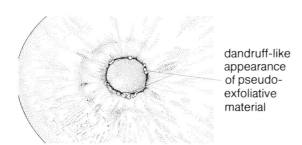

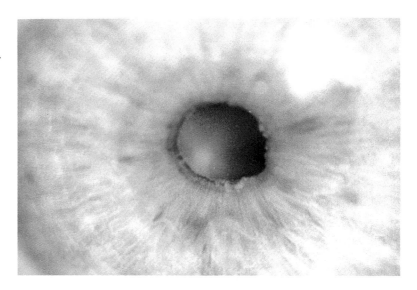

Fig. 7.30 Following mydriasis, the appearance of the abnormal material can be seen on the anterior lens surface. The peripheral lens and pupillary zone are coated with a white flaking membrane but the mid-zone has been swept free by the pupillary movements over the lens surface.

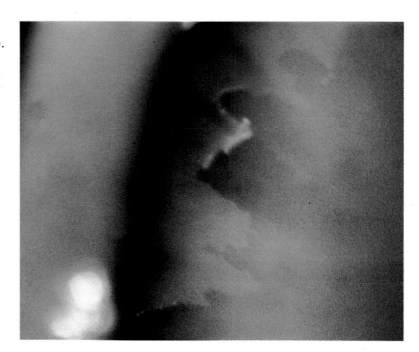

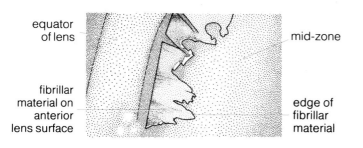

Fig. 7.31 Histology of an eye with pseudoexfoliation glaucoma shows the presence of the P.A.S. positive eosinophilic material on the anterior surface of the lens and the posterior surface of the iris.

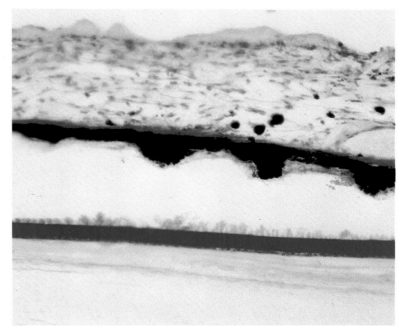

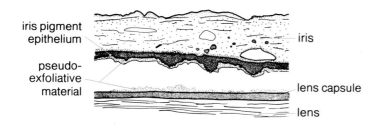

Fig. 7.32 The angle is open in pseudoexfoliation glaucoma but the meshwork contains more pigment than is usual together with the fibrillar material caught up in the meshwork. This material can also be found around the conjunctival vessels.

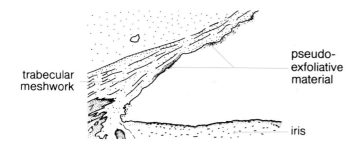

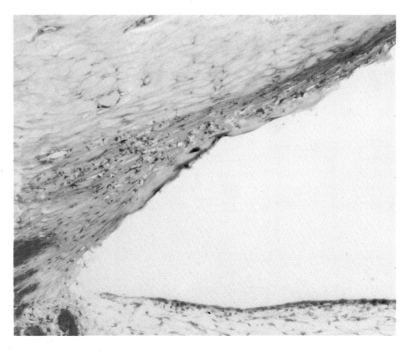

7.13

Fig. 7.33 Electron microscopy reveals the characteristic fibrillar material in the intertrabecular spaces.

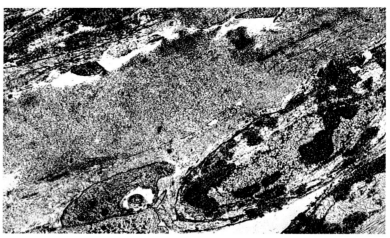

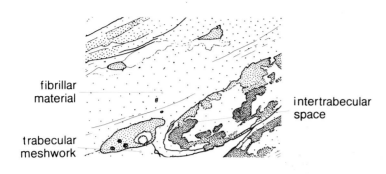

Treatment of Chronic and Simple Glaucoma
Fig. 7.34 Commonly prescribed drugs that are responsible for an increase in aqueous outflow.

Drugs which Increase Aqueous Outflow

a. 'conventional' outflow – trabecular meshwork

parasympathomimetics	– pilocarpine
	– carbachol
anticholinesterases	– physostigmine
	– echothiphate iodide
	– demarcarium bromide
alpha-adrenergic agonists	– epinephrine

b. 'unconventional' outflow routes – uveoscleral and others

| beta-adrenergic agonists | – salbutamol |
| | – epinephrine |

Fig. 7.35 Commonly prescribed drugs that cause a decrease in aqueous production.

Drugs that Decrease Aqueous Production

carbonic anhydrase inhibitors	– acetazolamide
	– dichlorophenamide
cardiac glycosides	– ouabain, digoxin
beta-adrenergic blockers	– timolol
	– propranolol
	– etc

Fig. 7.36 Following a trabeculectomy, this patient has developed a limbal filtration bleb on to his eye at the twelve o'clock position. Notice the relatively avascular central area and surrounding blood vessels indicating a successfully established bleb. Vascularization of the whole bleb is usually a sign of failure with loss of control of intraocular pressure.

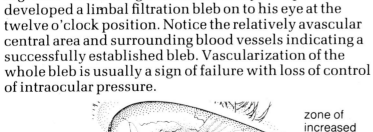

drainage bleb (avascular zone)

zone of increased vascularity around drainage bleb

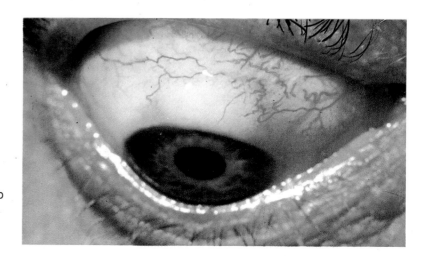

ACUTE CLOSED ANGLE GLAUCOMA

Acute closed angle glaucoma presents a dramatically different clinical picture to that of chronic open angle glaucoma. It usually occurs in the elderly and is not often seen in patients under fifty-years years of age. It is much more common in females and, like open angle glaucoma, there is a familial tendency to develop the condition.

Pathophysiology

The basic mechanism for the development of acute angle closure is an increase in the relative pupil block brought about by contact of the pupillary margin with the anterior lens surface through semimydriasis. This produces a pressure difference between the posterior and anterior chamber with a consequent bowing forwards of the iris periphery to occlude the angle of the anterior chamber, if the chamber is shallow. The important factor, therefore, is the depth of the anterior chamber, which tends to be shallower in hypermetropia and in the elderly because of increasing lens size. It is unusual for angle closure to occur if the anterior chamber depth is greater than 2.5mm.

Angle closure in a predisposed eye can be precipitated by a variety of mechanisms, such as pupillary dilatation in conditions of dim illumination or with emotion. A wide variety of provocative tests have been devised to diagnose susceptible eyes: none of these have been entirely satisfactory. Seating a patient in the dark or lying prone will lead to significant pressure rises in some patients: similarly mydriasis can initiate an attack, and an acute attack is sometimes initiated following pupillary dilatation for funduscopy. Miotics cause a forward movement of the lens-iris diaphragm and will also produce angle closure on rare occasions. A combination of phenylephrine and pilocarpine drops produces angle closure in sixty percent of eyes with acute angle closure in the fellow eye and can be used as a provocative test.

Angle closure may be transient, acute or chronic. Many patients with acute glaucoma will have a history of prodromal attacks over the previous weeks or months. At these times, they may notice blurring of acuity due to corneal oedema, ocular pain and aching or redness of the eye. The more observant may notice rainbow coloured haloes around a polyspectromatic white light source. This effect is due to the prismatic effects of the corneal oedema. An established attack of acute glaucoma produces loss of visual acuity with intense pain and redness of the eye and is an ocular emergency; irreversible visual loss will occur within hours unless the pressure is relieved.

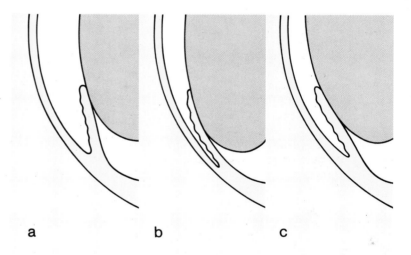

Fig. 7.37 Anterior chamber profile in normal (a) and angle closure glaucoma before (b) and after (c) peripheral iridectomy. Note the marked difference in the axial anterior chamber depth between the normal and the angle closure glaucoma eye. Note also that in the angle closure glaucoma eye, the axial anterior chamber depth does not alter following peripheral iridectomy. However, there is a marked change in the configuration of the iris periphery following iridectomy, with deepening of the periphery and widening of the anterior chamber angle. Widening of the angle follows removal of pupil block and allows peripheral iridectomy to confer protection against the subsequent development of acute angle closure glaucoma.

Clinical Features

Fig. 7.38 During an attack of acute angle closure glaucoma, the rise in intraocular pressure is associated with infarction of the iris tissue with an associated inflammatory response. There is decompensation of the corneal epithelium with the development of corneal oedema, which can be seen by the irregular scatter of light from the corneal surface.

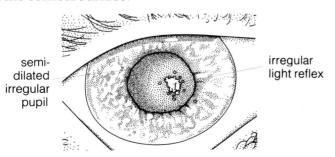

semi-dilated irregular pupil

irregular light reflex

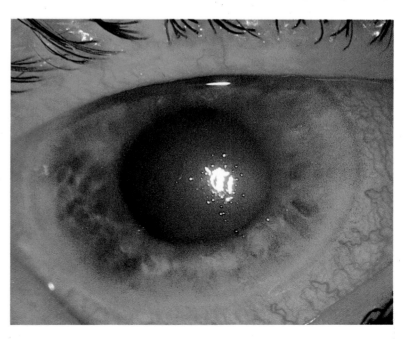

Fig. 7.39 During an acute attack of angle closure glaucoma the pupil is semi-dilated. The oval appearance results from the infarction of iris tissue and sectorial atrophy with spiralling of the stromal fibres.

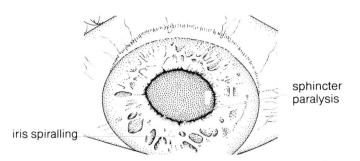

iris spiralling

sphincter paralysis

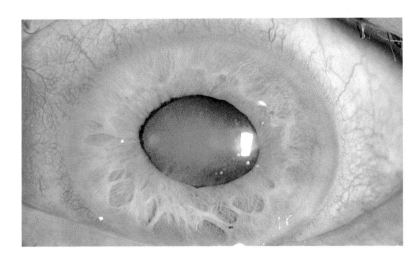

Fig. 7.40 Following an acute attack of angle closure glaucoma the iris atrophy remains with changes which are suggestive of previously raised pressure. This patient has had a peripheral iridectomy: the pupil is irregular following sectorial infarction of the iris with spiralling of the remaining viable fibres and depigmentation secondary to atrophy of the iris stroma.

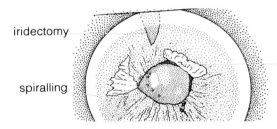

iridectomy

spiralling

depigmentation secondary to iris atrophy

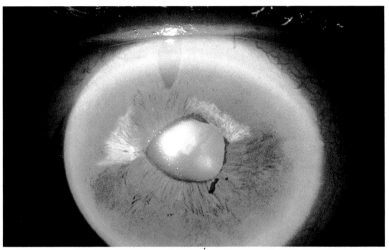

Fig. 7.41 Raised intraocular pressure may cause necrosis of the anterior lens epithelium. Following an acute attack of angle closure glaucoma, diffuse small white opacities (glaucomfleken) are often seen in the anterior subcapsular region. Within time, these opacities are covered by new normal lens cortex and appear to sink into the growing lens. (cf. The Lens – Chapter 11).

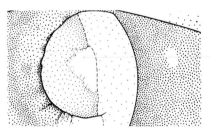

descrete granular glaucomfleken

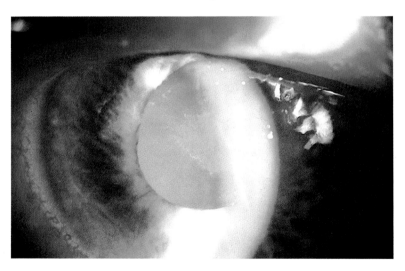

Fig. 7.42 A high-power view of glaucomfleken shows its irregular amoeboid shape. Glaucomfleken are virtually diagnostic of a previous attack of acute angle closure glaucoma.

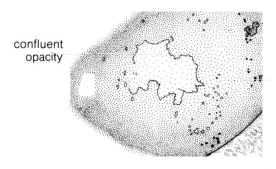

confluent opacity

scattered subcapsular opacities

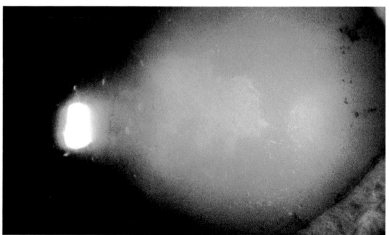

Fig. 7.43 A histological section of lens with glaucomfleken shows foci of epithelial cell necrosis.

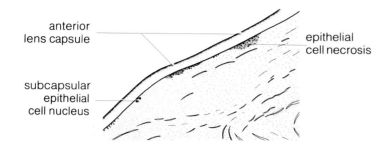

Fig. 7.44 An oedematous corneal epithelium can be cleared with glycerol drops for scrutiny of the optic disc and this should be an essential part of the clinical assessement following an attack of acute glaucoma. This rather hazy view shows a normal optic disc with no previous signs of raised intraocular pressure or neuronal damage. After the raised intraocular pressure had been controlled, further examination revealed that the optic disc was slightly swollen, the central cup smaller, and a haemorrhage had developed inferiorly. These changes are probabaly due to venous engorgement and hypotony.

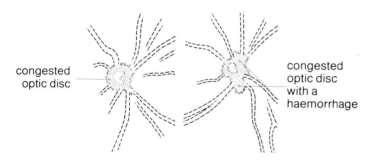

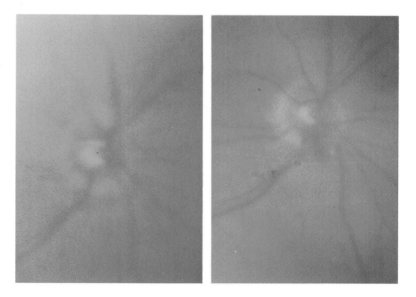

Fig. 45 Six months later, the optic disc shown in Fig. 7.44 appears normal. This is usually the case, providing the attack of raised intraocular pressure has been rapidly controlled, otherwise sufficient damage occurs producing visible optic atrophy and corresponding field loss. This type of optic atrophy is different in appearance from chronic simple glaucoma in that it looks like a flat optic neuropathy and is not associated with pathological enlargement of the optic cup.

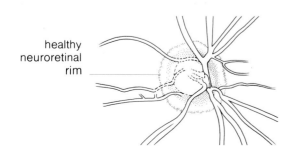

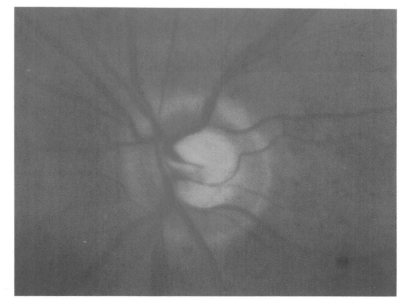

Fig. 7.46 Six months after an attack of acute glaucoma. Comparison of the normal left and involved right eye of another patient demonstrates the 'flat' optic atrophy which indicates neuronal and vascular damage to the disc, from the acute attack, with associated field loss. Should ocular pressure continue to remain elevated following the acute attack, the optic nerve takes on an appearance indistinguishable from that seen in chronic simple glaucoma.

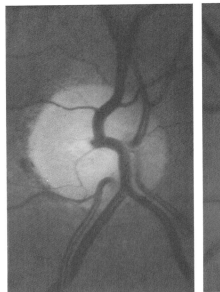

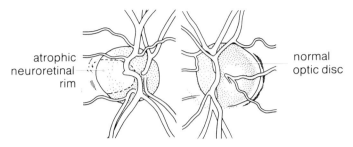

atrophic neuroretinal rim

normal optic disc

Treatment

Fig. 7.47 The treatment of acute angle closure glaucoma lies in reducing the intraocular pressure with acetazolamide and/or hyperosmotic agents such as oral glycerol. Pilocarpine may re-open the angle and re-establish outflow, but a peripheral iridectomy must be performed to relieve pupil block and prevent further attacks. A prophylactic iridectomy is always performed on the fellow eye as the risk of this eye developing an acute glaucomatous attack over a ten year follow-up period is about seventy percent. Slit image photography of the anterior chamber illustrates the deepening of the periphery of the anterior chamber and the consequent increase in angle width following peripheral iridectomy.

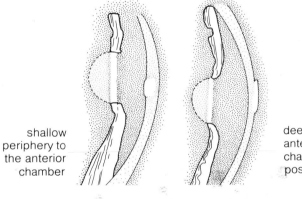

shallow periphery to the anterior chamber

deeper anterior chamber post-iridectomy

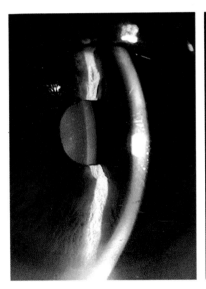

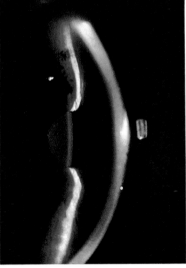

Fig. 7.48 Gonioscopic appearance of the angle of the anterior chamber before iridectomy in an eye with acute angle closure glaucoma. There is only a 'chink' of angle visible. (Same eye as illustrated in Fig. 7.47.)

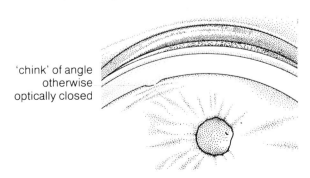

'chink' of angle otherwise optically closed

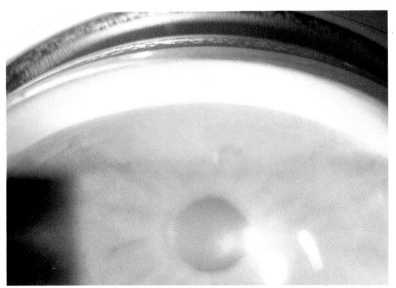

Fig. 7.49 Gonioscopic appearance of the angle of the anterior chamber in the same eye as Fig. 7.48 following iridectomy. The structures within the angle are much more apparent after the angle has been widened.

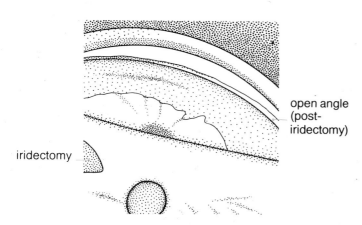

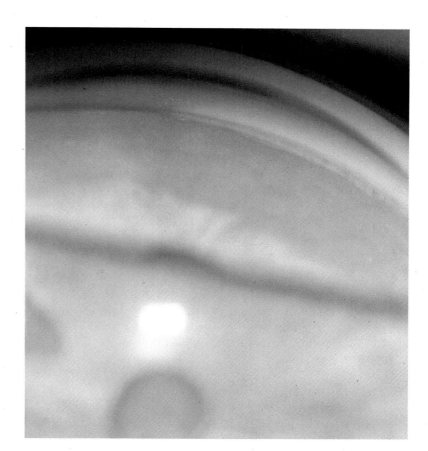

Fig. 7.50 This gonioscopic view demonstrates, post-iridectomy, the appearance of peripheral anterior synechiae following a prolonged attack of acute angle closure glaucoma. The long-term prognosis for intraocular pressure control depends upon the extent of trabecular meshwork damage from ischaemia or the formation of synechiae during the acute attack. It must also be remembered that open angle glaucoma can coexist in an eye with closed angle glaucoma.

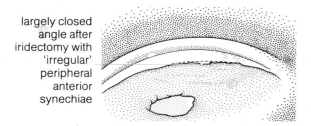

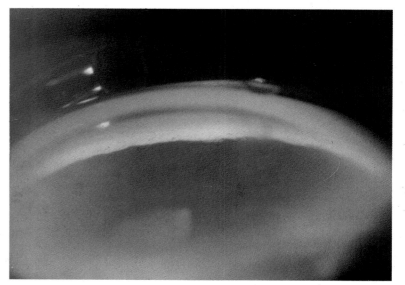

Fig. 7.51 Histological section demonstrates adhesions between the anterior iris surface and the trabecular meshwork which have occluded the angle in this eye with chronic closed angle glaucoma.

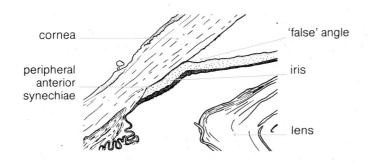

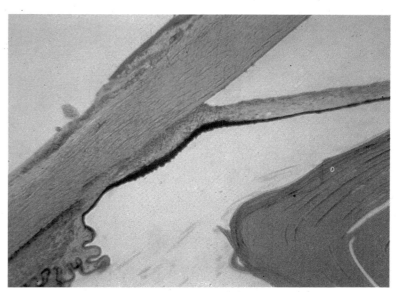

CONGENITAL GLAUCOMA

Congenital glaucoma is rare and usually considered to be the result of maldevelopment of the angle of the anterior chamber with obstruction by a mesodermal membrane. Juvenile and adult eyes react differently to raised intraocular pressure: the sclera of the younger eye is able to stretch more and high intraocular pressures can produce ocular enlargement known as buphthalmos (ox eye).

The hallmarks of buphthalmos are corneal oedema, increased corneal diameter (reflecting overall ocular enlargement), and splits in Descemet's membrane. The intraocular pressure is usually raised, but the extent of this depends on how far the scleral expansion has compensated for the increased pressure. It is important to assess the optic disc, but the typical changes associated with raised intraocular pressure may not be seen until scleral expansion stops at about three years of age.

Buphthalmos may occur as an isolated defect in one or both eyes, and is more common in male infants, or as part of a syndrome with associated defects. Goniotomy forms the basis of initial treatment, supplemented by topical therapy or filtering surgery at a later stage. Buphthalmic eyes have large refractive errors, and accurate refraction and control of amblyopia play an important part in the visual outcome. The measurement of intraocular pressure in babies is difficult and usually has to be performed as part of an examination under anaesthesia, which will have its own effects upon intraocular pressure.

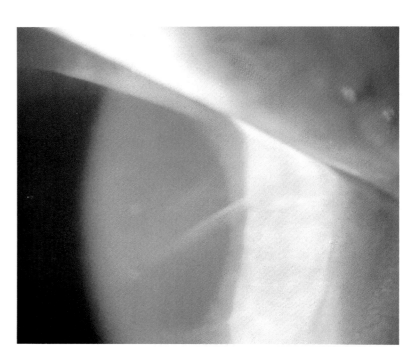

Fig. 7.52 This small boy has corneal enlargement and oedema typical of buphthalmos. Lacrimation and intense photophobia are the usual presenting symptoms. The child will often bury its head in a pillow to avoid the light from a window.

Fig. 7.53 A high-power view of the cornea demonstrates the appearance of 'splits' in Descemet's membrane, which are probably caused by tearing of the membrane associated with an enlargement of the cornea, and are characteristic of buphthalmos. The splits usually develop during the first eighteen months following birth and are a sign of uncontrolled intraocular pressure. They are sometimes associated with transient stromal oedema which invariably subsides with the reconstitution of Descemet's membrane. Similar 'splits' can be seen in the normal eye from birth trauma.

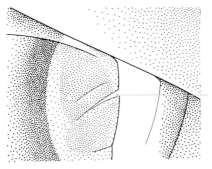

'split' in Descemet's membrane

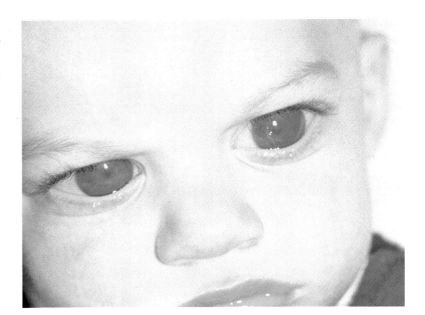

Fig. 7.54 Examination of the eye in buphthalmos may reveal maldevelopment of the iris, abnormal adhesions between the peripheral iris and the trabecular meshwork associated with maldevelopment of the angle, and, in some instances, anomalies of the cornea and lens. This histological section of the angle demonstrates the abnormal anterior insertion of the iris together with poorly formed trabecular structures.

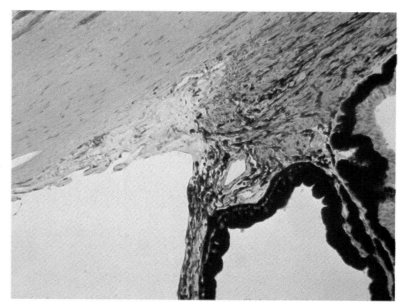

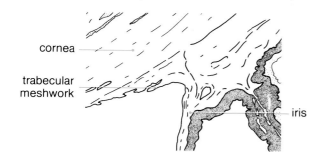

Anterior Chamber Cleavage Syndromes

This is a group of conditions in which there is a developmental defect of the angle of the anterior chamber. Posterior embryotoxon is the term given to an unusual prominence of Schwalbe's line which rotates outwards to be seen as a white band inside the limbus. It occurs in about fifteen percent of normal people and is considered to be hyperplasia of mesodermal tissue on the posterior cornea near the angle and is of no pathological significance.

Fig. 7.55 Drawing of the anterior chamber angle in a patient with Axenfeld's anomaly. Notice the characteristic multiple abnormal iris processes extending anteriorly to be inserted into Schwalbe's line.

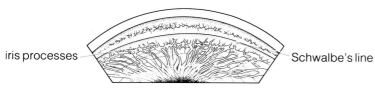

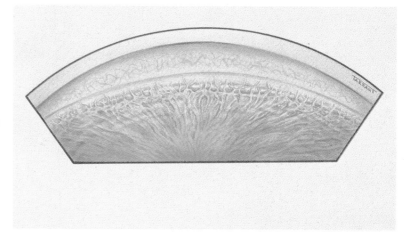

Fig. 7.56 Rieger's syndrome is associated with iris hypoplasia, posterior embryotoxon, and angle anomalies. Glaucoma may present in infancy but is more usual in the first to third decades of life. Associated defects include maxillary hypoplasia and dental deformities. Notice the grossly abnormal iris with hypoplasia of the anterior iris surface and distortion of the pupil (iris pigment epithelium may be seen at the temporal margin).

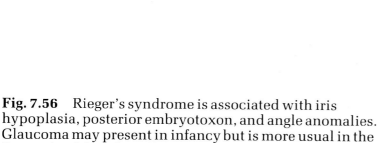

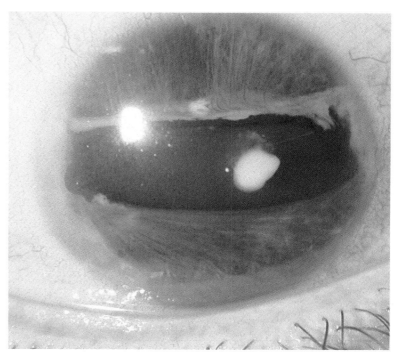

7.21

Fig. 7.57 Abnormal dentition in a patient with Reiger's syndrome.

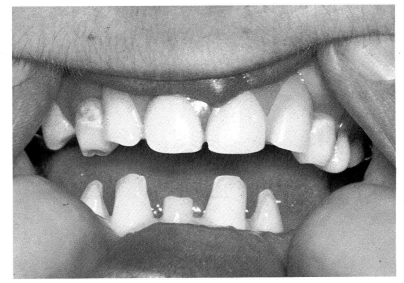

Fig. 7.58 Aniridia is a bilateral developmental anomaly in which the iris extends forwards from the iris root as a small cuff, which may form peripheral synechiae and occlude the angle. Early glaucoma occurs in about thirty percent of patients. Cases may occur sporadically or be inherited as an autosomal dominant trait associated with deletion of the shorter arm of chromosome eleven. Sporadic cases show a high incidence of nephroblastoma and all affected infants should be screened with intravenous pyelography (see Uveal Tract, Chapter 9).

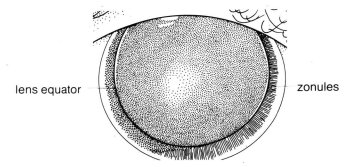

lens equator — zonules

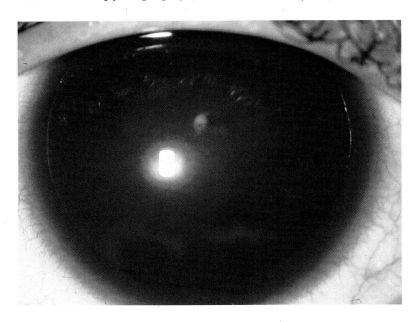

Fig. 7.59 Gonio-photograph of an eye with aniridia demonstrates the formation of peripheral anterior synechiae which lead to the development of intractible glaucoma. Other ocular anomalies found with aniridia include hyperplastic optic discs and maculae, and corneal scarring and cataracts.

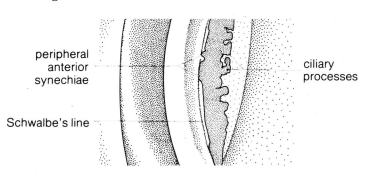

peripheral anterior synechiae — ciliary processes

Schwalbe's line

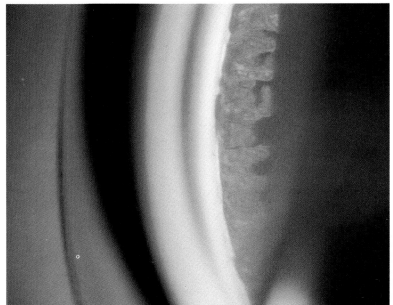

8. Secondary Glaucoma

R. A. Hitchings

Introduction

Glaucoma arising secondary to other ocular conditions is responsible for only a small proportion of all cases of glaucoma, but frequently produces the most difficult problems in diagnosis and management.

Secondary glaucoma arises from two basic mechanisms: either by the development of adhesions (peripheral anterior synechiae) between the iris root and the inner surface of the trabecular meshwork, which occlude the angle (secondary closed angle glaucoma); or by direct damage to the trabecular meshwork, which increases resistance to aqueous flow (secondary open angle glaucoma).

Secondary closed angle glaucoma may occur with or without pupil block. The presence of pupil block or a flat anterior chamber for more than a few days will, in itself, produce peripheral anterior synechiae and this can be responsible for the failure of the peripheral iridectomy to control raised intraocular pressure following an attack of acute closed angle glaucoma.

SECONDARY ANGLE CLOSURE GLAUCOMA WITH PUPIL BLOCK

Inflammation of the anterior segment, producing posterior synechiae and occluding the pupillary aperture, is the most common cause of secondary angle closure glaucoma with pupil block, although the use of topical steroids and mydriatics have been effective in reducing its incidence. Pupil block may develop insiduously in low grade iritis following gradual occlusion of the pupil, or suddenly, with acute iritis. Treatment is aimed at preventing occlusion of the pupil but for the established condition, laser or surgical iridectomy with topical steroids and mydriatics is used to break the pupillary block. Peripheral iridectomy is performed routinely during most intraocular surgery in order to avoid pupil block post-operatively.

Pupil block glaucoma may also be produced by changes in the lens. Intumescence will cause rapid shallowing of the anterior chamber facilitating angle closure and producing signs and symptoms similar to those seen with acute angle closure glaucoma. It is important to remember that the elderly patient may be unaware of visual loss in the cataractous eye prior to the onset of glaucoma – his attention will be drawn to the increasing blindness, however, by the pain resulting from the glaucoma. Glaucoma due to lens intumescence must be distinguished from phacolytic glaucoma (cf Fig. 8.39) but the treatment for both conditions is lens extraction.

Both subluxation or anterior dislocation of the lens may create pupil block and also produce secondary angle closure glaucoma. These conditions can occur either spontaneously in patients with congenital dislocation of the lens, or secondary to traumatic subluxation of the lens. Incipient glaucoma may be identified prior to the attack by unilateral shallowing of the anterior chamber together with phakodenesis. Unilateral shallowing of the anterior chamber is an important sign which enables a differentiation to be made between secondary pupil block and primary angle closure glaucoma.

Pupil block in aphakia may occur acutely, with inflammation, in the first few days following cataract extraction or, less commonly, a number of days or weeks following the operation. The diagnosis is suggested by a combination of raised intraocular pressure and peripheral shallowing of the anterior chamber. Aphakic pupil block usually occurs with a flat anterior chamber and little prolapse of the vitreous gel, but it may present with apparently normal axial anterior chamber depth, the pupil and chamber itself being filled with prolapsed vitreous. The established condition can be treated either by laser iridotomy or by division of the posterior synechiae from the anterior hyaloid face, both manoeuvres recreating communication between the posterior and anterior chambers of the eye and allowing spontaneous retroplacement of the iris periphery.

Angle closure glaucoma typically occurs in hypermetropic eyes which have a small anterior segment. There are a number of other ocular conditions where the eye itself is considerably smaller than normal, such as congenital high hypermetropia (nanophthalmos), mucopolysaccharidoses and congenital syphilis. Angle closure glaucoma occurs frequently in these rare conditions and often responds poorly to open surgical iridectomy because the anterior chamber fails to reform, the eye developing malignant glaucoma. Laser iridotomy is now, therefore, the preferred method of treatment to break the pupil block in these unusual cases.

Glaucoma may persist after an attack of pupil block from any cause if a large proportion of the angle has been closed by the peripheral anterior synechiae which have formed during the attack.

Pupil Block with Uveitis

Fig. 8.1 Examination of the anterior segment of a patient with chronic uveitis reveals a diffuse scattering of light from aqueous flare and clearly visible circumferential peripheral anterior synechiae. The pupil is occluded by posterior synechiae and iris bombé is present.

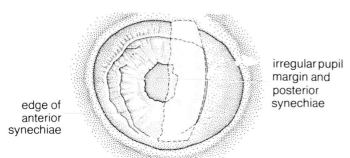

edge of anterior synechiae

irregular pupil margin and posterior synechiae

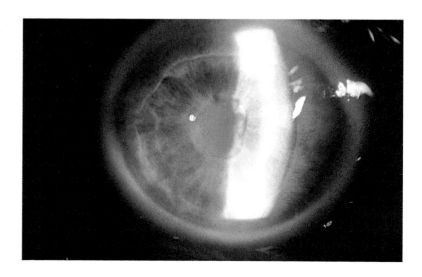

Fig. 8.2 These two slit-image photographs show the same patient before and after treatment. Peripheral anterior synechiae are again evident as is pupil block and iris bombé. A deepening of the peripheral part of the anterior chamber is clearly evident following laser iridotomy (right).

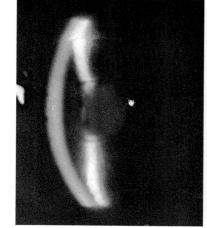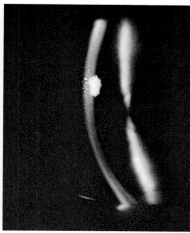

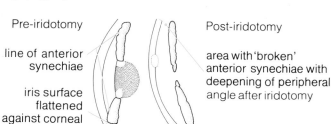

Pre-iridotomy — line of anterior synechiae — iris surface flattened against corneal endothelium

Post-iridotomy — area with 'broken' anterior synechiae with deepening of peripheral angle after iridotomy

Pupil Block with Lens Changes

Fig. 8.3 Acute angle closure glaucoma secondary to intumescence of the lens. In addition to the cataractous lens, this eye has other features which are suggestive of a raised intraocular pressure: these include a hazy corneal reflex from corneal oedema, a semi-dilated and fixed pupil from iris infarction, and circumlimbal injection signifying inflammation.

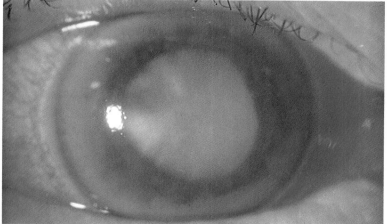

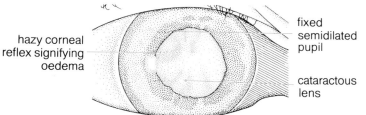

hazy corneal reflex signifying oedema — fixed semidilated pupil — cataractous lens

Fig. 8.4 A slit image photograph of the same patient shows evidence of corneal oedema and opacification of the lens. Notice the shallowing of the anterior chamber. Some uveitis may be present because of ischaemia and this must be differentiated from the large accumulations of lens material and macrophages seen in the deep anterior chamber of phacolytic glaucoma.

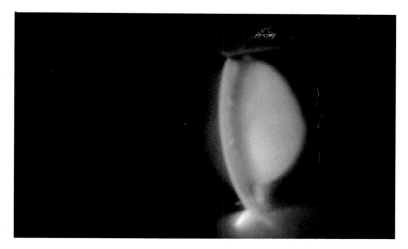

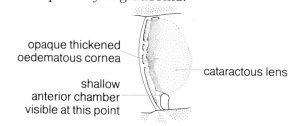

opaque thickened oedematous cornea — cataractous lens — shallow anterior chamber visible at this point

Fig. 8.5 Slit image photography of the left and right eye of this patient demonstrates a subluxed lens in the left eye. The anterior chamber is shallow and further examination shows that the anterior lens surface is closer to the posterior corneal surface inferiorly than superiorly.

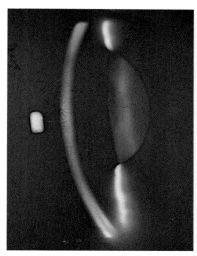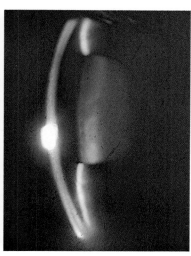

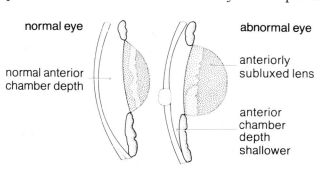

normal eye — normal anterior chamber depth

abnormal eye — anteriorly subluxed lens — anterior chamber depth shallower

Fig. 8.6 Occasionally, pupillary dilatation during routine funduscopy allows a subluxated lens to swing into the pupil and block communication between the posterior and anterior chambers. Careful positioning of the patient and miotics usually allow the lens to be repositioned safely. Notice the nuclear cataract in this lens.

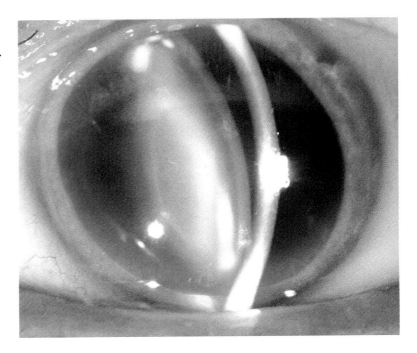

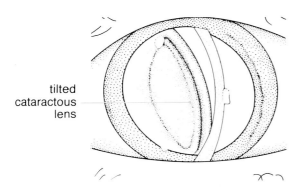

tilted
cataractous
lens

Fig. 8.7 Pupil block glaucoma following traumatic anterior dislocation of the cataractous lens.

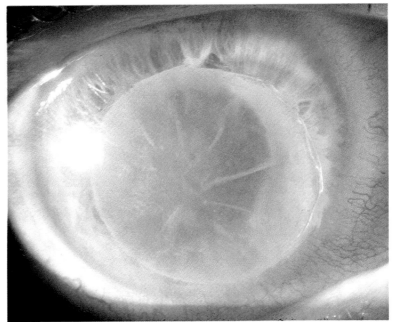

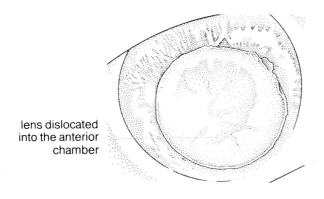

lens dislocated
into the anterior
chamber

Fig. 8.8 The slit image view of the same patient as Fig. 8.7 demonstrates how the pupil is totally blocked by the lens while the iris is convex anteriorly.

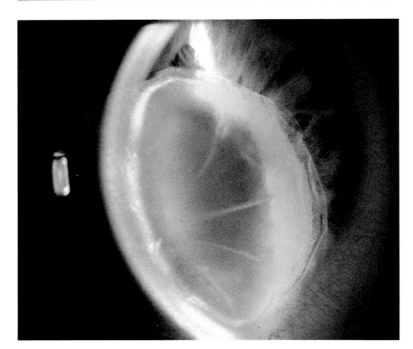

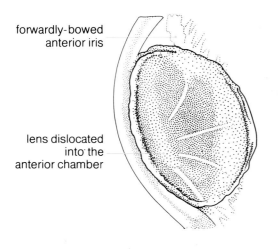

forwardly-bowed
anterior iris

lens dislocated
into the
anterior chamber

Pupil Block in Aphakia

Pupil block in aphakia may occur acutely (with inflammation) in the first few days following cataract extraction or, less commonly, a number of days or weeks following an operation. The diagnosis of post-operative aphakic pupil block is usually suggested by a combination of raised intraocular pressure and shallowing of the anterior chamber.

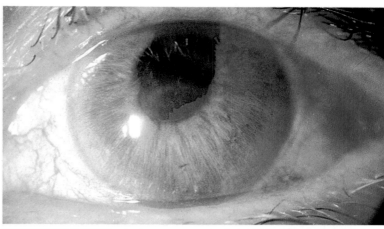

Fig. 8.9   In this patient, adherence of the pigment epithelium of the iris to the anterior hyaloid face by posterior synechiae is seen following attempted mydriasis as a pigmented adhesion from the pupil margin onto the anterior hyaloid face (top). A slit image photograph of the same patient (bottom) shows anterior iris convexity together with a shallow anterior chamber. The extent to which the vitreous gel fills or is prolapsed into the anterior chamber determines the depth of the central part.

Treatment is by intensive mydriasis but if this fails to break the synechiae to the hyaloid face, a posterior synechotomy or laser iridotomy is indicated.

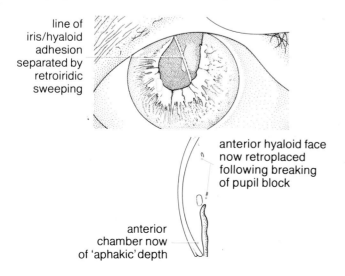

iris pigment epithelium adherent to the anterior hyaloid face, 'left behind' in attempted pupillary dilatation

shallow anterior chamber and iris bombé

anteriorly convex anterior hyaloid face

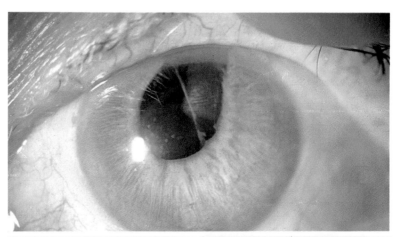

Fig. 8.10   Following a synechotomy procedure in the same patient as in Fig. 8.9, an oblique pigmented line can be seen crossing the anterior hyaloid face with opacification of one half of the face and an optically clear zone in the other half (top). This iris pigment remained after the division of adhesions between the anterior hyaloid face and the pupil margin. The optically clear zone represents the anterior hyaloid face which has been exposed following successful surgical treatment and subsequent mydriasis. A slit image photograph demonstrates the deepening of the anterior chamber seen following resolution of the block (bottom).

line of iris/hyaloid adhesion separated by retroiridic sweeping

anterior hyaloid face now retroplaced following breaking of pupil block

anterior chamber now of 'aphakic' depth

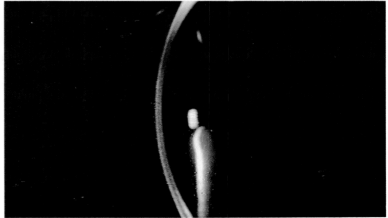

Angle Closure in Small Eyes

Fig. 8.11 A small shallow anterior chamber predisposes to secondary glaucoma with pupil block and this is occasionally seen in patients with congenital syphilis. In this patient, the millimetre scale demonstrates a horizontal corneal diameter of less than 9 mm (the eye has had an iridectomy and a cataract is also present.)

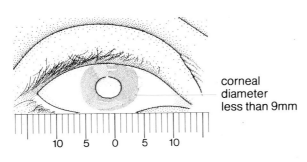

corneal diameter less than 9mm

10 5 0 5 10

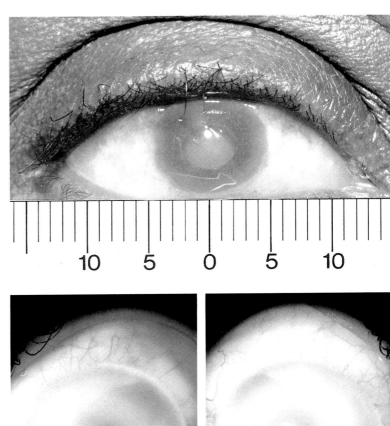

10 5 0 5 10

Fig. 8.12 Other conditions which result in small eyes and increase the risk of angle closure glaucoma include retrolental fibroplasia, high hypermetropia (nanophthalmos) and the mucopolysaccharidoses (as in this patient with the cloudy corneas of Maroteaux — Lamy syndrome who has also had bilateral broad optical iridectomies.)

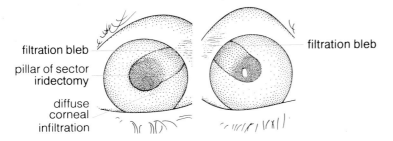

filtration bleb

pillar of sector iridectomy

diffuse corneal infiltration

filtration bleb

SECONDARY ANGLE CLOSURE GLAUCOMA WITHOUT PUPIL BLOCK

The mechanisms by which the angle may close without pupil block can be subdivided into three groups:—
  i) Changes in the posterior segment which push the lens-iris diaphragm forwards.
 ii) Changes in the anterior segment which result in loss of the anterior chamber and the formation of peripheral anterior synechiae.
iii) Cellular proliferation within the anterior chamber with occlusion of the angle.

Posterior Segment Space-Occupying Lesion Producing Secondary Angle Closure

Tumours form the most important group of conditions which are responsible for space-occupying lesions of the posterior segment. Other conditions which can cause an increase in the volume of the posterior segment include choroidal effusions arising either spontaneously or secondary to intraocular surgery, encircling straps used in retinal detachment surgery, posterior scleritis, and an increase in fluid in the posterior segment following a breakdown of the blood-retinal barrier which may be seen following panretinal photocoagulation or after occlusion of the central retinal vein.

Fig. 8.13 This patient had a long-standing blind right eye and presented with recent onset of pain, conjunctival oedema, and haemorrhage into the anterior chamber.

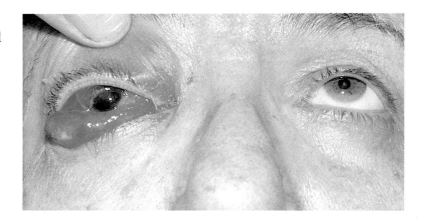

Fig. 8.14 An ultrasound scan of the same patient as in Fig. 8.13 illustrates posterior segment echoes which are suggestive of a tumour mass.

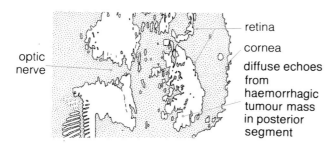

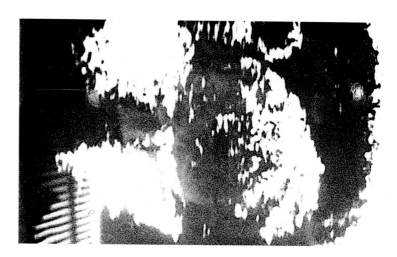

Fig. 8.15 Hemisection of the enucleated eye shows a large haemorrhagic choroidal melanoma together with an anteriorly displaced lens and loss of the anterior chamber.

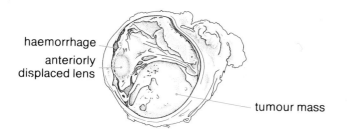

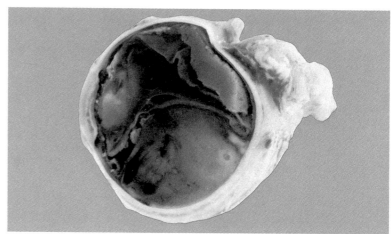

Fig. 8.16 Posterior scleritis may be associated with annular choroidal effusion causing a forward rotation of the ciliary body about the scleral spur and a corresponding forward movement of the lens-iris diaphragm to produce angle closure glaucoma. This photograph shows an eye with diffuse scleritis.

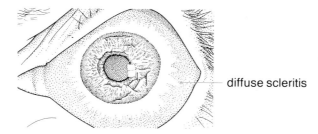

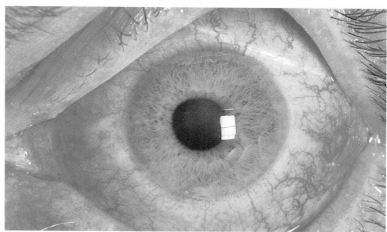

Fig. 8.17 Slit image photographs of each eye of the same patient show a considerable difference in anterior chamber depth between the two eyes with angle closure in the affected eye.

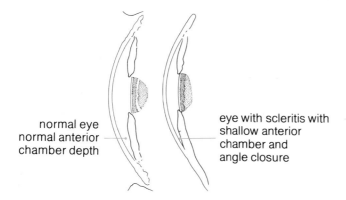

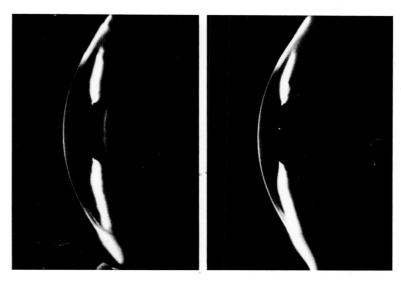

8.7

Fig. 8.18 A fundus painting of the same patient as in Fig. 8.17 reveals a massive annular choroidal effusion which was confirmed by a B-scan ultrasonography (Fig. 8.19).

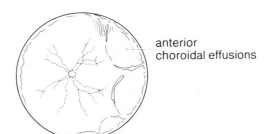

anterior
choroidal effusions

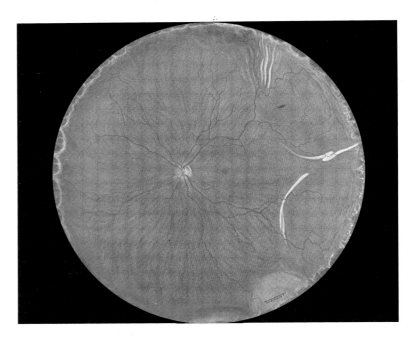

Fig. 8.19 B-scan ultrasound showing choroidal effusion. Management requires investigation for the cause of the scleritis and anti-inflammatory therapy such as systemic phenylbutazone or systemic steroids. As treatment of the scleritis is followed by spontaneous resolution of the effusions with deepening of the anterior chamber, antiglaucoma therapy involves acetazolamide, topical beta-blockers, sympathomimetics for the raised intraocular pressure, and cycloplegics to dilate the pupil and deepen the anterior chamber, together with topical steroids. Should the angle remain closed for longer than a few days, a laser iridotomy will help in limiting the development of peripheral anterior synechiae.

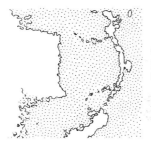

echo marking
position of anterior
choroidal effusions

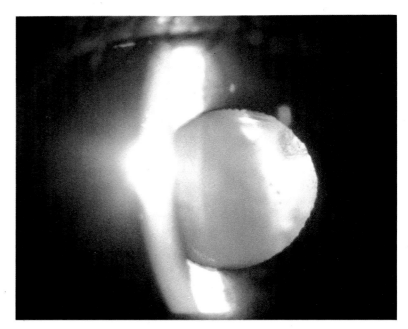

Fig. 8.20 Persistent hyperplastic primary vitreous can produce a contracting retrolental mass with forward rotation of the ciliary body and lens-iris diaphragm, pushing the iris forwards to occlude the angle. The anterior chamber is often shallow in these eyes making angle occlusion more likely. This slit image photograph shows a shallow anterior chamber and retrolental mass.

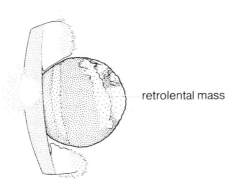

retrolental mass

Fig. 8.21 Following mydriasis, elongated ciliary processes may be seen adhering to the mass (top). Gonioscopy further demonstrates the traction on the ciliary body with elongation of the ciliary processes (bottom).

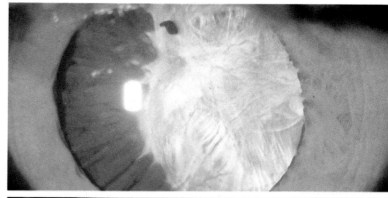

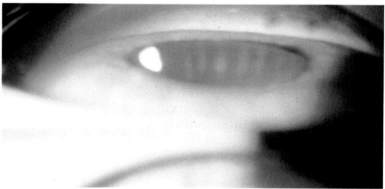

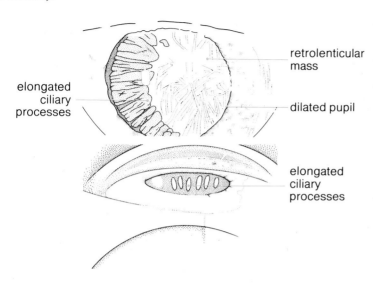

Loss of the Anterior Chamber Following Changes in the Anterior Segment

Changes in the anterior segment, which result in a loss of the anterior chamber, may occur following surgery, perforating injury or corneal ulceration. These produce an aqueous leak from the anterior chamber sufficient to allow iris trabecular apposition, which will lead to the formation of peripheral anterior synechiae. Treatment is by sealing the leak with cycloplegics to dilate the pupil and deepen the anterior chamber and topical steroids. Should the angle remain closed for longer than a few days, peripheral synechiae develop. The rate at which such synechiae develop depends to a large extent upon the amount of inflammation within the anterior chamber: they may develop within a space of days in the case of an inflamed eye although this process normally takes longer if there is no inflammation present. Normally, such aqueous leaks seal spontaneously and the anterior chamber reforms. A rare complication following closure of a wound leak, however, is a failure of the anterior chamber to reform. When this occurs, aqueous humour collects behind the lens to produce malignant glaucoma.

Fig. 8.22 These two slit-image photographs of the anterior segments of both eyes from one patient demonstrate a shallow anterior chamber in one eye while the fellow eye has no anterior chamber. This particular eye has recently undergone filtering surgery which led to the loss of the anterior chamber and the development of malignant glaucoma.

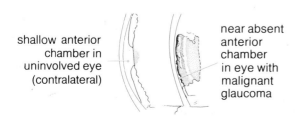

MALIGNANT GLAUCOMA

Malignant glaucoma is the term used to describe eyes with very high pressure, absent or shallow anterior chamber, and retrolenticular accumulation of aqueous humour in the absence of pupil block. The most common cause of this rare condition is filtration surgery in an eye with a shallow anterior chamber. Surgery on the fellow eye may be followed by the same result. The primary process appears to be an obstruction to forward movement of aqueous humour in the presence of a flat anterior chamber, causing loculation in the posterior segment.

The term 'malignant' was originally used because the eye did not respond to, and appeared to be made worse by, treatment with pilocarpine. Initial treatment involves the use of atropine drops (to relax the ciliary muscle and pull the lens-iris diaphragm posteriorly) and hyperosmotic agents (to dehydrate the vitreous and reduce its volume). If this fails, decompression of the retrolenticular aqueous pool by pars plana vitrectomy combined with reformation of the anterior chamber is usually successful. Alternatively vitreous aspiration and reformation of the anterior chamber (Chandler's operation) or cataract extraction have been largely superseded.

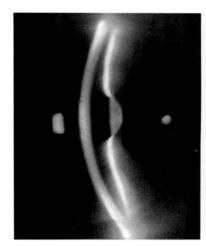
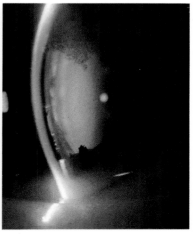

8.9

Fig. 8.23 The ultrasound B scan demonstrates retrolenticular accumulation of aqueous humour in a neglected case of malignant glaucoma.

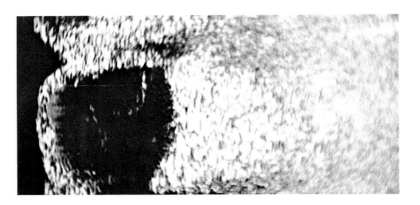

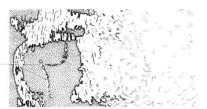

retroplaced anterior hyaloid face from retrolenticular aqueous pooling

Cellular Proliferation with Angle Occlusion
Several different processes may be responsible for obstructing the angle by cellular proliferation.

NEOVASCULARIZATION
Neovascularization (rubeosis) of the iris and angle, with accompanying fibrous tissue formation, is the most common cause of cellular proliferation with angle occlusion and occurs most frequently in diabetic eyes or those central retinal vein occlusions in which there is extensive retinal capillary non-perfusion. Iris neovascularization is seen less commonly with diffuse retinal vascular disease, carotid ischaemia, long-standing retinal detachment, or intraocular tumours. In all these diseases, retinal hypoxia seems to stimulate the formation of some unknown neovascular factor which stimulates neovascular growth on the retina, optic disc or iris. Rubeosis of the iris is seen initially around the pupil margin. Fronds of neovascular tissue extend from the

pupil over the iris stroma and on to the iris root and trabecular meshwork where they insinuate and occlude the trabecular meshwork and Schlemm's canal. Neovascularization of the angle usually causes progressive angle occlusion and elevated intraocular pressure (thrombotic glaucoma), which in time leads to blindness. Occasionally, however, this process may cease to leave partial angle closure while, in some cases (such as that seen in heterochromic cyclitis), peripheral anterior synechiae are not produced at all. During the development of neovascularization of the anterior segment there may be a sudden breakdown in the blood aqueous barrier. The resulting inflammatory process produces the sudden onset of pain and redness with which the patient presents. In such cases topical anti-inflammatory treatment usually controls the symptoms, even though the intraocular pressure may still be extremely high.

Fig. 8.24 An anterior segment photograph of an eye with thrombotic glaucoma. The patchy corneal reflex signifies corneal oedema. The eye also has an irregular dilated pupil and evidence of rubeosis iridis. Contraction of fibrovascular tissue is responsible for pulling the iris in to the trabecular meshwork and this can totally occlude the angle within a week. At the pupillary margin, the same process produces ectropion uveae.

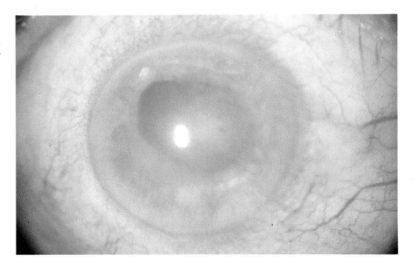

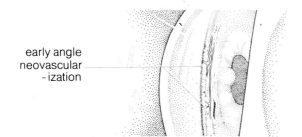

irregular and semidilated pupil

dilated episcleral vessels

diffuse corneal cloudiness secondary oedema

dilated abnormal iris vessels

Fig. 8.25 Goniophotograph of a patient with thrombotic glaucoma demonstrates neovascularization in the open angle.

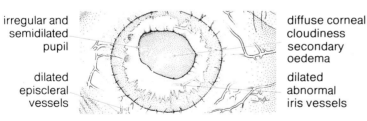

early angle neovascular -ization

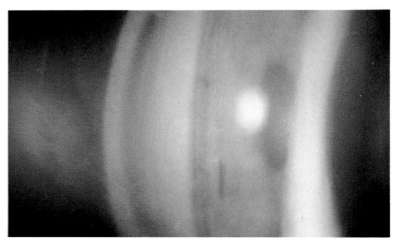

Fig. 8.26   This second goniophotograph shows new vessels on the anterior iris surface and in the 'false' angle of a patient with peripheral anterior synechiae formation.

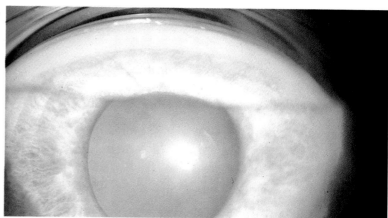

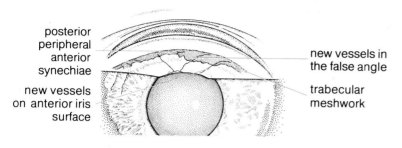

posterior peripheral anterior synechiae

new vessels on anterior iris surface

new vessels in the false angle

trabecular meshwork

Fig. 8.27   Following a central retinal vein occlusion, this fundus shows resolving retinal haemorrhages and disc swelling. The extensive full-thickness retinal haemorrhage indicates the likelihood of massive capillary closure and non-perfusion of the retina. This is confirmed by the fluorescein angiogram (right), which demonstrates closure of the normal retinal capillary bed with leakage from the retinal vessels in the hypoxic retina. Such an eye has a substantial risk of developing rubeosis within three months of initial venous occlusion. Peripheral panretinal ablation at the stage of early rubeosis with laser or cryotherapy can prevent the progression to neovascular glaucoma and sometimes salvage some remaining vision in the eye. Conventional drainage surgery is unsuccessful in these eyes because of neovascularization within the sclerostomy and fibrosis in the drainage bleb (Chapter 14).

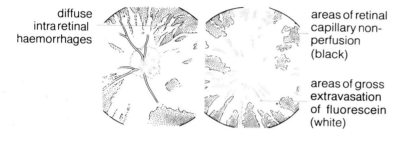

diffuse intra retinal haemorrhages

areas of retinal capillary non-perfusion (black)

areas of gross extravasation of fluorescein (white)

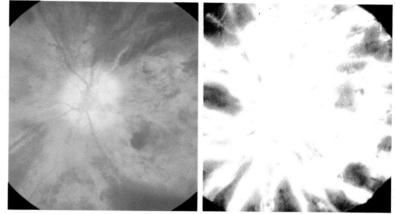

Fig. 8.28   Histology of the iris in neovascular glaucoma demonstrates a fibrovascular membrane on the anterior iris surface (top). Following occlusion of the angle, endothelial slide occurs from the corneal surface over the false angle formed on the iris surface creating new basement membrane across the angle (bottom). (Separation between Descemet's membrane and the corneal stroma is an artefact.)

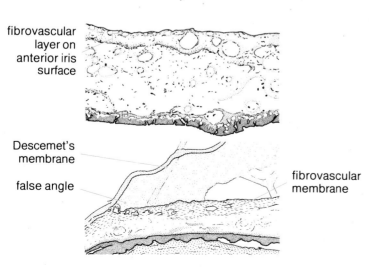

fibrovascular layer on anterior iris surface

Descemet's membrane

false angle

fibrovascular membrane

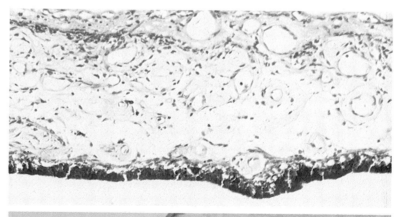

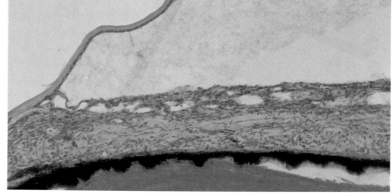

THE PROLIFERATIVE ENDOTHELIAL SYNDROMES

Essential iris atrophy, Chandler's syndrome, and the iris naevus (Cogan-Reese) syndrome have in common a primary disorder of the corneal endothelium: they may in fact be different parts of the same disease spectrum. The basic defect appears to be a cellular proliferation of the corneal endothelium with formation of Descemet's membrane spreading across the angle and onto the anterior iris surface (see The Cornea, Chapter 6.)

Chandler's syndrome is considered a variant of essential iris atrophy. It is unilateral, occurs mainly in females, and is characterized by corneal endothelial cell decompensation, which causes early presentation with haloes. The glaucoma produced is often quite mild: peripheral anterior synechiae and corectopia (eccentric pupil) are seen.

The iris-naevus syndrome is again unilateral with heterochromia. Iris nodules, which are really foci of remaining normal iris tissue surrounded by endothelial cells, are seen on the anterior iris surface. This endothelial traction also produces ectropion uveae and peripheral anterior synechiae.

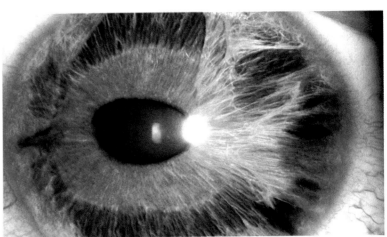

Fig. 8.29 Essential iris atrophy is a rare syndrome which is characterized by unilateral glaucoma, corectopia, pseudopolycoria, and peripheral anterior synechiae formation. In the early stages, there is thinning of the iris stroma in the mid-periphery and eccentricity of the pupil progressing to full-thickness hole formation.

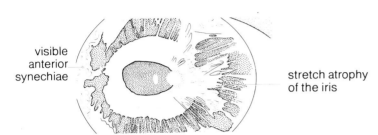

visible anterior synechiae

stretch atrophy of the iris

Fig. 8.30 In severe cases of essential iris atrophy, there is full-thickness hole formation and ectropion uveae. Characteristically, the pupil is drawn towards the site of peripheral anterior synechiae formation while 'stretch atrophy' of the iris in the opposite quadrants leads to the iris hole formation. Peripheral anterior synechiae eventually encircle the angle. In this photograph, notice that pseudopolycoria and ectropion uveae lie in opposite quadrants, giving credence to the theory of iris stretch 'pulling' its pigmented iris epithelium as well as the pupil towards one part of the angle.

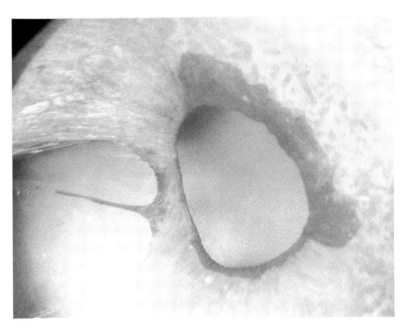

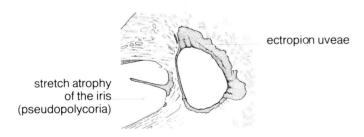

ectropion uveae

stretch atrophy of the iris (pseudopolycoria)

Fig. 8.31 A goniophotograph of a patient with essential iris atrophy illustrates the formation of the peripheral anterior synechiae. The glaucoma is usually out of all proportion to the extent of peripheral anterior synechiae formation and probably reflects endothelial cells covering the trabecular meshwork in those areas where the angle still appears open.

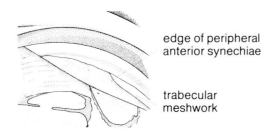

edge of peripheral anterior synechiae

trabecular meshwork

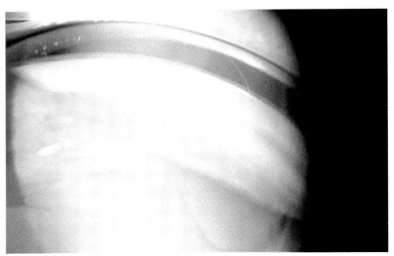

Fig. 8.32 The appearance of the angle and anterior iris surface under the light microscope in a patient suffering from essential iris atrophy shows ectropion uveae, formation of a Descemet's-like membrane on the anterior iris surface, and peripheral anterior synechiae.

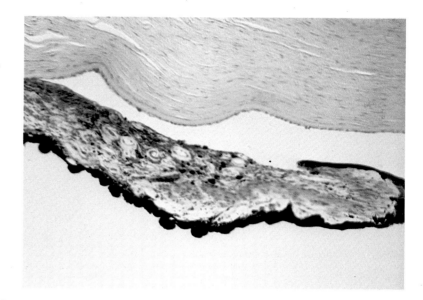

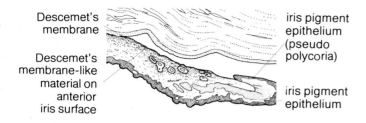

Descemet's membrane

Descemet's membrane-like material on anterior iris surface

iris pigment epithelium (pseudo polycoria)

iris pigment epithelium

Fig. 8.33 This patient with Chandler's syndrome shows a bullous keratopathy (which is a prominent feature of the syndrome) together with corectopia and iris atrophy (both of which are less marked than in essential iris atrophy). The glaucoma is frequently quite mild. Peripheral anterior synechiae tend to be less extensive than in essential iris atrophy.

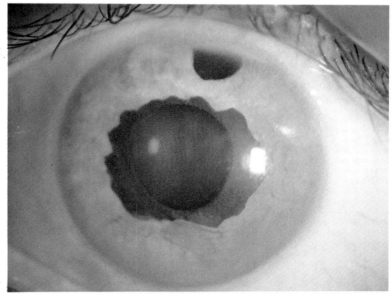

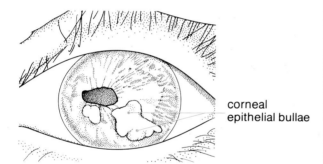

corneal epithelial bullae

Fig. 8.34 In the iris-naevus syndrome, iris atrophy is less visible than in the typical case of essential iris atrophy while there is more corneal oedema. The anterior surface of the iris is covered by a sheet of Descemet's membrane-like material through which normal nodules of iris tissue protrude. These have been mistaken for iris melanomas which in the past have led to enucleation. Ectropion uveae is common. In this photograph, note the extensive development of ectropion uveae together with loss of the usual appearance of the anterior iris. The patient has a surgical peripheral iridectomy.

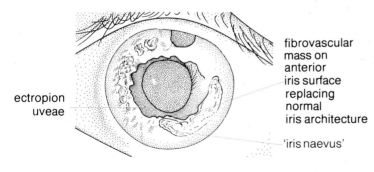

ectropion uveae

fibrovascular mass on anterior iris surface replacing normal iris architecture

'iris naevus'

EPITHELIALIZATION OF THE ANTERIOR CHAMBER

This results from poorly repaired perforating injuries or surgical incisions.

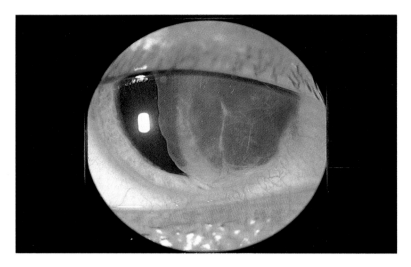

Fig. 8.35 In this example, epithelialization has spread as a cyst from a traumatic perforation at the limbus.

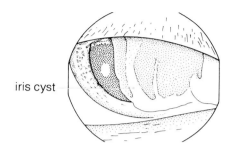

iris cyst

Fig. 8.36 Glaucoma results from occlusion of the angle by the traumatic iris cyst, or from direct spread of epithelial cells over the inner surface of the trabecular meshwork. Treatment involves total removal of the epithelial cells.

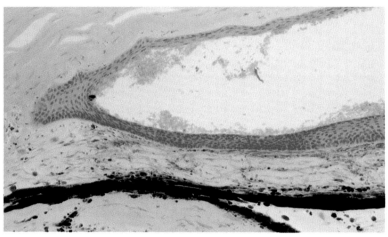

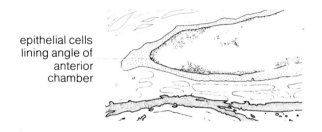

epithelial cells lining angle of anterior chamber

SECONDARY OPEN ANGLE GLAUCOMA

Outflow of aqueous humour (the outflow facility) may be reduced in the presence of an open angle if there has been disruption to the anatomical structure of the trabecular meshwork (as in traumatic angle recession), if the trabecular meshwork becomes clogged by cells or debris, or if there is an increased episcleral venous pressure.

Traumatic Angle Recession

A blunt injury to the eye compresses the globe and the shock wave transmitted through the anterior chamber tears the ciliary muscle at its insertion into the scleral spur. Gonioscopic examination shows recession of the angle as

posterior displacement of the ciliary band. Such injuries are common after blunt trauma, especially if a hyphema is present. Angle recession may be the only visible sequel to such a contusion injury, or may coexist with signs of such an injury on one or more of the intraocular structures. Glaucoma occurring soon after trauma is probably related to coincidental uveitis or hyphema. Extensive angle recession can be followed by glaucoma years later and is thought to be a non-specific trabecular degeneration from the initial trauma. Such eyes require prolonged follow-up. The possibility of a retinal dialysis or subsequent traumatic cataract must also be borne in mind.

Fig. 8.37 Gonioscopy in a patient with angle recession can show a widening of the ciliary band, or, on occasion following a complete tear of the ciliary muscle, widening of the angle together with a white strip of sclera. These goniophotographs show the temporal aspect of the anterior chamber in both the normal and involved eye. An artificially wide angle with pigmentation can be seen in the affected eye at the recessed site.

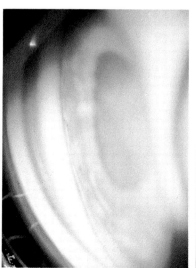
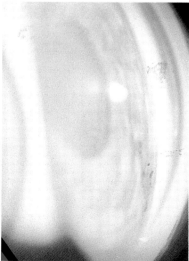

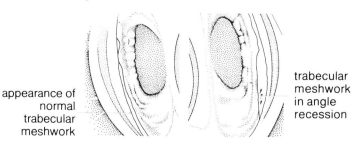
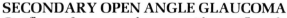

appearance of normal trabecular meshwork

trabecular meshwork in angle recession

Fig. 8.38 The light microscopic appearance shows recession of the angle with inflammation of the sclera and pigmentation of the trabecular meshwork. Pigment granules are also seen on the anterior iris surface.

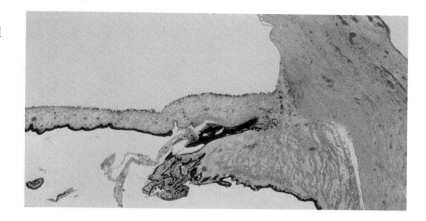

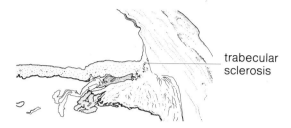

trabecular sclerosis

Lens Induced Glaucoma (Phacolytic Glaucoma)

Two different types of cellular response, are seen in eyes with a degenerate lens. Under certain conditions, the lens capsule of an hypermature cataract leaks denatured cortical material. This in turn excites a macrophage response, and the macrophages, gorged with lens material, accumulate around and clog the trabecular meshwork causing a secondary open angle glaucoma known as phacolytic glaucoma.

Fig. 8.39 Photomicrographs demonstrate the swollen macrophages obstructing the trabecular meshwork. Clinically large accumulations are seen floating in the anterior chamber of an eye with a cataractous lens and acute glaucoma. Characteristically, keratic precipitates do not form and cataract extraction cures the condition.

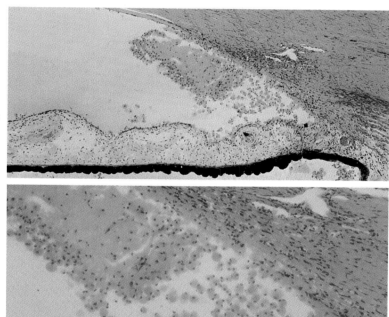

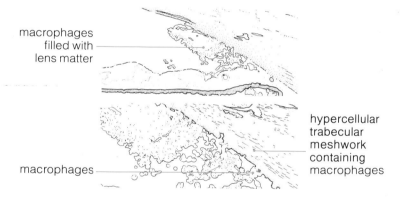

macrophages filled with lens matter

macrophages

hypercellular trabecular meshwork containing macrophages

Phacoanaphylactic Uveitis

Under normal conditions, lens protein is sequestrated in foetal development from the systemic immune system. Sensitization of this immune system by the lens protein may cause phacoanaphylactic endophthalmitis. In this situation, a granulomatous inflammation occurs secondary to rupture of the lens capsule and a chronic inflammatory response ensues, usually accompanied by raised intraocular pressure. Histological examination reveals invasion of the lens cortex and uvea by these inflammatory cells. Resolution follows removal of the lens material if that is possible.

Fig. 8.40 A massive inflammatory response with extensive fibrosis may be seen between the posterior iris and anterior lens surface. The anterior lens capsule has been ruptured and inflammatory cells present beneath the capsule adjacent to and interspersed with the lamellae of the anterior lens stroma.

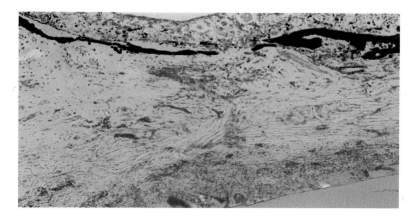

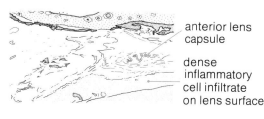

anterior lens capsule

dense inflammatory cell infiltrate on lens surface

Haemolytic Glaucoma

Blood cells and their products of degeneration may produce secondary open angle glaucoma. Under normal conditions, healthy red blood cells pass through the trabecular meshwork to enter Schlemm's canal. A hyphema represents the accumulation of red blood cells at a faster rate than they can be removed by the normal process. If the trabecular meshwork becomes clogged by these cells, intraocular pressure will increase. With a healthy angle, elimination of the hyphema is followed by return of intraocular pressure to normal.

Haemolytic glaucoma should be suspected when open angle glaucoma is discovered in an eye with a long-standing vitreous haemorrhage and a minimal uveitis with yellowish discolouration within the anterior and posterior chambers, especially if it is aphakic. Phase contrast microscopy may be used to identify these degenerate red blood cells (ghost cells) from fluid removed at the time of an aqueous tap. It is considered that the lack of maleability of ghost cells renders them more likely to occlude the pores within the trabecular system.

Fig. 8.41 The histological appearance of the trabecular meshwork in haemolytic glaucoma shows degenerate red blood cells (ghost cells) on the trabecular spaces and within macrophages.

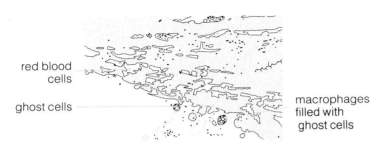

red blood cells

ghost cells

macrophages filled with ghost cells

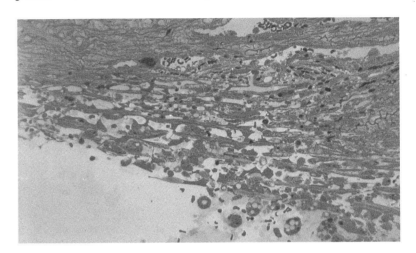

Siderosis

Siderosis results from the widespread deposition of iron throughout the eye which diffuses from a retained ferrous ocular foreign body. Glaucoma occurs secondary to sclerosis of the trabecular meshwork, and is thought to

result from a direct toxic effect. Clinically, eyes with siderosis demonstrate mydriasis, heterochromia, retinal degeneration with optic atrophy, as well as raised intraocular pressure.

Fig. 8.42 The right eye of this patient shows evidence of siderosis with brown-green discolouration of the iris from iron deposition.

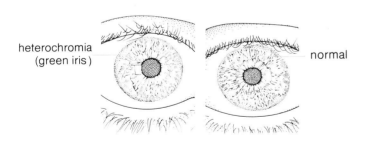

heterochromia (green iris)

normal

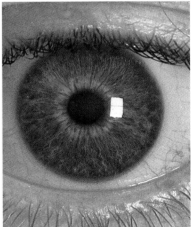

Fig. 8.43 Histology shows iron deposition within the meshwork and Schlemm's canal.

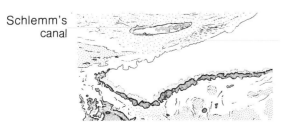

Schlemm's canal

blue staining iron in fibrosed trabecular meshwork

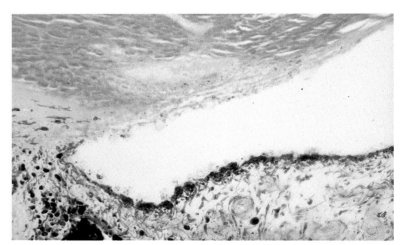

Tumour Infiltration

Secondary open angle glaucoma can occur with tumours of the anterior segment. It may be seen with either seeded malignant melanoma cells or other tumour cells which block the angle mechanically. Less commonly, a malignant melanoma may arise directly from the iris root and ciliary body and invade the angle directly. Affected eyes required enucleation. On rare occasions, a melanomalytic glaucoma arises secondary to trabecular obstruction by macrophages engorged with melanin released by the tumour.

Fig. 8.44 This eye has an amelanotic iris melanoma which, on gonioscopy (bottom) is seen to be infiltrating the angle.

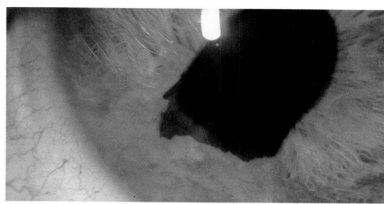

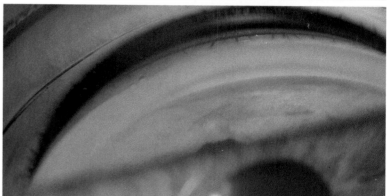

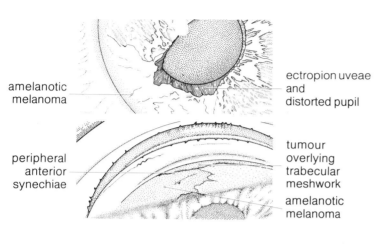

Fig. 8.45 Light microscopy of the angle in a patient with glaucoma secondary to iris melanoma shows that malignant melanoma cells have blocked the angle mechanically.

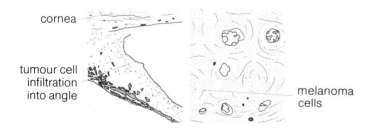

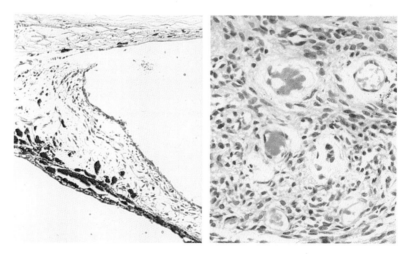

Fig. 8.46 Melanomalytic glaucoma arises secondary to trabecular obstruction by macrophages engorged with melanin released by a localized tumour.

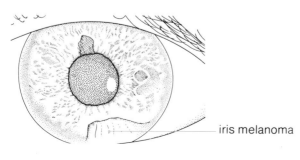

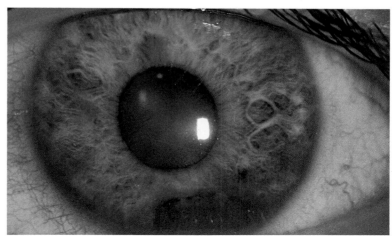

Fig. 8.47 Gonioscopic view of the same patient shows heavy pigmentation within the angle. Local excision of the tumour in this case was followed by resolution of the coincidental glaucoma.

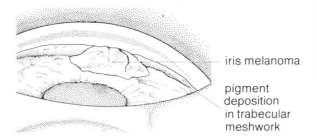

iris melanoma

pigment deposition in trabecular meshwork

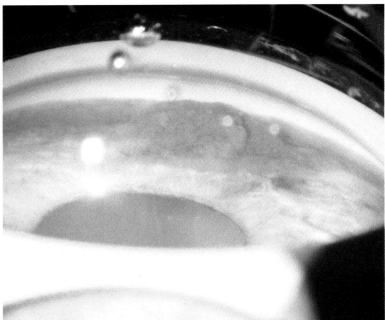

Uveitis and Glaucoma

Uveitis producing posterior synechiae, iris bombé, and angle closure has already been demonstrated (cf. Figs. 8.1 and 8.2). A secondary open angle glaucoma is very commonly seen with an anterior uveitis of any cause and is due, at least in part, to mechanical obstruction of the trabecular meshwork by inflammatory cells which resolves with the attack. Chronic uveitis can result in glaucoma either as a result of peripheral anterior synechiae formation or trabecular sclerosis (in which case the angle appears normal on gonioscopy). Two specific syndromes in which uveitis and glaucoma are associated are the Posner-Schlossman syndrome and Fuchs' heterochromic cyclitis.

Fig. 8.48 Slit image and gonioscopic photographs demonstrate the development of peripheral anterior synechiae in chronic uveitis (without loss of the anterior chamber). Although usually confined to the inferior angle, such synechiae can extend circumferentially. A variant of this process occurs with sarcoidosis where trabecular granulomas form as focal lesions around the circumference of the angle and, if untreated, these granulomas produce small areas of peripheral anterior synechiae. These gonioscopic appearances would be identical to those seen after loss of the anterior chamber from whatever cause.

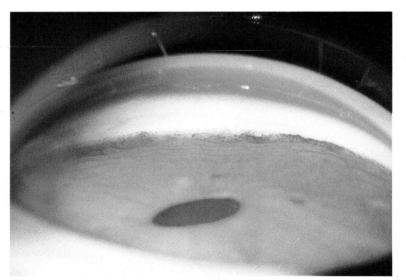

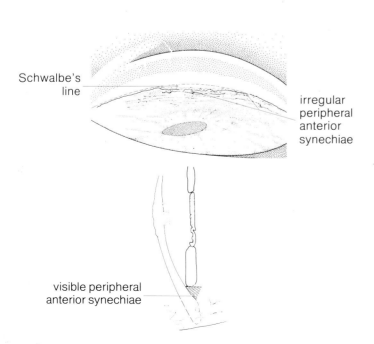

Schwalbe's line

irregular peripheral anterior synechiae

visible peripheral anterior synechiae

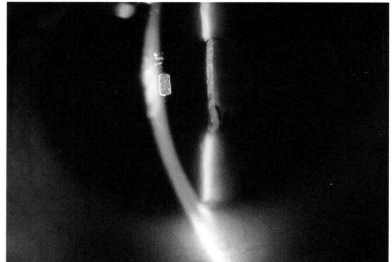

The Posner-Schlossman Syndrome (Glaucomatocyclitic Crises)

This unusual condition is typically seen in young adult males who develop very high levels of intraocular pressure with minimal anterior uveitis. The syndrome is usually uniocular but either eye can be involved in the attacks. Patients present with symptoms from corneal oedema due to intraocular pressures in the 40-60 mm Hg range. The uveitis is minimal, posterior synechiae do not form, and optic nerve damage does not usually occur. Occasionally, following many attacks. chronic elevation of intraocular pressure occurs; it is thought that then permanent damage to the meshwork has occurred either directly from the disease process or secondary to raised intraocular pressure causing degenerative changes in the meshwork. Whatever the mechanism, a condition clinically indistinguishable from chronic simple glaucoma develops. Typically, acute attacks last days to weeks. In between such attacks, the occasional 'sentinel' keratitic precipitates can be found.

Fig. 8.49 The 'sentinel' keratic precipitates seen during the quiescent phase. There is some evidence of crises being associated with high levels of aqueous humour prostaglandins, although treatment with anti-prostaglandins has not been of use in aborting or preventing the attacks.

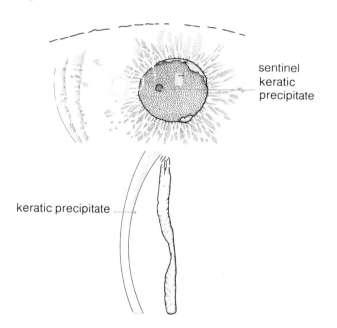

sentinel keratic precipitate

keratic precipitate

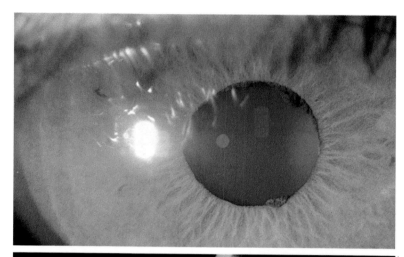

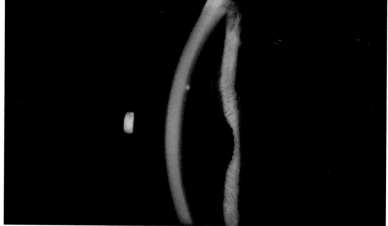

Fuchs' Heterochromic Cyclitis

About seventy percent of Fuchs' heterochromic cyclitis is unilateral. Iris atrophy (the affected iris stroma showing anterior stromal atrophy and a lighter colour); fine keratic precipitates, cataract, glaucoma, and occasionally a fine neovascularization of the angle are all seen in an established case (see Chapter 10.)

Neither anterior nor posterior synechiae develop.

The glaucoma responds to conventional medical or surgical treatment and the eye responds well to cataract surgery should it be indicated.

Fig. 8.50 A patient with heterochromic cyclitis of the right eye. The iris is lighter than the left and a cataract is present.

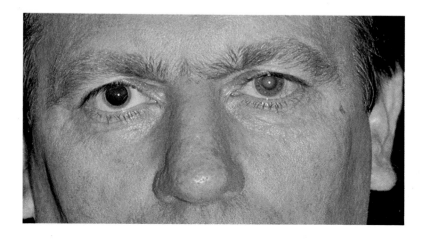

Steroid Induced Glaucoma

Topical steroids cause raised intraocular pressure in a small proportion of patients. There is some evidence that this population is genetically controlled and may be similar to those at risk from chronic simple glaucoma. The glaucoma usually appears after a few weeks of treatment and this complication must be borne in mind in any patient on topical steroid therapy. Different steroid preparations vary in their ability to produce this phenomenon but this may be related to their potency and penetration of the cornea. The mechanism is uncertain. In some cases the intertrabecular spaces have been found blocked by a fibrillar material of unknown aetiology. The fact that in most cases intraocular pressure falls to normal on cessation of the topical steroid suggests that the drug plays an active part in metabolism of the cells within the anterior chamber angle.

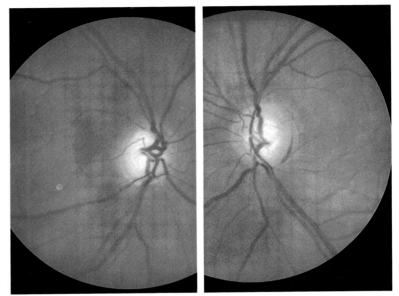

Fig. 8.51 Gross glaucomatous cupping is seen in this patient who had used topical steroids without supervision for treatment of mild ocular irritation associated with contact lens wear.

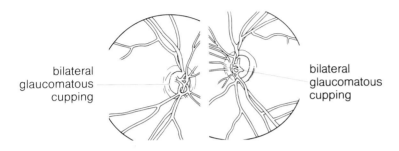

bilateral glaucomatous cupping

bilateral glaucomatous cupping

Fig. 8.52 The visual fields of the same patient show the gross field loss which caused her to present. Visual acuities were 6/9 in each eye.

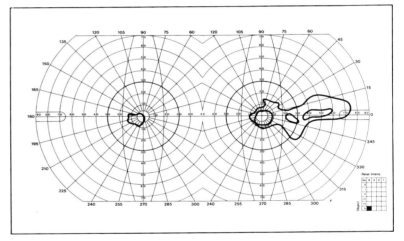

Fig. 8.53 Electron micrograph of the trabecular meshwork in the patient whose optic discs were shown in Fig 8.51. Fibrillar material occludes the intertrabecular spaces and it is speculated that this may produce the glaucoma.

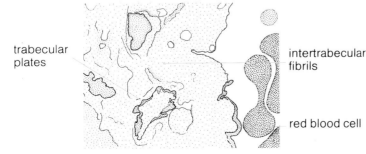

trabecular plates

intertrabecular fibrils

red blood cell

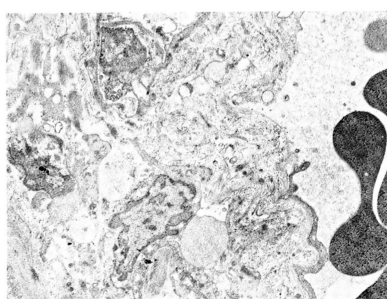

Raised Episcleral Venous Pressure

This is usually caused by a shunting of arterial blood to the orbital veins by a carotico-cavernous fistula, but is occasionally seen with gross cor pulmonale, the Sturge-Weber syndrome or superior vena cava obstruction. Any increase in episcleral venous pressure will cause an increase in intraocular pressure so as to maintain the pressure gradient across the trabecular meshwork.

With fistulae between the carotid artery and cavernous sinus where the shunt is usually of high flow, the diagnosis is obvious from the dramatic neuro-ophthalmic signs (see Chapter 20.) However, coexistent ocular hypoxia complicates this picture and even in the presence of rubeosis iridis (which is not infrequently present in these

eyes) the intraocular pressure may be low. Arterio-venous communications within the dural vessels are frequently of low flow and these patients present with red eyes, arterialized conjunctival vessels, and glaucoma without the other signs of bruits, or proptosis seen with carotico-cavernous fistulae. Apart from the glaucoma, these dural shunts usually have a benign prognosis. The glaucoma may vary in severity: those cases with high intraocular pressure respond poorly to medical treatment. Filtration surgery is usually successful, but in the Sturge-Weber syndrome, a coexisting choroidal haemangioma may massive intraocular haemorrhage.

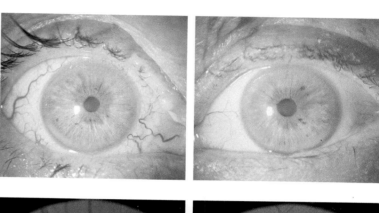

Fig. 8.54 Arterialized vessels are seen in the conjunctiva of a patient with a dural arterio-venous fistula.

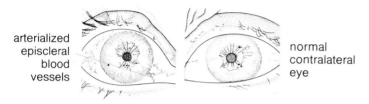

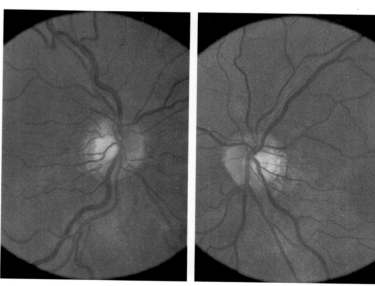

Fig. 8.55 Retinal veins are engorged in the right eye but at this stage the optic discs do not show glaucomatous changes.

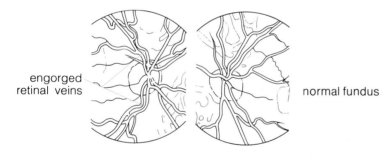

Fig. 8.56 More obvious vascular changes can be seen in the conjunctival vessels of this patient with a high volume flow in the shunt (left). The carotid angiogram (right) demonstrates the fistula within the cavernous sinus and a grossly dilated superior ophthalmic vein. Orbital ultrasonography can also be used to demonstrate the dilated superior orbital vein.

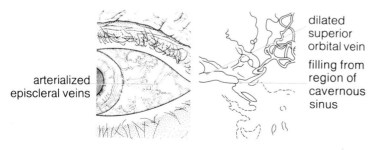

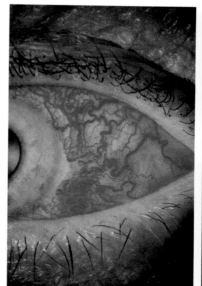

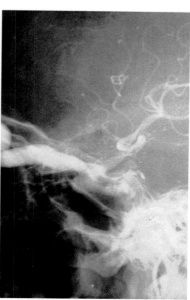

8.21

Sturge-Weber Syndrome

Fig. 8.57 These goniophotographs compare the normal and abnormal eyes of a patient with the Sturge-Weber syndrome. Blood can be seen within Schlemm's canal in the affected eye and this is a common finding in the presence of raised episcleral venous pressure.

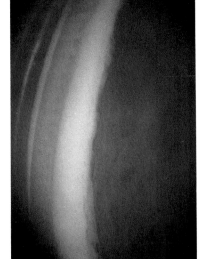
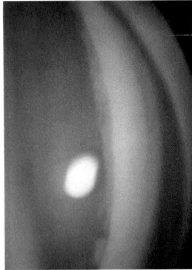

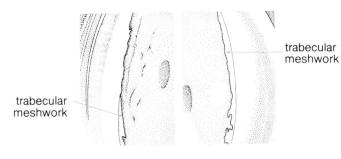

trabecular meshwork

trabecular meshwork

9. The Uveal Tract

D. J. Spalton

NORMAL ANATOMY

The uveal tract is a pigmented vascular layer lying between the retina and sclera and consists of the iris, ciliary body, and choroid, each lying in continuity. Apart from the specialized muscular structure of the iris and ciliary body, the uveal tract is concerned with nutrition of the eye through the secretion of aqueous humour by the ciliary epithelium of the ciliary body, and the maintenance of the outer retina from the choroidal circulation.

Embryologically, the uveal tract is derived from both neuroectoderm and mesoderm. Neuroectoderm of the optic cup forms the muscles and the pigmented epithelium of the ciliary body, while the surrounding mesoderm forms the uveal stroma. Melanocytes from the neural crest are scattered throughout the tract and there is both an inter-individual and inter-racial difference in their relative concentration. Such differences account for the colour of the iris and the degree of fundus pigmentation

The Iris

The iris controls the degree of retinal illumination through the tone of the sphincter and dilator muscles which are under parasympathetic and sympathetic neuronal control respectively. The pigment epithelium on the posterior surface prevents entry of extraneous non axial light and so refines the optics of the eye (the absence of this may contribute to the poor visual acuity of ocular albinos).

The stroma forms the anterior surface of the iris. This fibrovascular tissue is anterior to the constrictor and dilator muscles that lie on the pigment epithelial surface which is, in fact, a double layer of densely pigmented cells. About 1-2 mm from the pupillary margin on the anterior surface, there is a frill known as the collarette. This is the site of the embryological pupillary membrane, which atrophies in the eighth month of gestation, and the minor arterial circle of the iris.

The iris derives its blood supply from anastomosis of the posterior and anterior ciliary circulations at the major arterial circle, which lies in the root of the ciliary body and sends radial branches to the incomplete minor circle at the level of the collarette. Iris blood vessels have tight endothelial junctions and thick vascular walls to withstand compression by iris dilatation.

Fig. 9.1   A normal iris.

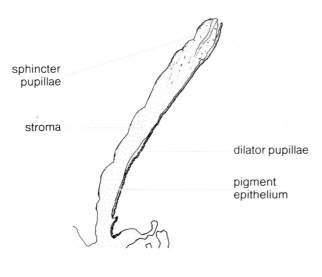
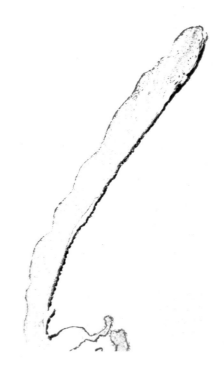

sphincter pupillae

stroma

dilator pupillae

pigment epithelium

The Ciliary Body

A precise knowledge of the position of the ciliary body is important in the positioning of surgical incisions for vitreous surgery. The surface markings of the ciliary body from the corneal limbus are 1.5 to 8 mm on the temporal side, and 1.5 to 7 mm on the nasal side. The anterior third (2 mm) contains the ciliary muscle and ciliary processes and is known as the pars plicata. The posterior two-thirds, the pars plana, inserts posteriorly into the ora serrata of the retina. There is a dense attachment of the vitreous base over this area and onto the anterior equatorial retina.

The ciliary muscle controls accommodation and in transverse section has a triangular shape. The outermost fibres run longitudinally, inserting into the scleral spur; more internally, the muscle fibres are radial with the innermost fibres running circumferentially. Contraction of the external longitudinal fibres transfers tension indirectly to the trabecular meshwork through the scleral spur and may explain the mechanism of the pressure-lowering effect of pilocarpine.

Overlying the ciliary muscle, the epithelium and stroma are thrown up into about eighty ciliary processes. These have a vascular stroma and are covered by two layers of pigment epithelium which are continuous with the iris pigment epithelium anteriorly and with the retinal pigment epithelium and neurosensory retina posteriorly. The inner or superficial epithelial layer is nonpigmented and has tight intercellular junctions. Aqueous humour is secreted through these cells (cf. Primary Glaucoma – Chapter 7). As in the choroid, the capillaries in the ciliary processes are fenestrated. The zonular fibres supporting the lens run radially from the troughs between the ciliary processes.

Fig. 9.2 A posterior view of the lens and anterior segment shows the insertion of the retina into the pars plana at the ora serrata and the folds of the pars plicata. A few remaining zonular fibres can be seen supporting the cataractous lens.

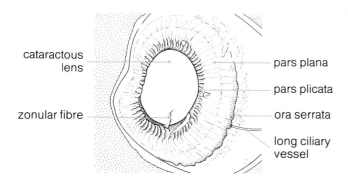

cataractous lens — pars plana

pars plicata

zonular fibre — ora serrata

long ciliary vessel

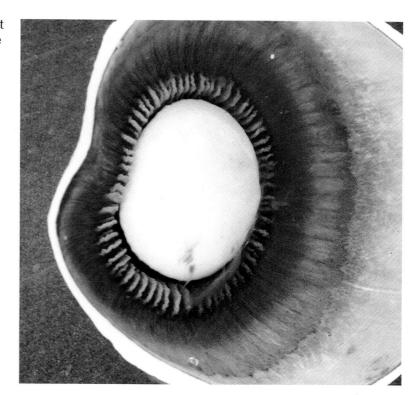

Fig. 9.3 The normal ciliary body is seen extending from the scleral spur to the ora serrata. Under higher power the details of the pars plicata are more clearly seen. Notice the two layers of ciliary epithelium, the zonular fibres and the major arterial circle of the iris.

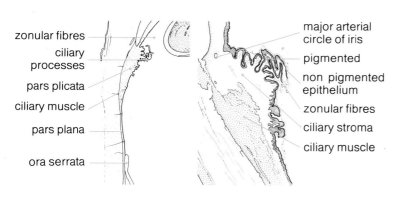

zonular fibres

ciliary processes

pars plicata

ciliary muscle

pars plana

ora serrata

major arterial circle of iris

pigmented

non pigmented epithelium

zonular fibres

ciliary stroma

ciliary muscle

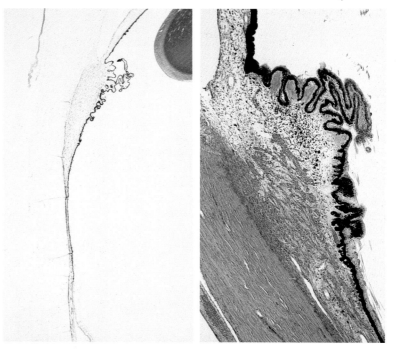

Fig. 9.4 At the ora serrata, the neuroretina becomes attenuated and cystic and terminates as the inner nonpigmented epithelium of the ciliary body. The retinal pigment epithelium is continued as the outer pigmented layer of the pars plana.

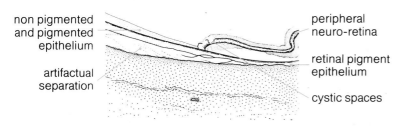

non pigmented and pigmented epithelium

artifactual separation

peripheral neuro-retina

retinal pigment epithelium

cystic spaces

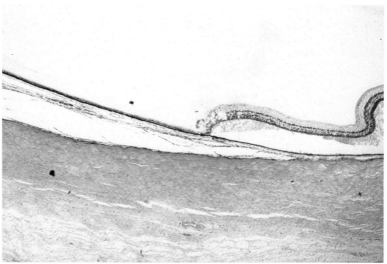

The Choroid

The lamina suprachoroidia is an area of delicate connective tissue which forms a potential space immediately beneath the sclera. The long ciliary vessels and nerves lie in this space and it is in this area that choroidal effusions collect. The choroid has an extensive vascular bed: the larger vessels are the most external and give rise to a network of fenestrated capillaries, the choriocapillaris, which lies directly under Bruch's membrane and supplies the vascular needs of the outer retina through the retinal pigment epithelium. The stromal tissue contains melanocytes, collagen fibres and lymphocytes.

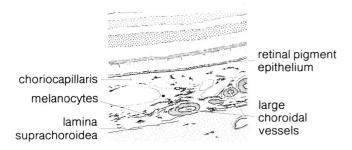

Fig. 9.5 The normal choroid is a highly vascular tissue whose macroscopic appearance is black due to pigmentation from stromal melanocytes.

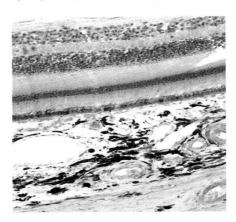

Blood Supply

The uveal tract, and especially the choroid, has an exceptionally high blood flow (677 mg/min) and for this reason only about three percent of the oxygen carried is extracted. The choroid supplies oxygen to the retinal pigment epithelium and photoreceptors by diffusion and, in the monkey, about sixty-five percent of the oxygen consumed by the retina comes from this source. Other metabolites are transported through the pigment epithelium to the retina by active transport processes.

The vascular supply of the uveal tract is derived from the posterior ciliary circulation anastomosing anteriorly with the anterior ciliary arteries. The short posterior ciliary arteries leave the ophthalmic artery posteriorly in the orbit (cf. The Orbits and Lacrimal System – Chapter 20) and run forwards to penetrate the sclera circumferentially around the optic disc as twelve to fifteen branches. These branches supply the disc (cf. The Optic Disc – Chapter 17) and the choroid. At the disc, two long posterior ciliary branches run forwards medially and laterally in the lamina suprachoroidia to anastomose with the anterior ciliary arteries adjacent to the major circle of the iris. The anterior ciliary arteries are also derived from the ophthalmic artery.

They lie on the external ocular muscles (two arteries on the medial, inferior and superior recti, one on the lateral) and penetrate the sclera at the muscle insertions to contribute to the supply of the iris, ciliary body and anterior choroid. Long posterior ciliary arteries can frequently be seen in the horizontal meridians of a normal eye if the retinal pigmentation is not too dense. The choroidal venous return drains into the orbital veins by the four vortex veins, one lying in each quadrant of the equatorial sclera.

The choroidal arteries lie under the scleral surface and divide rapidly to form the inner choriocapillaris, a network of large diameter capillaries lying beneath Bruch's membrane. These capillaries have fenestrations between the endothelial cells allowing plasma to leak readily into the extracellular space. While there are anatomical anastomoses between the choroidal vessels, the choriocapillaris seems to function physiologically on a 'lobular' supply basis. This is sometimes revealed in the early phases of a fluorescein angiogram and is seen clinically as choroidal infarcts such as Elschnig's spots or Siegrist's streaks.

Fig. 9.6 Diagram showing the vascular supply of the choroid by the anterior and posterior ciliary circulations. (Further details of the anterior ciliary and conjunctival circulations are described in Chapter 5.)

Fig. 9.7 The microcirculation of the choriocapillaris seems to function on a physiological lobular basis although there are anatomical junctions between the physiological boundaries.

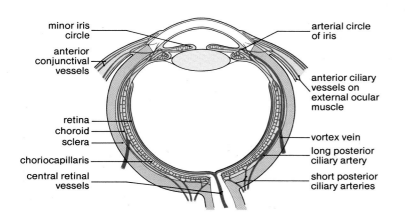

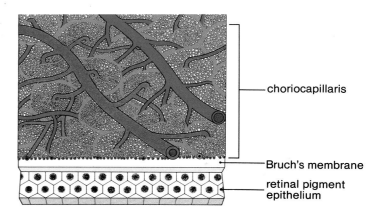

Fig. 9.8 Frequently, a fluorescein angiogram shows patchy delayed filling of the choroidal bed in the earliest phase which supports the concept of a lobular choroidal supply. These hypofluorescent patches may represent single lobules or groups of separate lobules. Some researchers have postulated that the size and distribution of lobules is relatively consistent in human eyes.

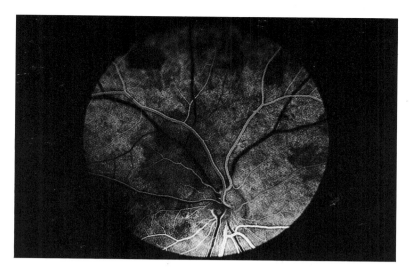

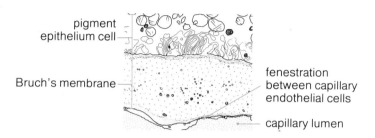

areas of delayed
choriocapillaris
filling

retinal artery

Fig. 9.9 Choriocapillaris capillaries have a wider diameter (20-30 mm) than is usual elsewhere. Electron microscopy demonstrates the fenestrations between endothelial cells.

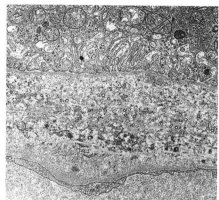

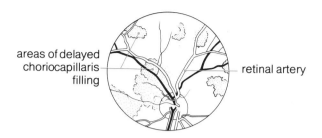

pigment
epithelium cell

Bruch's membrane

fenestration
between capillary
endothelial cells

capillary lumen

CONGENITAL ANOMALIES OF THE UVEAL TRACT
Colobomas
Colobomas are formed by defects of closure of the optic cup which occur at seven to eight weeks of foetal life (cf. The Optic Disc – Chapter 17) and can present as a sectorial deficiency varying from the trivial to the gross. They are typically found infero-nasally and may involve the iris, choroid and retina, or optic disc.

Fig. 9.10 Defects of the iris are sometimes associated with segmental absence of the lens zonules causing a localized indentation of the lens, or with defects in the choroid and retina. This child with bilateral iris colobomata also has a divergent left eye due to a large chorioretinal coloboma involving the macula.

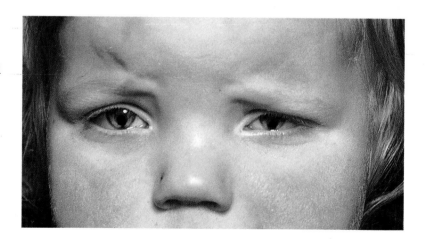

Aniridia
Aniridia occurs either as a familial autosomal dominant disease or sporadically. The autosomal dominant condition is associated with glaucoma, nystagmus, corneal opacities and photophobia, while sporadic cases

usually have a high incidence of nephroblastoma (Wilm's tumour) and all such children require screening by intravenous pyelography. A vestigial iris remnant can usually be seen as a frill on gonioscopy.

Fig. 9.11 Retroillumination of the eyes in a child with aniridia shows the lens and zonular gap. The iris remnant remains as a frill which forms peripheral anterior synechiae to obstruct the angle.

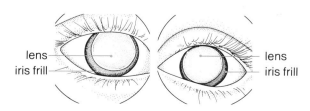

lens
iris frill

lens
iris frill

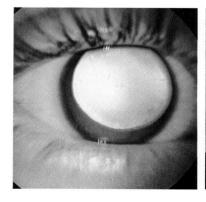
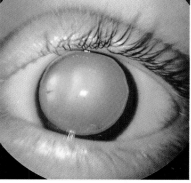

Fig. 9.12 An intravenous pyelogram from a child with sporadic aniridia shows a large tumour replacing the right kidney.

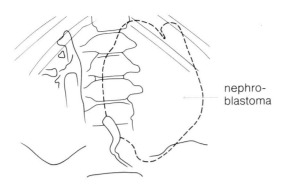

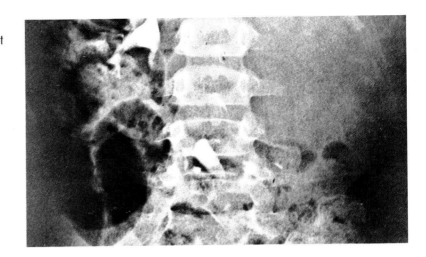

nephro-
blastoma

Albinism

Albinos have a deficiency of melanin within the uveal tract and the disorder occurs in both systemic (autosomal recessive) or purely ocular forms (usually X-linked, but rarely recessive) when cutaneous pigmentation is normal. Purely cutaneous albinos have no ocular complication. By hair follicle analysis oculocutaneous albinos can be divided into those who have a complete absence of pigmentation (tyrosinase negative), and those who are tyrosinase positive. Tyrosinase positive subjects can be more difficult to diagnose as they have a more normal cutaneous and ocular pigmentation. Such patients usually have reddish or lighter hair and paler skin pigmentation than other members of the family, although all

pigmented with age. Ocular albinos have normal skin and hair pigmentation but markedly translucent irides. Skin biopsy, however, demonstrates structural anomalies in the melanosomes of these patients.

Apart from increased iris transillumination and hypopigmented fundi, albinos with ocular involvement have congenital nystagmus, a high incidence of squint and amblyopia, and a curious anomaly of the chiasm in which the majority of optic nerve fibres from each eye decussate. This neuroanatomical abnormality may help to explain the nystagmus and occasionally produces interesting field defects or pupillary abnormalities in the rare instances when albinos also have chiasmal lesions.

Fig. 9.13 An oculo-cutaneous tyrosinase negative patient with congenital nystagmus and a right convergent squint. Notice the white eyelashes.

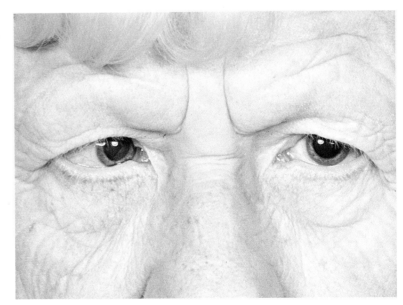

Fig. 9.14 Retroillumination of the iris through the pupil demonstrates the gross lack of iris pigmentation. Fundus photography in the same patient shows the lack of retinal and choroidal pigmentation. Large choroidal vessels are clearly seen.

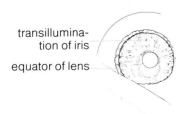
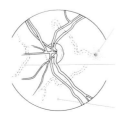

transillumina-
tion of iris

equator of lens

abnormal
macular reflex

prominent
choroidal
vessels

hypo-
pigmented
fundus

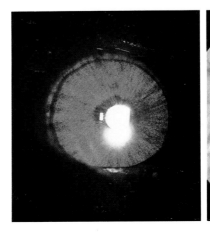
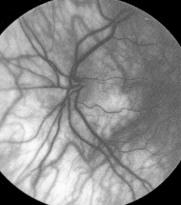

TUMOURS OF THE UVEAL TRACT

Uveal melanocytes are derived from the neural crest while other pigmented structures in the eye have their origins in the neuroectoderm of the optic cup. Malignant change in these pigmented structures is rare whereas naevi and melanomas form the most common group of intraocular tumours. The smooth muscle or vascular components of the uveal tract may produce a tumour on rare occasions but these are usually benign.

Iris Tumours

Melanotic tumours are by far the most common lesion but a variety of other primary tumours or metastases are occasionally seen in the iris.

Iris Naevi

Naevi are very common in people with light-coloured irides and are seen as flat or slightly raised localized swellings on the anterior iris stroma. Benign iris naevi are more common in neurofibromatosis. They are usually multiple and often have a pearly white or slightly pigmented appearance and are known as Lisch nodules. These are seen in most adults with the disease and are a useful confirmatory sign in making the diagnosis.

Iris Malignant Melanomas

Iris melanomas often arise from a pre-existing naevus and, while they may occur anywhere on the iris, the most common site is the pupillary area or mid-periphery. Elevation and distortion of the iris architecture are said to indicate invasion and malignant change but these tumours rarely metastasise. The tumours usually consist of spindle cells which have a slow growth rate and low grade malignant potential. Iris melanomas are comparatively rare, comprising about five percent of all intraocular tumours.

In the absence of angle involvement or glaucoma, iris melanomas can be left alone for many years. Spread towards the angle is treated by excision biopsy.

Juvenile Xanthogranuloma

Juvenile xanthogranuloma of the iris is a rare iris lesion seen in infants and usually presents with a spontaneous hyphema. The lesion is a histiocytic granuloma and is part of the spectrum of the histiocytosis X diseases which are non-malignant histiocytic proliferations that probably result from a defect in thymic regulation of T cells. Intraocular lesions are treated by local radiotherapy.

Fig. 9.15 Multiple iris naevi seen in a patient with neurofibromatosis.

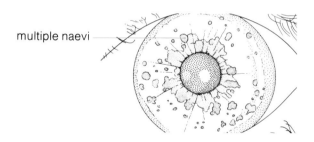

multiple naevi

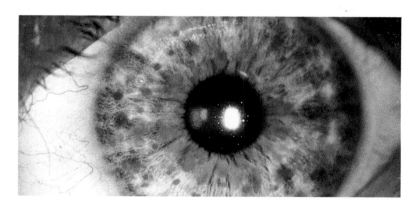

Fig. 9.16 More unusually, the neurofibromatos tissue forms a sheet on the iris stroma with traction on the pupillary margin producing ectropion uveae. (This patient had also had surgery for congenital glaucoma.)

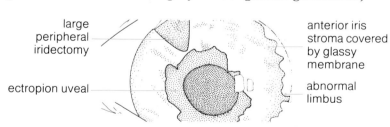

large peripheral iridectomy

ectropion uveal

anterior iris stroma covered by glassy membrane

abnormal limbus

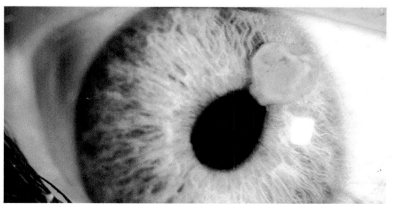

Fig. 9.17 An elevated brownish melanoma distorts the iris architecture and produces some ectropion uveae. This lesion had remained unchanged for several years.

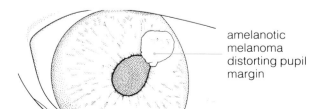

amelanotic melanoma distorting pupil margin

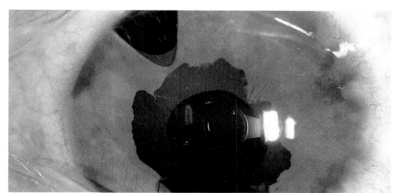

Fig. 9.18 Peripheral melanomas may arise from the iris but the ciliary body must be carefully scrutinized for posterior invasion or, alternatively, a primary ciliary body tumour extending anteriorly. Many of these lesions can be treated by a localized cyclo-iridectomy procedure.

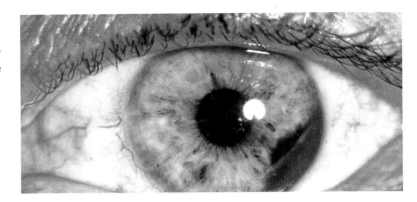

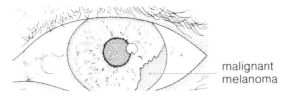

malignant melanoma

Fig. 9.19 Pathology of a surgically removed naevus shows that the anterior surface of the iris near to the pupil is slightly elevated by an increased number of heavily pigmented dendritic melanocytes.

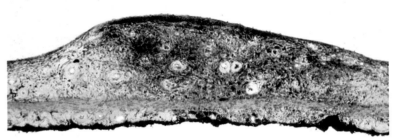

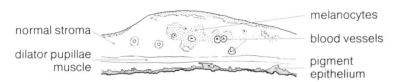

normal stroma — melanocytes — blood vessels

dilator pupillae muscle — pigment epithelium

Fig. 9.20 A yellowish raised patch on the iris typical of juvenile xanthogranuloma. The infant should be examined for other bony or soft tissue lesions of histiocytosis X.

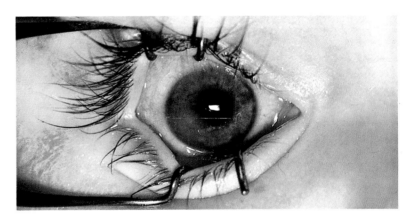

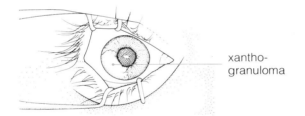

xantho-granuloma

CHOROIDAL TUMOURS

Melanotic lesions are by far the most common type of choroidal tumour and can be divided into benign naevi or malignant melanomas. The amount of pigment contained in both naevi or melanomas can produce a range of appearance which varies from a dense black lesion to virtually complete amelanosis. Both naevi and melanomas are much rarer in negroes, the incidence being 15:1, white to blacks.

Choroidal Naevi

Choroidal naevi are common and occur in about ten percent of the Caucasian population, most commonly in the posterior pole. They have a low malignant potential, the change to malignancy being about 1 in 5000 per year.

Fig. 9.21 Choroidal naevi vary in size and shape but typically have a slate-grey colour with well defined borders. About five percent are amelanotic. Multiple or bilateral naevi are often seen in neurofibromatosis. A diameter of over 10 mm, or more than minimal elevation of the overlying retina, suggests malignant change within a naevus.

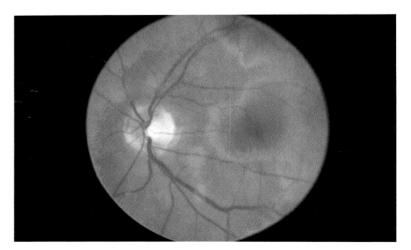

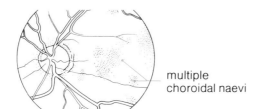

multiple choroidal naevi

Fig. 9.22 Drusen are frequently seen overlying a naevus and a small serous detachment is not uncommon.

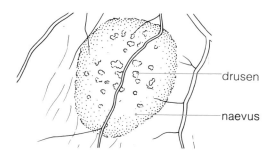

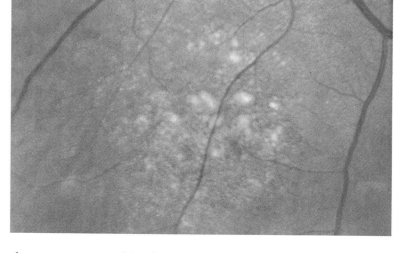

Fig. 9.23 The appearance on fluorescein angiography will depend on whether the naevus involves the choriocapillaris (producing choroidal hypofluorescence) and if there is a disturbance of the overlying retina producing leakage from retinal pigment epithelial

changes, serous detachment, or staining of drusen. This angiogram of the same patient shown in Fig. 9.23 shows early masking of choroidal fluoresence and staining of the drusen in the later stages. No intrinsic vascularization is seen within the naevus.

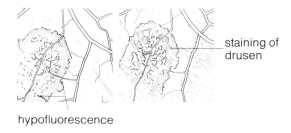

staining of drusen

hypofluorescence

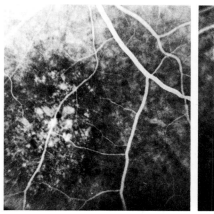

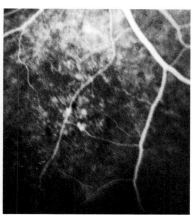

Fig. 9.24 Pathological examination of a donor eye shows an asymptomatic naevus in the equatorial fundus. Histology of the same specimen shows a thin placoid lesion (artifactually separated) involving the whole thickness of the choroid. The lesion contains plugs of densely pigmented benign melanocytes and which are covered by normal retinal pigment epithelium.

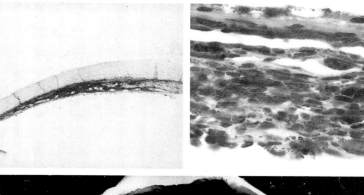

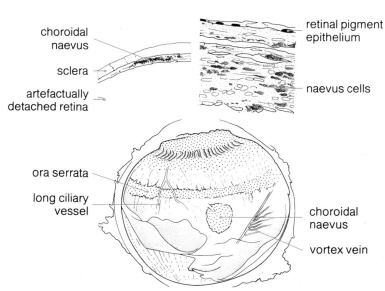

choroidal naevus

sclera

artefactually detached retina

retinal pigment epithelium

naevus cells

ora serrata

long ciliary vessel

choroidal naevus

vortex vein

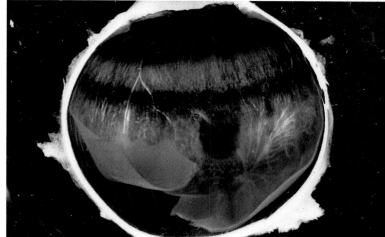

Choroidal Malignant Melanomas

Malignant change may arise in a pre-existing naevus or *de novo* in the choroid. Most patients present with loss or disturbance of vision from involvement of the retina or macula by tumour or subretinal fluid and, less frequently, with vitreous haemorrhage, absolute glaucoma, uveitis, or extra scleral spread. Some tumours may be discovered as a coincident finding on routine ocular examination. Unsuspected malignant melanomas are found in about four percent of blind eyes enucleated for other reasons.

Size, elevation, haemorrhage, significant serous retinal detachment, and especially documented growth all suggest malignancy (although choroidal naevi may be slightly elevated and have overlying serous detachment), and there is no substitute for fundus photography to document these changes. Orange pigmentation, thought to be lipofuscin, is seen frequently on the tumour surface and is helpful in making the diagnosis.

Melanomas must be distinguished from choroidal naevi, choroidal haemangiomas, metastases, pigment epithelial hamartomas of the disc (cf. The Optic Disc – Chapter 17), and choroidal neovascularization or haemorrhages.

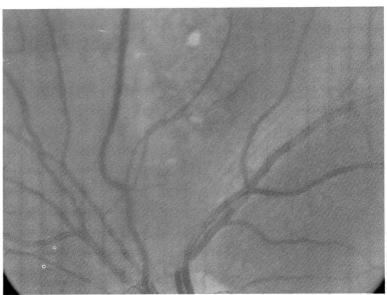

Fig. 9.25 Small or diffuse flat melanomas cause the greatest difficulty in diagnosis. This small slightly elevated lesion, just above the optic disc, shows orange pigmentation on its surface. This is thought to be lipofuscin derived from degenerating retina and is a helpful pointer to malignancy.

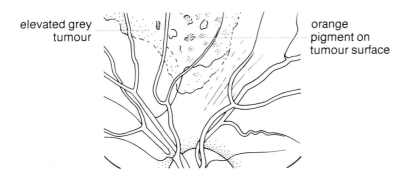

elevated grey tumour

orange pigment on tumour surface

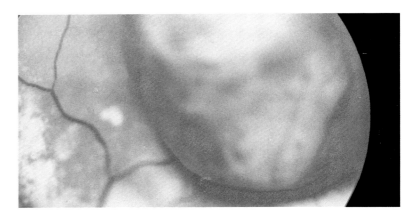

Fig. 9.26 More characteristically, larger melanomas tend to break through Bruch's membrane at a focal point to lie under the retina. This gives the tumour a typical 'collar stud' appearance, as seen with this rather amelanotic tumour.

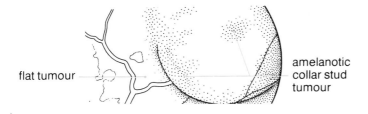

flat tumour

amelanotic collar stud tumour

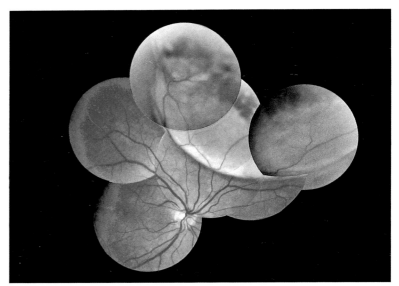

Fig. 9.27 This composite photograph of a large peripheral melanoma shows the collar stud appearance with haemorrhage on the tumour surface. Large choroidal vessels can often be seen within the superficial tumour substance.

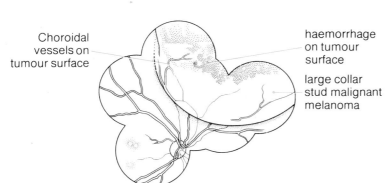

Choroidal vessels on tumour surface

haemorrhage on tumour surface

large collar stud malignant melanoma

DIAGNOSIS OF CHOROIDAL MALIGNANT MELANOMAS

Careful indirect ophthalmoscopy and biomicroscopy will usually diagnose a malignant melanoma although there is no substitute for clinical experience. Other investigative techniques such as scleral transillumination of the lesion, ultrasonography and fluorescein angiography are all of proven value in substantiating the diagnosis.

Measurement of tumour uptake of radioactive phosphorus (P32 Test) is used in some American centres. Melanomas normally produce a field defect since retinal function is disturbed over the lesion. This is not diagnostic as other lesions such as choroidal haemorrhages will also cause a field defect but such defects do help, however, in differentiating between small naevi and melanomas.

Fig. 9.28   Transillumination of a posterior segment lesion is an easily performed clinical examination. It is easiest if the lesion lies anterior to the equator so that the conjunctiva does not have to be opened. A bright light source is placed under the lesion which is viewed through a dilated pupil in a dark room, or alternatively, the eye may be illuminated through the pupil and the lesion viewed against the trans-scleral glow. Malignant melanomas do not transilluminate whereas other lesions such as choroidal haemorrhages or haemangiomas readily light-up.

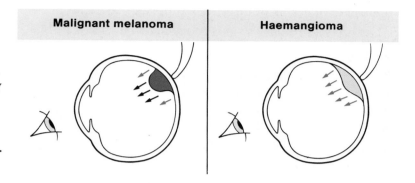

Fig. 9.29   An ultrasonic B-scan demonstrates a protruding 'collar stud' tumour in the posterior segment with a small low density area posteriorly within the mass. This acoustically quiet area is a common finding in melanomas and represents a more homogenous area within the tumour where cells are tightly packed and have little variation in density to reflect sound.

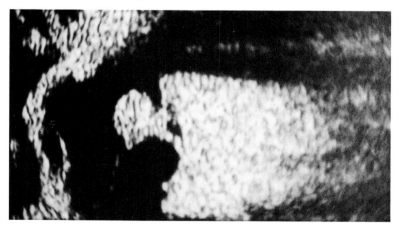

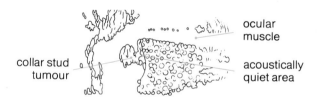

collar stud tumour — ocular muscle — acoustically quiet area

Fig. 9.30   Fluorescein angiography is a useful aid in documenting a malignant melanoma but the changes seen in the angiogram are not diagnostic. Typical findings are masking of background, choroidal fluorescence from involvement of the chorio capillaris, a vascular supply within the tumour and disturbance of the overlying retinal pigment epithelium.

The angiogram of the lesion shown in Fig. 9.26 shows masking of the background choroidal fluorescence with the spot of pigment epithelial atrophy shown as a window defect. In the arterial phase, areas of hyperfluorescence appear where the pigment epithelium is disturbed over the tumour and, in the later phases, these areas coalesce and stain fluid in the subretinal space. The degree of pigmentation within the tumour and its vascularity will vary from patient to patient and will influence the angiographic appearances.

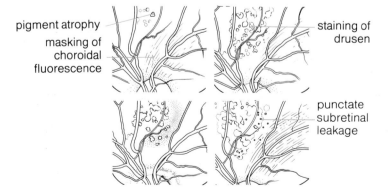

pigment atrophy
masking of choroidal fluorescence
staining of drusen
punctate subretinal leakage

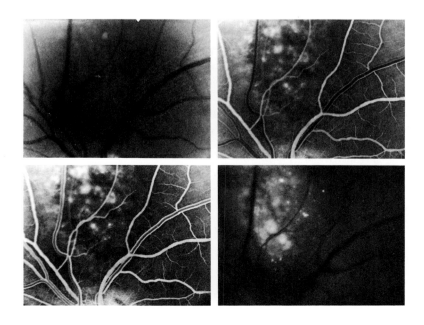

PATHOLOGY

Choroidal malignant melanomas consist of either spindle cells (types A and B), epithelioid cells, or a combination of these. These pathological distinctions are important as spindle cell tumours have an excellent prognosis (seventy-five per cent survival at five years), whereas the survival rate is lower for mixed spindle and epithelioid cell tumours (forty percent at five years), and pure epithelioid cell tumours (thirty percent at five years).

The size of the tumour is also important since large tumours have a worse prognosis, as do densely melanotic tumours.

Choroidal melanomas spread either by direct invasion of the sclera (especially along the vortex veins) or the optic nerve, and haematogenously, usually to the liver. The clinical presentation of diffuse flat tumours tends to occur at a later stage: such tumours are more difficult to diagnose and have a poorer prognosis.

Fig. 9. 31 The typical collar stud appearance is caused by rupture of Bruch's membrane, lying at the waist of the tumour. Clumps of pigmentation are seen within the tumour and the subretinal fluid stains eosinophils. Some serous retinal detachment is seen with almost all melanomas. An injection of the choroidal vasculature with fluorescent latex demonstrates the tumour circulation from the choroid of a similar collar stud tumour.

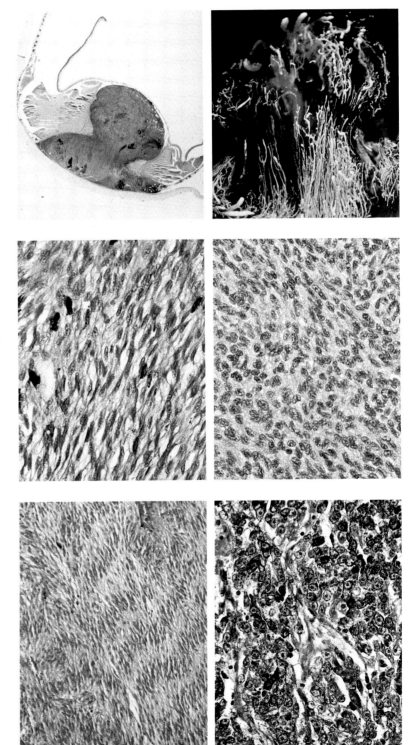

detached neuroretina

pigmented melanocytes

rupture of Bruch's membrane

choroidal vessels entering collar stud extension

Fig. 9.32 Spindle A cells (left) are characterized by a fusiform nucleus with a nuclear fold from infolding of the nuclear membrane with no nucleolus. Cell boundaries are indistinct and mitotic figures are rare. This cell type carries the best prognosis. Spindle B cells (right) are similar with indistinct boundaries but have a prominent nucleolus in a plumper nucleus. Mitotic figures are more common. The distinction between A and B cells is often arbitrary and tumours frequently have mixtures of both types.

Fig. 9.33 A fasicular arrangement of spindle B cells (left) is seen in some melanomas but this pathological finding does not appear to have clinical significance. Epithelioid cells (right) are noncohesive. Cell borders are distinct: the cells have abundant cytoplasm, large ovoid nuclei and conspicuous nucleoli. Mitotic figures are common. Pure epithelioid cell tumours are the rarest cell type but carry the worst prognosis.

Fig. 9.34 Mixed cell tumours are the most common type of tumour and consist of areas of epithelioid and spindle B cells juxtaposed to each other. Darkly pigmented tumours also tend to have a poor prognosis.

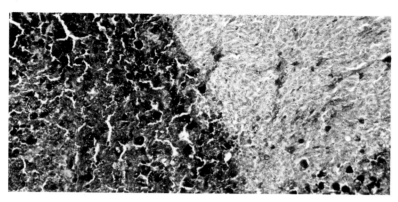

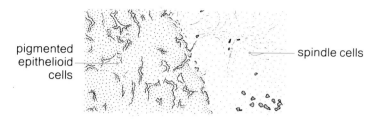

pigmented epithelioid cells — — spindle cells

Fig. 9.35 Scleral spread. A melanoma can be seen invading the sclera along the path of a blood vessel transversing the sclera.

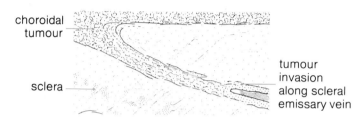

choroidal tumour

sclera

tumour invasion along scleral emissary vein

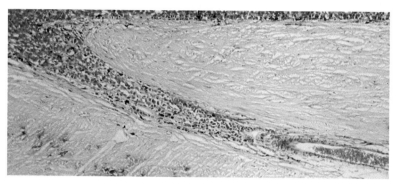

TREATMENT

The recent appreciation that some melanomas are relatively slow-growing and only metastasise late has led to a more conservative approach in their management. Standard enucleation procedures are followed by a peak in the death rate one-and-a-half to two years later and it seems likely that tumour cells may be disseminated by surgical manipulation of the eye at the time of enucleation. While eyes that have lost vision or have suspected optic nerve or scleral invasion should be enucleated, it seems safe to watch small lesions if the eye has useful vision until signs of growth are documented. Although C.T. scanning and ultrasonography will show macro invasion of the orbit, microscopic spread cannot be identified and the occasional melanoma will invade the sclera at an early stage. A reappraisal of the techniques of both localized excision or ablation, and the indications and method of enucleation, is currently under way.

Fig. 9.36 This ciliary body malignant melanoma has invaded the iris anteriorly and penetrated the sclera to produce hyperaemia of the conjunctival vessels. Scleral spread is usually accomplished either through the emissary vein or by direct scleral invasion. The eye was enucleated.

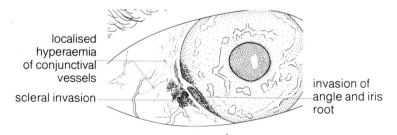

localised hyperaemia of conjunctival vessels

scleral invasion

invasion of angle and iris root

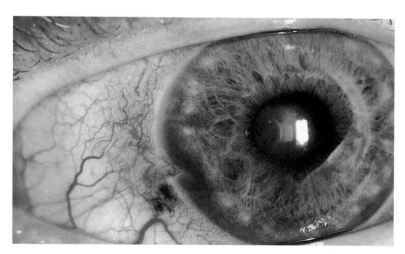

Fig. 9.37 Annual mortality rates from metastatic disease following enucleation of tumours of varying size. Large tumours carry the worst prognosis. A clear peak in the mortality rate is seen eighteen months to two years following enucleation and it is postulated that this is due to dissemination of tumour cells by surgical manipulation. Reproduced from L. E. Zimmerman et al, Ophthalmology *87* (6) 537-564 1980, courtesy of the Editors.

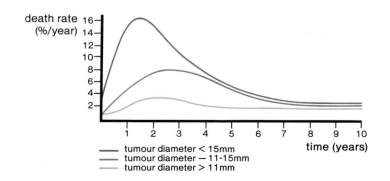

death rate (%/year)

time (years)

—— tumour diameter < 15mm
—— tumour diameter — 11-15mm
—— tumour diameter > 11mm

Choroidal Metastases

Choroidal metastases probably occur more often than is realised but, because of the short life expectancy of the patients, they are not referred for ophthalmic examination. The common primary sites are the breast and lung. Patients usually present with blurring or distortion of vision from macular involvement.

Metastases are frequently multiple or bilateral and usually have a slightly elevated appearance with rather indistinct boundaries. They tend to be relatively depigmented and to have less serous retinal detachment than a malignant melanoma. The growth rate is usually rapid. Globular or collar stud tumours with rupture of Bruch's membrane are uncommon. Most patients have a short life expectancy. Choroidal metastases are usually radiosensitive and this palliative treatment can improve vision by shrinking the tumour with absorption of subretinal fluid and so improve the quality of life during the terminal illness.

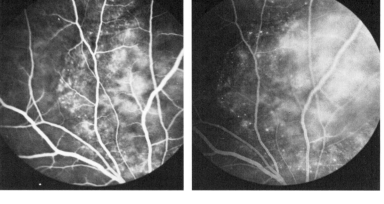

Fig. 9.38 These photographs show bilateral choroidal metastases in a patient with disseminated carcinoma of the breast. The tumours are slightly raised depigmented lesions with rather ill defined margins, invading the disc in the left eye. Serous retinal detachment is seen over both lesions.

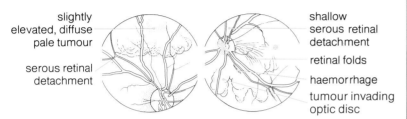

slightly elevated, diffuse pale tumour

serous retinal detachment

shallow serous retinal detachment

retinal folds

haemorrhage

tumour invading optic disc

Fig. 9.39 Fluorescein angiography shows changes similar to those seen with a malignant melanoma. There is masking of background fluorescence early in the run due to interference with the choriocapillaris. In the early arterio-venous phase, focal leakage of dye appears over the tumour and later forms pools in the subretinal space.

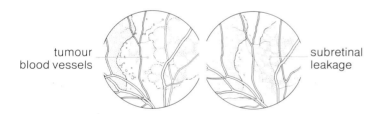

tumour blood vessels

subretinal leakage

Fig. 9.40 Occasionally, patients will present with an ocular metastasis in the absence of overt malignancy. Physical examination and systemic investigations demonstrate the extent of the disease. A radioisotope bone scan of the previous patient shows widespread disseminated 'hot' spots in the skeleton. Ultrasonography confirmed the presence of hepatic tumour deposits.

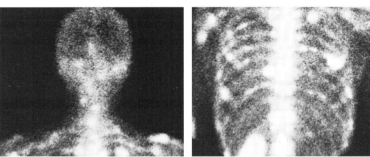

Fig. 9.41 Histology of another patient shows plump pleomorphic cells from a bronchial carcinoma invading the choroid. Bruch's membrane and the retinal pigment epithelium are still intact.

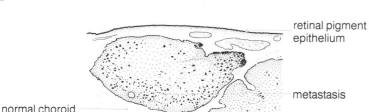

retinal pigment epithelium

metastasis

normal choroid

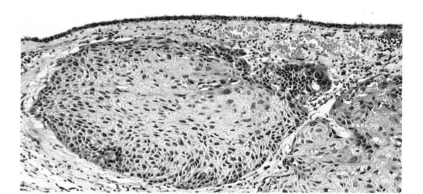

Choroidal Haemangioma

These occur as isolated lesions, or as part of the Sturge-Weber syndrome when they are associated with facial and meningeal angiomas, epilepsy, and glaucoma.

Isolated fundus lesions usually appear in the posterior pole as a focal reddish slightly raised lesion, with a width of several disc diameters. Overlying serous retinal detachment is common and frequently causes the presenting symptoms. Such detachment can be controlled, if necessary, by photocoagulation to the tumour surface. Choroidal haemangiomas are often

mistaken clinically for malignant melanomas but they transilluminate and have different appearances on ultrasonography and fluorescein angiography. Typically, fluorescein angiography demonstrates a coarse vascular pattern followed by diffuse leakage and localized mottling in the later phases. The vascular bed of the tumour is highly reflective to ultrasound.

In the Sturge-Weber syndrome, haemangiomas tend to be flat and diffuse, affecting the whole fundus and giving it a deep red 'tomato ketchup' appearance.

Fig. 9.42 A child with the typical naevus of the Sturge-Weber syndrome. Ocular involvement is said to be more common if the upper lid is involved by the naevus. Facial hemihypertrophy is a common feature, as in this patient.

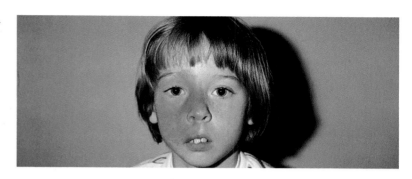

Fig. 9.43 This child was unusual in that he had a localized rather than diffuse choroidal haemangioma which is yellowish red, slightly raised, and involves the macula. Serous detachment is present. The vision was reduced to counting fingers in this eye. Fluorescein

angiography shows a diffusely even mottled appearance in the arterio-venous phase, which, in later phases, became coarser with areas of focal leakage and masking of fluorescence by the retinal pigment.

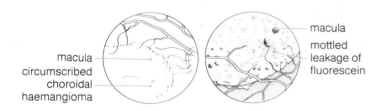

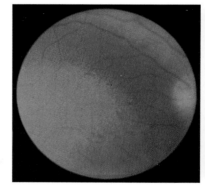

Fig. 9.44 ß-scan ultrasonography shows high density echoes from within the tumour due to the marked changes of tissue density.

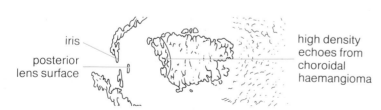

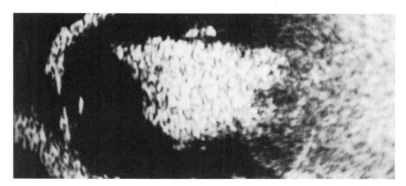

Fig. 9.45 C.T. scan of another patient with an intracranial angioma demonstrates meningeal calcification and hemicortical atrophy. The patient had epilepsy.

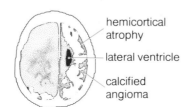

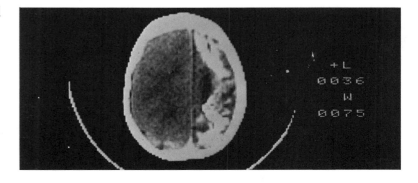

Fig. 9.46   Pathology shows large, thin walled blood vessels within the haemangioma. The overlying retina is degenerate due to accumulation of serous exudate in the outer plexiform layer.

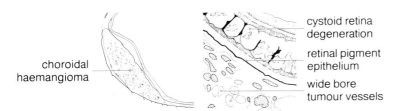

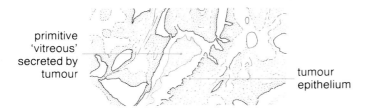

choroidal haemangioma

cystoid retina degeneration

retinal pigment epithelium

wide bore tumour vessels

Medulloepithelioma

This is a rare tumour of the ciliary epithelium which overlies the ciliary body, and is most commonly seen in childhood. The tumour tends to be benign or only locally invasive and has to be differentiated from a retinoblastoma or malignant melanoma of the ciliary body.

Fig. 9.47   Histology of a typical tumour shows a lacy network of polarized epithelium which secretes primitive vitreous. This appearance gave rise to the older name diktyoma (a network). Some tumours have a tetratoid change and may contain cartilage or muscle elements.

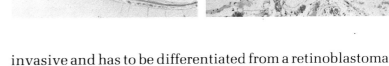

primitive 'vitreous' secreted by tumour

tumour epithelium

TRAUMA TO THE ANTERIOR SEGMENT

The management of ocular injuries requires the definition of the structures involved with the extent of their damage, and the management depends upon whether or not there has been perforation to the globe. Injuries to the posterior segment carry a poorer prognosis and are discussed in Chapter 12. Injuries to other structures in the eye are discussed in their relevant volumes.

Blunt Injuries – Hyphemas

Blood lying within the anterior chamber usually remains fluid and does not clot. Hyphemas are commonly seen following blunt injury to the eye and are the result of ruptures of the iris sphincter or recession of the iris root by the shock wave transmitted through the aqueous humour. There is usually an associated uveitis and ocular hypertension or hypotension, depending on whether the predominant effects of the trauma have been to obstruct the angle or damage the ciliary body and inhibit aqueous secretion (cf. Primary Glaucoma and Secondary Glaucoma – Chapters 7 and 8). Most hyphemas absorb over a period of days; patients have a substantial risk of a concomitant retinal dialysis or later development of cataract or glaucoma. All patients require gonioscopy and careful fundoscopy when the hyphema clears.

Occasionally, bleeding recurs from a hyphema a few days after the injury; this is especially common in children. Should this haemorrhage be severe, the anterior chamber fills with blood, the angle is obstructed, and the intraocular pressure rises to produce an 'eight ball hyphema' (a term from the days of musketry, graphically describing a hard black eye). In this situation, the high intraocular pressure forces degenerate blood products into the corneal stroma: there is also a risk of central retinal artery occlusion. The bloodstaining of the cornea will usually clear spontaneously over several months.

Fig. 9.48   Following a blunt injury, the anterior chamber is filled with a fresh hyphema that is settling to produce a fluid level inferiorly which, with rest, should absorb over a few days. The intraocular pressure needs monitoring and secondary uveitis, which contributes to the pain and redness of the eye, has to be controlled.

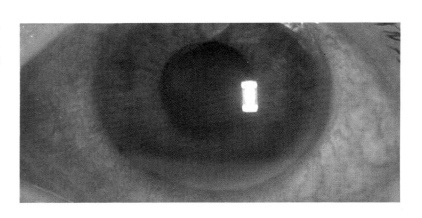

Fig. 9.49 Eight ball hyphema. This eye has suffered a severe rebleed with concomitant increase in intraocular pressure. These eyes present a considerable management problem. Operative decompression is difficult as the haemorrhage often clots, so inhibiting its removal and obscuring the view of the intraocular contents. Ultrasound is invaluable in locating the intraocular contents and is essential for a full assessment of the patient.

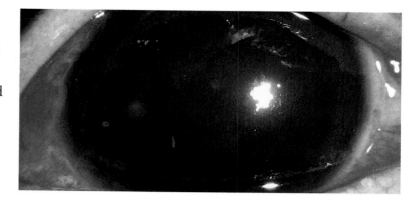

Fig. 9.50 Iris injury. Blunt trauma can cause a rupture of the iris root (an iris dialysis), which is usually associated with cataractous lens changes. Cataractous changes are not inevitable, however, as in this patient, a racing car driver, who was hit in the eye twenty years earlier by a flying stone. A localized lens opacity can be seen in the iris dialysis.

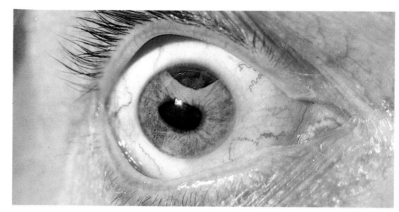

Perforating Injuries

Following perforation, the iris plugs leaks within the anterior segment where it appears as a sinister black nodule protruding in the wound. Unless it is replaced within hours, the uveal tissue rapidly becomes ischaemic and necrotic and must be excised. Delay in surgical repair rapidly increases the risk of infection and long-standing delay will increase the risk of sympathetic uveitis. The appreciation of these problems has led to the early repair of ocular wounds with complete microscopical exploration of the wound, excision of prolapsed uveal tissue, wound toilet, and accurate apposition of wound edges. Both

endophtalmitis and sympathetic uveitis are fortunately rare if ocular injuries are treated properly and promptly.

Wounds to the posterior segment prolapse the choroid and the vitreous gel. Some degree of vitreous haemorrhage is common and there is a substantial risk of early retinal detachment with severe wounds, or some time later in more moderate cases from vitreous fibrosis and traction. Ultrasonic evaluation and early vitrectomy are invaluable in salvaging visual potential for a number of these severely traumatized eyes (cf. Vitreous and Vitreoretinal Surgery – Chapter 12).

Fig. 9.51 A fresh penetrating injury from a broken bottle. The superior laceration involved the full thickness of the upper lid and the levator tendon. The globe is perforated through the cornea and extending into the ciliary body. Fresh iris tissue is prolapsed, and the lens has almost certainly been damaged.

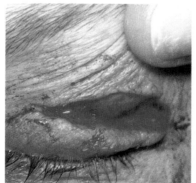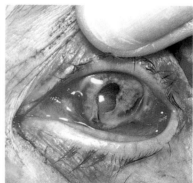

Fig. 9.52 This iris prolapse followed a burst corneoscleral section after cataract surgery. The iris is seen medially as a black nodule covered by conjunctiva, which usually contains prolapsed vitreous gel. Treatment lies in excision of the prolapsed iris tissue, anterior vitrectomy to clear the prolapsed vitreous from the wound, and resuturing of the wound.

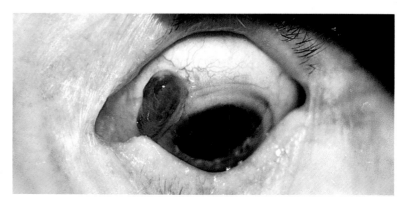

Sympathetic Ophthalmitis

Sympathetic ophthalmitis is usually seen in eyes with perforations involving prolapse of uveal tissue, especially if this has been present for any length of time. It is a rare and devastating complication of ocular trauma which has become much less common with the recognition of the need for prompt microsurgical repair of ocular perforations and the meticulous removal of prolapsed uveal tissue from the wound. The incidence is thought to be of the order of 0.1 percent of ocular traumatic perforations but this may have increased recently as vitreous surgeons have attempted to retain and repair more seriously traumatized eyes; very rarely the condition can be seen after a non perforating injury. Anecdotal evidence suggests that purulent endophthalmitis following perforation protects the patient from developing sympathetic ophthalmitis.

Frequently, the injured eye never really settles down following the injury but with the onset of sympathetic ophthalmia, both the fellow eye and the traumatized eye develop a granulomatous panuveitis. This usually occurs two weeks to three months following the initial event and the majority of cases have occurred within a year of injury. In rare situations, however, new cases have been reported to start many years later. Enucleation of the eye at the time of injury prevents the development of sympathetic ophthalmitis but once the disease occurs, enucleation no longer affects the course of events. Vision is lost in the fellow eye from cataract, glaucoma, macular oedema, vitreous opacification, and retinal detachment. The previously poor prognosis has been improved by intensive treatment with high doses of steroids and cytotoxic drugs.

The rarity of the disease with reference to the large number of perforating injuries seen, has still to be explained. The aetiology seems to be related to immunological sensitization to the retinal S or soluble antigen, which is released from the photoreceptors. Sensitivity to melanin pigment from the uveal tract does not appear to be important.

Lens induced uveitis (cf. Secondary Glaucoma – Chapter 8) results from auto-sensitization to lens protein, either as a result of trauma or surgery but, like sympathetic uveitis, the strange feature is the comparative rarity of the disease given the number of potential patients. Patients usually have a granulomatous anterior uveitis which can be distinguished from sympathetic ophthalmitis clinically or ultrasonically by the absence of choroidal involvement. In about twenty-five percent of cases, however, the two conditions co-exist. Removal of the lens, if feasible, cures the condition.

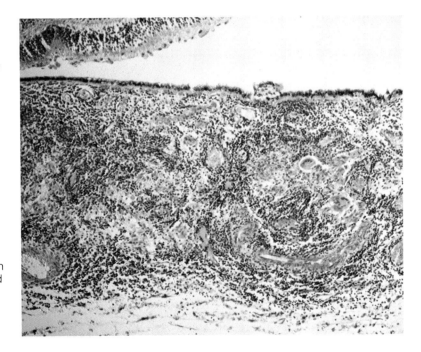

Fig. 9.53   The pathology of sympathetic ophthalmitis is the same in both eyes. This specimen shows granulomatous inflammation of the choroid with conspicuous multinucleated giant cells. On the surface of Bruch's membrane there is a small focal aggregation of metaplastic pigment epithelium (early Dalen-Fuch's nodule) and, while these are characteristically seen in sympathetic uveitis, they occur in other granulomatous types of uveitis and are therefore not diagnostic.

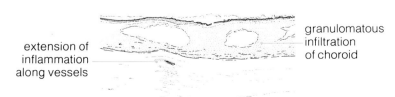

Fig. 9.54   This specimen shows choroidal granulomatous inflammation manifested by focal accumulations of histiocytes surrounded by lymphocytes; there is also some characteristic extension of the process along vascular channels into the sclera. Eosinophils are seen frequently within the lesion.

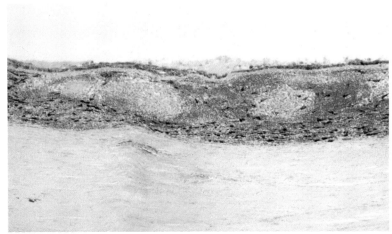

10. Intraocular Inflammation

D. J. Spalton

Introduction

The uveal tract consists of the iris, ciliary body, and choroid in continuity. Inflammation in this tract is known generically as uveitis. There have been many attempts to classify uveitis using clinical features such as the site of maximum inflammation, its rapidity of onset, or the appearance of the keratic precipitates (KP): an aetiological categorization has also been used which defines whether the uveitis is the result of perforating or non-perforating stimulus (exogenous or endogenous uveitis). None of these classifications has been entirely satisfactory and, while the aetiology of some types of uveitis can be diagnosed from their ocular morphology, little is known about the basic underlying immunological processes of any particular type. It is useful, however, in the management of each patient, to know the principal sites of inflammation, but as the uveal tract is one continuous structure it is not surprising for inflammation in one part to be associated with changes elsewhere. For example, a severe anterior uveitis can produce a cellular infiltration of the vitreous (some authorities would then term this an iridocyclitis), or a posterior uveitis can produce variable inflammatory changes in the anterior chamber. Inflammation throughout the eye is known as panuveitis.

The onset of the uveitis may be acute or chronic: acute inflammation produces pain and redness and photophobia, whereas chronic inflammation can occur in an entirely white eye. This distinction is not exclusive and the clinical appearance can change with time so that acute symptoms may be followed by chronic uveitis and *vice-versa*. Until fairly recently, granulomatous uveitis was differentiated from the non-granulomatous type by the appearance of the KP, being large, pale, and greasy (mutton fat KP) in granulomatous uveitis. This clinical classification is not really helpful as there is often a considerable overlap in the appearance of KP, and some diseases, such as sarcoidosis, may present with either granulomatous or non-granulomatous KP.

More recent concepts of immunology have highlighted the particularly unusual features of the eye. The avascularity of the cornea and vitreous and the physiological blood-aqueous and blood-retinal barriers normally isolate the eye from the general immune system and alter any ocular inflammatory response. Lens antigens are sequestrated from the systemic circulation in early foetal life and do not gain access to the systemic immune system in significant quantities unless there is damage to the lens and its capsule. The absence of ocular lymphatic drainage means that the afferent arc of the ocular immune response must occur through the blood and therefore stimulates the lymph nodes, liver and spleen indirectly. In some ways, the uveal tract can react rather like a lymph node, retaining immunocompetent cells from a previous inflammatory reaction (or from elsewhere), and then mounting a localized response when stimulated either as part of a generalized systemic response, or locally by a specific antigen. Damage to the ocular blood barriers or abnormal vascularization within the eye will result in a leakage of antigens into the eye, and the relative avascularity of the cornea and vitreous will then discourage their removal: such retention will stimulate and prolong the inflammatory reaction.

While uveitis is often thought of as a distinct entity, a secondary uveitis frequently plays an important role in many other ocular diseases and can be responsible for many postoperative complications. Uveitis will produce visual loss through damage to and loss in clarity of the ocular media, glaucoma from angle damage, defective secretion of aqueous humour resulting in hypotony, retinal or choroidal destruction, and neovascularization.

SIGNS OF UVEITIS

Inflammation within the eye produces damage to the vascular endothelium of the intraocular vessels with consequent breakdown of the blood-ocular barrier and exudation of leucocytes and plasma into the eye. The signs of this process within the eye will depend upon the region most affected, the rapidity of onset, its severity, and its duration.

Fig. 10.1 Ciliary injection is seen in its classical form as a dusky red circumlimbal vasodilatation in the area where the ciliary and scleroconjunctival circulations anastomose and reflects inflammation of the anterior uveal tract. Such an appearance is not necessarily always seen, however, and the condition is sometimes difficult to distinguish from the diffuse appearance of conjunctival inflammation.

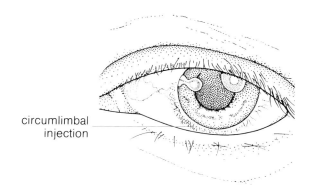

circumlimbal injection

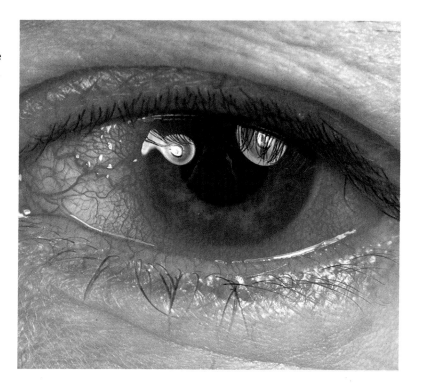

Fig. 10.2 Cells in the anterior chamber are a sign of active inflammation within the eye. They consist of clumps of leucocytes which have crossed the inflamed vascular endothelium to agglutinate and float within the aqueous humour. In the slit-lamp beam, they have an appearance similar to particles of dust in a sunbeam. They are best seen by a narrow high density beam directed obliquely across the anterior chamber.

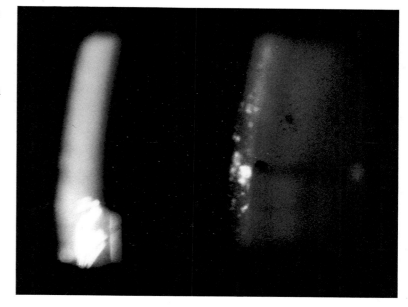

Fig. 10.3 A flare within the aqueous humour is the result of an abnormally high concentration of plasma proteins from the leaking intraocular blood vessels. It defines the slit-lamp beam within the anterior chamber rather like a car headlight cutting through a foggy night. A flare will usually be found in the presence of cells, although it often remains within the aqueous humour for some time after the cells have disappeared and then represents persisting vascular damage rather than active inflammation.

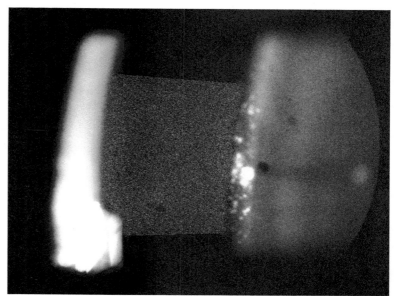

Fig. 10.4 Severe vascular damage, usually seen with really acute inflammation, infection, or following surgery, will allow even the largest plasma proteins to exude into the aqueous humour. Such exudation is manifested by fibrin which clots in the anterior chamber to produce the 'plastic' uveitis so typical of HLA B27 – associated acute anterior uveitis.

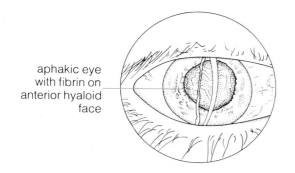

aphakic eye with fibrin on anterior hyaloid face

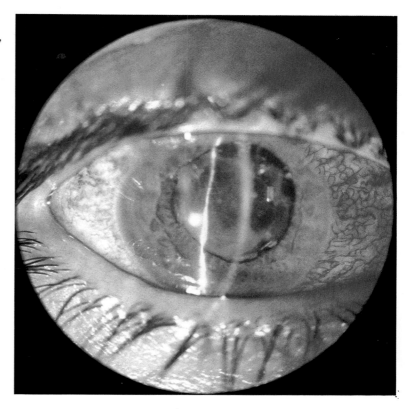

Fig. 10.5 Cells within the anterior chamber agglutinate and circulate through the aqueous humour to become deposited on the corneal endothelium. They are then known as keratic precipitates (KP) and are one of the classical signs of anterior uveitis. KP are typically seen in the inferior quadrant of the cornea, probably because of the effect of gravity and convection currents within the aqueous humour. They will, however, vary in distribution and number, and in size, colour and shape.

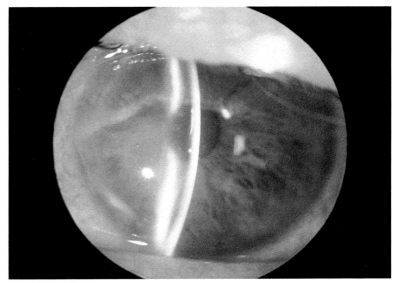

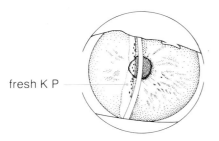

fresh K P

Fig. 10.6 With resolution of the uveitis through treatment or time, the KP either disappear or persist and become pigmented, so demonstrating their chronicity.

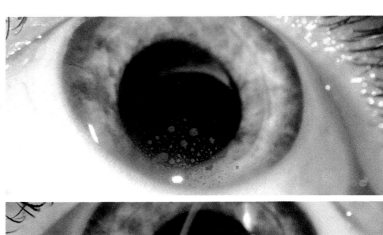

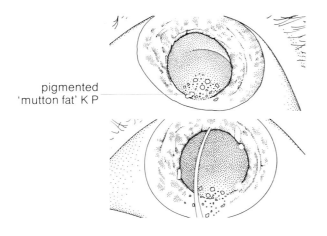

pigmented 'mutton fat' K P

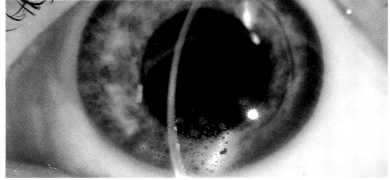

Fig. 10.7 Pathological specimens of KP consist of a mixture of leucocytes, polymorphs, macrophages and lymphocytes. Polymorphs predominate in fresh KP while macrophages and lymphocytes are deposited later. The time-honoured clinical distinction between granulomatous and non-granulomatous uveitis, which was made on the appearance of KP, was formerly thought to have aetiological implications. This is not necessarily so, however, and it is often difficult to make the clinical distinction: some diseases such as sarcoidosis can present in either way. The appearance of the KP more probably reflects differences in the antigen to antibody ratio.

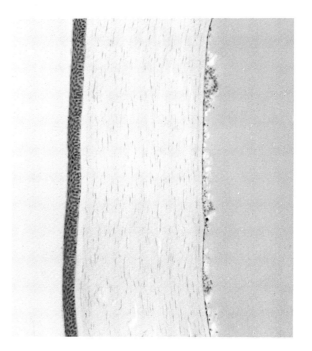

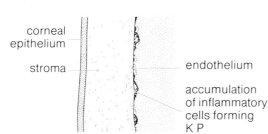

corneal epithelium

stroma

endothelium

accumulation of inflammatory cells forming K P

10.4

Fig. 10.8 A massive leucocytic response with an acute anterior uveitis can occur with precipitation of the cells as pus and is known as a hypopyon. This is typical of Behçet's disease, but is also seen occasionally with other causes of severe anterior uveitis. A retinoblastoma or reticulum cell sarcoma may sometimes present in this way (as, of course, does intraocular infection).

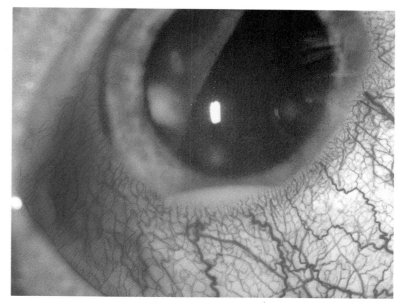

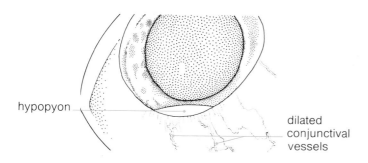

Fig. 10.9 Posterior synechiae are adhesions between the pupillary margin and anterior lens surface and always reflect a previous anterior uveitis. Pupillary dilatation retracts the iris from contact with the anterior lens capsule and prevents their formation. This is one of the objects of mydriasis in the treatment of uveitis which will sometimes break weak adhesions to leave tell-tale pigment on the lens. Ring adhesions will seclude the pupil and prevent aqueous humour flow from forming an iris bombé (cf. Secondary Glaucoma – Chapter 8).

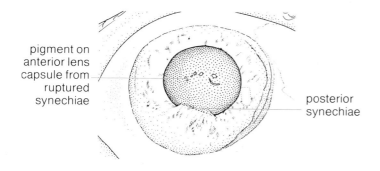

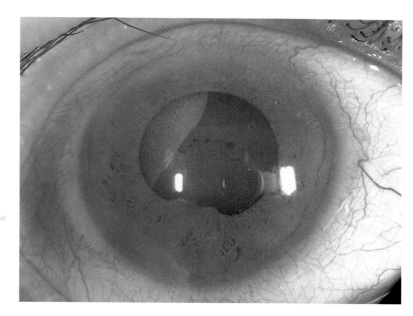

Fig. 10.10 Iris nodules are accumulations of leucocytes which lie on the iris surface. At the pupil margin they are known as Koeppe nodules, and on the anterior iris stroma as Busacca nodules.

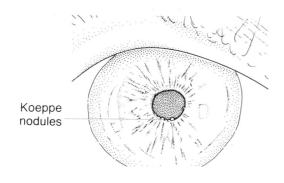

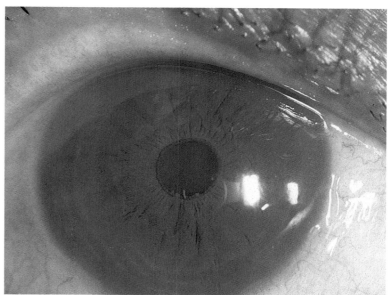

10.5

Fig. 10.11 Granulomas within the iris substance are seen occasionally. The iris of this patient with sarcoidosis appears swollen and thickened locally by granulomatous infiltrations between six to eight o'clock positions, with dilatation of the overlying blood vessels.

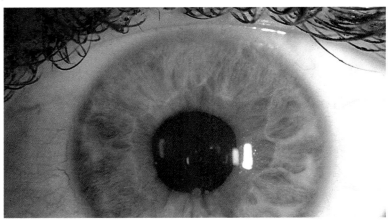

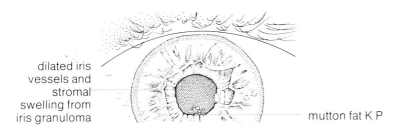

dilated iris vessels and stromal swelling from iris granuloma

mutton fat K P

Fig. 10.12 Posterior uveitis produces a cellular vitreous infiltration, analogous to the anterior chamber infiltration, but, because of the viscosity and structure of the vitreous gel, the cells tend to have a more restricted circulation. As a result of this limited circulation, cells are sometimes seen in localized areas – over the ciliary body, the optic disc, or a focus of chorioretinitis, for example. Cells may lie in small clumps, larger groups known as 'snowballs', and as retrohyaloid precipitates on a detached posterior vitreous face. In pars planitis (intermediate uveitis) cells lie inferiorly as a 'snow bank' over the pars plana and ora serrata. Persistent vitreous inflammation leads to collapse and detachment, with haze and debris in the gel.

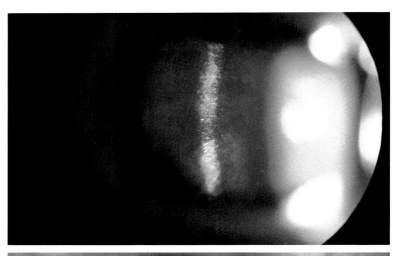

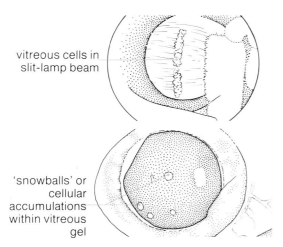

vitreous cells in slit-lamp beam

'snowballs' or cellular accumulations within vitreous gel

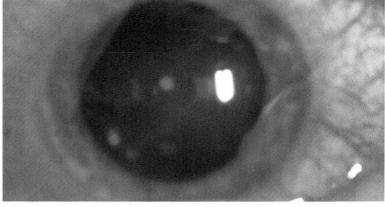

Fig. 10.13 Macular oedema can be seen with a posterior uveitis of any type or severity. While mild degrees can be compatible with normal vision, it is frequently responsible for loss of acuity. Depending on the duration and severity, it will resolve with the uveitis leaving a normal macula, or progress to cystoid changes and macular damage with persisting poor acuity. If the uveitis resolves, visual acuity may improve slowly over a period of many years.

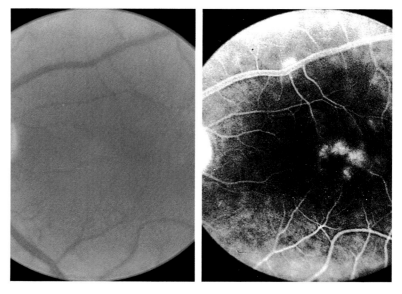

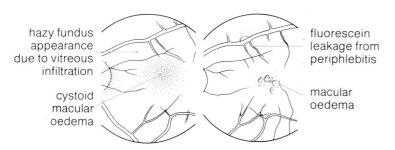

hazy fundus appearance due to vitreous infiltration

fluorescein leakage from periphlebitis

cystoid macular oedema

macular oedema

CAUSES OF UVEITIS

The causes of uveitis are legion, but it is helpful to divide them into three broad groups – those associated with known infections (e.g., syphilis, herpes simplex or zoster, toxoplasmosis); those with known systemic disease (sarcoidosis, Still's disease); and the largest group of all, idiopathic uveitis. For convenience, this final group is broken down into different morphological categories (e.g., acute anterior uveitis, pars planitis, heterochromic cyclitis), but many of these syndromes have broad overlapping clinical features and, as yet, many of these categories have little underlying immunological basis.

Acute Anterior Uveitis

The causes of acute anterior uveitis are numerous but, in the absence of systemic signs or symptoms, it is unusual to find a specific cause. It is therefore reasonable to restrict the initial investigation of a patient with idiopathic anterior uveitis to a routine screening of chest x-ray, blood count and erythrocyte sedimentation rate (ESR), plasma urea, electrolytes and proteins, with x-rays of the sacroiliac joints and syphilis serology where indicated.

The prevalence of acute anterior uveitis in a predominantly Caucasian population is about 12 per 100,000 population per year. The most common systemic associations of acute anterior uveitis in Great Britain are sarcoidosis, ankylosing spondylitis and Reiter's disease. These latter two conditions are very strongly associated with the presence of the HLA B27 tissue antigen. This antigen is present in about eight percent of a normal population and about fifty percent of all new cases of acute anterior uveitis. The way in which HLA B27 is linked to uveitis is unknown, although it seems probable that a linkage with other genes which control the immune response is the likely cause. Other factors must also be involved, since about twenty-five percent of patients with ankylosing spondylitis will suffer an attack of uveitis, whereas only one percent of the population with HLA B27 will be affected by uveitis during their lifetime. The presence of HLA B27 does not alter the clinical features of the uveitis but its presence correlates with the severity, uniocular involvement, and joint disease, especially in men. Considerable speculation has recently been given to whether there might be molecular mimicry between HLA B27 and bacterial *Klebsiella pneumoniae* antigens, (a normal bowel inhabitant).

Ankylosing Spondylitis

This disease predominantly affects young adult males but females can be affected in a male:female ratio of 3:1. Ninety-six percent of patients have HLA B27. Attacks of anterior uveitis occur acutely, usually in one eye, and are not related to exacerbations of joint disease or its severity, or any other known predisposing factor. The attacks usually subside over several weeks and, with treatment, do not usually produce residual ocular damage. Most patients can expect several attacks of acute anterior uveitis in either eye before the disease burns out in later life, but the degree to which any one patient is affected is extremely variable.

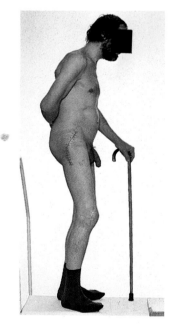

Fig. 10.14   This patient has the typical kyphoscoliotic posture of ankylosing spondylitis and has had a total hip replacement for ankylosis of the joint.

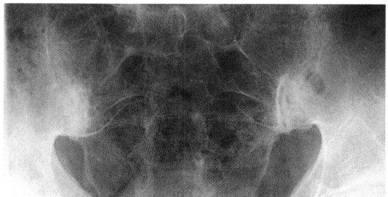

Fig. 10.15   The changes of ankylosing spondylitis are seen in their earliest form in the sacroiliac joints. There is sclerosis of the periarticular bone with narrowing and irregularity of the joint space progressing eventually to ankylosis. Similar changes are seen in the spine.

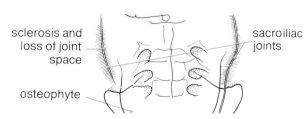

sclerosis and loss of joint space

sacroiliac joints

osteophyte

Reiter's Disease

This syndrome is a triad of arthritis, urethritis and acute anterior uveitis. Typically, a seronegative arthritis affects large peripheral joints such as the knees but the spine is also involved, especially the sacroiliac joints, and follows a few weeks after bacterial dysentery or a non-specific urethritis. Conjunctivitis and uveitis occur in thirty to fifty percent of patients. Other systemic features are plantar fasciitis and keratoderma blennorhagica on the penis, palms or soles of the feet. Aortic incompetence is rarely seen as a late complication. Males are usually affected, HLA B27 is present, and there is strong evidence that the disease is related to chlamydial genital infection if it follows a non-specific urethritis. Partial manifestations of the syndrome are common. Most patients recover over a few weeks but the arthritis sometimes progresses to chronic joint destruction.

Fig. 10.16 Typical keratoderma blennorrhagica of the penis.

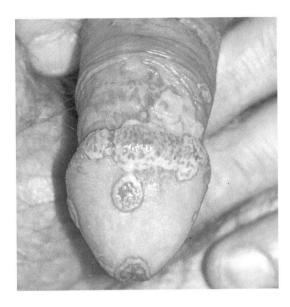

Herpes Zoster Ophthalmicus

Keratitis and anterior uveitis are common features of herpes zoster ophthalmicus and may occur independently of each other. It has been said that keratitis and uveitis are particularly frequent if the vesicles appear along the side of the nose – the cutaneous distribution of the nasociliary nerve which also innervates the iris and dilator pupillae – but this is not invariable clinically.

The uveitis is frequently acute in onset and coincident with keratitis, and usually persists for many months. Sector atrophy of the iris is commonly seen and is due to a vasculitis of the iris vessels: retroillumination of the iris shows sectorial translucency to advantage. Corneal anaesthesia commonly persists, ocular nerve palsies and optic neuritis are also seen occasionally, and post-herpetic neuralgia can be disabling in a minority of patients.

Fig. 10.17 Herpes zoster ophthalmicus with involvement of the nasociliary nerve along the lateral border of the nose. Cutaneous lesions may vary in severity from confluent vesicles to the occasional punctate lesion.

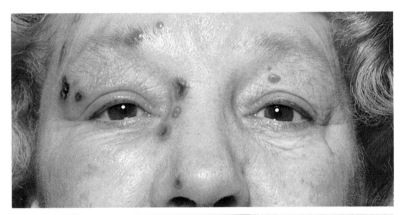

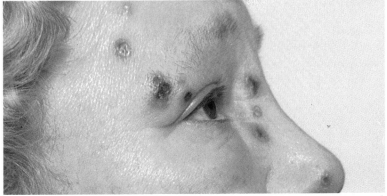

Fig. 10.18 Sectorial iris atrophy following herpes zoster uveitis. Retroillumination of the iris would show loss of iris pigment epithelium.

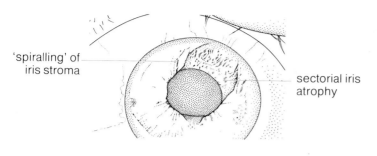

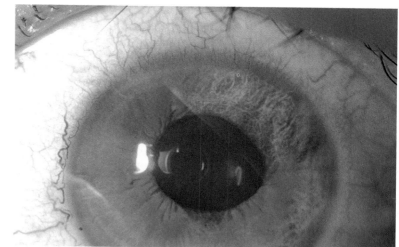

Chronic Anterior Uveitis

Still's disease is a seronegative arthritis occurring before the age of sixteen years. It frequently starts as a systemic illness with fever, a maculo-papular skin rash, and lymphadenopathy. The pauci-articular form, in which less than four joints are involved and which has an equal sex incidence, seems to be most commonly associated with a chronic anterior uveitis, especially if antinuclear antibodies are present in the blood. Knee, ankle and elbow joints are most commonly involved. The uveitis in these children is difficult to diagnose in its early stages and they require careful and frequent ophthalmological care.

Children with chronic iridocyclitis tend to have HLA DW5.

Vision is usually lost insidiously in an entirely white eye, from a chronic anterior uveitis which gradually produces cataract, glaucoma and eventual phthisis bulbi. Band keratopathy frequently develops during the disease and may be difficult to remove satisfactorily. Cataract surgery in these eyes has frequently hastened the visual deterioration but it now seems that concomitant lensectomy and total vitrectomy produce a much quieter eye and better visual prognosis.

Fig. 10.19 This boy has bilateral arthritis in the knees, ankles and elbows from Still's disease. Seen next to a normal child of the same age, he is below normal height due to treatment with systemic steroids.

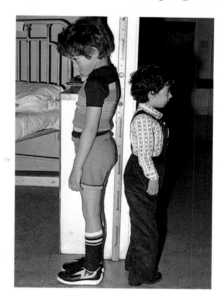

Fig. 10.20 This eye shows the typical features of chronic anterior uveitis in Still's disease. There is a moderately advanced band keratopathy with posterior synechiae and a dense cataract. There is no conjunctival injection.

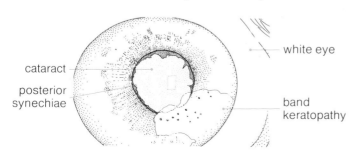

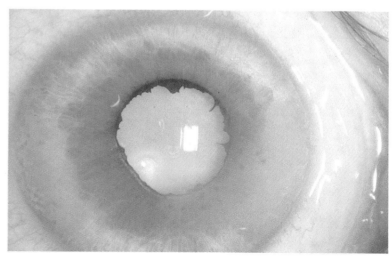

Sarcoidosis

Sarcoidosis is a multisystem disorder and causes about five percent of all cases of anterior uveitis, whereas ocular involvement is seen in about twenty-five percent of all patients with systemic sarcoidosis. About seventy-five percent of patients presenting with ocular sarcoidosis will have positive chest x-ray findings, bilateral hilar lymphadenopathy in the acute form, and pulmonary interstitial fibrosis in the chronic stage. Although the chest x-ray changes are good circumstantial evidence of sarcoidosis, the diagnosis should, where possible, be confirmed histologically by demonstrating non-caseating granulomas in biopsy tissue. To some extent, bronchial biopsy is superseding the Kveim test, although this still has its uses in the more difficult cases. The serum lysozyme and angiotensin converting enzyme are raised in patients with systemic sarcoidosis but appear to be an index of granuloma mass; their role as a diagnostic tool has yet to be fully assessed.

Anterior uveitis and posterior uveitis with retinal vasculitis are the most common features of ocular sarcoidosis. The anterior uveitis may be acute or chronic and either granulomatous or non-granulomatous. Patients should also be examined for granulomas in other common sites such as the lacrimal glands, lids or conjunctiva, where biopsy is easy to perform and readily confirms the diagnosis. A secondary glaucoma from trabecular involvement with granuloma formation and peripheral anterior synechiae formation is not uncommon.

Retinal vasculitis and posterior uveitis occur in the absence of anterior uveitis in a minority of patients. Typically, a creamy white exudation ('candle wax') is seen around equatorial retinal veins: more subtle changes are more easily seen on fluorescein angiography, which shows areas of segmental leakage along the retinal veins. This periphlebitis occasionally leads to vascular occlusion, peripheral vascular closure, and neovascularization, and this is the most serious complication of ocular sarcoidosis. Focal pigment epithelial changes are seen in some patients. Macular oedema contributes to the visual loss.

Optic disc swelling may result from local oedema, infiltration by sarcoidosis granuloma or, occasionally, from raised intracranial pressure with disease of the central nervous system. The finding of a vitreous cellular infiltrate in cases of obscure optic disc swelling is a helpful diagnostic finding which indicates a local ocular inflammatory condition and thus makes neurological investigations unnecessary.

The morphological appearance of Eales' disease (idiopathic retinal vasculitis) is usually similar to that of retinal sarcoidosis.

Fig. 10.21 Positive findings of sarcoidosis are seen on the chest x-ray of about seventy-five percent of patients with ocular disease. Trans-bronchial biopsy confirms the diagnosis. Pulmonary interstitial fibrosis is probably an indication for systemic steroid therapy, regardless of the findings in the eye, but hilar lymphadenopathy usually resolves spontaneously.

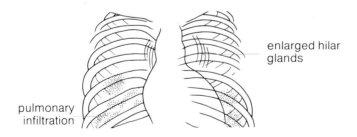

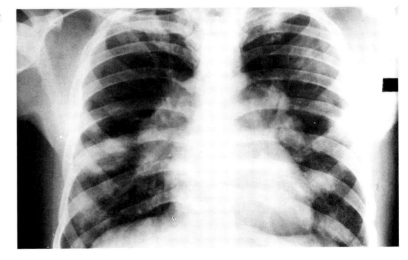

Fig. 10.22 Sarcoidal granulomas are seen along the lid margin and on the tarsal conjunctiva. Blind biopsy of normal appearing conjunctiva with multiple sections will sometimes demonstrate non-caseating granulomas, but the great majority of these patients will have more obvious changes elsewhere.

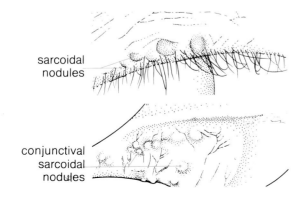

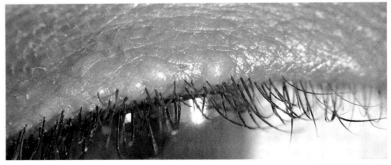

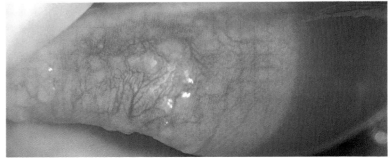

Fig. 10.23 Lacrimal gland infiltration is not uncommon. Sarcoidosis is particularly common in American blacks.

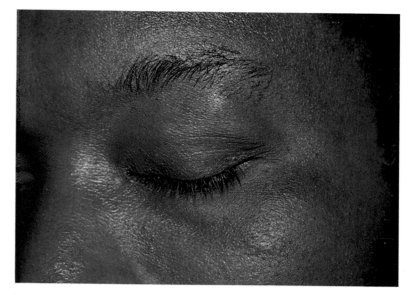

Fig. 10.24 Biopsy of the lacrimal gland of this patient shows multinucleated giant cells and marked granuloma formation without caseation. The patient also had infiltration of the external ocular muscles.

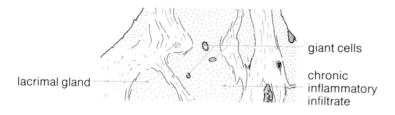

Fig. 10.25 'Candle wax' exudate around a peripheral retinal vein. Fluorescein angiography demonstrates the vascular leakage from the lesions.

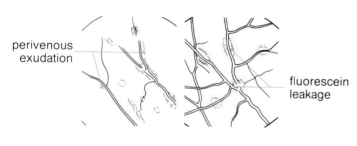

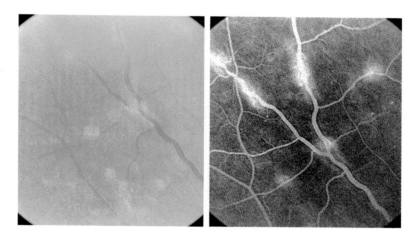

Fig. 10.26 Severe periphlebitis can lead to occlusion and peripheral vascular closure followed by neovascularization at the same site which, like new vessel formation from other causes, presents a serious threat to vision. The neovascularization is amenable to laser therapy, providing that intraocular inflammation has been adequately suppressed prior to photocoagulation.

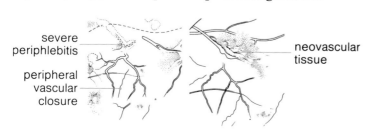

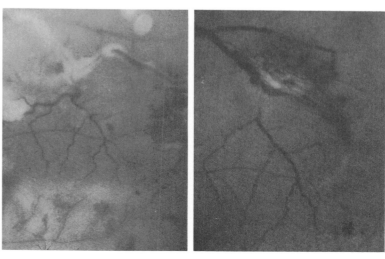

10.11

Fig. 10.27 Optic disc swelling with acute sarcoidal posterior uveitis. This is probably the result of a combination of infiltration and local oedema. The optic discs returned to normal with systemic steroid therapy without residual optic nerve damage. Cerebrospinal fluid was normal throughout.

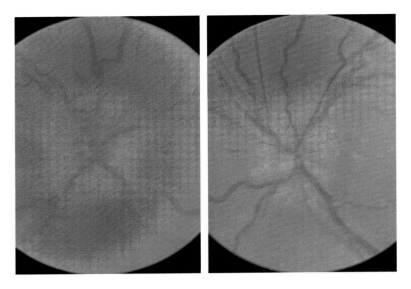

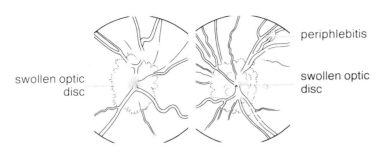

Fig. 10.28 Atrophic pigment epithelial changes seen in the posterior pole following resolution of sarcoidosis are due to granuloma formation at the level of the retinal pigment epithelium or choroid.

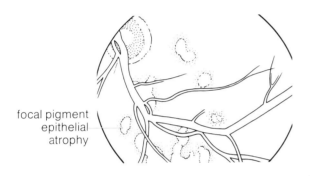

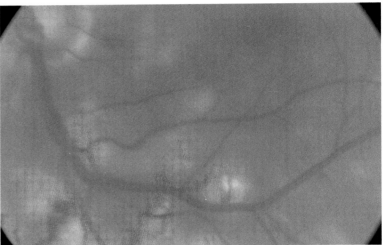

Behçet's Disease

This disease was originally described in males of Eastern Mediterranean origin but it is increasingly being recognized in less dramatic forms in females and in other racial groups. The diagnosis is always made on the clinical signs and is based on the triad of uveitis with oral and genital ulceration. Arthritis, erythema nodosum, skin pustules, venous thrombosis, and neurological signs are also seen. Ocular involvement occurs particularly if the patient has the HLA B5 antigen. Intensive treatment with steroids and cytotoxic agents has greatly improved what was previously an appalling visual prognosis. There is good evidence that Behçet's disease is produced by abnormal circulating immune complexes with abnormalities of phagocytosis; an underlying viral aetiology is suspected.

Fig. 10.29 Mouth ulcers are painful and episodic and cannot be distinguished clinically or pathologically from aphthous ulceration. Their presence often pre-dates other symptoms.

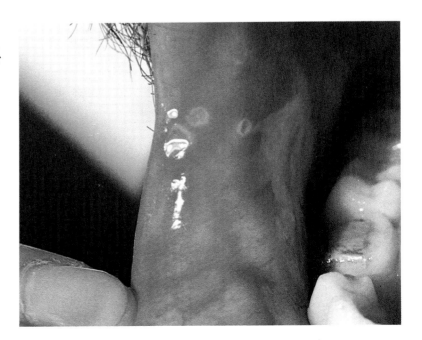

Fig. 10.30 Genital ulcers are not seen as frequently as mouth ulcers. This patient has active ulceration but white scars can be seen at sites of previous ulcer formation. Genital symptoms occur more frequently in males.

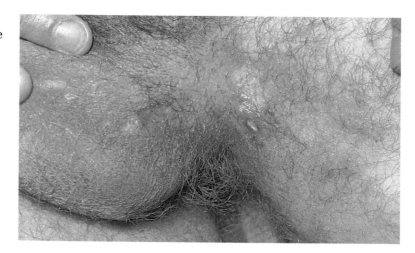

Fig. 10.31 Recurrent hypopyon is one of the widely recognised features of severe Behçet's disease with uveitis. It occurs with a brisk uveitis in eyes which are severely damaged. There is frequently some disparity between the lack of intensity of conjunctival injection and the intraocular signs.

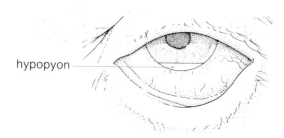

hypopyon

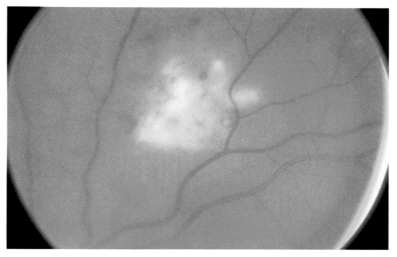

Fig. 10.32 The posterior uveitis of Behçet's disease is diffuse and may be asymmetrical or even unilateral. There is diffuse vascular leakage throughout the fundus: focal periphlebitis, as seen in sarcoidosis, is not a feature of Behçet's disease. This patient shows posterior uveitis with both optic disc oedema and retinal oedema in one eye: the fellow eye was normal.

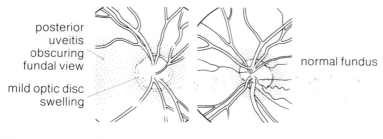

posterior uveitis obscuring fundal view

mild optic disc swelling

normal fundus

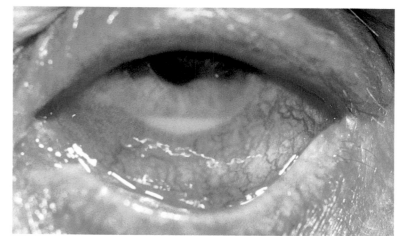

Fig. 10.33 White necrotic infiltrates of the inner retina sometimes with intraretinal haemorrhage, occur during the active phases of Behçet's disease. These resolve over a period of two to three weeks to leave a relatively undisturbed retinal pigment epithelium and retinal vasculature.

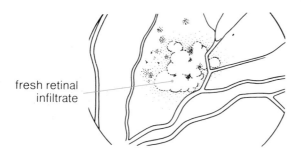

fresh retinal infiltrate

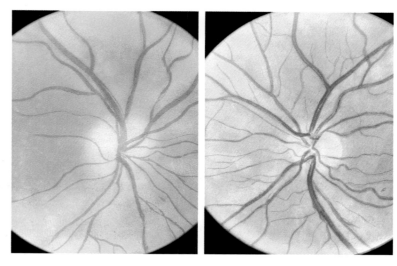

10.13

Fig. 10.34 Occlusions of major retinal veins are a feature of Behçet's disease and are frequently followed by neovascularization, as in this patient. A retinal infiltrate is seen inferiorly in the viable retina.

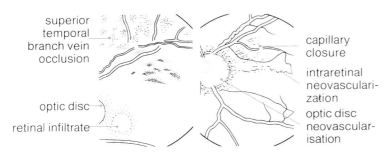

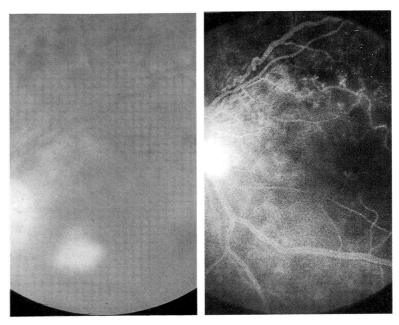

Fig. 10.35 Major vascular occlusions are seen elsewhere in Behçet's disease. This patient had an inferior vena cava thrombosis with a caput medusae due to venous bypass through the cutaneous veins of the abdominal wall.

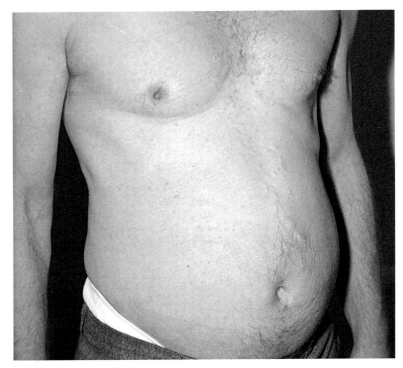

Fig. 10.36 In the terminal phase, the retina and its vasculature are destroyed with secondary optic atrophy the retinal arteries are then seen merely as white threads Although there is some disturbance at the macula, pigmentary changes are comparatively sparse for the severity of the disease.

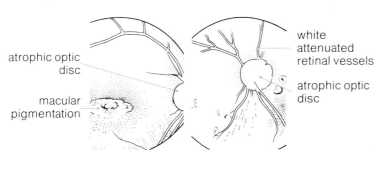

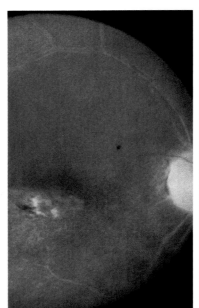

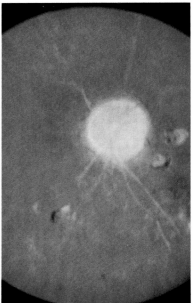

Toxoplasmosis

Ocular toxoplasmosis is virtually always of congenital origin, and ocular toxoplasmosis is one of the few specific causes of uveitis that can usually be diagnosed from the fundal appearance. The organism crosses the placenta during an acquired maternal infection of a non-immunized person and has a predilection for neurological tissue. The animal reservoir is in the cat.

Toxoplasmosis does not cause anterior uveitis in the absence of lesions in the fundus. Pigmented, circum-scribed scars are usually seen in the posterior poles of one or both eyes and visual acuity is lost if the macula or its axons are involved: field defects occur from lesions elsewhere. The parasite persists in an encysted state for many years following infection. The fundal lesions remain quiescent but have a tendency to become reactivated in adults between twenty and forty years of age, producing a fluffy white retinal lesion in the area of previous chorioretinal scarring with a posterior uveitis. If the lesion is small, vitreous infiltration may be localized to this area. The activity of the lesion subsides over several months with further retinal scarring. This reactivation appears to be due to a proliferation of toxoplasma organisms released from their encysted state by decreasing levels of host immunity. Many authorities recommend treatment with sulphonamides and pyrimethamine or clindamycin to destroy the organism together with steroids to suppress the inflammatory response.

A severe intracranial infection of a foetus can produce intracranial calcification, hydrocephalus, mental retardation and epilepsy. A positive toxoplasma dye test indicates previous infection with toxoplasma but does not necessarily correlate with ocular disease activity.

Fig. 10.37 This is a typical quiescent toxoplasma scar in the posterior pole. It is sharply circumscribed with retinal pigmentation and pigment epithelial atrophy. Note the associated nerve fibre defect.

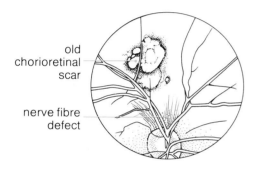

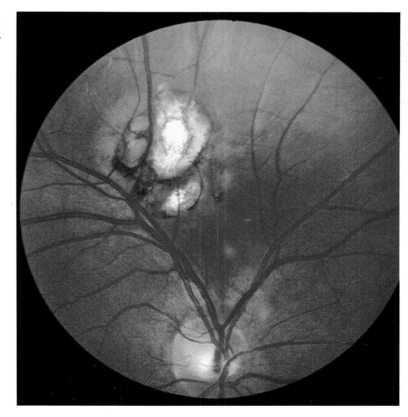

Fig. 10.38 The fellow eye of the same patient shows reactivation in an area of previous scarring. A few weeks later, after treatment, the fresh creamy retinal exudate subsided to leave further retinal destruction and pigment atrophy. The primary pathology is in the retina with secondary choroidal scarring. Note the associated posterior vitreous detachment.

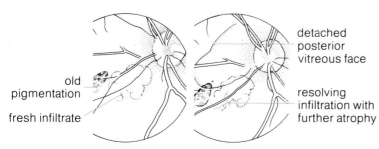

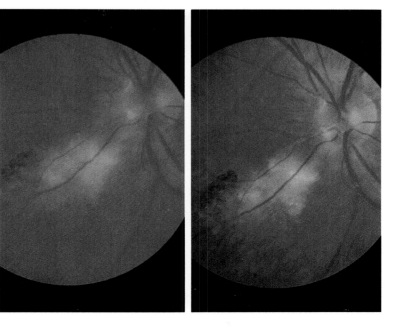

10.15

Fig. 10.39 Pathology of toxoplasmosis. The parasite remains encysted and intracellular in the retina for many years following infection as inactive bradyzoites. At some stage, possibly due to decreasing antigenic stimulus and falling levels of antibody, the cyst ruptures to release the active tachyzoites. These proliferate, and are then taken up intracellularly once again, so producing a necrotic retinitis.

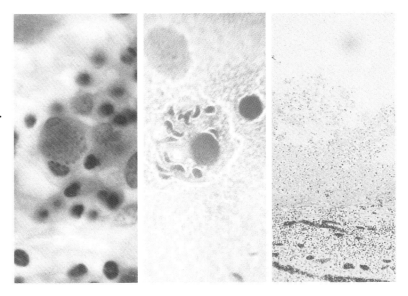

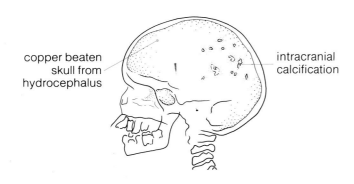

Fig. 10.40 Typical intracranial calcification seen in a child with severe congenital toxoplasmosis.

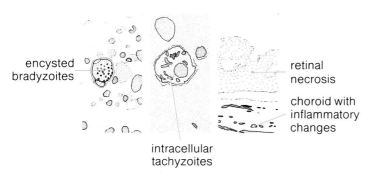

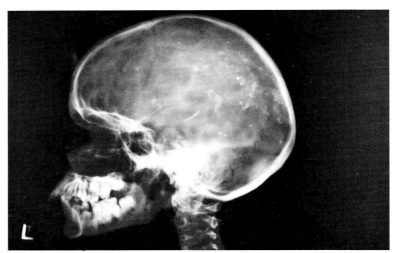

Toxocara

This nematode has its reservoir in dogs, especially young puppies, and the ova persist for long periods in contaminated soil: it infests the eyes of children, especially if they have a tendency to eat dirt. Ocular toxocariasis is produced in two forms – a massive exudative white lesion containing the nematode in the posterior pole, (sometimes presenting in a child as a poorly-sighted eye with leucoria), and a peripheral form with smaller white lesions in the equatorial retina with bands of retinal traction – the disease is usually uniocular. Affected eyes are white and inflammatory signs are confined to the vitreous gel.

A pulmonary infiltrate and transient eosinophilia is sometimes found in the acute stages of toxocariasis (visceral larva migrans): complement fixing antibodies are useful in making the diagnosis. An enzyme-linked immunosorbent assay (ELISA test) has recently been devised which is highly specific and sensitive and can be performed on aqueous humour.

Fig. 10.41 This is the fundus appearance of a three-year-old black child who presented with a six month history of unilateral non-progressive visual loss. There is a large white central granuloma present, with retinal traction. Visual acuity was counting fingers: the ELISA test was strongly positive and the family owned a young puppy.

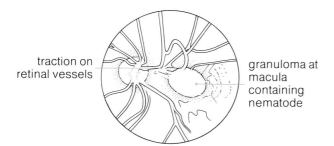

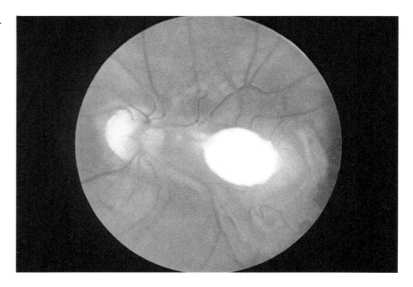

Fig. 10.42 Histology demonstrates a granuloma in the posterior pole of an infected eye. Serial sections and higher power demonstrate the encysted nematode.

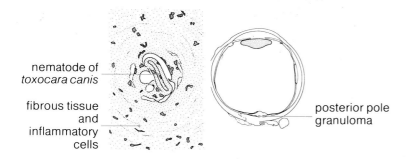

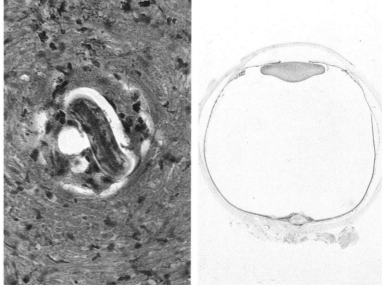

nematode of *toxocara canis*

fibrous tissue and inflammatory cells

posterior pole granuloma

Syphilis

Syphilitic infection during pregnancy infects the foetus and produces a retinopathy with a pepper and salt appearance of diffuse pigmentation and atrophy in the peripheral retina. Active lesions are rarely seen but are said to be focal yellowish spotty pigment epithelial changes with periarteritis and periphlebitis. Following congenital syphilis, interstitial keratitis appears between the ages of five and twenty-five years of age. Patients may have other stigmata of infection such as nasal and dental deformities or nerve deafness. Progressive neurological deficit, however, is uncommon.

Secondary syphilis, although rare, is again becoming more common and should be searched for in any atypical intraocular inflammation, whether anterior or posterior, both because of the ease of treatment and the serious sequelae of missing the diagnosis. The absorbed

fluorescent treponemal antibody test (FTA-ABS) is highly specific, and active infection can be distinguished from treated or latent infection by demonstrating IgM or IgG antibodies.

Secondary syphilis is usually associated with a typical cutaneous maculo-papular rash on the limbs and trunk, hands and feet. Acute iritis may be present with iris papules (roseata) and can be associated with a diffuse chorioretinitis. Inflammation may resolve to leave a picture resembling retinitis pigmentosa with arteriolar narrowing, disc pallor and pigment atrophy, and bone corpuscular intraretinal pigmentation. Visual fields and function are usually better than would be expected with a tapetoretinal degeneration and there is often more pigmentary atrophy than one would expect with an inherited retinal dystrophy.

Fig. 10.43 This patient was known to have had congenital syphilis. The optic disc is pale, retinal vessels are attenuated and there is widespread chorioretinal atrophy. The equatorial retina of the fellow eye shows large clumps of intraretinal pigmentation: these are larger

than is usually seen. Such patients often have surprisingly good visual function in spite of their retinopathy. Visual loss is usually due to the keratitis and subsequent cataract formation.

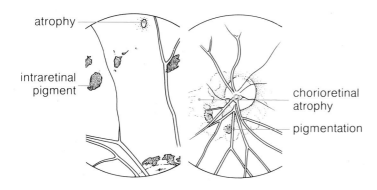

atrophy

intraretinal pigment

chorioretinal atrophy

pigmentation

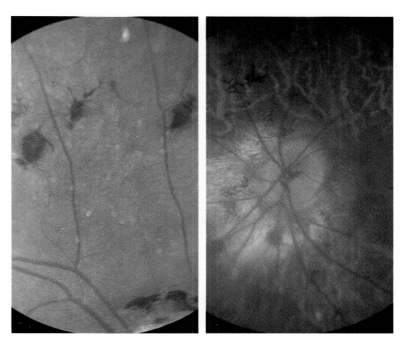

Fuchs' Heterochromic Cyclitis

This is a distinctive entity with many features atypical to any other form of anterior uveitis. The findings are of small diffuse KP scattered over the whole of the corneal endothelium with a fluffy or feathery appearance at their border, which is different from the usual well-circumscribed KP seen in other conditions. The eye is usually white. The superficial stroma of the iris has a characteristic moth-eaten appearance and becomes depigmented, having a bluish tinge in Caucasian patients. Fuchs' heterochromic cyclitis is usually unilateral, but bilateral cases are seen although they are more difficult to diagnose; it is the cause of a substantial minority of cases of anterior uveitis seen in a uveitis clinic. Posterior synechiae never form but glaucoma is not uncommon and is caused by a fine neovascularization of the angle. Cataracts are common and are hastened by steroid therapy, the indications for which are dubious in this condition. The aetiology is suspected to be some form of vascular degenerative process, possibly involving sympathetic nerve fibres and iris pigment.

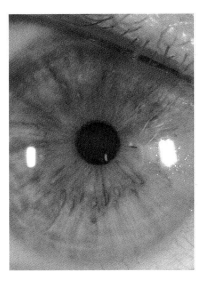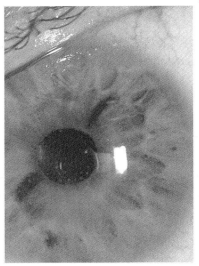

Fig. 10.44 The right eye of this patient is normal but the left shows depigmentation of the iris and fine K.P. on the corneal endothelium. Loss of detail of the anterior iris surface is seen and some lens opacity is present.

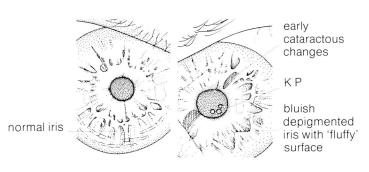

normal iris

early cataractous changes

K P

bluish depigmented iris with 'fluffy' surface

Intermediate Uveitis (Pars Planitis)

This is a definite but rather amorphous syndrome, the required clinical features of which vary considerably between different ophthalmologists. There is always a cellular vitreous exudate, especially in the anterior vitreous gel, together with the formation of 'snowballs' (accumulations of cells) which are usually seen inferiorly in the peripheral anterior gel.

A 'snow bank' or massive infiltrate is sometimes seen inferiorly over the pars plana and peripheral retina and, not infrequently, there is a mild peripheral periphlebitis, or small patches of peripheral pigment epithelial atrophy present. Macular oedema and mild disc swelling are common.

Pars planitis tends to affect young adults and is usually bilateral. Patients present with floaters (from vitreous debris), or blurred vision of gradual onset (from macular oedema), in white eyes. The response to steroids can be variable, but the condition tends to burn out over a number of years. Most cases have no apparent aetiology, but sarcoidosis, Crohn's disease, Whipple's disease and multiple sclerosis can produce similar pictures.

There is little pathology available on these eyes, but available material shows that the 'snowballs' are granulomatous in nature and that there is little uveal inflammation with more marked reaction in the retinal vessels and vitreous. The 'snow bank' is composed of collapsed vitreous gel with proliferating retinal astrocytes, sometimes with neovascularization.

Fig. 10.45 This fundus painting shows cystoid macular oedema and an extensive 'snow bank' inferiorly, more marked than is frequently seen. In the inferior equatorial area there are focal patches of pigment atrophy and vitreous 'snowballs'.

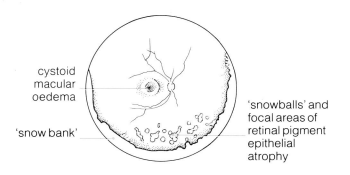

cystoid macular oedema

'snow bank'

'snowballs' and focal areas of retinal pigment epithelial atrophy

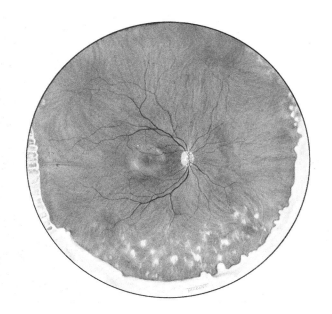

Fig. 10.46 This forty-two-year-old man presented with uniocular symptoms but had bilateral signs. The optic disc is normal, but there is wrinkling of the internal limiting membrane and a trace of macular oedema producing blurring of vision in this eye.

There was a low grade cellular vitreous infiltration and, inferiorly, 'snowballs' could be seen within the gel, in addition to a low grade periphlebitis of the equatorial retinal veins. The patient was systemically well and all investigations were normal.

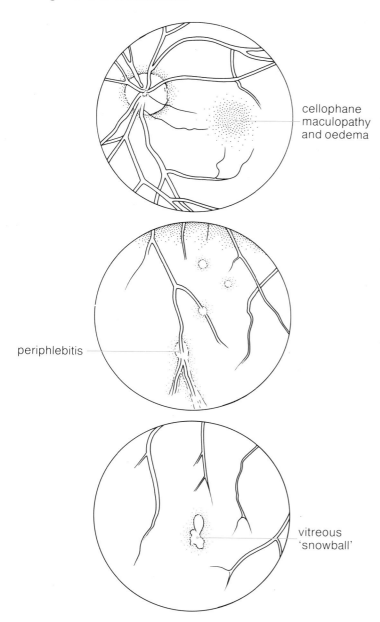

cellophane maculopathy and oedema

periphlebitis

vitreous 'snowball'

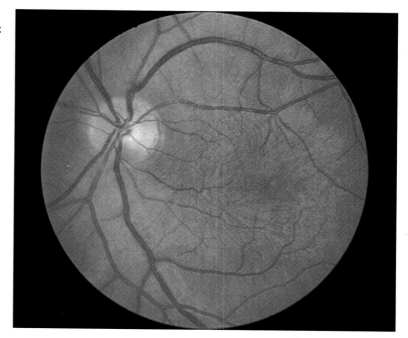

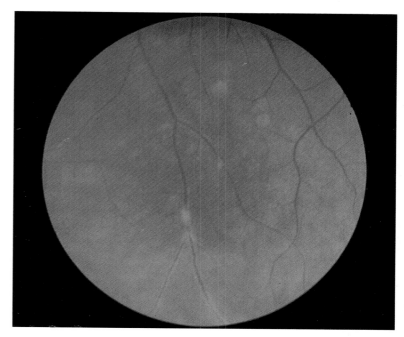

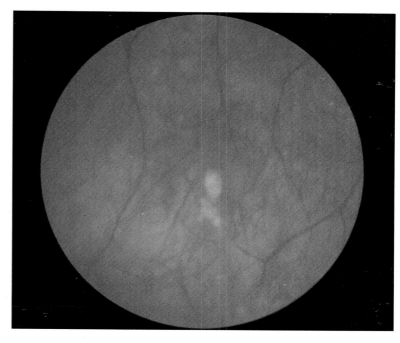

THE PIGMENT EPITHELIOPATHIES

Pigment epitheliopathies are a group of conditions where the primary pathology seems to occur in the retinal pigment epithelium or choriocapillaris. They are characterized by a deep, pale swelling of the pigment epithelium, which masks fluorescence early in the angiogram, with staining only occurring in the later stages. The lesions heal with scarring, and inflammatory signs can be variable. The aetiology is presumed to be either a vasculitic or ischaemic lesion of the choriocapillaris with infarction of the overlying pigment epithelium, or possibly, an immunological response directed at the pigment epithelium. It is not known whether the various varieties of fundus morphology and clinical presentation represent distinct conditions or different parts of the spectrum of the same basic disorder. Certainly, acute multifocal placoid pigment epitheliopathy, the Vogt-Koyanagi-Harada's syndrome, and sympathetic uveitis have morphological features in common and some patients seem to be hybrids of the distinct syndromes. While the milder types are usually restricted to the eye, systemic vasculitis can be seen with all types.

Acute Multifocal Placoid Pigment Epitheliopathy (AMPPE)

This syndrome usually occurs in young or middle-aged adults and is usually bilateral. There is often a history of preceding flu-like illness or respiratory infection which has been treated with antibiotics and it has been suggested that some type of immune reaction to a virus or these antibiotics may be the cause of the syndrome.

Patients present with blurred vision of fairly rapid onset. There is a vitreous infiltrate and a variable amount of acute anterior uveitis. Focal pale swollen areas, with a fluffy border of about half a disc diameter, are seen deep to the neuroretina and are thought to represent areas of oedematous and swollen pigment epithelial cells. These produce characteristic appearances on fluorescein angiography. The lesions are hypofluorescent early in the angiogram, masking the background choroidal fluorescence. At this stage, a large choroidal vessel can sometimes be seen within the lesion and this is thought to indicate blockage of the choriocapillaris circulation with preservation of the larger choroidal vessels, either through vasculitis or ischaemia of a lobular vessel. Later in the angiogram, the lesions leak and stain with fluorescein.

The lesions of AMPPE all appear and evolve in phase. Over two to three weeks, the acute phase of the condition resolves with subretinal pigmentary scarring and, usually, a return to near normal acuity. Treatment does not influence the outcome.

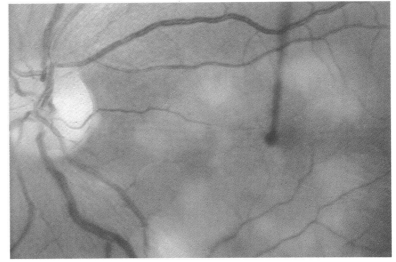

Fig. 10.47 Acute placoid lesions are seen as these typical creamy white subretinal lesions, about a quarter to a half a disc diameter in size and scattered throughout the posterior pole. In this patient there is mild serous retinal detachment with retinal folds at the macula.

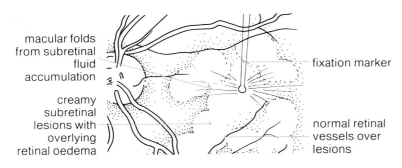

Fig. 10.48 Early and late fluorescein angiograms show the typical masking of background fluorescence in the early stages with later leakage and staining of the lesion.

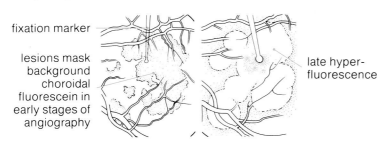

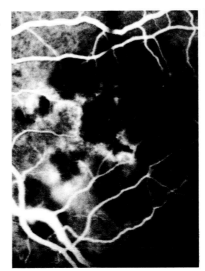
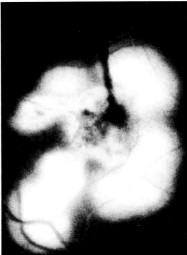

Fig. 10.49 Three months later, the acute lesions healed to leave irregular atrophy and scarring of the retinal pigment epithelium. Vision returned to normal.

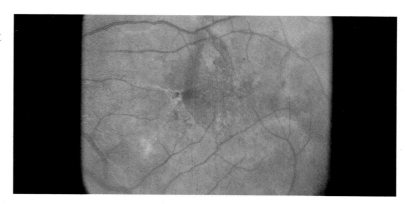

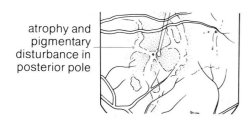

atrophy and pigmentary disturbance in posterior pole

Fig. 10.50 Fluorescein angiography demonstrates the extensive pigmentary disturbance.

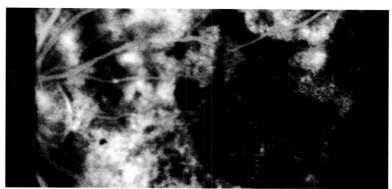

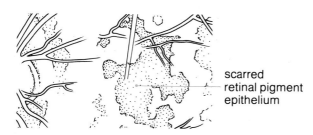

scarred retinal pigment epithelium

Serpiginous or Geographic Choroiditis

This condition usually occurs in middle-aged patients and is bilateral, although frequently asymmetrical, and the changes in one eye may precede the other by many years. The eyes are white and there is relatively minimal vitreous infiltration. The characteristic early lesion is an area of pale pigment epithelial atrophy in the posterior pole in the vicinity of the disc, which has a relapsing and remitting course. Relapses are seen as an area of greyish subretinal

swelling at the edge of a lesion which spread equatorially in a serpiginous fashion. In the active state, fluorescein angiography shows early masking followed by late leakage in the same area. The lesion resolves over several weeks with destruction of the overlying retina, to reappear elsewhere on the border at a later date. Visual acuity is lost if the macula is affected. No treatment seems to affect the course of the disease.

Fig. 10.51 Colour photographs demonstrate the typical fundus picture of this forty-six-year-old man who presented with unilateral disturbance of vision. There is extensive serpiginous scarring of the posterior pole in the right eye with atrophy and hyperpigmentation. Visual acuity was good as the macula was not involved, but the patient noticed a dense paracentral ring scotoma.

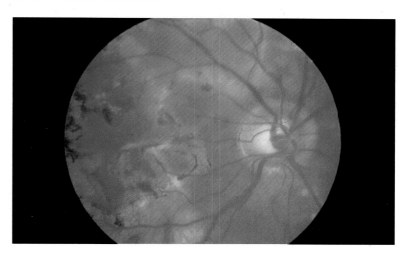

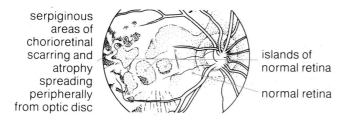

serpiginous areas of chorioretinal scarring and atrophy spreading peripherally from optic disc

islands of normal retina

normal retina

Fig. 10.52 The left eye was asymptomatic but early disease can be seen in the posterior pole.

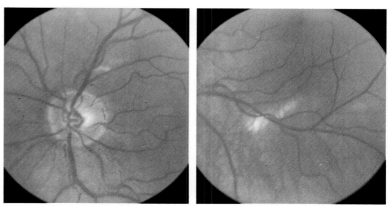

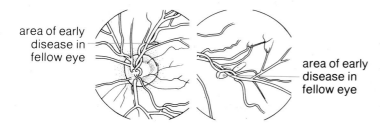

area of early disease in fellow eye

area of early disease in fellow eye

Fig. 10.53 A few months later, active disease can be seen at the periphery of an area of previous scarring in the right eye as pale soft white subretinal lesions.

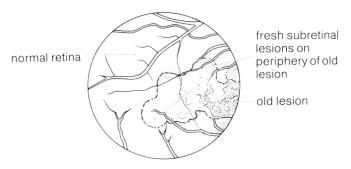

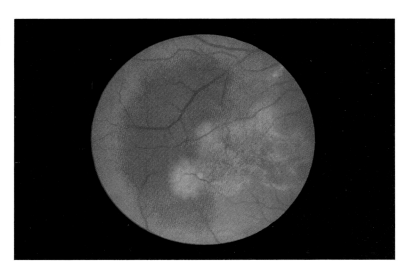

Fig. 10.54 A fluorescein angiogram demonstrates the extensive disease in the posterior pole with masking of background fluorescence by the new lesions.

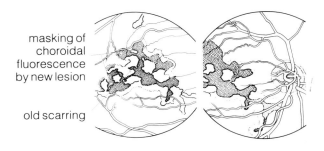

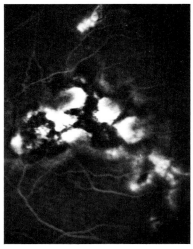
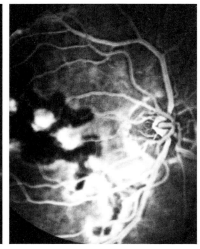

Vogt-Koyanagi-Harada's Syndrome

Harada's disease (posterior uveitis and cerebrospinal fluid pleocytosis) and the Vogt-Koyanagi syndrome (posterior uveitis, dysacousia and vitiligo) appear to be part of the same disease. The aetiology of the condition is unknown, but there is a strong racial influence, in that it is much more common in the Far East and accounts for six to seven percent of all cases of uveitis in Japan. Recent studies have shown a strong relationship with HLA D locus antigens and there are strong similarities to experimental allergic uveitis induced by the retinal 'S', or soluble antigen, located in the photoreceptor outer segments identified as rhodopsin kinase. Pathologically, Vogt-Koyanagi-Harada's Syndrome is similar to sympathetic ophthalmitis although the visual prognosis seems to be better. (cf. Chapter 9 – The Uveal Tract.)

Young or middle-aged adults are affected. There is sometimes a short preceding illness of headache and mild malaise or meningism. Both eyes are affected. There is always some posterior uveitis, but the amount of anterior uveitis can vary from minimal to severe panuveitis. Discrete and well-circumscribed retinal detachments of varying size are seen over the posterior pole with mottling and scarring of the underlying pigment epithelium. In the active stages, fluorescein angiography shows multifocal leakage through the pigment epithelium.

Patients usually respond to steroids. In the acute stages, patients may have pleocytosis of the cerebrospinal fluid and dysacousia which tends to recover quite rapidly. Alopecia, vitiligo, and poliosis may follow weeks to months later.

Fig. 10.55 This Indian lady has substantial vitiligo following the onset of the Vogt-Koyanagi-Harada's syndrome many years before. The only normal skin pigmentation remains on her cheeks. Poliosis of the eyelashes can be seen.

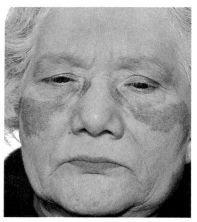
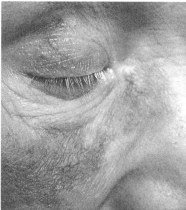

Fig. 10.56 In another patient with acute disease, there is mild optic disease swelling, localized serous retinal detachments with subretinal fluid accumulation around the disc and in the periphery of the fundus, and evidence of pigment epithelial disturbance.

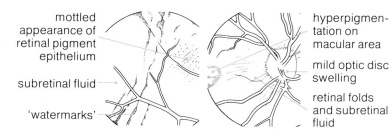

mottled appearance of retinal pigment epithelium

subretinal fluid

'watermarks'

hyperpigmen-tation on macular area

mild optic disc swelling

retinal folds and subretinal fluid

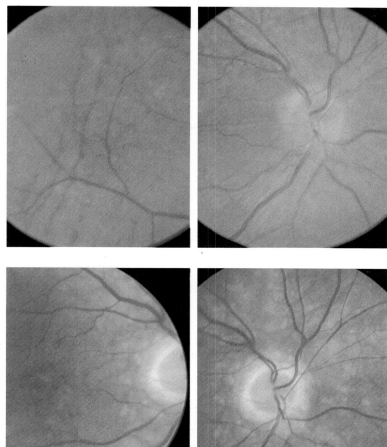

Fig. 10.57 Several months later and following treatment with steroids, the active inflammation and serous detachments have subsided, to reveal widespread scarring of the retinal pigment epithelium throughout the fundus. Vision returned to normal. Relapses and further episodes of uveitis are not uncommon.

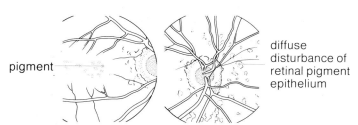

pigment

diffuse disturbance of retinal pigment epithelium

PRESUMED OCULAR HISTOPLASMOSIS SYNDROME

This is a rather poor name for a syndrome similar to that seen in the United States of America, which is due to infection of the choroid by the *histoplasmosis capsulatum* yeast. This organism is not found in Britain, but eyes are occasionally seen with an identical fundal appearance, presumably due to infection by a similar but unknown organism. Affected eyes are white and without vitreous infiltrate. The condition is usually bilateral.

The components of the syndrome are peripapillary atrophy and punctate pigmented or atrophic lesions in the posterior pole and equatorial retina. Acuity is lost from disciform degeneration, which arises from scars in the macular area. This is particularly tragic as the disease is most common in active middle-age.

Experimental work in animals with histoplasma capsulatum shows that injection of organisms is followed by transient fungaemia and is associated with a variable degree of clinical or subclinical systemic disease. The fungaemia clears over three to four weeks. Small inflammatory foci are left within the choroid, with or without overlying change in the retinal pigment epithelium. Although these foci do not contain active organisms, the inflammatory cells can be reactivated at a later date by some non-specific response to produce further changes in the previously normal overlying retinal pigment epithelium. If these occur in the macular area, there is a substantial risk of stimulating choroidal neovascularization and a disciform scar.

Fig. 10.58 Peripapillary atrophy and typical punctate lesions are seen in the right eye of a patient with a disciform neovascular scar at the macula.

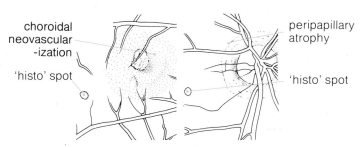

choroidal neovascular-ization

'histo' spot

peripapillary atrophy

'histo' spot

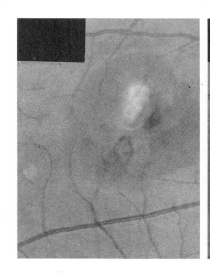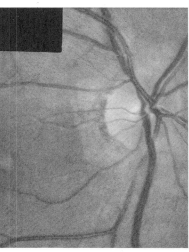

Fig. 10.59 A photograph of another patient shows fibrosis under the macula, pigmentation and atrophy around the disc, and punctate atrophic areas nasal to the disc. Similar lesions but without disciform changes, are seen around the left macula. This eye has a substantial risk of developing a disciform lesion at a later date.

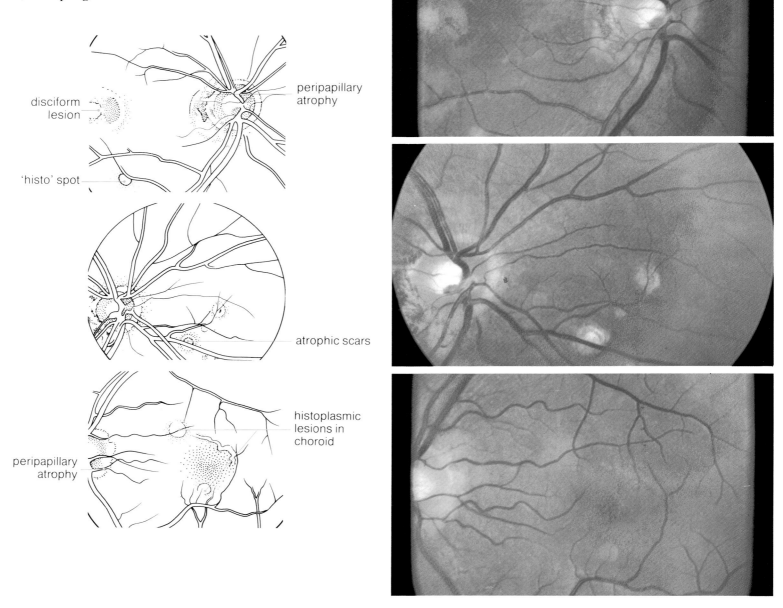

11. The Lens

N. A. Phelps Brown

THE NORMAL LENS, ITS DEVELOPMENT AND AGEING

The normal lens contains about sixty-five percent water, thirty-five percent protein and traces of minerals common to other body tissues. The protein is of two categories – the insoluble albuminoid (denatured protein that increases with age), and the soluble crystallines α, β, and γ which are found in varying concentrations within different areas of the lens. Lens proteins are organ specific but not species specific. Glucose metabolism is conducted via anaerobic pathways. If a slit lamp beam is used to transilluminate the lens, the beam is broken up into a number of zones or bands of differing brightness. The zones categorize the various parts of the lens although they do not necessarily correspond with the surgical anatomy.

Fig.11.1 The lens placode differentiates from the surface ectoderm at the 4mm stage (about three weeks after conception). By 14mm (six weeks) it has separated from the surface ectoderm to form the lens vesicle and the embryonic lens nucleus then begins to form. The lens is supported by the tunica vasculosa lentis, which is derived from the hyaloid vascular system. This blood supply is fully formed by three months gestation, after which it begins to atrophy, and has disappeared by the end of the seventh month of gestation.

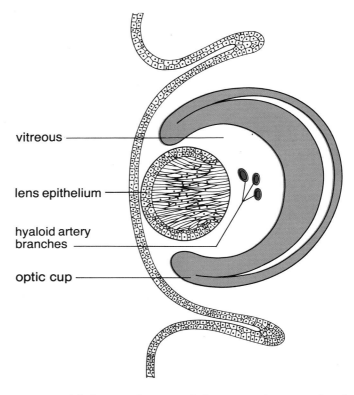

vitreous

lens epithelium

hyaloid artery branches

optic cup

Fig.11.2 In the normal lens, the zones or bands of discontinuity between the fibres are most evident around the age of forty-five years. These zones are not static features like the growth rings of a tree trunk, but can be likened more to the waves or ripples in a stream. The lens fibres comprising each zone are continuously being pushed centrally by the formation of new fibres under the capsule and so form the nucleus. In youth, the nucleus is more flexible than the cortex, but it becomes harder than the cortex with increasing age. It is convenient to take the dividing line between cortex and nucleus as the point of sudden reduction in brightness of the slit image view. There is no colour difference between anterior and posterior cortex although the anterior cortex appears blue as the shorter wavelengths of light are the first to be scattered. Other constant features are the subcapsular clear zone and zone of disjunction.

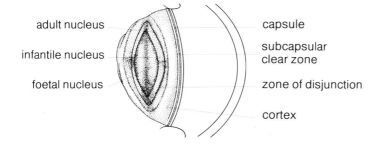

adult nucleus

infantile nucleus

foetal nucleus

capsule

subcapsular clear zone

zone of disjunction

cortex

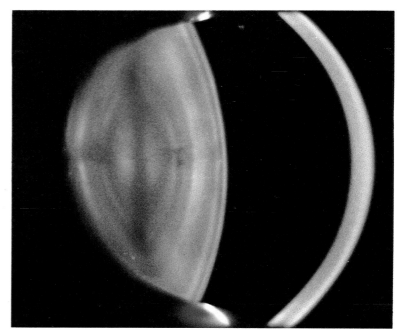

Fig.11.3   In this ten-year-old child, the lens is composed largely of nucleus, the cortex being represented only by a thin bright band. The rate of growth in the width of the lens is linear from the age of ten years. The observed growth is the sum of growth processes by surface accretion and central compaction. If growth ceases, for any reason, compaction continues and contributes to the small lens size often observed in cataract (cf. Fig.11.5).

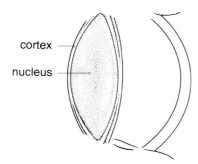

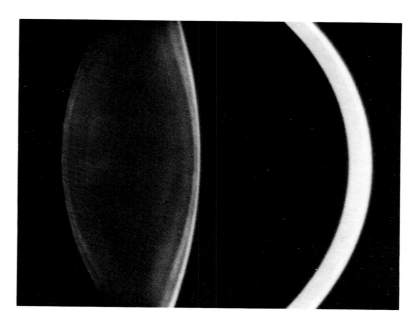

Fig.11.4   The lens in the aged is greatly increased in sagittal width compared with that in childhood.
This increase is due almost entirely to growth of the cortex with the nucleus remaining almost unchanged.
The scattering properties of the lens are greatly increased in the elderly so that it appears to be brighter. The radii of curvature of its surfaces, particularly the anterior surface are reduced so that the lens becomes more convex (it was formerly believed that the lens became flatter on ageing).

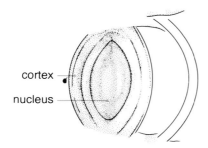

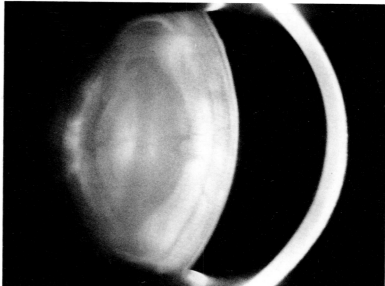

Fig.11.5   In a normal lens there is an increase in sagittal width with age which is largely the result of cortical growth.

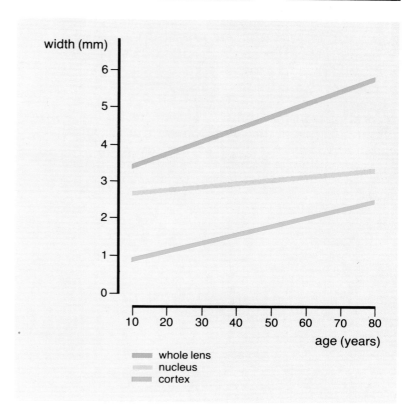

Fig.11.6 The radius of curvature of the anterior surface of the lens becomes progressively shorter with age. The lens therefore becomes more spherical.

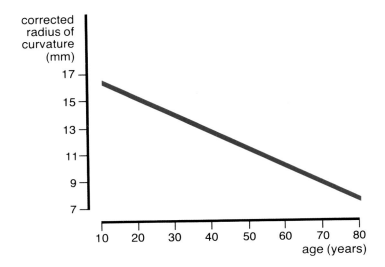

Fig.11.7 In patients of a similar age, lenses which develop cataract, particularly in the subcapsular region, tend to be smaller than normal. The small size is largely accounted for by a reduction in the normal width of the cortex, the nucleus being much the same size. While a reduction in width implies a slower growth rate, it could also be the result of central compaction. (This should be distinguished from the process of maturation of a cataractous lens where the lens may swell as a result of osmotic forces.)

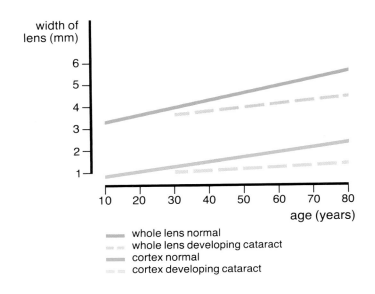

whole lens normal
whole lens developing cataract
cortex normal
cortex developing cataract

Fig.11.8 This histological section shows the anterior surface of the lens near to the equator. The capsule appears structureless and stains weakly. The epithelium, which is only present anteriorly, is composed of a single layer of nucleated cells. It is responsible for the continual production of new lens fibres which are seen to be separating from the epithelial layer in the lower part of the picture. Although the young fibres are nucleated, they eventually lose their nuclei as they sink into the cortex. The epithelium and young nucleated fibres together comprise the anterior subcapsular clear zone (cf. Fig.11.2).

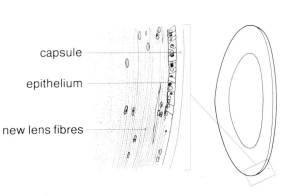

capsule

epithelium

new lens fibres

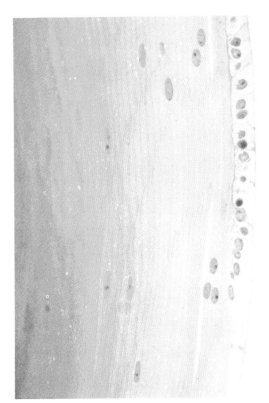

Fig.11.9 Lens fibres are hexagonal in cross-section and lie in layers, rather like the skin of an onion. There are no lens sutures with the embryonic nucleus, but the suture lines of the foetal nucleus are easily seen in the adult as an erect Y anteriorly and an inverted Y posteriorly.
With increasing age the sutures become a more complex branching system in the cortex, each lens fibre running antero-posteriorly across the equator of the lens and interdigitating with its neighbours.

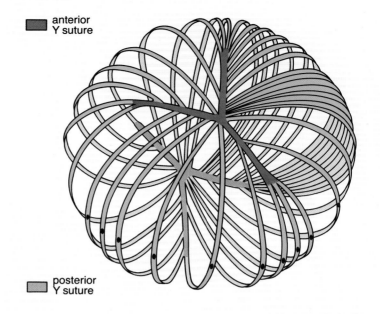

anterior
Y suture

posterior
Y suture

Fig.11.10 The anatomical arrangement of lens fibres is demonstrated by a sutural cataract. Opacities form as the tips of the growing lens fibres reach the suture line. This may either produce a few punctate opacities along the sutures or a densely opaque 'Y'-shaped cataract. The opacities may increase in size during development of the lens and then remain static. Their effect on vision is usually slight, although on occasions they can be more severe.

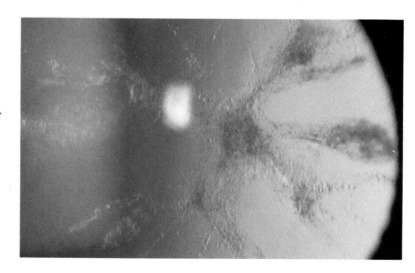

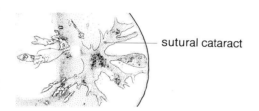

— sutural cataract

Accommodation
By contraction of the ciliary muscle (under para-sympathetic III nerve supply) the lens changes shape and increases its diopteric power to focus near objects on to the retina. The increase in diopteric strength of the lens is largely accounted for by a reduction in radius of curvature of the central part of the anterior surface, which also moves forward slightly. The curvature of the lens, which at rest is close to spherical, becomes more conoid

on accommodation. This aspherical change appears to be brought about by a difference in behaviour between the nucleus and the cortex; the nucleus undergoing the greater change and distending the anterior axial capsule which is comparatively weaker. The force required to change the shape of the lens comes from the capsule which tends to mould the lens as the tension from the suspensory zonule on the capsule is relaxed.

Fig.11.11 These slit-image photographs show the changes in a thirty-year-old lens focussed at infinity (left) and exerting ten dioptres of accommodation (right). The increased curvature of the anterior lens surface and its slight anterior postioning can be clearly seen.
The posterior lens surface remains relatively unchanged.

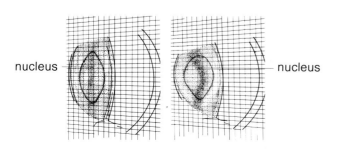

nucleus — | — nucleus

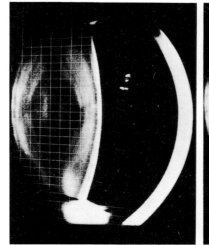 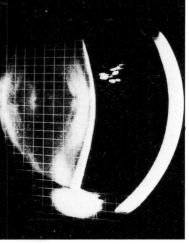

11.5

Fig.11.12 The mechanism of accommodation was first demonstrated by the observation of the Purkinje-Sansom images. These are produced by reflection of light from the anterior and posterior lens surfaces which act as convex and concave mirrors respectively. Accommodation is measured in dioptres, thus one dioptre of accommodation is needed to focus from infinity to one metre, or three dioptres to focus at thirty-three centimetres. A child has as much as fourteen dioptres of accommodation, but by sixty years of age this has virtually disappeared.

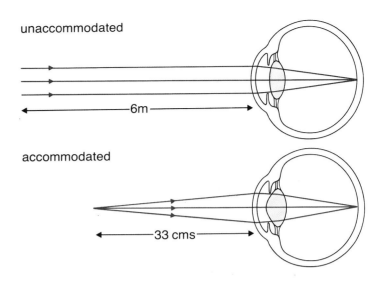

unaccommodated

←————6m————→

accommodated

←————33 cms————→

Anomalies of Shape and Position

Anomalies of lens shape are extremely rare disorders which are usually congenital and may be genetically determined in which case there may be other systemic abnormalities. The position of a lens may be altered either as a result of trauma or because of an inherent weakness in the zonule resulting from genetic error. In the absence of trauma, subluxated or dislocated lenses are usually associated with systemic signs.

Fig.11.13 This is a young lens with posterior lenticonus, a conical deformity usually situated at the posterior pole. A very slight amount of cortical cataract is seen in the fibres subjacent to the cone and is quite usual in this condition. Posterior lenticonus may be inherited in a dominant manner and can also occur in association with Alport's syndrome, the main systemic features of which are hereditary haemorrhagic nephritis and nerve deafness. Refraction through the lens is uneven and results in axial myopia and irregular astigmatism.

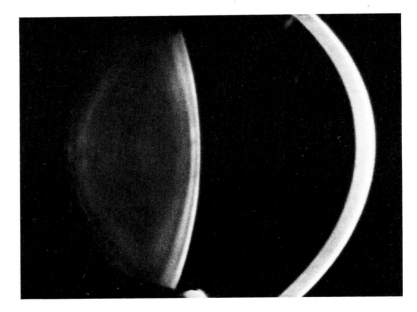

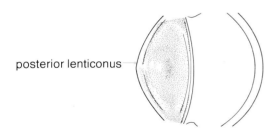

posterior lenticonus

Fig.11.14 Spherophakia defines a number of conditions in which the lens has an abnormally short radius of curvature and may also be exceptionally small (microphakia). It may be seen in conditions in which the zonule is defective as in this patient with the Marchesani syndrome. Extreme myopia results. Although this lens is normally situated, there is usually a tendency for lenses to subluxate and dislocate anteriorly.

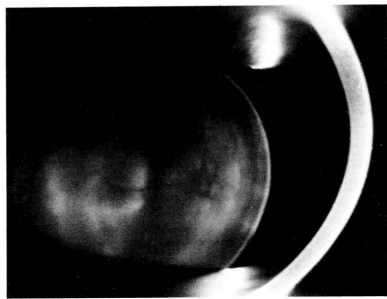

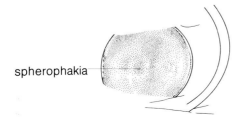

spherophakia

Fig.11.15 The Marchesani syndrome is inherited recessively and characterized by short stature, stubby fingers (top) and toes (bottom) which have stiff joints. Spherophakia, lenticular myopia of ten-to-twenty dioptres, and lens dislocation are common. Heterozygotes can show a milder form of the disease.

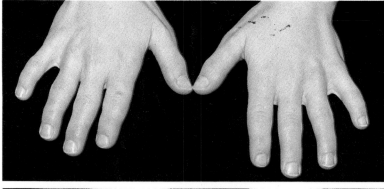

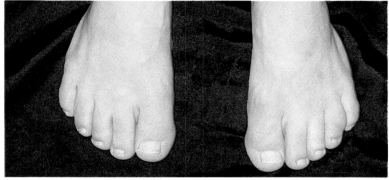

Fig.11.16 Lens subluxation is demonstrated in this slide. The lens is displaced from its axial position although it remains behind the iris and is attached to the zonule in at least one place. The photograph on the right shows the edge of a medially displaced lens visible in the pupillary area in a patient with Marfan's syndrome. The slit-view of a different patient (left) shows a lens displaced upwards (as is more usual in Marfan's syndrome). A zonular fibre is still attached below in the region where the zonule is degenerate. This lens shows spherophakia with zones of discontinuity running parallel with the capsule, unlike those seen in the normal lens. The condition results in myopic astigmatism.

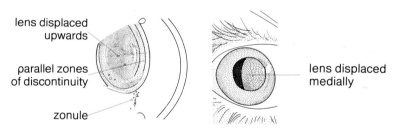

lens displaced upwards

parallel zones of discontinuity

zonule

lens displaced medially

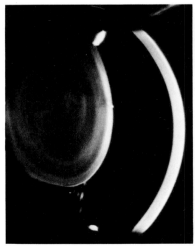

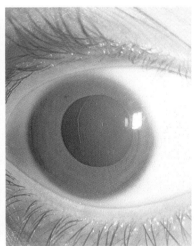

Fig.11.17 Marfan's syndrome is a dominantly inherited disease of the connective tissue which combines disorders of the skeleton, eye, and cardiovascular system. Patients have an arm span greater than height. Arachnodactyly is consistent and can be measured by the metacarpal index. Death frequently results from dissection of an aortic aneurysm.

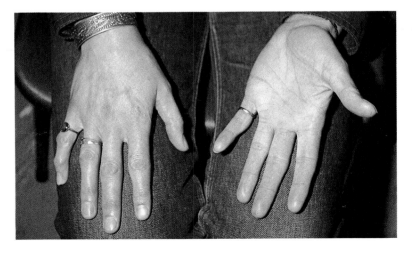

Fig.11.18 This previously normal lens was dislocated into the anterior chamber by blunt trauma. Corneal oedema is seen and is the result of pupil block glaucoma, a common complication of lens subluxation or dislocation (cf. Glaucoma – Volumes 7 and 8). Lenses can dislocate posteriorly and come to lie either in the vitreous or on the retinal surface without causing any apparent damage for a number of years.

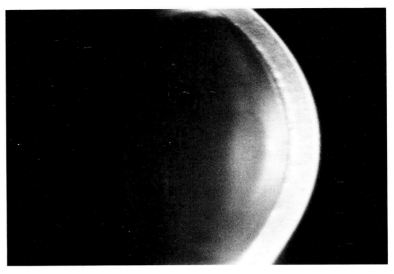

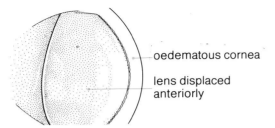

oedematous cornea

lens displaced
anteriorly

CATARACT

Cataracts can be classified according to their position within the lens and the degree of maturity or opacity produced. If lens damage is insufficient to progress to maturity, a localized opacity is produced in the injured region which becomes surrounded by new lens fibres as they are laid down beneath the capsule. Damaged lenses do not grow as quickly as normal. Lens opacities usually originate in either the capsular and subcapsular regions, the cortex, or the nucleus.

Fig.11.19 This diagram illustrates the different morphological characteristics of cataract together with their depth and location within the lens. The following illustrations demonstrate clinical examples of these anatomical entities.

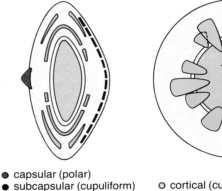

● capsular (polar)
● subcapsular (cupuliform)   ○ cortical (cuneiform)   ● sutural
○ supranuclear (coronary)   ○ nuclear (lamellar)   ○ nuclear

Capsular Cataract

Capsular cataracts are a relatively uncommon type of cataract whose origin may be either congenital or, less frequently, acquired in later-life. Those involving the anterior pole seldom require treatment as they are unlikely to interfere with vision to any great extent.

Fig.11.20 Capsular opacities occur at the lens poles and are commonly congenital; a persistent pupillary membrane or lenticonus may occasionally be associated. Subjacent lens fibres are affected and growth may produce an appearance similar to a stack of plates. Pyramidal cataract is a form of capsular opacity which projects forward as a hard white cone. Anterior polar opacities do not affect visual acuity as severely as those in the posterior pole which are formed nearer to the nodal point of the eye.

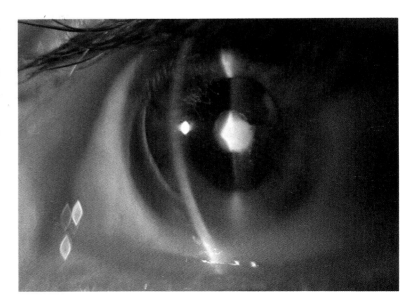

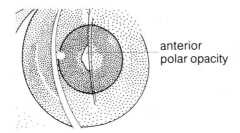

anterior
polar opacity

Fig.11.21 True capsular damage of the lens is rarely seen in the adult but trauma, especially infrared radiation (glass blowers' cataract), may cause capsular splitting and peeling. White fibrillary material on the lens capsule, pupil margins, and zonule are typical signs of pseudo lens exfoliation (cf. Glaucoma – Volumes 7 and 8). Mercury (as preservative in eye drops or from chronic industrial exposure) may be precipitated as a grey deposit on the capsule while chlorpromazine exposure leads to the formation of white granules. Following prolonged use of chlorpromazine in psychiatric treatment, a characteristic star-shaped cataract often develops consisting of numerous white dots in the capsule and anterior cortex. The opacities are probably composed either of the drug or a metabolite derived from it.

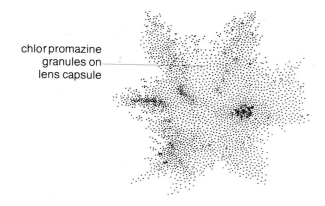

chlorpromazine granules on lens capsule

Subcapsular Cataract

Subcapsular cataracts are a common form of lens opacity which may produce a devastating effect on the vision when affecting the posterior pole of the lens. They may arise either as a result of senile changes or as secondary conditions to other ocular disease.

Fig.11.22 Complicated cataracts result from ocular disease, usually inflammatory, but also dystrophic conditions such as retinitis pigmentosa or degenerations such as high myopia. These cataracts (such as the one shown here in retroillumination) are typically posterior subcapsular, but they may also be found anteriorly when resulting from anterior segment disease.

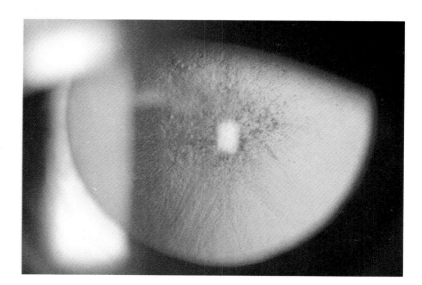

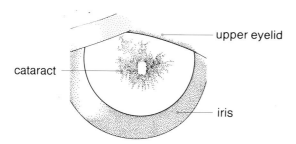

upper eyelid

cataract

iris

Fig.11.23 The subjacent cortex often contains opacities which help to differentiate this condition from senile cupuliform cataract. These deeper cortical opacities are only seen in long-standing eye disease and were themselves subcapsular at the time of their formation. A number of drugs and poisons have been implicated in causing cataract, and by far the most common is that following prolonged use of systematic or local steroids.

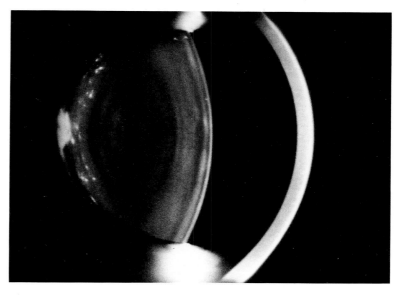

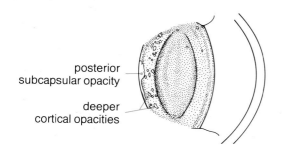

posterior subcapsular opacity

deeper cortical opacities

Fig.11.24 Senile cupuliform cataract appears as a collection of opacities and cysts in the posterior subcapsular region at the posterior pole. It often has a discrete margin giving it a cup shape.

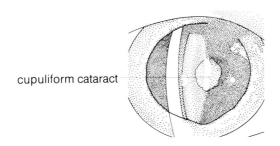

cupuliform cataract

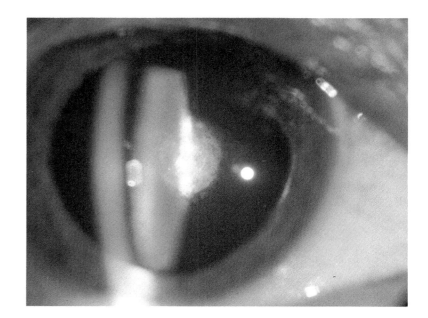

Fig.11.25 The opacities do not extend into the overlying cortex as in the complicated cataract (cf. Fig.11.23). The earliest sign of anterior subcapsular opacity is loss of the subcapsular clear zone.

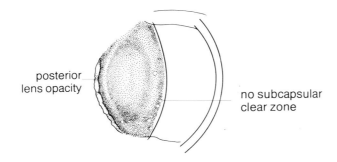

posterior
lens opacity

no subcapsular
clear zone

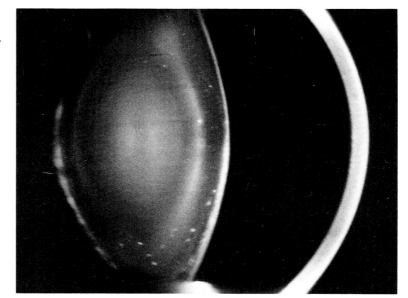

Fig.11.26 The position of a posterior subcapsular cataract on the optical axis of the lens near the nodal point of the eye (n) has a very destructive effect on vision (Ray ana'). Pupillary constriction in bright light enhances this effect because the reduced aperture prevents access by light rays which normally bypass the nodal point (Ray abca'). This effect can be alleviated in some patients by mydriasis.

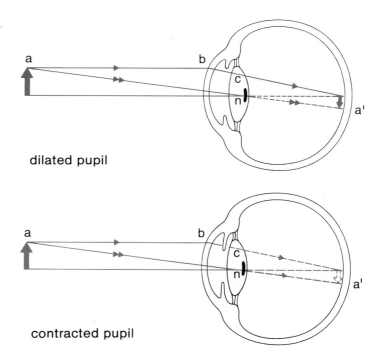

dilated pupil

contracted pupil

Traumatic Subcapsular Changes

A variety of physical agents will lead to cataract formation in the injured lens over a variable period of time. Direct trauma to the lens (as, for example, in a penetrating eye injury) may produce changes within hours, whereas the effects of indirect trauma (such as in a blunt eye injury) may not be apparent for many years.

The anterior subcapsular region is also affected to a lesser degree. After severe irradiation, the cataract deteriorates to maturity, but following more minor irradiation the cataract eventually becomes a static discrete opacity, which comes to lie deeper in the lens with time (right).

Fig.11.27 Radiation cataract results from injury to the lens by ionizing radiation, (X-rays, β-rays, γ-rays and neutrons), about 400 rads being sufficient to produce a cataract. It begins as a centripetal streaming of granular particles in the posterior subcapsular clear zone (left) which form a plaque of opacities at the posterior pole.

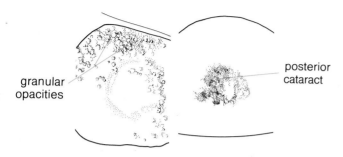

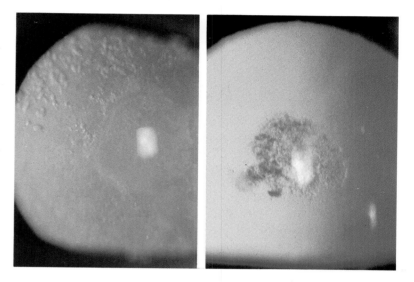

Fig.11.28 Traumatic cataract results from blunt or penetrating injury to the lens. The injured fibres are initially vacuolated rather than opaque and the primary changes may therefore be missed by examination with focal illumination. The lens sutures are clearly seen by retroillumination in this example of early traumatic cataract due to a metallic foreign body.

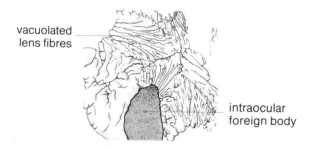

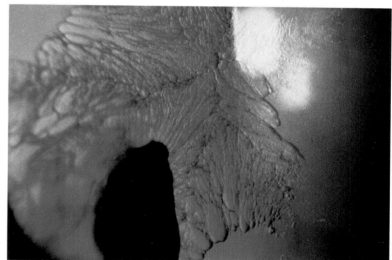

Fig.11.29 If the injury is insufficient to cause major lens damage the traumatic cataract usually settles to a compact white star-shaped opacity, and eventually comes to lie at a deeper level within the lens. The cataract shape is determined by the anatomy of the lens fibres and sutures. While both anterior and posterior subcapsular regions are usually affected, the anterior defect is more obvious.

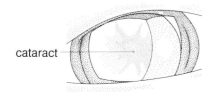

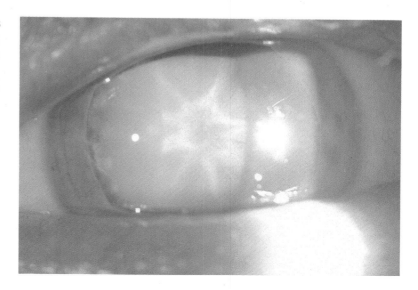

Dystrophia Myotonica

Fig.11.30 Dystrophia myotonica is commonly associated with cataract. Characteristically there is an early appearance of polychromatic glistening granules in the subcapsular and cortical areas which progress to posterior subcapsular changes and maturity.

These opacities can be a useful genetic marker for this autosomal dominant condition although the lens is sometimes unaffected in people who have overt disease.

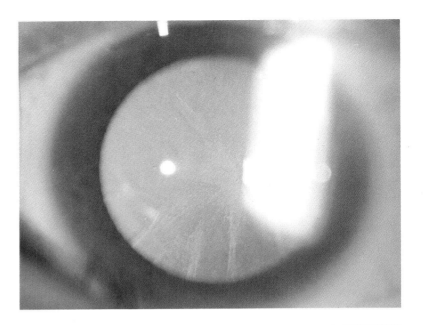

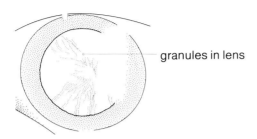

granules in lens

Fig.11.31 This patient, who has recently had cataract surgery to the right eye, has an appearance typical of dystrophia myotonica. Notice the frontal balding, wasting of the temporalis muscles, and evidence of external ocular myopathy with bilateral ptosis. In addition, some patients have a pigmentary retinopathy which contributes to their visual loss. Myopathy of the respiratory muscles can make general anaesthesia hazardous.

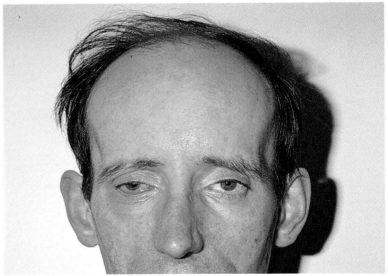

Cortical Cataracts

Cortical cataracts are the most common variety of lens opacity and may be found in all ages. Their size and position means they often produce little visual impairment, other than through the effects of light scatter, and progression of such cataracts is often very slow.

Fig.11.32 Punctate opacities form discrete dots which are often coloured brown or blue (blue-dot opacities). They are either congenital or developmental in origin and are laid down down gradually in increasing number as lens growth continues.

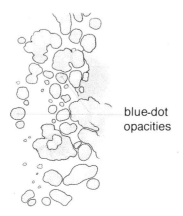

blue-dot opacities

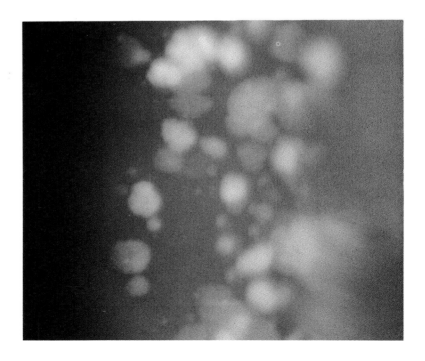

Fig.11.33 While punctate cataracts are usually situated in the cortex, they may also be seen within the nucleus if opacity formation began either *in utero* or in infancy. Punctate opacities are relatively common and accumulation is seldom sufficient to interfere with vision.

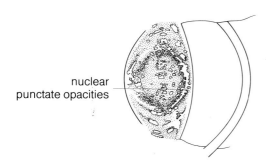

nuclear
punctate opacities

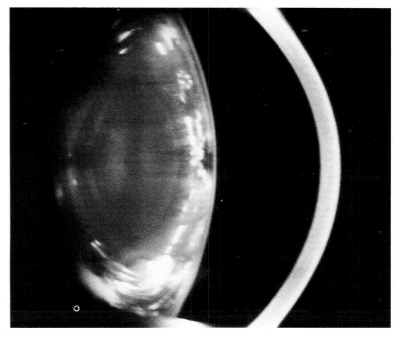

Fig.11.34 The coronary cataract often occurs in association with punctate opacities. When viewed by retroillumination, the cataract is seen to form a crown (corona) around the nucleus. The opacities are distributed radially with a rounded club or petal-shaped appearance.

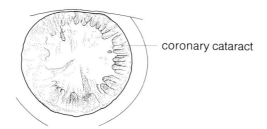

coronary cataract

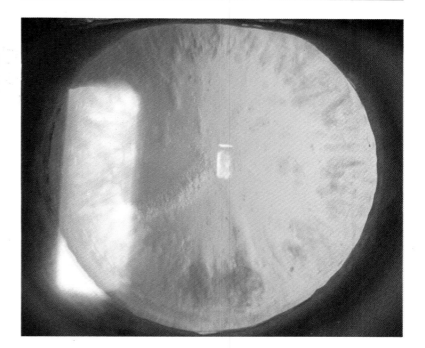

Fig.11.35 The depth of coronary cataract within the lens is shown by focal illumination. In this example, the anterior cortex is also affected by punctate opacities.

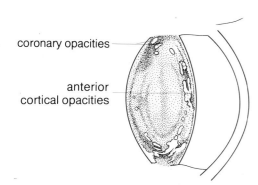

coronary opacities

anterior
cortical opacities

Fig.11.36 Cuneiform cataracts are a relatively common form of senile opacity which lie in radial wedge shapes at about mid-depth in the cortex. They form peripherally and sometimes extend into the pupillary area.

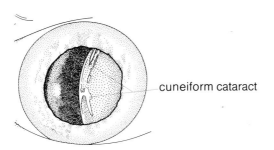

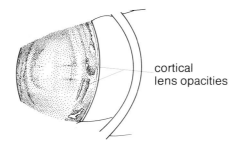

cuneiform cataract

Fig.11.37 When viewed on the slit lamp, cuneiform cataracts appear as dark wedges by retroillumination. They usually have little effect on acuity, but occasionally encroach onto the visual axis and then cause blurring or distortion of vision. They may also affect the quality of vision due to their light scattering effect.

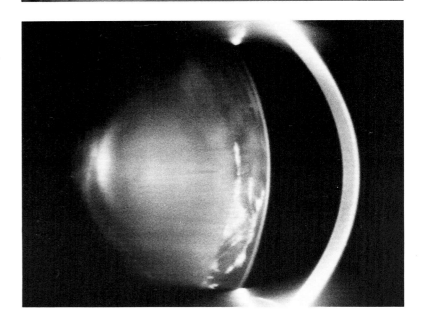

cortical lens opacities

Nuclear Cataract

Nuclear cataracts occur at the two extremes of life: in the very young they are rare, and their effect on vision may diminish with time if normal clear lens is laid down around the cataract. In old-age, small amounts of nuclear

sclerosis may actually aid vision by inducing a degree of myopia, enabling the reading spectacles of middle-age to be thrown away.

Fig.11.38 The extent to which the nucleus is affected by congenital cataract depends on the duration of cataract formation *in utero*. The embryonal nuclear cataract, *(cataracta centralia pulverulenta)* (left) consists of minute star-shaped opacities which affect only the central interval (embryonal nucleus). It is bilateral, often dominant in inheritance, and does not interfere with vision. In the total nuclear cataract (right), the whole of the embryonic and foetal nucleus is affected, but the cortex remains clear.

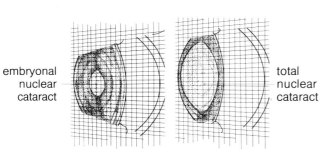

embryonal nuclear cataract   total nuclear cataract

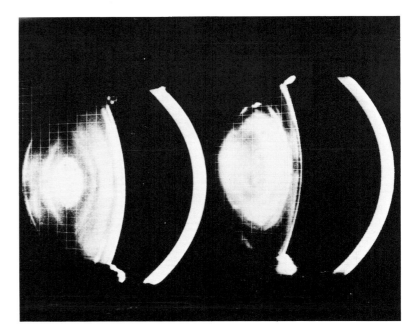

Fig.11.39 While lamellar cataract is usually nuclear and congenital in origin, it is not a nuclear cataract by definition. It is an opacity which usually affects just one lamella of the lens fibres surrounding the nucleus anteriorly and posteriorly. When the precipitating cause is not removed immediately, however, some overlying fibres are also affected and are called riders.

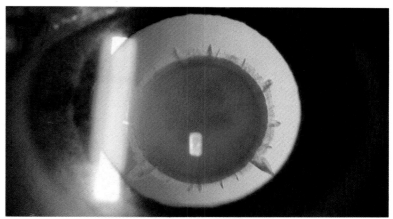

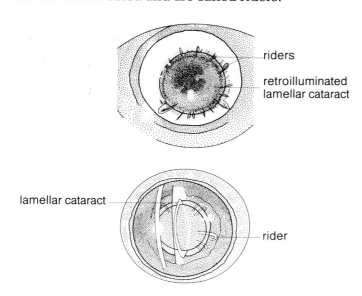

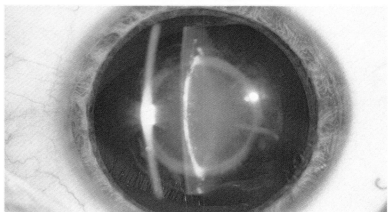

Fig.11.40 When lamellar cataract occurs in the child, it is initially subcapsular and passes centrally with age. This example shows two concentric affected lamellae. Genetic, metabolic, and infective causes should be sought.

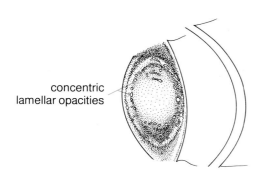

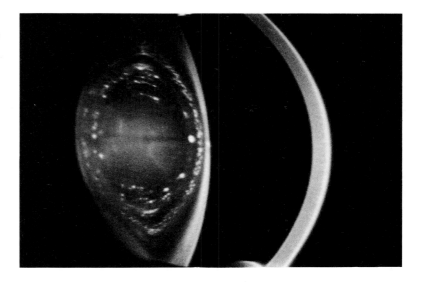

Fig.11.41 By far the most common cause of congenital cataracts is maternal rubella occurring during the first trimester of pregnancy. The incidence of this condition, however, is now declining through the increased use of immunization and monitoring of maternal antibodies in early pregnancy. Affected infants will have raised titres of rubella antibody. Other signs of the disease are frequently present as in this two-year-old infant who had bilateral nerve deafness, microcephaly, severe mental retardation, and a congenital heart defect.

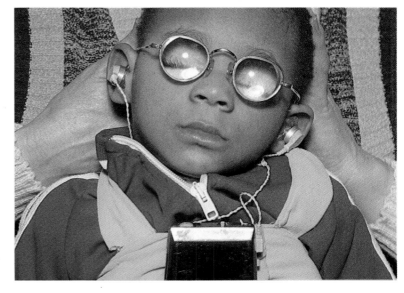

Fig.11.42 The common nuclear sclerotic cataract is either yellow or brown. These colours gradually darken with development of the cataract and lead to loss of colour discrimination for the patient. This is said to account for the increasing predominance of oranges, reds, and browns in the later paintings of many artists such as Rembrandt and Turner.

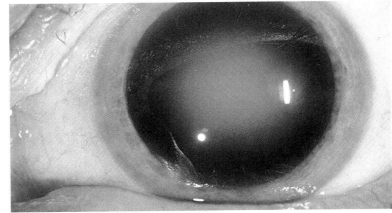

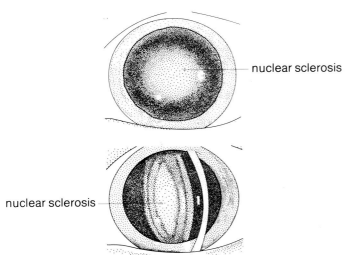

nuclear sclerosis

nuclear sclerosis

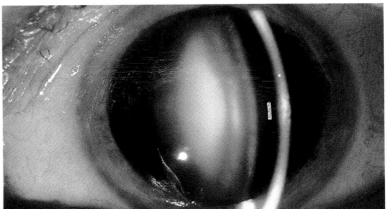

Fig.11.43 Senile nuclear sclerosis causes relatively little light scatter and sight is first affected by myopia resulting from the increasing refractive index of the nucleus. Subcapsular cataract may form later leading to a rapid deterioration in vision.

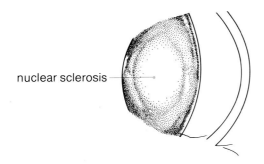

nuclear sclerosis

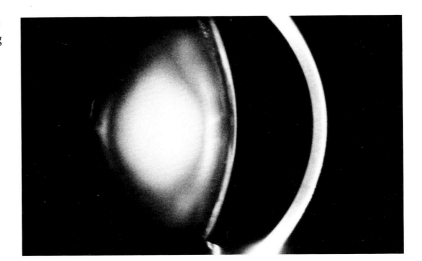

Fig.11.44 The increasing compaction of lens fibres into the nucleus with age leads to an increase in the refractive index of the nucleus and lenticular myopia. While the normal ageing process can account for changes of up to 0.5 dioptres a year, the process can be greatly enhanced by a nuclear cataract.

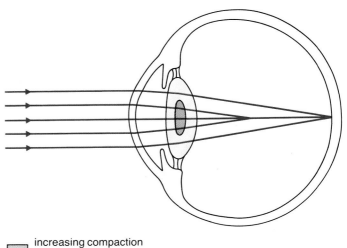

increasing compaction or nuclear cataract

PROGRESS AND PROGNOSIS OF CATARACT

Opacities which are intially subcapsular sink into the lens when normal lens fibre growth resumes and when the cause has not been so severe or prolonged as to lead to the formation of a mature cataract. The degree of visual blurring will depend on the site of the opacity within the lens and its proximity to the nodal point. Glare is produced by scatter of light, and monocular diplopia results from changes in refractive index within the lens. In addition, irregular refraction will produce monochromatic haloes and distortion, and brunescence will affect the patient's colour discrimination. Lenses affected by cataract, particularly subcapsular cataract, are commonly small for the subject's age (cf. Fig.11.7). The small size of the affected lens appears to be due to loss of cortex with a consequent increase in curvature of the pupillary zone, which further contributes to the myopia caused by nuclear sclerosis.

Fig.11.45 This slit photograph shows a traumatic cataract affecting the same lamella both anteriorly and posteriorly in a fifty-eight-year-old man who had received a blunt injury to the lens twenty years previously.

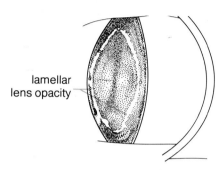

lamellar lens opacity

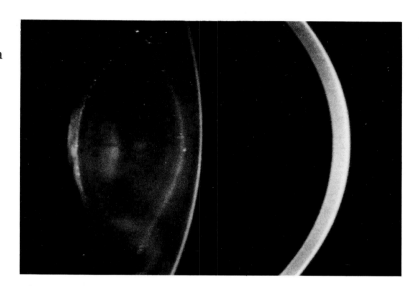

Fig.11.46 Reformation of the subcapsular clear zone superficial to the opacity indicates that lens growth has been resumed and prognosis is therefore good. This slit photograph shows glaucoma flecks one year after an attack of acute glaucoma; the subcapsular clear zone is completely reformed. Vision is unaffected and the opacities have not increased in size or number.

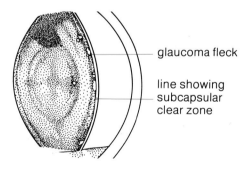

glaucoma fleck

line showing subcapsular clear zone

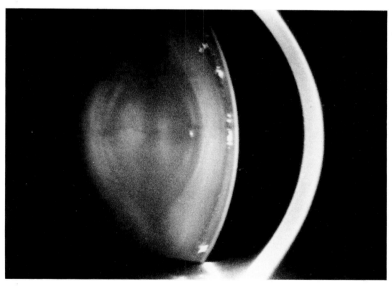

Fig.11.47 The severely traumatized lens may show thinning. This lens of a ten-year-old child sustained trauma eight weeks previously; there is an obvious posterior subcapsular cataract and thinning of the posterior cortex. These are bad prognostic signs and the cataract progressed rapidly to maturity.

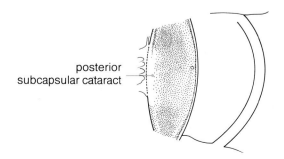

posterior subcapsular cataract

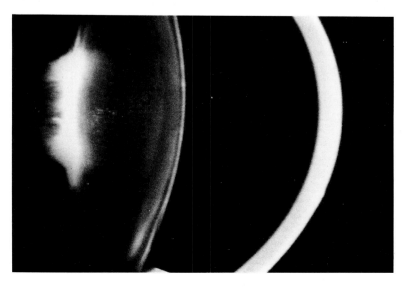

Fig.11.48 A cataract is said to be mature when all fibres are opacified up to the capsule. This is associated with water-entry into the lens by osmosis, and swelling. Water clefts can be seen as dark areas in this lens of a young subject with anorexia nervosa. The lens size and shallow anterior chamber would be normal for a subject of eighty years.

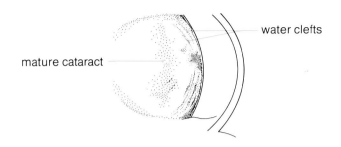

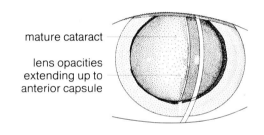

Fig.11.49 The slit lamp appearance of a similar subject shows the extent of opacification.

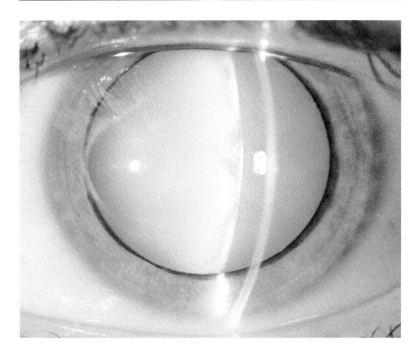

Fig.11.50 The maturing lens, even in young subjects, can become intumescent to a degree that causes shallowing of the anterior chamber, pupil block, and closed angle glaucoma. This is possible when the anterior chamber and produce a phakolytic glaucoma. (cf. Glaucoma – Volumes 7 & 8).
of the cataract, there is a gradual liquefaction of the lens cortex which may leak out of the capsule to leave behind a shrunken lens with a wrinkled capsule: this is then known as a hypermature cataract.

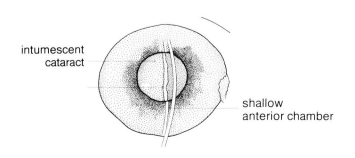

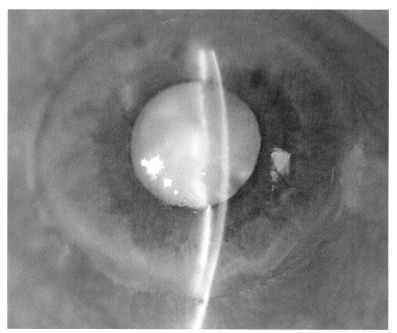

Fig.11.51 If some liquid cortex remains, the nucleus may then sink inferiorly (Morgagnian cataract) and can be mistaken for a subluxated lens. Soft lens material can seep out through the capsule at this stage. This is taken up by macrophages which may obstruct the angle of the anterior chamber and produce a phakolytic glaucoma. (cf. Glaucoma – Volumes 7 & 8).

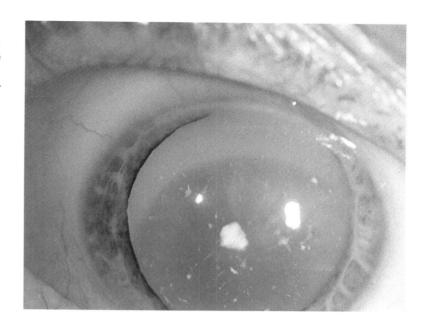

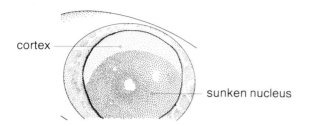

UNILATERAL CONGENITAL CATARACT IN CHILDHOOD

These can result from maternal infection, trauma or other ocular disease. They may also be present as inherited diseases and other ocular anomalies are frequently present.

Fig.11.52 As well as the cataract, the right eye of this child was convergent, microphthalmic and had a rubella retinopathy. In this situation, sucessful visual results from surgery are negligible because of the associated amblyopia from unilateral aphakia.

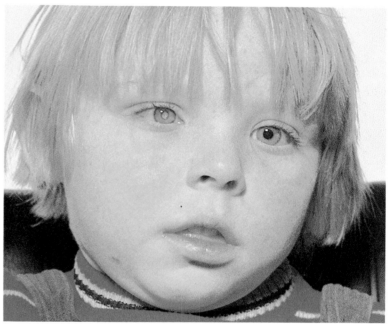

APHAKIA

Surgical removal of all or part of the lens eliminates the contribution of the lens to the overall refraction of the eye.

The normal eye then becomes markedly hypermetropic and requires optical correction with either spectacles, contact lens or intraocular lens.

Fig.11.53 Following extracapsular extraction there may be further proliferation of lens fibres from the remaining lens epithelium. These pearly excrescences are known as Elschnig's pearls.

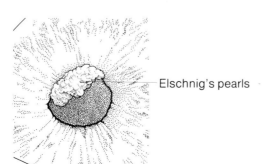

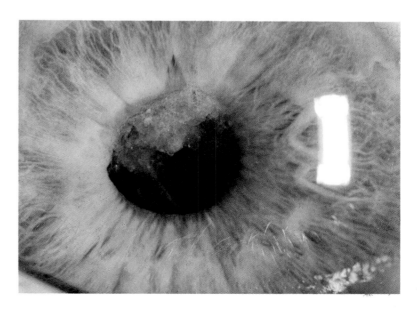

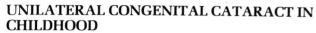

11.19

Fig.11.54 Elschnig's pearls are usually associated with thickening and fibrosis of the posterior capsule and, as these remnants lie near the nodal point, their effect on acuity is severe. Capsulotomy removes the problem.

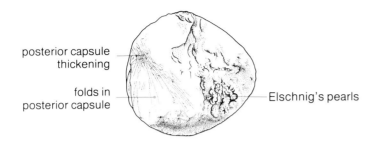

posterior capsule thickening

folds in posterior capsule

Elschnig's pearls

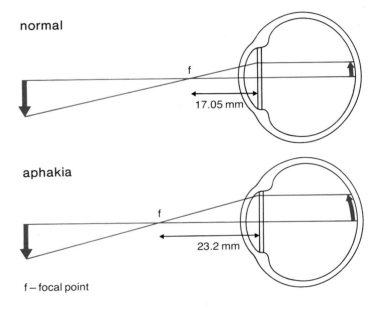

Fig.11.55 The removal of the crystalline lens means that the eye becomes a single refracting surface at the corneal interface. The optical consequences of this can be illustrated by studying the reduced eye. The anterior focal distance increases from 17.05mm in the phakic eye to 23.2mm in the aphakic eye. The anterior principal focus, which is normally 15.7mm in front of the cornea, is thus moved further forward. Rays of light passing through this point emerge, after refraction, parallel to the visual axis to form the retinal image. The size of the retinal image will be proportional to the angle of the ray through the anterior principal focus; in aphakia the retinal image will thus be larger as this point is further from the cornea. The increase in image size will be in the ratio 23.2: 17.05 or 1.36: 1.

normal

f

17.05 mm

aphakia

f

23.2 mm

f – focal point

Fig.11.56 As a convex lens moves closer to the cornea it loses effectivity and the retinal image size decreases. A contact lens will produce a magnification of six to seven percent which in the case of unilateral aphakia can be fused with the retinal image of the phakic eye. Anterior segment intraocular lenses magnify by two percent, posterior chamber lenses are emmetropic. Other optical problems with aphakic spectacles are a small field of vision, spherical aberration, and the roving scotoma produced by the high spherical power of the spectacle lens and its prismatic effects.

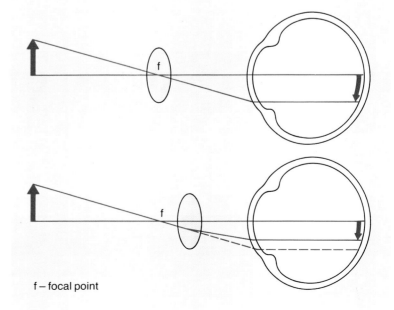

f

f

f – focal point

12. Vitreous and Vitreo-retinal Disorders

D. McLeod

Introduction

The vitreous cavity is the space within the eye bounded anteriorly by the lens and its zonular fibres, and more posteriorly by the ciliary body, retina and optic disc. Its volume is usually about 4 mls, though this may increase to as much as 10 mls in highly myopic eyes. Normally, the space is entirely occupied by vitreous gel, a virtually acellular viscous fluid with a ninety-nine percent water content; the low molecular and cellular content is essential for the maintenance of transparency. The major molecular constituents of the vitreous gel are hyaluronic acid and immature collagen fibrils whose physico-chemical interrelationship is responsible for its viscoelastic properties. The gel is of no importance in maintaining the shape or 'tone' of the eye. Indeed, apart from its role in oculogenesis, the vitreous has no well-substantiated function so that an eye devoid of gel is not adversely affected. Nevertheless, the physical relationship between the vitreous gel and the retina is the basis of a variety of serious sight-threatening pathological conditions.

EMBRYOLOGY OF THE VITREOUS

During early development, the invaginated optic vesicle (optic cup) contains the primary vitreous, a vascularized tissue supplying the lens and retina (both of which have an ectodermal origin). During the third month of gestation, the primary vitreous gradually loses its vascularity and is compressed axially by the development of the secondary vitreous which is avascular and derives mainly from the anterior retina and ciliary body. The principal remnant of the primary vitreous is Cloquet's canal.

Fig. 12.1 Light micrograph of a section through the eye of a 13 mm human foetus showing primary and secondary vitreous and artefactual re-establishment of optic vesicle (silver stain).

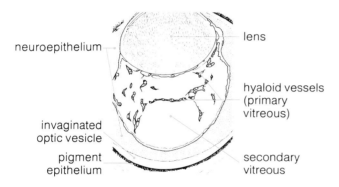

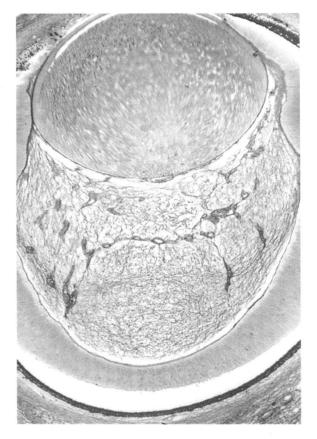

ANATOMY OF THE VITREOUS AND RETINA

The retina terminates anteriorly at the ora serrata which has a scalloped margin and is located approximately 8 mm posterior to the corneoscleral limbus (along a line marked externally by the extra-ocular muscle insertions). The part of the ciliary body immediately anterior to the ora serrata is relatively featureless and is termed the pars plana.

The cortical part of the vitreous gel has a higher content of hyaluronic acid and collagen compared with the less dense central gel. In addition, the gel exhibits 'condensations' both within its substance and along its boundaries. The boundary condensations are termed the anterior and posterior hyaloid 'membranes', while the more central gel is divided into 'tracts'. Cloquet's canal, a remnant of the primary vitreous, is a tubular axial tract stretching sinuously between the lens anteriorly and the optic disc posteriorly.

During oculogenesis and subsequently, important zones or points of attachment are established between the vitreous gel and surrounding structures. These 'developmental' attachments form the basis of much vitreo-retinal pathology. The vitreous base is an annular zone of adhesion some 3-4 mm wide which straddles the ora serrata: the strength of the adhesion between the basal gel and the most peripheral retina and posterior pars plana is such that they cannot be separated (even by severe trauma). The anterior border of the vitreous base is the posterior site of insertion of the anterior hyaloid membrane, while the posterior border of the vitreous base marks the anterior limit of potential separation between the gel and retina. Irregularities of the posterior border of the vitreous base are important in retinal tear formation.

Weiger's ligament is an annular zone of adhesion some 8-9 mm in diameter between the gel and the posterior lens capsule. It also marks the junction between the anterior hyaloid membrane and the expanded anterior portion of Cloquet's canal. This adhesion is broken down during intracapsular cataract extraction. An exaggerated vitreopapillary adhesion marks the junction of the posterior hyaloid membrane and the slightly expanded posterior limit of Cloquet's canal around the margin of the optic disc. The associated glial cell membrane ('epipapillary gliosis') is a primary vitreous remnant which often becomes avulsed from the edge of the disc during posterior vitreous detachment.

Exaggerated vitreo-retinal adhesions are also present in relation to two important developmental degenerations of the retina: lattice degeneration and cystic retinal tufts. Lattice degeneration comprises oval or elongated areas of thinning and vascular sclerosis in the peripheral retina. The lesions are generally orientated circumferentially but may be radially directed along the post-equatorial course of retinal veins. Lattice degeneration is found in approximately seven percent of normal eyes, and the glial proliferations and vitreo-retinal adhesions around the margins of the degenerate areas are frequently the basis of tearing of the retina. Cystic retinal tufts are focal areas of gliosis and vitreo-retinal adhesion located equatorially

which form the basis of 'operculated' tear formation. Some eyes also demonstrate abnormally strong vitreo-retinal adhesions along the course of retinal veins ('para-vascular adhesions') which may result in retinal tear formation.

Elsewhere, the cortical gel constituting the posterior hyaloid membrane is adherent to the retina via the 'inner limiting lamina' which is the basal lamina (basement membrane) of the Müller's cells. Gel fibrils insert into the most superficial part of the smooth internal aspect of the basal lamina, and this is the plane of cleavage of the gel from the retina in posterior vitreous detachment.

Fig. 12.2 Diagram of normal vitreoretinal anatomy showing the macroarchitectural features of the gel and important sites of vitreoretinal attachment.

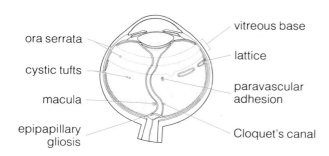

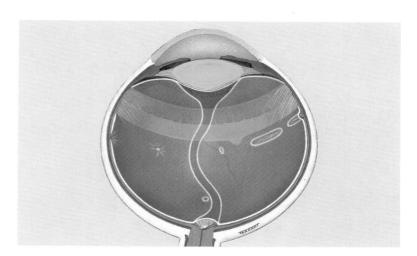

Fig. 12.3 Electron micrograph of the vitreoretinal juncture outside the various areas of exaggerated vitreoretinal adhesion.

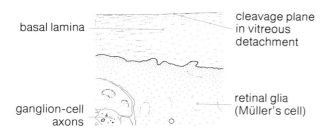

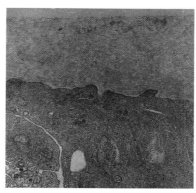

CONGENITAL VITREO-RETINAL ANOMALIES
Normal eyes show persistence of primary hyaloid tissue as Cloquet's canal and epipapillary gliosis. A mild exaggeration of glial proliferation on the disc is seen in 'Bergmeister's papilla', while a Mittendorf's dot is a frequent primary vitreous remnant on the posterior lens capsule. The hyaloid artery may occasionally persist as a vascular channel growing into the central gel from the optic disc or a glial plaque may persist on the posterior lens capsule. The most

frequent severe developmental anomaly is persistent hyperplastic primary vitreous which usually presents in infancy as a microphthalmic squinting eye with leukocoria. Pupil dilatation may demonstrate dragging of the ciliary processes towards a central plaque of fibrovascular tissue which invades the lens posteriorly and ultimately causes a complete cataract and secondary angle closure glaucoma (cf. Secondary Glaucoma – Chapter 8).

Fig. 12.4 Fundus photograph of a persistent hyaloid artery, and slit-beam photograph of anterior primary vitreous remnants behind the lens.

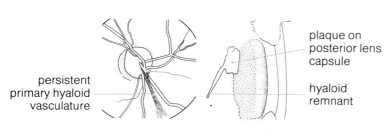

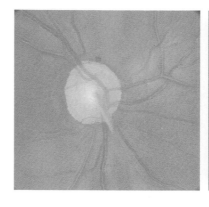

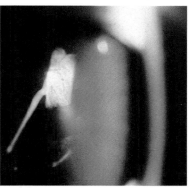

Fig. 12.5 Horizontal B-scan sections; the normal vitreous is acoustically empty with no echoes from Cloquet's canal or other gel architecture (left). Ciliary dragging, cataract and a primary hyaloid remnant are seen in an eye with persistent hyperplastic primary vitreous (right).

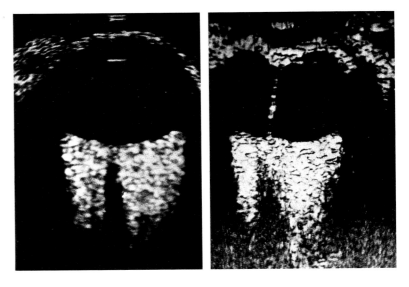

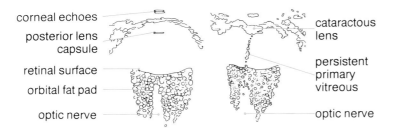

corneal echoes
posterior lens capsule
retinal surface
orbital fat pad
optic nerve

cataractous lens
persistent primary vitreous
optic nerve

DEGENERATIONS AND NON-PROLIFERATIVE INVASIONS OF THE GEL

By virtue of its avascular and acellular nature, the vitreous gel has an extremely limited repertoire of pathological change unless invaded by cells or molecules from surrounding structures. The architectural features of the gel which are apparent in childhood, gradually disappear with time owing to a breakdown in the physicochemical interrelationship between hyaluronic acid and collagen molecules (syneresis; lacunar degeneration; vitreous collapse). This process is accelerated in aphakic and myopic eyes. As the gel degenerates, the collagen fibrils tend to aggregate (giving rise to 'floaters' or 'muscae volitantes'), and spaces devoid of any collagen sub-architecture ('lacunae') develop in the gel. With ageing, the fluid contents of a premacular lacuna may break through a

dehiscence in the posterior vitreous cortex to separate the gel from the retina and start a 'posterior vitreous detachment with collapse'. The detached posterior hyaloid membrane becomes wrinkled and usually separates completely from the retina up to the posterior border of the vitreous base (or up to the posterior aspect of any other exaggerated vitreo-retinal adhesions which may be present). Epipapillary glial tissue can become avulsed from the disc margin during vitreous detachment and may be seen ophthalmoscopically as a small ring of tissue attached to the posterior gel boundary ('Weiss's ring'). Patients often notice this floater after vitreous detachment. It is often described as a 'cobweb' or circle and moves alarmingly with eye movements.

Fig. 12.6 Slit-beam photographs of syneretic gel showing a clear space (lacuna) behind the immediate retrolental gel (left), and a detached posterior hyaloid membrane with characteristic wrinkling of the gel condensation (right).

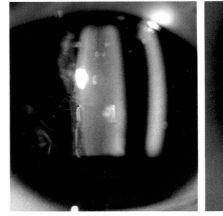

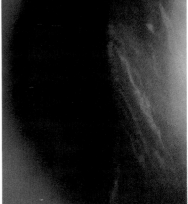

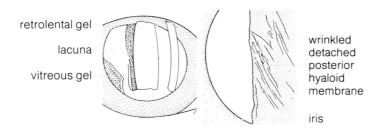

retrolental gel
lacuna
vitreous gel

wrinkled detached posterior hyaloid membrane
iris

Fig. 12.7 Light micrograph of detached gel showing wrinkled posterior hyaloid membrane bounding a mass of gel, and photograph of avulsed epipapillary gliosis (Weiss's ring) attached to the detached posterior hyaloid interface.

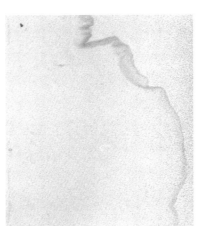

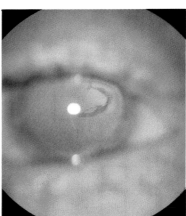

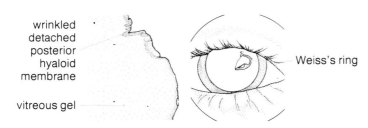

wrinkled detached posterior hyaloid membrane
vitreous gel

Weiss's ring

Asteroid Hyalosis

Asteroid hyalosis is a specific form of gel degeneration in which globules of calcium soaps aggregate on vitreous fibrils and move with the gel on eye movement. When dense, asteroid bodies may preclude ophthalmoscopic visualization of the retina, though they rarely impair the patient's vision. They are not associated with any systemic condition.

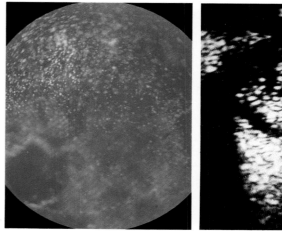 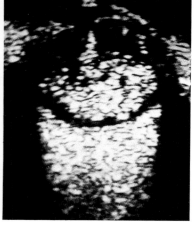

Fig. 12.8 Fundus photograph of yellow and white asteroid bodies (seen against a background of retrohyaloid haemorrhage) (left), and B-scan ultrasound section showing high amplitude (bright) echoes from asteroid bodies in a detached gel ('posterior vitreous detachment without collapse') (right).

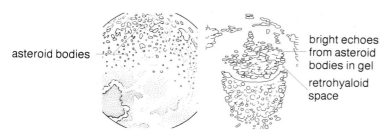

asteroid bodies

bright echoes from asteroid bodies in gel

retrohyaloid space

Amyloidosis

Amyloidosis of the vitreous is a rare condition usually associated with the primary or familial (dominantly inherited) form of amyloidosis. Proteinaceous material, probably derived from the retinal circulation, becomes coated on the collagenous framework of the gel bilaterally to produce a 'glass-wool' opacification; associated cellular invasion is conspicuous by its absence.

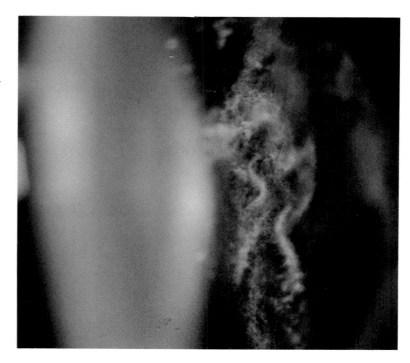

Fig. 12.9 Slit photograph of vitreous amyloidosis showing 'pseudopodia lentis', that is proteinaceous material coating retrolental vitreous fibrils.

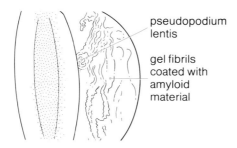

pseudopodium lentis

gel fibrils coated with amyloid material

Inflammatory Infiltration

Invasion of the vitreous cavity by inflammatory cells occurs in a variety of circumstances including exogenous and endogenous infections, inflammations, and in response to retained reactive foreign bodies. The infiltration may be diffuse and low grade (as in pars planitis), diffuse and severe (as in bacterial endophthalmitis), or more focal with large clumps of inflammatory cells ('snow balls'). All such infiltrations tend to be associated with exaggerated syneretic degeneration and, ultimately, detachment of the vitreous gel.

Fig. 12.10 Fundus photograph (left) of clumps of inflammatory cells in attached cortical vitreous, and similar inflammatory precipitates on a detached posterior hyaloid interface demonstrated by retroillumination (right).

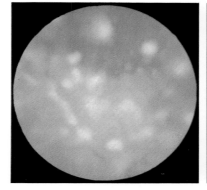 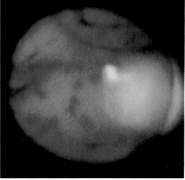

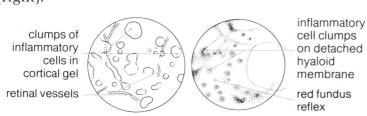

clumps of inflammatory cells in cortical gel

retinal vessels

inflammatory cell clumps on detached hyaloid membrane

red fundus reflex

Vitreous Haemorrhage

Haemorrhage within the vitreous cavity may be due to trauma or may arise spontaneously. The principal causes of spontaneous vitreous haemorrhage are retinal tears and extraretinal neovascularization secondary to retinal ischaemia. In both instances, the haemorrhage is usually associated with (and is initiated by) posterior vitreous detachment.

Blood in the vitreous gel initially forms a localized fibrinous clot, but subsequent fibrinolysis causes dispersion of the haemorrhage throughout the gel. The blood then undergoes a form of haemolysis whereby the biconcave erythrocytes lose most of their enclosed haemoglobin and change to spheroidal erythroclasts.

Biodegradation of the released haemoglobin produces pigments which often stain the gel an ochre-yellow or orange colour. Such staining of a detached erythroclast-clogged vitreous cortex produces an 'ochre membrane'.

The blood products also cause an exaggerated syneresis of the gel so that, in those eyes where the vitreous haemorrhage was not initially associated with posterior vitreous detachment (e.g., trauma and Terson's syndrome), vitreous separation usually follows in a matter of days or weeks. The mechanisms of spontaneous absorption of vitreous haemorrhage have not been clearly elucidated, though phagocytosis by macrophages, outflow of cells through the trabecular meshwork, and syneretic disintegration of the gel play a part. One rare consequence of vitreous haemorrhage is 'synchisis scintillans', which is a localized form of cholesterolosis bulbi. It is characterized by the presence of cholesterol crystals in the vitreous cavity which tend to sediment inferiorly, but may be seen to scatter and shower throughout the vitreous cavity after eye movement.

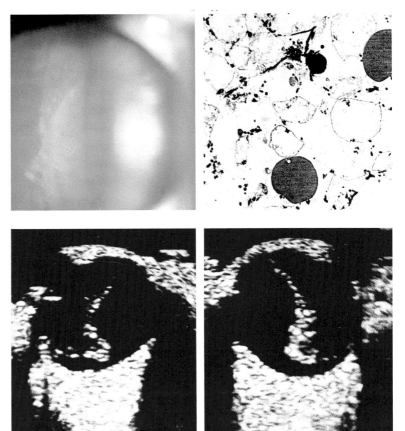

Fig. 12.11   Slit photograph of ochre stained anterior gel from long-standing vitreous haemorrhage (left), and electron micrograph showing erythrocytes and erythroclasts (right).

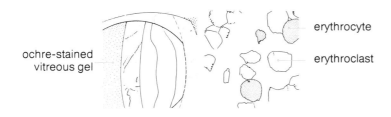

ochre-stained vitreous gel

erythrocyte

erythroclast

Fig. 12.12   B-scans of vitreous haemorrhage with the eye looking left and right. Echoes from haemorrhage in the vitreous cortex are seen outlining a detached and collapsed gel which moves, suspended from its basal attachments, during eye movement.

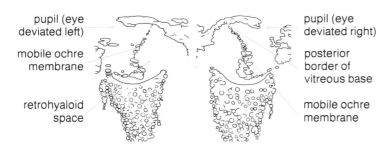

pupil (eye deviated left)

mobile ochre membrane

retrohyaloid space

pupil (eye deviated right)

posterior border of vitreous base

mobile ochre membrane

Fig. 12.13   Fundus photograph of polychromatic cholesterol crystals in an eye which had previously undergone vitrectomy for an ochre membrane and macular retinal detachment secondary to haemoglobin-SC disease; the crystals were literally 'dripping' from retained haemorrhage in the basal gel (synchisis scintillans).

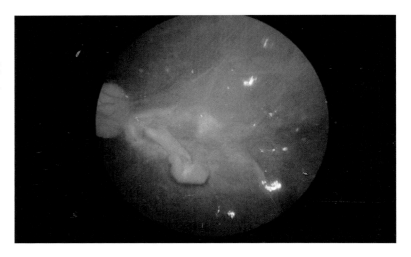

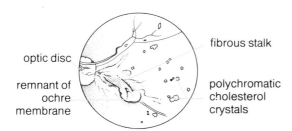

optic disc

remnant of ochre membrane

fibrous stalk

polychromatic cholesterol crystals

RHEGMATOGENOUS RETINAL DETACHMENT

Strictly speaking, 'retinal detachment' is a misnomer. The term is used to denote separation of the neuroepithelium from the pigment epithelium (rather than detachment of the retina from the choroid) and therefore implies re-establishment of the space between the original layers of the embryonic optic cup. The most common cause of retinal detachment is the formation of a 'break' or full-thickness discontinuity in the neuroepithelium with recruitment of fluid from the vitreous cavity into the subretinal space via the break – 'rhegmatogenous retinal detachment'. Classically, breaks are subdivided into 'tears' (secondary to dynamic vitreo-retinal traction) and 'holes' (secondary to localized retinal disintegration or atrophy), though the term 'hole' is sometimes used synonymously with break. Most retinal tears occur in association with posterior vitreous detachment by the operation of 'dynamic vitreous traction'. This term denotes the transmission of rotational energy (generated by saccadic contraction of the extraocular muscles) to the contents of the vitreous cavity through the coats of the eye (sclera, choroid and retina). While the vitreous remains attached to the retina, this energy transmission is dispersed throughout the total area of vitreo-retinal contact. After posterior vitreous detachment, however, the rotational forces are essentially concentrated within the area of residual vitreo-retinal attachment at the vitreous base or more posteriorly.

Dynamic vitreo-retinal traction operating in relation to a localized posterior extension of the vitreous base, to a relatively short segment of lattice degeneration, or to a paravascular vitreo-retinal adhesion results in a 'flap-tear' (arrow-head tear, U-tear or horseshoe tear). The tractional forces are such that the 'arrow' always points posteriorly with the gel attached to the anterior aspect or flap of the tear. Variants of flap tears are sometimes seen in relation to extensive lattice lesions. Tears based on lattice degeneration occur especially in myopic eyes while tiny flap breaks at the posterior border of the vitreous base are particularly associated with aphakia. Tearing of the retina is often accompanied by haemorrhage (sometimes recurrently from bridging vessels), initially experienced entoptically as a 'tadpole' floater in the appropriate part of the visual field; there may be associated photopsia from traction on the retina.

Dynamic vitreo-retinal traction operating in relation to a cystic retinal tuft usually produces an 'operculated' tear where a small piece of neuroepithelium is completely avulsed from the retina, coming to lie in the vicinity of the round retinal break but attached to the overlying detached posterior hyaloid membrane.

Dynamic vitreo-retinal traction is also said to be the cause of 'dialysis' of the retina. Spontaneous dialyses are usually situated inferotemporally and differ from flap-tears in that the gel is attached to the posterior margin of the break. Dialyses are not normally associated with posterior vitreous detachment (at least in the early stages) and since the break is situated at the ora, some form of 'splitting' of the basal gel is implied. Dynamic vitreous traction is not implicated in the aetiology of atrophic holes, which occur equatorially in otherwise normal appearing retina or within areas of lattice degeneration, especially in myopes.

Fig. 12.14   Diagram illustrating the concept of dynamic vitreo-retinal traction after posterior vitreous detachment with collapse; generation of a flap-tear and an operculated tear is also shown.

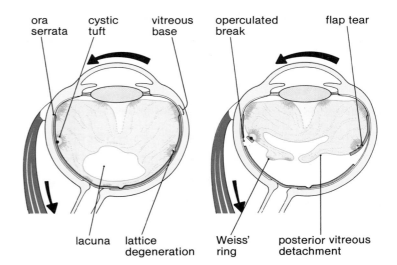

Fig. 12.15   Fundus paintings of lattice degeneration (left) and snail-track degeneration (right) (a variant of lattice degeneration) showing typical circumferential orientation of equatorial and pre-equatorial lesions.

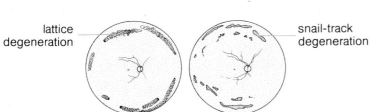

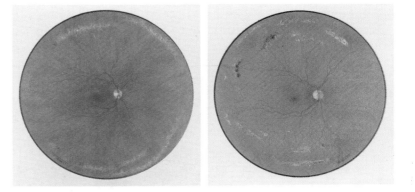

Fig. 12.16 Composite painting of the various types of retinal break – tears, holes and dialysis. Those breaks in the right half of the painting are associated with lattice degeneration.

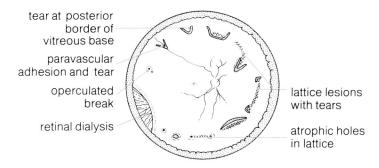

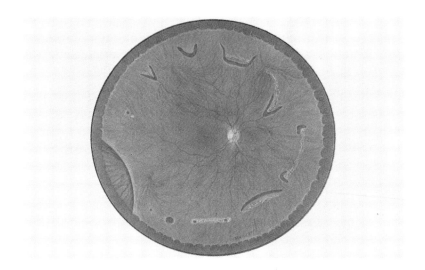

Subretinal Fluid Accumulation

Dynamic vitreo-retinal traction has a role not only in the pathogenesis of retinal tears but also in the process of progression to retinal detachment. Separation of the neuroepithelium from the pigment epithelium occurs first in the immediate vicinity of the break, and as more subretinal fluid is recruited from the vitreous cavity (from the retrohyaloid space or from syneretic gel), the area and elevation of retinal separation increases. Nevertheless, if the globe is completely immobilized at an early stage, the retina may partially or even completely reattach as the effect of dynamic vitreo-retinal traction is eliminated.

Gravitational forces play a major role in determining the distribution of subretinal fluid. A retinal detachment which becomes total soon after its onset is generally caused by a tear between the 11 and 1 o'clock meridians. Other tears above the horizontal meridian (3 o'clock to 9 o'clock) tend to cause subtotal detachments, recruited fluid progressing downwards on the same side as the tear at first and then upwards on the opposite side of the disc (but to a level lower than that on the side of the tear). As the fluid rises, it tends to form a 'recurved' or convex meniscus between the equator and ora serrata whereas the meniscus on the side of the tear is concave. Inferior subretinal fluid from a superior tear tends to separate partially into two bullae with a cleft or 'cleavage' of less elevated retina in the 6 o'clock meridian. Subretinal fluid recruited through a break located below the horizontal meridian tends to accumulate more slowly compared with that descending from above. The upper limits of detachment form recurved edges on each side, the higher edge indicating the side of the break. No cleavage fold is seen with inferior breaks. These factors aid the localization of breaks.

Subretinal fluid accumulates more quickly if fluid is recruited from the retrohyaloid space (e.g., via a flap-tear after posterior vitreous detachment) compared with breaks occurring without posterior vitreous detachment (e.g., atrophic holes and dialyses) when potential recruitment of fluid from syneretic gel may be limited. As a retinal detachment progresses, the patient notices an increasing field defect corresponding to the detached area; central vision is distorted and diminished as the macula detaches.

The detached neuroepithelium tends to be less transparent than normal, especially in cases with marked oedema and folding of the deep retinal layers internal to the external limiting membrane (outer retinal shagreen). Under the external limiting membrane, the outer segments of the rods and cones are shed from the detached area, and the photoreceptor nuclei may eventually degenerate. Restoration of vision after retinal reattachment is dependent upon the reversal of retinal oedema and the regeneration of receptor outer segments.

The vitreous gel also shows characteristic changes after retinal tearing and detachment. In addition to vitreous haemorrhage, retinal tear formation is often associated with the release of pigment epithelial cells from Bruch's membrane and their dispersion within the vitreous cavity. Thus, the presence of pigment cells in the retrolental gel in a phakic eye strongly implies the presence of a retinal break. Dedifferentiation of these cells into fibroblast-like cells and synthesis of new collagen within the gel and on the posterior hyaloid interface results in retraction and immobilization of the gel. Such changes are frequently associated with the proliferation and contraction of cellular membranes on the retinal surface.

Fig. 12.17 Photograph of a flap-tear based on lattice degeneration causing a retinal detachment (left), and photograph of an oral dialysis causing a shallow retinal detachment (right).

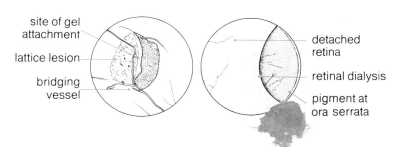

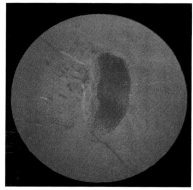

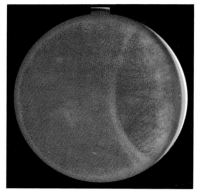

Fig. 12.18 Fundus photographs of rhegmatogenous retinal detachments. The configuration of the bullous detachment on the left changed with eye movement, indicating a mobile retina. A detached macula is seen on the right with characteristic folding of the outer retina resulting from oedema. This appearance is known as outer retinal shagreen.

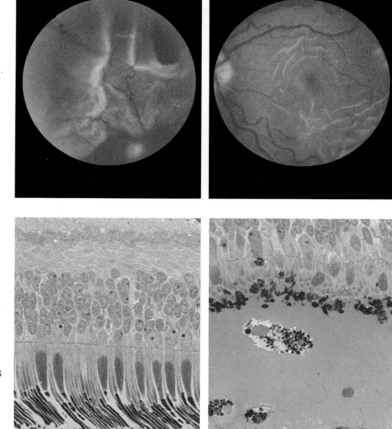

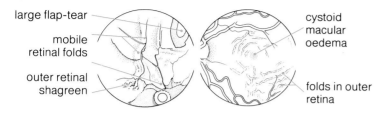

large flap-tear
mobile retinal folds
outer retinal shagreen
cystoid macular oedema
folds in outer retina

Fig. 12.19 A comparison of light micrographs of normal attached retina and detached retina demonstrates shedding of the outer segments of photoreceptors after retinal detachment. The subretinal fluid, recruited from the vitreous cavity through a break, contains pigment cells and macrophages.

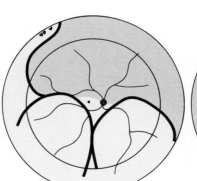

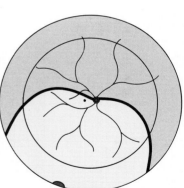

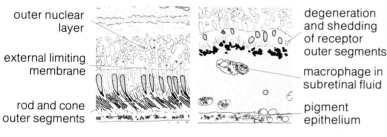

outer nuclear layer
external limiting membrane
rod and cone outer segments
degeneration and shedding of receptor outer segments
macrophage in subretinal fluid
pigment epithelium

Fig. 12.20 Diagrams demonstrating the influence of gravity in determining progression of subretinal fluid accumulation (pink-attached; blue-detached retina).

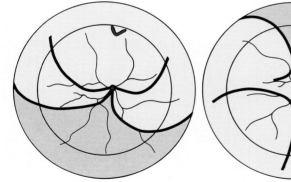

Fig. 12.21 Slit-beam photograph of the anterior gel after retinal break formation showing pigment cells ('tobacco dust') (left), and slit-beam photograph showing aggregation of pigment cells into larger clumps together with fibroblast proliferation and collagen synthesis within the gel (right).

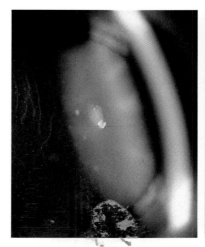

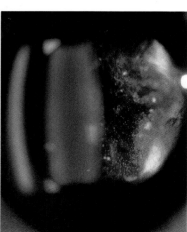

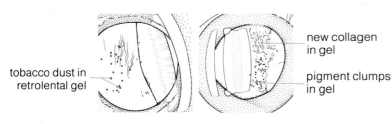

tobacco dust in retrolental gel
new collagen in gel
pigment clumps in gel

NATURAL HISTORY OF RHEGMATOGENOUS RETINAL DETACHMENT

If the retina remains detached for many months, it becomes progressively atrophic. The pigment epithelium beneath the detachment also atrophies, and reactive pigment epithelial proliferation at the margin of a subtotal retinal detachment produces a 'high-water mark' or demarcation line, which may limit further extension of the detachment to a greater or lesser degree. Multiple high-water marks in detached retina indicate recurrent

extension of the detachment. Other indices of long-standing detachment include retinal cysts (secondary schises), peripheral neovascularization and 'shifting' subretinal fluid (that is, marked displacement of viscous subretinal fluid according to the patient's posture). Occasionally, the retina reattaches spontaneously leaving a puddle of subretinal fluid around the original break and marked pigmentary changes.

Fig. 12.22 Long-standing detachment secondary to an inferonasal dialysis with high-water marks, smooth atrophic detached retina, macular hole, retinal cyst and peripheral neovascularization, and a spontaneously reattached temporal detachment secondary to an atrophic hole in lattice degeneration.

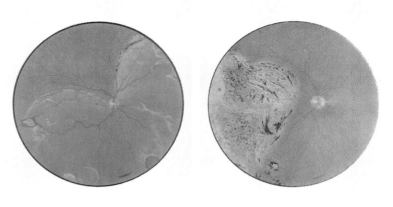

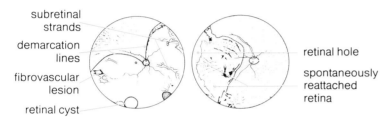

Extraretinal Proliferation

Many detachments are complicated by proliferation of fibroblasts on the retinal surface to form 'epiretinal membranes'. The fibroblasts may arise from dispersed pigment epithelial cells, from glial cells growing out through dehiscences in the inner limiting lamina, or from other sources. The cells contract and the 'tangential' or 'surface' traction so produced initially causes striation of the inner retina progressing to full-thickness fixed folding of the underlying retina. The cellular contraction is thereafter stabilized or consolidated by collagen synthesis.

The contractile process may be focal (for example macular pucker or star-folding) or more generalized (massive preretinal retraction). In the latter case, the resulting immobile configuration of detachment is demonstrable by B-scan ultrasound, with features including thickening and straightening of the retinal leaves, high equatorial elevation of the retina and retraction of the detached posterior hyaloid membrane ("Triangle sign"). Vitreous gel sometimes herniates posteriorly through a central hiatus in this coronal membrane.

Fig. 12.23 Electron micrograph of a fibroblast from an epiretinal membrane showing contractile intracellular filaments (stress cables) and extruded collagen fibres.

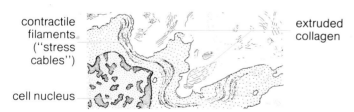

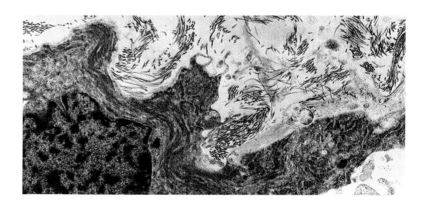

Fig. 12.24 Fundus photograph showing full-thickness folding of detached retina (star-fold) secondary to contraction of an epiretinal membrane.

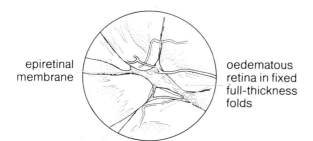

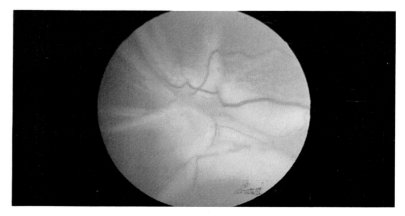

Fig. 12.25 Fundus photographs from an eye with a total retinal detachment and massive preretinal proliferation. The immobilized central retina is drawn into a funnel-shaped configuration, while stretching of the the peripheral retina distorts and immobilizes the original flap-tear.

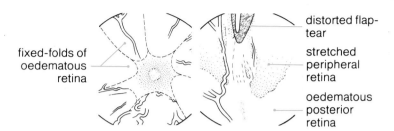

fixed-folds of oedematous retina

distorted flap-tear

stretched peripheral retina

oedematous posterior retina

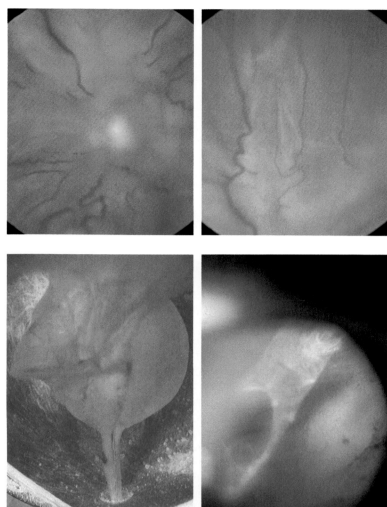

Fig. 12.26 Macro-photograph of a dissected globe with massive preretinal retraction shows an extremely narrow funnel configuration of retinal detachment posteriorly and a large secondary retinal schisis (left). A slit photograph from an eye with massive preretinal retraction shows herniation of gel through a large hiatus in the coronal vitreous membrane, and high equatorial folding of the retina posterior to the vitreous membrane (right).

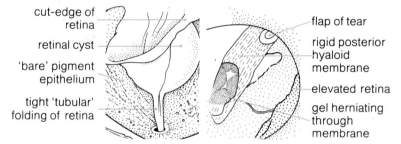

cut-edge of retina

retinal cyst

'bare' pigment epithelium

tight 'tubular' folding of retina

flap of tear

rigid posterior hyaloid membrane

elevated retina

gel herniating through membrane

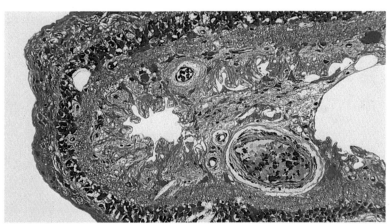

Fig. 12.27 Histology of a fixed retinal fold showing striation of the retinal surface and maintenance of full-thickness folding by surface proliferations bridging between the retinal leaves.

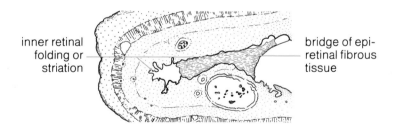

inner retinal folding or striation

bridge of epi-retinal fibrous tissue

Fig. 12.28 B-scans of eyes with massive preretinal retraction; the typical 'triangle' sign (left), and (right) an unusual configuration with gross retinal folding and closure of the retinal leaves in front of the optic disc.

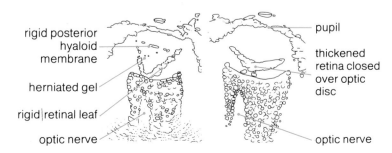

rigid posterior hyaloid membrane

herniated gel

rigid retinal leaf

optic nerve

pupil

thickened retina closed over optic disc

optic nerve

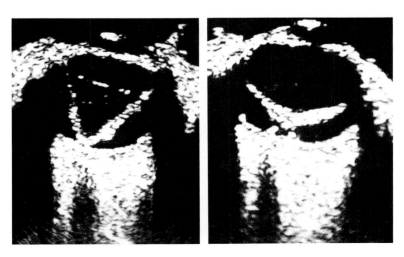

DIFFERENTIAL DIAGNOSIS OF RETINAL DETACHMENT

The majority of retinal detachments are rhegmatogenous in origin, that is they are caused by a break in the retinal neuroepithelium. Others (referred to as 'traction' detachments) reflect the development of 'static' traction forces within the vitreous gel, along the detached posterior hyaloid membrane or on the retinal surface. Massive preretinal retraction is a type of 'combined rhegmatogenous and traction detachment' wherein cellular proliferation and contraction on the retinal surface and along the detached posterior hyaloid membrane occurs subsequent to retinal break formation and retinal detachment. In other 'combined' detachments, tangential traction from epiretinal proliferation is the primary event with subsequent retinal break formation, such as in proliferative diabetic retinopathy.

Two other broad groups of retinal detachments are recognized – 'solid' detachments (for example due to a choroidal malignant melanoma) and 'serous' detachments (in central serous retinopathy, Harada's disease and the uveal effusion syndrome, etc.). Retinal detachments must also be distinguished from other disturbances in the coats of the eye which may simulate detachment of the retina. Thus, scleral infolding (e.g., from hypotony), scleral swelling (e.g., from posterior scleritis), ciliochoroidal detachment, pigment epithelial detachment and retinoschisis may all mimic a retinal detachment.

The term retinoschisis refers to a process whereby fluid accumulates within the retinal neuroepithelium to form a large intraretinal cyst. The cyst cavity has an inner (or vitreal) leaf and an outer leaf, and breaks may develop in one or both of these leaves. When fluid passes through an outer leaf break, the outer layer detaches from the pigment epithelium and the schisis is said to have progressed to a retinal detachment. Retinoschises are classically divided into 'infantile' and 'senile' varieties, though some schises present in young adults (presenile schisis).

Infantile retinoschisis is a rare disorder with a 'sex-linked' mode of inheritance; it therefore affects young males. A common presentation is vitreous haemorrhage, while central vision may be impaired by associated 'foveal schisis'. The inner leaf of the cyst is extremely thin with large breaks between the retinal vessels (hence the old term – 'congenital vascular veils'). Progression to a retinal detachment through an outer leaf break is unusual.

After middle-age, bilateral retinoschises are frequently discovered during routine examination of the peripheral fundus, and tend to be located inferotemporally. The outer leaf of the schisis often has a grey translucency with a mottled pattern. Outer leaf breaks tend to be large with rolling-over of their edges, while inner leaf breaks are usually small.

The uveal effusion syndrome is an unusual condition often mistaken for either a rhegmatogenous detachment complicated by ciliochoroidal detachment, or a 'ring melanoma' of the anterior choroid. It is characterized by deep ciliochoroidal detachments and a serous retinal detachment which exhibits marked 'shifting fluid'. Following resolution over a period of months, characteristic mottling of the pigment epithelium may be observed.

Fig. 12.29 Fundus painting of an eye with infantile retinoschisis complicated by temporal retinal detachment (which is uncommon) (left). Peripheral 'senile' schisis with frosting of the post-oral retina is seen on the right.

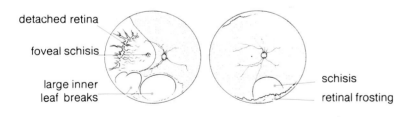

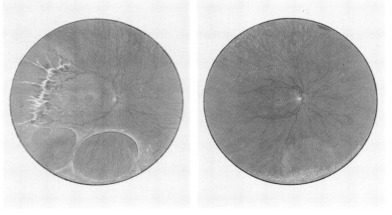

Fig. 12.30 Fundus painting of a 'senile' retinoschisis with typical large outer-leaf breaks, a small inner-leaf break and pigment demarcation around a localized retinal detachment (left). A painting of a similar senile schisis shows progression to an extensive inferotemporal retinal detachment (right).

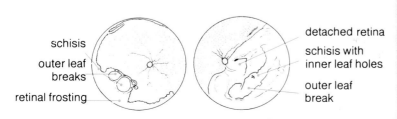

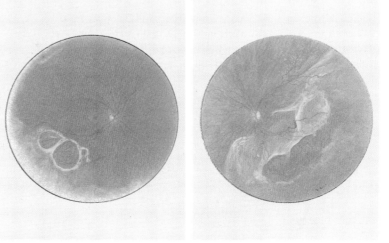

Fig. 12.31 Fundus painting of an eye with the uveal effusion syndrome with large ciliochoroidal detachments and serous retinal detachment (left). A 'healed' uveal effusion (right) shows typical extensive pigmentary changes which can sometimes be confused with genetically-determined retinitis pigmentosa.

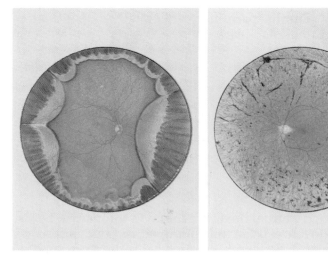

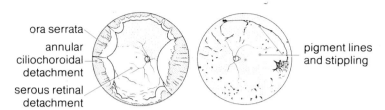

ora serrata

annular ciliochoroidal detachment

serous retinal detachment

pigment lines and stippling

SPECIAL RHEGMATOGENOUS DETACHMENTS

Certain rhegmatogenous detachments pose special problems in management owing to the unusual size or location of the retinal break. While most breaks are located between the equator and the ora serrata, more posterior breaks are sometimes seen. These may be related, for example, to posterior paravascular vitreo-retinal adhesions or to radially orientated post-equatorial lattice degeneration. This is especially true of detachments associated with a dominantly inherited vitreoretinal anomaly termed Wagner's disease or Stickler's syndrome. The anomaly is characterized by myopia, paravascular pigmentary changes, dragging of the major vessels at the optic disc, 'veils' or condensations of cortical vitreous around large lacunae or dehiscences in the gel, and multiple posterior vitreo-retinal adhesions. Systemic associations include cleft palate, characteristic facies with a long philtrum, and arthalgia.

Highly-myopic eyes with posterior staphylomata are prone to posterior breaks, especially at the macula or nasal to the optic disc. Macular breaks probably represent 'operculated' tears consequent upon posterior vitreous detachment and may themselves cause detachment of the posterior retina, or extensive detachment extending up to the ora serrata when accompanied by peripheral breaks.

Other breaks are distinguished by their great size. Giant retinal breaks are located immediately post-orally or, less frequently, at the equator. They are a variant of flap tears and result from the operation of dynamic vitreous traction (the gel mass being attached to the anterior margin of the break). The posterior flap moves independently of the gel, essentially under the influence of gravity, and there may be posterior extensions of the breaks, especially at their upper limit. Satellite U-tears are often seen, and the giant tear may extend from 90° up to 360°. Giant tears are especially associated with congenital myopia and trauma, and have a marked propensity to massive preretinal retraction.

Fig. 12.32 Fundus photographs from a patient with Stickler's syndrome showing a condensation of cortical gel with a retinal break, and paravascular pigmentary changes.

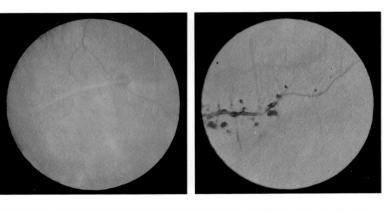

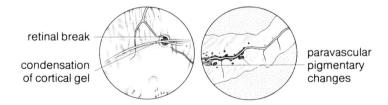

retinal break

condensation of cortical gel

paravascular pigmentary changes

Fig. 12.33 Fundus photograph of a myopic eye with a macular break and retinal detachment.

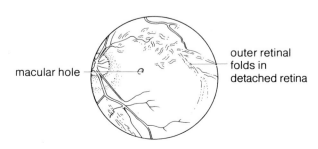

macular hole

outer retinal folds in detached retina

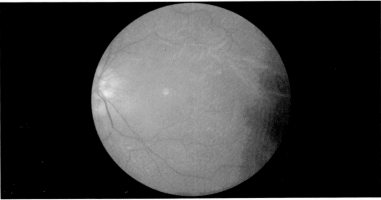

Fig. 12.34 Fundus paintings of eyes with giant retinal breaks and small flap tears.

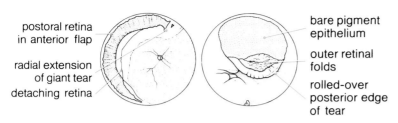

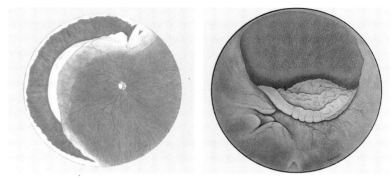

TRAUMA

Many types of retinal break are found in traumatized eyes; they may develop at the time of impact or penetration or subsequently. Inferotemporal dialyses sometimes appear to be traumatic in origin, while the term 'disinsertion' is usually applied to a less severe variety of oral break which involves single, or multiple, elevations of individual oral bays. Flap tears and irregular impact site breaks may also occur, and a macular hole may appear in association with posterior commotio retinae. There is, however, a specific type of peripheral break which is pathognomonic of blunt trauma and this is most commonly located superonasally. It is characterized by 'avulsion of the vitreous base'

comprising a strip of ciliary epithelium, ora serrata, and immediately post-oral retina into which the basal vitreous gel remains inserted. This 'bucket-handle' often hangs down in the vitreous cavity and the free posterior edge of torn retina may become detached.

Retinal disinsertions and dialyses also develop in the vicinity of penetrating injuries involving the pars plana or peripheral retina, especially when there is significant incarceration of basal gel into the wound. If vitreous loss through the wound is more severe, such oral breaks may occur in the quadrant opposite to the site of injury.

Fig. 12.35 Composite fundus painting demonstrating some of the types of retinal break seen after blunt or penetrating trauma.

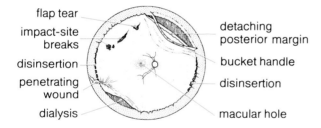

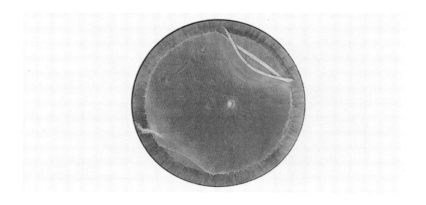

Intraocular Foreign Bodies

Penetration of the posterior segment by a high energy foreign body can result in severe vitreoretinal complications. Diagnosis of ocular retention of a small foreign body depends on careful attention to the details and circumstances of the injury and close scrutiny for evidence of ocular penetration, such as a small entry site in the anterior sclera and signs of vitreous disturbance. Immediate posterior segment damage after foreign body penetration is generally restricted to the site of ultimate impaction or through and through penetration. In most hammer and chisel accidents, high velocity ferrous material penetrates the cornea or limbal sclera, the lens and vitreous, and impacts in the retina. Initially, local tissue coagulation may be visible, together with bleeding into the cortical gel in the vicinity of the impact site and along the 'track' or path of the foreign body's penetration through the gel. If the foreign body is 'reactive', the overlying gel may become liquified.

The integrity of the retina is usually secured by chorio-retinal scarring around the foreign body, but a small retinal break, subsequently causing retinal detachment, may develop if the foreign body ricochets off the retina rather than impacting within it. Subsequently, fibroblast prolifera-tion may occur either locally at the impact site (encapsu-

lating the foreign body or puckering and distorting the underlying and adjacent retina) or along the haemorrhagic track to form a trans-gel traction band. Visual loss depends on the particular site of impaction (macular, papillary or peripheral), on opacities in the media (cataract or vitreous haemorrhage), or retinal detachment.

Surgical removal of the foreign body may be indicated because of the risk of generalized posterior segment complications such as severe vitritis and endophthalmitis (from bacterial or toxic chemical penetration along with the foreign body, or acute chalcosis) or metallic deposition (siderosis bulbi, or chronic chalcosis). Siderosis results from the chemical destruction and ocular absorption of retained ferrous material. The effects start to appear several months after injury and include glaucoma and cataract (cf. Primary and Secondary Glaucoma – Chapters 7 and 8, and The Lens – Chapter 11), and destruction of the retinal photoreceptors which produces characteristic ERG changes that are useful in assessing the visual potential of such eyes.

Radio-opaque intraocular foreign bodies are best detected by x-ray examination using a double exposure 'eye-mover' lateral x-ray film. Various methods are available for precise radiological localization of the foreign body relative to the ocular coats, including CAT scanning, but accurate localization is now required less frequently because of the advent of closed intraocular microsurgical techniques for foreign body removal from eyes with opaque media. Ultrasound examination may be valuable for detecting radiolucent foreign bodies, but is a relatively inefficient method for detecting small metallic foreign bodies, especially if they are embedded in the

ocular coats. Foreign bodies can give rise to high amplitude echoes provided they are appropriately orientated to the sound beam; a variety of artefacts arising from metallic particles aid in their identification and localization, but the main value of ultrasound is in determining the vitreoretinal complications of foreign body impaction.

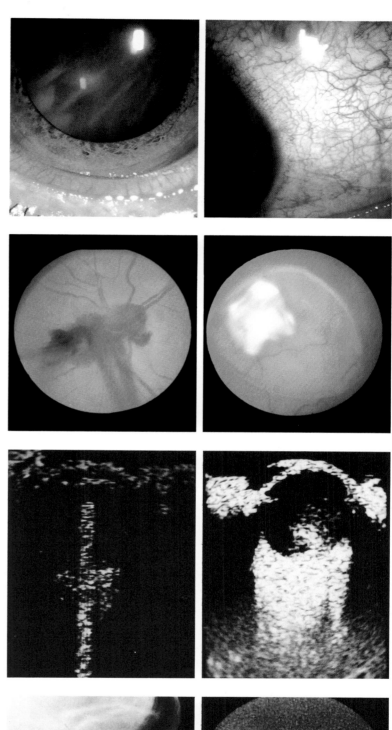

Fig. 12.36 Photograph of haemorrhage and 'stress lines' in the vitreous orientated towards the superotemporal region, where a foreign body entry site is located with prolapse of a small knuckle of vitreous gel.

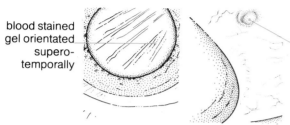

blood stained gel orientated supero-temporally

bead of gel prolapsing through foreign body entry site

Fig. 12.37 Fundus photograph of a foreign body impact site with pre-papillary haemorrhage in the cortical gel and along the track of the foreign body. A lacuna of syneretic gel overlying a large reactive foreign body on the retinal surface, seen some days after injury.

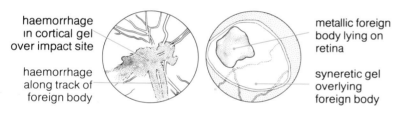

haemorrhage in cortical gel over impact site

haemorrhage along track of foreign body

metallic foreign body lying on retina

syneretic gel overlying foreign body

Fig. 12.38 B-scan ultrasound section at low gain showing multiple reflection artefacts from a foreign body located in the anterior gel (left), and posterior vitreous haemorrhage in another eye secondary to foreign body impaction near the optic disc (right).

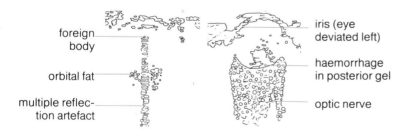

foreign body

orbital fat

multiple reflec-tion artefact

iris (eye deviated left)

haemorrhage in posterior gel

optic nerve

Fig. 12.39 Radiological detection and localization of a foreign body by an 'eye mover' lateral film (left), and by CAT scanning (right).

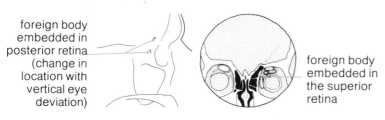

foreign body embedded in posterior retina (change in location with vertical eye deviation)

foreign body embedded in the superior retina

EXTRARETINAL NEOVASCULARIZATION

This vascularized epiretinal membrane proliferation, developing in response to ischaemia of the inner retina, may be complicated by vitreous haemorrhage, vitreoretinal traction and retinal detachment. Causes of extraretinal neovascularization include retinal vasculitis (Eales disease), retinal vein occlusion and haemoglobin SC disease, but the most common context of such vasoproliferation is diabetic retinopathy.

Ischaemic diabetic retinopathy characteristically affects the mid-peripheral retina outside the major temporal vascular arcades and nasal to the optic disc. Neovascularization generally develops near the posterior limit of the ischaemia, i.e., at the optic disc and along the major vascular arcades. Vascular mesenchyme, arising from intraretinal venules, grows out through the inner

limiting lamina and proliferates within the most cortical part of the vitreous gel as a vascularized epiretinal membrane ('flat new vessels'). The vessels do not grow into the central gel except occasionally within Cloquet's canal. The membranes incarcerate the gel in which they are proliferating, causing exaggerated vitreoretinal adhesions.

As in other epiretinal membranes, fibroblasts within the vascularized membranes contract and the tangential traction so produced is stabilized and consolidated by collagen synthesis. The tangential traction results initially in striation and folding of the inner retinal layers (inner limiting lamina and nerve fibre layer), and can then progress to full-thickness folding of the retina and traction retinal detachment.

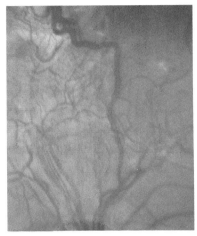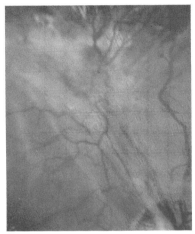

Fig. 12.40 Photograph of extensive fibrovascular epiretinal proliferation superotemporal to the optic disc before (left) and one month after (right) panretinal laser photocoagulation. A reduction in the vascular component of the membrane is evident but development of tangential traction and folding of the underlying retina has also occurred.

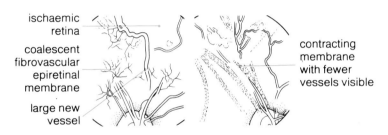

Fig. 12.41 Light microscopic section of diabetic retina demonstrates a fibrovascular epiretinal membrane causing inner retinal striation and progression towards traction detachment.

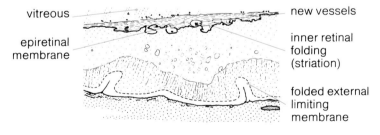

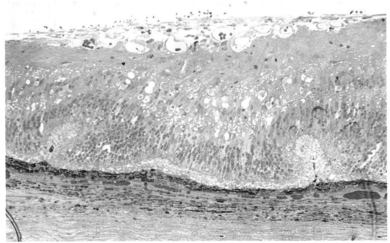

Diabetic Vitreous Haemorrhage

Bleeding into the vitreous from new vessels usually occurs at the time of posterior vitreous detachment which is 'incomplete' owing to the exaggerated vitreoretinal adhesions at sites of epiretinal vasoproliferation. The edges of the vascularized membranes tend to become avulsed from the retinal surface and come to lie in the same plane as the detached vitreous cortex. Fibrovascular tissue may thereafter proliferate forwards towards the vitreous base along the detached posterior hyaloid membrane ('forward new vessels'). Haemorrhage from the fragile new vessels invades the detached gel or (more commonly) the retrohyaloid space which is loculated by the epiretinal vasoproliferation. Lysed blood can thus form a 'red-carpet'

over the retina posterior to the vitreous base and surrounding islands of fibrosis. Retrohyaloid haemorrhage tends to clear more quickly than intra-gel haemorrhage.

Lysed red cells clogging the cortical gel may produce an ochre-membrane which tethers to the retina at sites of vasoproliferation and outlines the incomplete vitreous detachment on B-scan ultrasound examination. Erythrocytes in the retrohyaloid space often separate from the plasma (just like blood in a Westergren tube for ESR estimation), and the fluid level between plasma and red cells produces a line of high amplitude echoes by specular reflection on B-scan examination.

Fig. 12.42 Macro-photograph of a hemisected diabetic globe showing retinal ischaemia and fibrovascular proliferation along the posterior vitreous face, which is incompletely detached and bound tightly to the optic disc and temporal parapapillary retina.

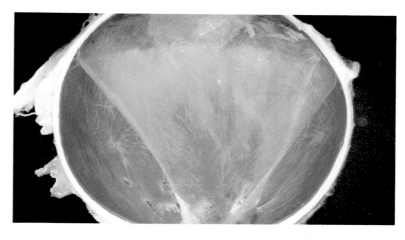

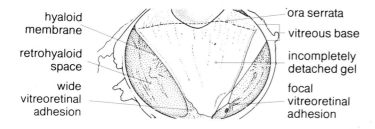

Fig. 12.43 Fundus photographs of bleeding into the vitreous gel (left) and into the retrohyaloid space (right).

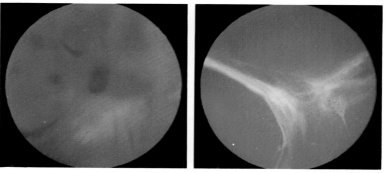

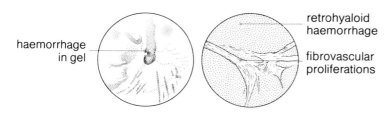

Fig. 12.44 B-scan ultrasound sections of diabetic eyes showing an ochre membrane tethering to disc new vessels (left) and fluid level from sedimented blood in the retrohyaloid space (right).

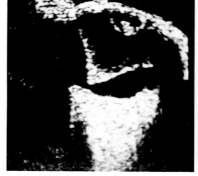

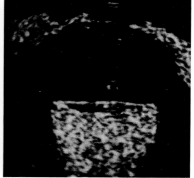

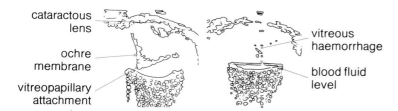

Diabetic Retinal Detachment

Three elements of vitreo-retinal traction combine to produce a traction retinal detachment in diabetes — tangential traction, anteroposterior traction, and bridging traction. Tangential traction results from contraction within vascularized epiretinal membranes; other traction forces are exerted along the rigid incompletely detached posterior hyaloid membrane. Anteroposterior traction refers to traction between the vitreous base anteriorly and fibrovascular tissue posteriorly, while bridging traction refers to traction between individual fibrovascular membranes. The retina is thus drawn forwards from the pigment epithelium by the traction system. The retinal configuration is anteriorly concave with truncation of the apex of the retinal elevation at the attachment of the posterior vitreous face. Such detachments seldom extend peripherally beyond the equator.

During avulsion of the edge of a fibrovascular membrane from the retina, a small oval 'operculated' break may develop in the immediate vicinity of the membrane. Because of this rhegmatogenous component, the detachment may take on a bullous configuration (retina anteriorly convex) and often extends to the ora serrata.

Fig. 12.45 Fundus paintings of diabetic 'pure traction' detachment (left), and bullous 'combined rhegmatogenous and traction' detachment (right).

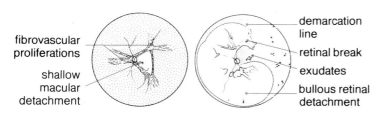

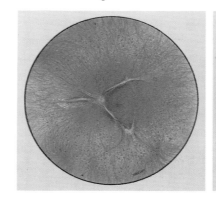

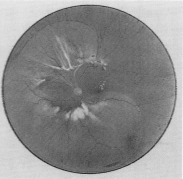

Fig. 12.46 B-scan ultrasound sections of diabetic traction retinal detachments.

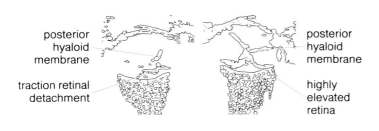

posterior hyaloid membrane

traction retinal detachment

posterior hyaloid membrane

highly elevated retina

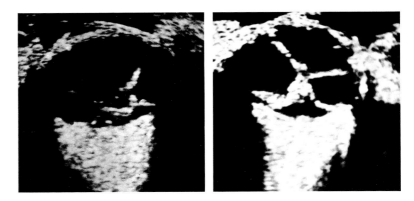

Non-diabetic Neovascularisation

Similar pathogenic mechanisms may operate to cause vitreous haemorrhage and retinal detachment in other proliferative retinopathies. In Eales' disease and haemoglobin SC retinopathy, for example, the ischaemia is generally more peripheral than in diabetes and the neovascularization is usually equatorial.

Fig. 12.47 Fundus paintings of eyes with complications of haemoglobin SC disease showing 'pure traction' detachment (left), and 'combined rhegmatogenous and traction' detachment (right).

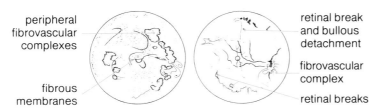

peripheral fibrovascular complexes

fibrous membranes

retinal break and bullous detachment

fibrovascular complex

retinal breaks

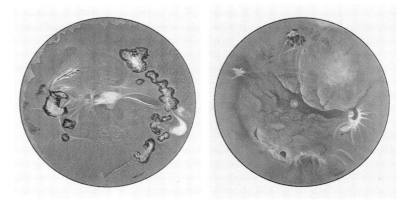

PRINCIPLES OF TREATMENT

The surgical manoeuvres employed in the management of vitreoretinal disorders can be broadly subdivided into four categories – retinal coagulation; scleral buckling; intraocular gas tamponade; and closed intraocular microsurgery – used singly or in combination according to the presenting problem. To these may be added 'drainage of subretinal fluid', though this in itself is ineffective as it does not influence the cause of detachment.

Retinal Coagulation

The purpose of retinal coagulation is to stimulate a reparative retino-choroidal reaction and thereby seal retinal breaks. Methods currently employed include transcleral cryopexy, diathermy through partial thickness sclera, and photocoagulation using laser or Xenon arc sources. Neuroepithelial necrosis can only be achieved by photocoagulation if the pigment epithelium and neuroepithelium are in apposition. Tissue necrosis may be induced in the pigment epithelium alone or in both the neuroepithelium and pigment epithelium, the latter giving rise to a stronger ultimate chorioretinal adhesion. Breaks are sealed by formation of a glial scar provided the neuroepithelium and pigment epithelium remain in contact during the several days required for adhesion. In the treatment of a flap-tear, a single row of contiguous cryocoagulations or a double row of argon laser burns around the break is generally sufficient.

Retinal coagulation alone is used in prophylaxis against break formation and to prevent an established tear progressing to a retinal detachment. Once subretinal fluid accumulates, retinal coagulation must be combined with other measures designed to restore contact between the neuroepithelium and pigment epithelium in the vicinity of the tear, such as scleral buckling or gas tamponade.

Fig. 12.48 Painting showing treatment of a flap-tear without detachment. The initial retinal opacification around the tear may be induced by cryopexy or laser photocoagulation, and the ultimate pigmentary reaction implies the break is sealed.

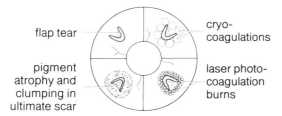

flap tear

pigment atrophy and clumping in ultimate scar

cryo-coagulations

laser photo-coagulation burns

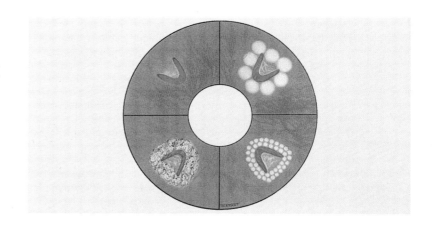

Fig. 12.49 Light micrograph of chorioretinal scar induced by laser photocoagulation; reparative glial tissue from the outer retina establishes direct connections with Bruch's membrane and pigment epithelial cells which have migrated into clumps.

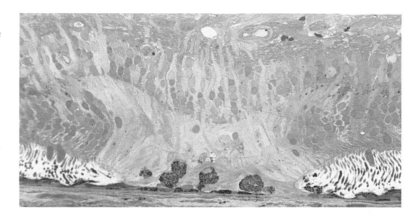

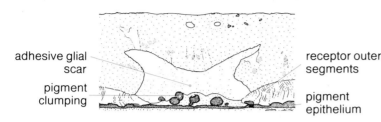

adhesive glial scar

pigment clumping

receptor outer segments

pigment epithelium

Closure of Retinal Breaks

Indentation of the sclera (so as to bring the pigment epithelium into closer contact with the detached neuroepithelium in the region of retinal tears) is achieved by scleral buckling. The buckle probably reduces local dynamic traction to such a degree that the tear closes spontaneously on the indentation; it has also been suggested that the buckle causes gel overlying the retinal tear to 'plug' the break. Various methods of indenting the sclera are available – some temporary, others permanent; some fixed onto the episclera, others implanted within a scleral pocket – but all depend upon the same principles to be effective. Episcleral explants are generally fashioned from cylinders of silastic sponge material ('plombs') or solid silicone tyres and bands. They are secured to the sclera by mattress stitches and may be sutured in a radial or circumferential orientation, the latter sometimes including the whole circumference of the globe (encirclement). Circumferentially orientated explants must be of sufficient width not only to close the posterior margin of a retinal break but also to elevate the anterior retina up to the ora serrata. This prevents redetachment from reopening of the anterior horns of the break. Eyes with multiple breaks in the same quadrant are especially suitable for treatment by circumferential explants, though there is a danger of 'fishmouthing' of the breaks, i.e., formation of a fold extending from the posterior margin of the break and causing posterior leakage of subretinal fluid. Encircling bands are utilized in order to maintain the height of underlying explants indefinitely, and also to militate against the continuing effects of vitreoretinal traction whether dynamic (such as in aphakic eyes) or static (as in eyes with peripheral surface proliferations).

Many simple rhegmatogenous detachments can be treated by scleral indentation alone without retinal coagulation or drainage of subretinal fluid. After some months, however, the buckle tends to reduce in height so tears may reopen and the retina redetach. Usually, therefore, tears are coagulated either at the time of buckling (using cryopexy) or postoperatively (using photocoagulation). Drainage of subretinal fluid is sometimes combined with scleral buckling and retinal coagulation in order to reduce the elevation of tears in a bullous detachment and so facilitate localization of the tear, trans-scleral cryopexy and accurate placement of the buckle. Subretinal fluid-drainage is particularly indicated if the retina in the vicinity of the tear is immobilized by epiretinal proliferation and contraction since spontaneous closure of the tear onto the buckle is less likely to occur.

Retinal breaks can also be closed internally in a relatively safe and elegant manner by 'gas tamponade'. Air is injected via the pars plana and the eye positioned post-operatively so that the arc of contact of the air bubble includes the region of the tear. This is the most efficient technique currently available for sealing breaks, but the bubble absorbs over a period of a few days, so tissue coagulation around the break must also be used in order to secure permanently the neuroepithelium to the pigment epithelium via a chorioretinal scar. Furthermore, measures designed to reduce or eliminate retinal traction in the area (scleral buckling or closed microsurgery) are also employed in most instances in order to ensure that the induced chorioretinal adhesive forces outweigh continuing vitreo-retinal traction forces.

Fig. 12.50 Fundus photographs of flap tears treated by cryopexy and episcleral explants. Circumferential plombage (left) may be complicated by 'fishmouthing' and failure of closure of the break, a problem seen much less frequently with radial explants (right).

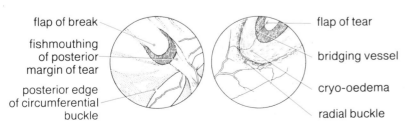

flap of break

fishmouthing of posterior margin of tear

posterior edge of circumferential buckle

flap of tear

bridging vessel

cryo-oedema

radial buckle

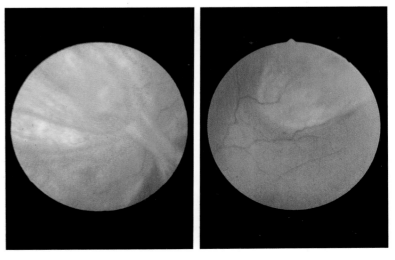

Fig. 12.51 Drawing of episcleral explants including an encircling band, a radial silastic plomb, and a circumferentially-orientated grooved tyre made of solid silicone.

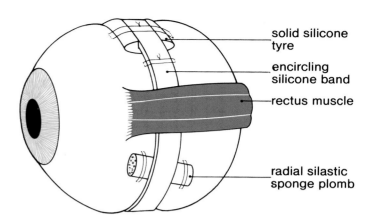

solid silicone tyre

encircling silicone band

rectus muscle

radial silastic sponge plomb

Fig. 12.52 Fundus painting of total retinal detachment caused by multiple breaks based upon lattice degeneration (left), and postoperative appearance after cryocoagulation, drainage of subretinal fluid and employment of the explants illustrated in Fig. 12.51 (right).

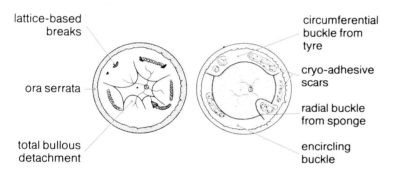

lattice-based breaks

ora serrata

total bullous detachment

circumferential buckle from tyre

cryo-adhesive scars

radial buckle from sponge

encircling buckle

Fig. 12.53 Fundus photograph of an intraocular air bubble employed to seal internally a superior break in an eye with diabetic retinopathy (left) and patient photograph emphasizing the importance of postoperative posture in maintaining internal closure of retinal breaks (right).

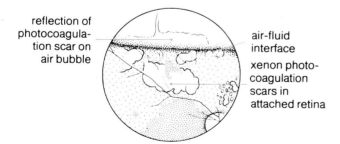

reflection of photocoagulation scar on air bubble

air-fluid interface

xenon photocoagulation scars in attached retina

Vitrectomy

Closed microsurgical techniques are employed to remove tissues from the vitreous cavity (such as gel, haemorrhagic debris or fibrous membranes) and to manipulate the retina (e.g., internal drainage of subretinal fluid, intraocular gas injection and hydraulic reattachment of the retina, or manipulation of the posterior flap of a giant tear).

Entry sites are fashioned in the pars plana near the base of the ciliary processes (so that the incisions are anterior to the vitreous base) some 3-4 mm from the limbus. An infusion system maintains the shape and pressure of the globe, fibre-optic devices provide reflex-free endoillumination, and surgical manoeuvres are generally

monitored by the surgeon using the optical system of the eye, a contact lens, and an operating microscope. A variety of implements are inserted through a third sclerotomy, including suction-cutters (which 'mince' the gel into tiny pieces prior to aspiration from the eye – vitrectomy), microscissors (to segment fibrous membranes, especially those proliferating on the retinal surface), and picks (to peel membranes off the retina). In most procedures, the whole of the gel (with any contained opacities) is removed apart from a frill of basal gel. Any connections between the basal gel and the posterior retina are thereby eliminated.

Fig. 12.54 Macrophotograph of the internal aspect of a healed pars plana entry site from an excised globe (left), and a diagram of common gauge microsurgery with three entry sites for infusion, endoillumination and a suction-cutter (right).

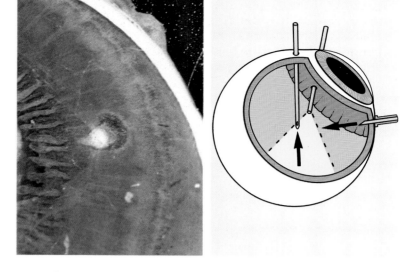

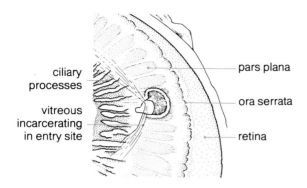

Fig. 12.55 Fundus painting of post-vitrectomy appearance in a diabetic eye with an ochre membrane originally tethering to new vessels from the optic disc . Scars from photocoagulation are scattered throughout the posterior pole and hard exudates are seen at the macula.

Visual acuity improved from light perception to 6/24 (left). In another eye with vitreous haemorrhage secondary to Eales disease, the central gel and an ochre membrane have been excised leaving islands of peripheral fibrovascular tissue. Vision improved from hand movements to 6/9 (right).

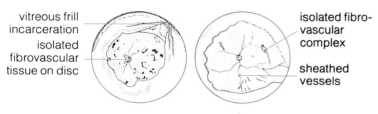

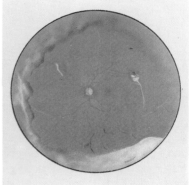

Fig. 12.56 Fundus paintings of post-vitrectomy appearances following closed microsurgery for vitreous haemorrhage secondary to retinal vein occlusion (left) and in Terson's syndrome (vitreous haemorrhage after subarachnoid haemorrhage) (right).

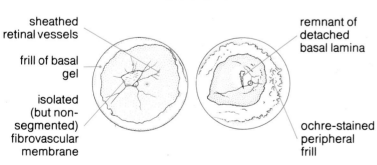

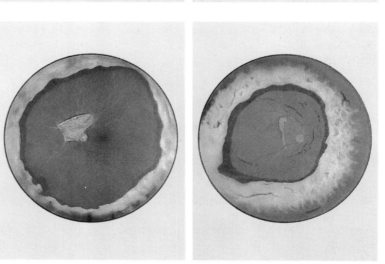

Simple vitrectomy techniques are also appropriate for the management of posteriorly located breaks and certain elements of vitreo-retinal traction such as transgel traction bands and traction exerted along the detached posterior hyaloid membrane (antero-posterior and bridging traction) as these are difficult to manage by conventional surgery. The majority of traction detachments, however, involve contracting epiretinal membranes (tangential traction) so that epiretinal dissection techniques with membrane peeling, membrane segmentation or delamination are necessary in order to permit retinal reapposition. In combined rhegmatogenous and traction detachments, such dissection must be combined with reattachment and sealing of retinal breaks, for example, by internal drainage of subretinal fluid, intraocular gas tamponade and retinal coagulation. With careful selection of cases, closed ocular microsurgery offers visual recovery for otherwise inoperable conditions.

Fig. 12.57 Fundus painting of posterior traction detachment secondary to impaction and subsequent magnet-extraction of an intraocular foreign body (left). Removal of gel and transgel traction bands permitted retinal reattachment (right) and visual improvement from $^6/_{24}$ to $^6/_9$.

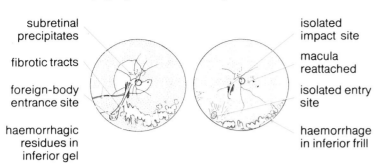

subretinal precipitates

isolated impact site

fibrotic tracts

macula reattached

foreign-body entrance site

isolated entry site

haemorrhagic residues in inferior gel

haemorrhage in inferior frill

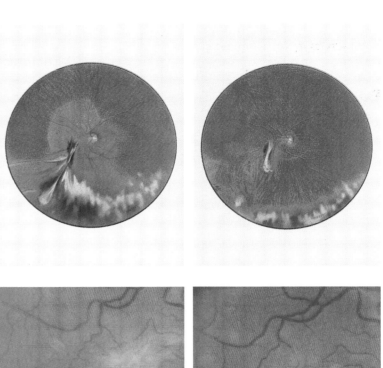

Fig. 12.58 Fundus photographs of a case of macular pucker illustrating the principle of membrane peeling. Epimacular fibrous membrane with distortion and full-thickness folding of the posterior retina (left) and post-operative appearance. Vision improved from $^6/_{60}$ to $^6/_5$.

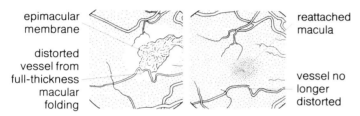

epimacular membrane

reattached macula

distorted vessel from full-thickness macular folding

vessel no longer distorted

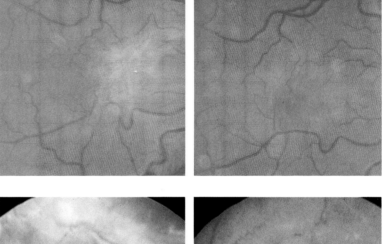

Fig. 12.59 Fundus photographs illustrating the principle of membrane segmentation for diabetic traction retinal detachment. Fibrovascular proliferation over the peripapillary retina with underlying traction detachment (left), and postoperative appearance with segmented islands of residual fibrovascular tissue and macular reattachment (right). Visual acuity improved from $^2/_{60}$ to $^6/_{12}$.

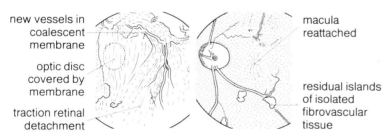

new vessels in coalescent membrane

macula reattached

optic disc covered by membrane

traction retinal detachment

residual islands of isolated fibrovascular tissue

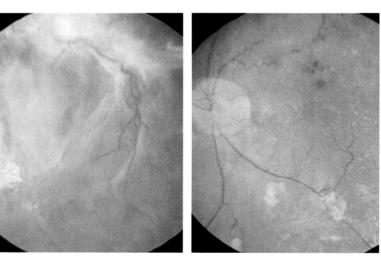

Fig. 12.60 Fundus painting of diabetic eye with vitreous haemorrhage and combined traction and rhegmatogenous detachment involving the macula (left). Following vitrectomy, cryocoagulation, internal drainage of subretinal fluid and conventional explant plombage, a postoperative painting shows clear axial vitreous and retinal reattachment (right).

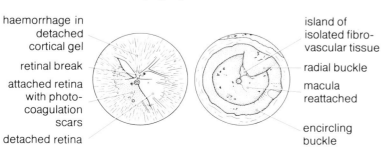

haemorrhage in detached cortical gel

island of isolated fibro-vascular tissue

retinal break

radial buckle

attached retina with photo-coagulation scars

macula reattached

detached retina

encircling buckle

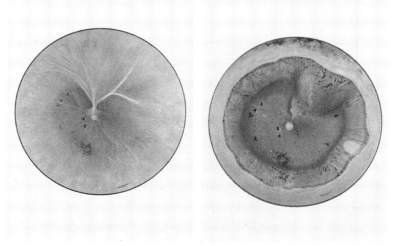

13. The Retina: Normal Anatomy and Physical Signs

D. J. Spalton
J. Marshall

EMBRYOLOGY

The optic cup develops from the optic vesicle in the first 6-7 weeks of gestation and consists of two layers of neuroectoderm separated by a space. The outer layer of cells will eventually form the retinal pigment epithelium and the inner layer the neurosensory retina, the potential space between them being re-established pathologically in later life in conditions such as rhegmatogenous retinal detachment or central serous retinopathy.

The inner layer of neuroectoderm (i.e. that adjacent to the vitreous gel) is initially about 10 cells deep. By three months of gestation it has proliferated into two layers, the inner and outer neuroblastic layers, separated by the transient layer of Chievitz. During the next two months of development the inner neuroblastic layer further differentiates: the ganglion cells appear first and migrate towards the inner retinal surface where they form the ganglion cell layer; the remaining cells migrate downwards to form the amacrine cells of the adult inner nuclear layer, and the inner plexiform layer of nerve fibres and synapses forms in between. Müller cells are differentiated early on from the inner neuroblastic layer and migrate downwards to lie in the inner nuclear layer. The outer neuroblastic layer also contributes to the inner nuclear layer by supplying the horizontal and bipolar cells; their migration obliterates Chievitz's layer.

The photoreceptors are the final layer to be differentiated. Some authorities believe they are derived from the neuroectoderm of the outer neuroblastic layer, but it is more likely that they are derived from the ependymal layer lining the primitive neural tube and optic vesicle. They are thought to be adapted from ciliated cells, and as such are analagous with those of the organ of Corti in the ear and others elsewhere in the nervous system. This common ancestory has been cited as a possible explanation of the association of blindness with deafness in some inherited retinal dystrophies.

The overall adult arrangement of retinal layers is present by five and a half months of gestation but retinal development is not uniform. For example, photoreceptors first differentiate at the macula, but then these cells are overtaken by those in all the other retinal areas so that at birth the macula is the only area not to have fully developed photoreceptor cells. The foveal photoreceptors are not completely developed until about 3 to 4 months after birth when the baby starts to fixate.

The retinal pigment epithelium starts to become pigmented at about 6 weeks of gestation and the process appears to be complete by 3 months when the epithelium is seen as a densely pigmented monocellular layer. Thus the retinal pigment epithelium is fully pigmented before the process of choroidal pigmentation has even begun.

Fig. 13.1 An axial section of the eye of a 20mm foetus (6 weeks gestation) shows the inner and outer layers of the optic cup which will form the neurosensory retina and retinal pigment epithelium, respectively. The primary vitreous and hyaloid vascular system are visible and the inner retina already shows signs of dividing into the inner and outer neuroblastic layers.

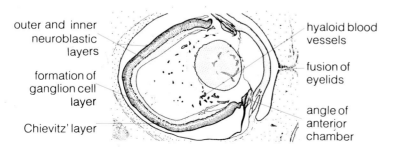

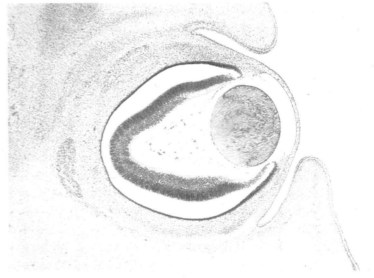

Fig. 13.2 An axial section of a 35mm (9-10 weeks gestation) embryo shows that the eye is very much larger and better developed. The inner and outer neuroblastic layers are well formed.

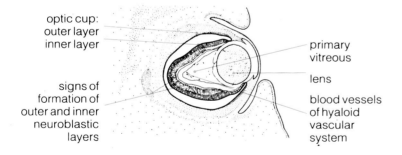

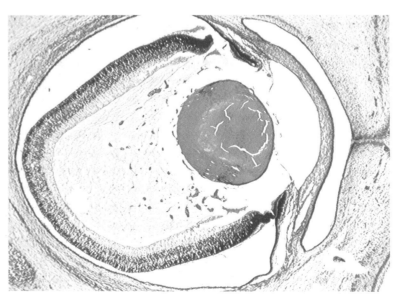

THE ANATOMY OF THE RETINA

The photoreceptors detect light and the retinal pigment epithelial cells provide their metabolic support. The inner retinal structure is supported by the Müller cells; the remaining neuroretinal tissue integrates and processes visual information so that by the time the visual signal reaches the axons in the optic nerve there has already been a considerable coding of information.

The retina consists of just four layers of cells and two layers of neuronal interconnections. In histological sections of the retina this simple six-layered structure is superficially lost and a far more complex multistratified appearance is seen which arises from the anatomical juxtaposition of similar parts of adjacent cells. For example, the photoreceptor cells alone give rise to five apparent layers.

The two so-called 'limiting membranes' are formed by components of the Müller cells, a type of retinal glial cell whose processes extend across all the retinal layers between the limiting membranes, and whose nuclei are found in the inner nuclear layer. The outer limiting membrane, lying midway along the inner segments of the photoreceptors, is not a real membrane, but an alignment of junctional complexes between Müller cells and photoreceptor cells. In contrast, the inner limiting membrane on the retinal surface is a tough acellular membrane, laid down by the Müller cells and into which fibres from the hyaloid membrane of the vitreous cortex insert.

The Pigment Epithelium

The retinal pigment epithelium (RPE) is a single layer of hexanocuboidal cells lying on Bruch's membrane. The function of the RPE is to service and maintain the overlying photoreceptor cells and in order to do this it sustains five major processes. These are the absorption of stray light, active transport of metabolites, the provision of a blood-retinal barrier, regeneration of visual pigments, and phagocytosis.

The cells contain fusiform granules of a browny-black melanin. This pigment absorbs light strongly between 400 and 800 nm and limits the amount of light that is reflected or scattered within the eye. Therefore, the photoreceptor cells are, to some extent, protected from image degradation by stimulation from randomly scattered light.

Electron microscopy of the border of the RPE cell adjacent to Bruch's membrane shows that the cell membrane is extremely convoluted and that large numbers of mitochondria reside in this portion of the cell These convolutions serve to increase the surface area of the cell which is covered with specific biochemical binding sites. Thus the RPE cells actively accumulate and transport the vital metabolites diffusing through Bruch's membrane from the underlying choriocapillaris, and actively excrete waste products. The retinal artery circulation does not contribute to the metabolic needs of the photoreceptors.

Free diffusion from the choriocapillaris into the neural retina is prevented by tight junctions, or zonular occludens, between the RPE cells. These are junctional complexes which extend around the entire circumference of each RPE cell and effectively bind them to their neighbours. The tight junctions and the active transport mechanisms together constitute the 'outer blood-retinal barrier', a mechanism whereby the photoreceptor cells are only exposed to required molecular species.

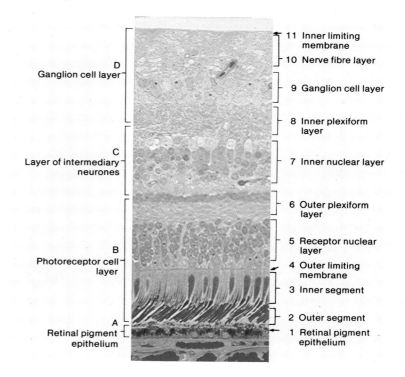

Fig. 13.3 The retinal cell layers are listed on the left and the apparent layers that these cells give rise to are shown on the right.

D Ganglion cell layer

C Layer of intermediary neurones

B Photoreceptor cell layer

A Retinal pigment epithelium

11 Inner limiting membrane
10 Nerve fibre layer
9 Ganglion cell layer
8 Inner plexiform layer
7 Inner nuclear layer
6 Outer plexiform layer
5 Receptor nuclear layer
4 Outer limiting membrane
3 Inner segment
2 Outer segment
1 Retinal pigment epithelium

The action of light on the visual pigments in the outer segments of the photoreceptor cells causes structural changes in the visual pigment so that the chromophore separates from the protein. In the rods this process is known as bleaching and results in the visual pigment rhodopsin being split into retinol and a protein called opsin. The enzymes required to allow these two to recombine into rhodopsin are situated in the RPE, therefore, these cells are essential for the maintenance of the visual cycle.

Each RPE cell functions as a static macrophage, in that throughout life it phagocytoses the tips of the overlying rods and cones. The engulfed particles, known as phagosomes, are progressively degraded intracellularly by the action of lysosomes. The breakdown products are then recycled for reincorporation into the photoreceptor cells or voided from the RPE into the choriocapillaris. With increasing age this system becomes less efficient and breakdown products may either become stored in the RPE as lipofuscin, or in Bruch's membrane as drusen. This accumulative process may well be responsible for many of the retinopathies of the elderly. Each RPE cell services up to 45 photoreceptors held in close physiological contact by receptor sheaths which extend from the surface of the cells. In addition microvillous processes from the RPE cell extend between the outer segment tips and these seem to play the major role in exchange of metabolites between the two cell layers. The extracellular space in this area of the retina is filled with a mucopolysaccharide intercellular ground substance called the inter-receptor matrix. There is no anatomical bond between the RPE cell and photoreceptor and this accounts for the ease with which these two layers can be pathologically separated.

Fig. 13.4 A flat preparation shows the monolayer of hexagonal RPE cells, and the natural colouration of their melanin granules. Electron microscopy demonstrates a zonular occludens junction between two RPE cells, and intracellular melanin granules and phagosomes. Mitochondria lie along the border with Bruch's membrane.

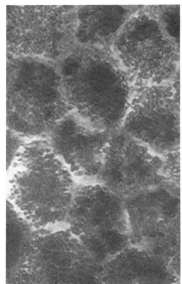
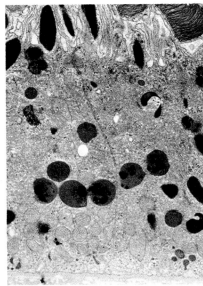
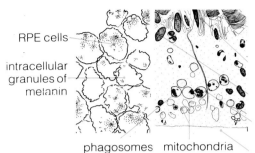

RPE cells

intracellular granules of melanin

phagosomes   mitochondria

outer segments of rods

villous processes of receptor sheaths

melanosomes

zonular occludens

Bruch's membrane

The Photoreceptor Cells

Although the photoreceptor cells are of two distinct types (rods and cones) both show the same basic structural organization. They are elongated and their cytoplasmic components are arranged in such a way that different functions take place at specific positions along their length. The photoreceptor cell transduces light by processes which are as yet not fully understood. The action of light on the photoreceptor surprisingly results in the 'switching off' of the cell. The sequence seems to start with photons being absorbed by the visual pigments in the outer segment which then undergo conformational changes. The molecular changes in the visual pigments cause the release of some type of internal transmitter from the discs, or nearby, which in turn passes to the boundary membrane of the cell inducing membrane alterations and hyperpolarization of the cell. This results in changes in the net flow of current around the photoreceptor and in turn this switches off the release of neurotransmitter at the cell's synapse. On returning to darkness the situation reverses and the neurotransmitter is switched on again. The structure of a photoreceptor consists of:

1. An outer segment which is the light-sensitive portion of the cell and consists of a stack of hollow coin-like membranes or discs and it is these disc membranes which contain the visual pigment molecules. In each rod there are about 1000 discs and each disc is separated from all the others and the boundary membrane of the cell. Therefore, rod outer segments can be thought of as analogous to a stack of coins in a tube. If the tube is broken and the stack disturbed individual coins will be lost. In cone cells, the outer segments differ in that all the 'discs' are joined to the boundary membrane with an aperture; it is through this hole that the discs are in contact with the extracellular space and, therefore, with each other. Consequently, it is not possible to isolate a single 'disc' from a cone outer segment.

2. A constricted region called the cilium, which resembles the structure of other cilia in that it contains a number of paired microtubules.

3. An inner segment which is the manufacturing portion of the rod or cone; in each case this is divided into two, an outer ellipsoid and an inner myoid. The ellipsoid contains mitochondria and provides energy for the transduction processes in the outer segment, and the myoid contains Golgi bodies and ribosomes to manufacture cell components and membranes.

4. An outer connecting fibre which runs from the inner segment to the nucleus. In cones this portion tends to be short as the nuclei are situated at the outside of the outer nuclear layer and close to the outer limiting membrane. For rods, the length varies with nuclear position.

5. A nucleus.

6. An inner connecting fibre which runs from the nucleus to the synaptic region. In cones, it is this structure that becomes elongated in the fovea, in order to make contact with the displaced intermediary neurones, and forms the fibre layer of Henlé.

7. A synaptic region. In rods this is sometimes called the rod spheral and in cones the cone pedicle. In both cells the synaptic region contains vesicles, and mediation of transynaptic information is by chemical agents. Both cells exhibit so-called invaginated connections with components from intermediary neurones deep to their synapse surface. These invaginated synapses are called 'triads' because they contain three processes; usually one from a bipolar cell, and two from horizontal cells. Rods have a single triad while cones may have up to twenty.

Unlike other neurones, photoreceptor cells are continually replacing a major portion of themselves throughout life and again this process differs between rods and cones. In rods, new discs are formed in the region of the cilium at the rate of about 1 to 5 an hour and, as each new disc is formed, older ones are progressively displaced towards the pigment epithelium. The oldest discs are shed from the tips of the outer segments in packets of about 30 at a time in a balanced process which does not radically alter rod length. The packets of rod discs are shed first thing in the morning, or, if in periods of prolonged darkness, at the onset of light. As previously stated the shed discs are phagocytosed by the RPE and in essence, therefore, the rod outer segment is entirely replaced every 8 to 14 days. Less is known about cone cells, although the best evidence to date suggests that their discs are also renewed, although the process is much slower than rods, taking about 9 months to 1 year to fully replace the outer segment. This time course is supported by observations on the recovery of cone function after retinal detachment surgery. In contrast to rods, cones shed their phagosomes at night.

Fig. 13.5 A diagram shows the intracellular anatomy of a rod and cone; this may be compared with the appearances seen on light microscopy of a horizontal section through the retina in the macula.

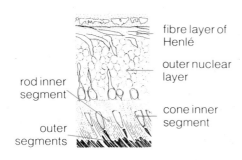

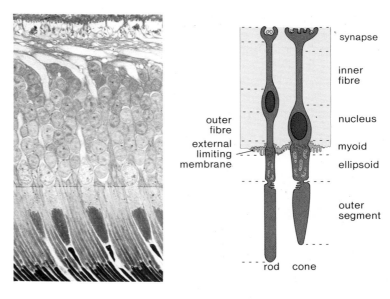

Fig. 13.6 Electron microscopy of the junction of the inner and outer segments of a rod and cone demonstrates the stacks of photoreceptor discs which, in the rod, are isolated from the boundary membrane but are connected to it in the cone. Mitochondria can be seen in the ellipsoid of each cell and the cilium of the rod is also visible. At the tip of the outer segment packets of photoreceptor discs are being phagocytosed by the RPE cell.

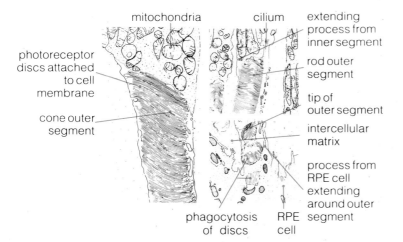

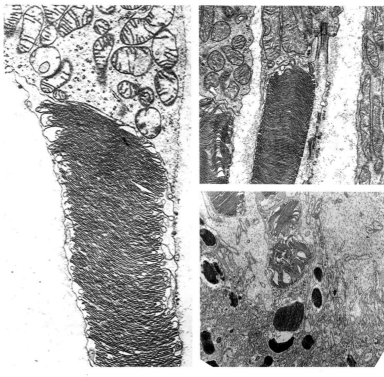

Fig. 13.7 The complex of a pigment epithelial cell and its photoreceptors is a highly metabolically active area. As yet, most of the metabolic pathways are unknown but it is likely that failures in specific processes account for the range of diseases seen in the inherited retinal dystrophies and that a general decrease in cellular efficiency produces the ageing changes in Bruch's membrane that lead to senile macular degeneration. The metabolic route to and from the photoreceptor can be broken down into eleven theoretical stages. The clinical importance of each of these pathways is not yet known.

Possible pathways of photoreceptor metabolism

A Systemic

1. transport defect

B Intraocular

2. receptor sites on RPE cell

3. transepithelial transport

4. donor mechanism

5. receptor sites (photoreceptor cell)

6. micro metabolism

7. membranogenesis

8. membrane stability

9. phagocytosis (membrane recognition)

10. lysis

11. voiding of lytic products

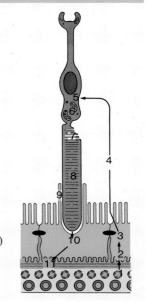

The Inner Retina

The inner nuclear layer contains the cell bodies of the bipolar cells, horizontal cells, amacrine cells and the Müller cells, which are a specialised type of glial cell. Until recently, the bipolar cell was thought to be the only retinal neurone to connect the outer plexiform layer with the inner plexiform layer thus effectively providing a channel for information from the photoreceptor cells to reach the ganglion cells. In reality the bipolar cells do not connect photoreceptors directly to ganglion cells because in the outer and inner plexiform layers respectively the horizontal and amacrine cell processes intervene. Thus, horizontal cells connect groups of photoreceptor cells together and modify their group output signal via the triads in the photoreceptor synapses before allowing the signal to be passed towards the inner plexiform layer by the bipolar cell. In the inner plexiform layer the bipolar cells commonly synapse with amacrine cells which in turn modify the signal before passing it on to groups of ganglion cells. We now know of the existence of one further neurone which has a position and connection array in the inner plexiform layer similar to an amacrine cell but which also possesses a long process which passes back to the outer plexiform layer. These cells are called interplexiform cells and as yet their relative importance in retinal function is unknown.

Müller cells are specialised glial cells which form the scaffolding of the retina. They expand in the inner retina as they approach the vitreous cortex to form the large area known as the footplate. These footplates can sometimes be seen clinically in the posterior pole as tiny reflecting dots which are known as Gunn's dots. The innermost portions of the Müllers fibres actively produce the fibrous acellular inner limiting membrane, which is a true membrane and extremely strong. The external limiting membrane is not a true membrane but rather the close alignment of specialised junctions of the Müller cells around the junction of the inner and outer segments of the photoreceptors.

Apart from supporting the retinal structure, Müller cells appear to be associated with nutrition of the photoreceptor inner segments and with the generation of neuronal impulses. They probably act as an ionic reservoir during hyperpolarization of the photoreceptor by light and this is reflected in their contribution to the B wave of the ERG. They also form the major element of scar tissue, or gliosis, which is the retina's characteristic response to cell death or disease.

The ganglion cell layer, together with its nerve fibre layer, is the innermost layer of the retina and by the time the neuronal signal is generated from these cells the information has been coded to a considerable extent. The retina responds to changes rather than to a steady state, therefore changes in contrast or movement of edges are important stimuli. Each neuronal cell in either the inner nuclear layer or ganglion cell layer will have its own receptive field (i.e. an ultimate connection with a group of photoreceptors) but receptive fields have been mostly studied at the ganglion cell level. Foveal cones have been said to have a 1:1:1 relationship with a bipolar cell and ganglion cell thereby producing a highly specific response. This arrangement was thought to be necessary to account for the resolution of the eye, however recent knowledge from the study and design of computerised reading machines now suggests that the lateral connectivity in the retina may provide sufficient communication channels between adjacent cells so that a strict 1:1 structure need not be adhered to. Outside the fovea the photoreceptors are grouped into larger receptive fields. If taken by average one ganglion cell would service 130 photoreceptors but, since the macular area is served by over 50% of the ganglion cells, receptive fields in this area probably control smaller groups of photoreceptors than those in the periphery.

Some ganglion cells are turned off by a bright light projected into the centre of their receptive field, others are turned on, in effect giving a response to white on black or black on white. Rods and cones can be integrated in receptive fields; some receptive fields will respond to a different colour or cone population when stimulated centrally or peripherally. Recently, some ganglion cells have been classified on the basis of their electrical responses in relation to projection of light on their photoreceptor cells. Some ganglion cells (X cells) give a sustained discharge if light is projected onto their photoreceptors, whereas others only fire transiently (Y cells) and others respond to a moving edge (W cells). There is good physiological evidence to link X cells to spatial discrimination and the production of visual acuity, whereas Y and W cells are probably concerned with detection of motion and its direction.

Fig. 13.8 This diagram illustrates the neuronal connections in the retina and the cells that participate. Each neuronal cell eventually relates to a group of photoreceptors – its 'receptive field'.

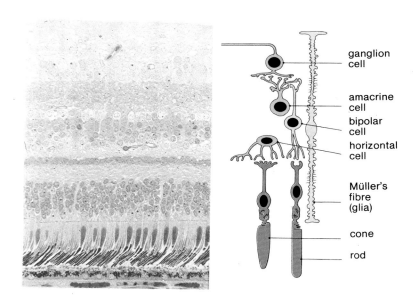

ganglion cell

amacrine cell

bipolar cell

horizontal cell

Müller's fibre (glia)

cone

rod

Topographical Changes in the Retina

The macula is seen clinically as an area of altered light reflex which lies 3.5 mm lateral and 1 mm inferior to the temporal edge of the optic disc. It appears darker than the surrounding retina, partly because of the presence of a yellow xanthophil pigment in the neural retina, and partly because the underlying RPE cells in this region are smaller and appear more densely pigmented. The exact margins are impossible to determine clinically and the definition used by the anatomist differs from that used by the clinician. The former defines its extent as that area of the retina centred on the fovea where the ganglion cell layer exceeds one layer, whilst the latter uses the altered light reflex criterion. Anatomically, the macula is about 5.5 mm across and at its centre is the fovea, a pit whose diameter is 1.9 mm. The floor of the pit is called the foveola, and is .35 mm in diameter. This is the only region of the fovea in which no rods are found. Cones are found in greatest density (15,000 mm^2) in the foveola decreasing to about 4000 to 5000 mm^2 in the periphery. In contrast, rods achieve their greatest density at about 20° from fixation (on the field isopter just peripheral to the optic disc). In total, the young adult retina contains about 120 million rods and 6 million cone cells.

Fig. 13.9 In the fovea the neural retina is about 90 μm thick compared to 350 μm in the perifovea. This thinning arises because the neurones of the inner retina, together with the ganglion cells, are displaced radially to allow incident light to fall on the highly specialised foveal cones without passing through a potentially light-scattering medium of neural retina and retinal capillaries. In order for the foveal cones to connect with the displaced inner retinal neurones the inner connecting fibres of the cones become very elongated and collectively form the fibre layer of Henlé. This layer is thought to be the location of the macular xanthophil pigment and a function of this may be to absorb blue light which is potentially harmful to the photoreceptors. Pathological oedema and exudation readily accumulate here because the inner connecting fibres are not tightly bound together. This is seen clinically as radially angled cystoid spaces with macular oedema or as a macular star with lipid exudation.

Fig. 13.10 Towards the far periphery the retina becomes thinner and the ganglion cell layer sparsely populated. In the elderly, the peripheral retina, adjacent to the ora serrata, may show cystic spaces within the attenuated neural retina. At the ora serrata the inner retinal layers are lost and the photoreceptors become shorter and fewer until finally the retina is lost to fuse with the unpigmented monolayer of the pars plana which runs forwards over the ciliary processes (see also Chapter 9).

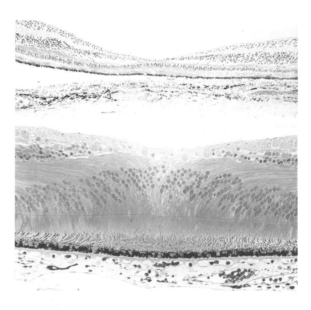

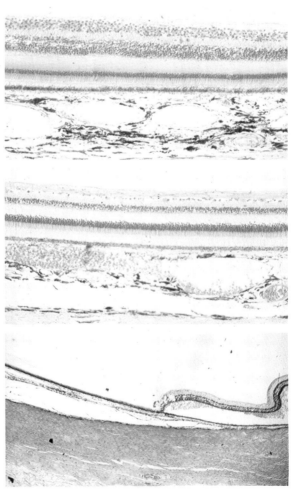

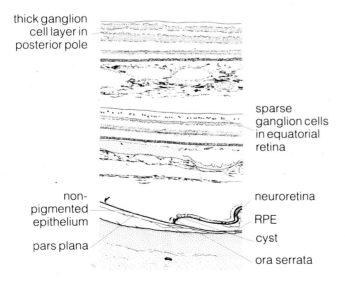

thick ganglion cell layer in posterior pole

sparse ganglion cells in equatorial retina

non-pigmented epithelium

pars plana

neuroretina

RPE

cyst

ora serrata

BLOOD SUPPLY OF THE RETINA

The central retinal artery supplies all the cells of the neural retina with the exeception of the photoreceptor cells. These receive their metabolic supply from the choroid by active transport through the retinal pigment epithelium (see 13.7). The central retinal artery is a true artery and as such can suffer atherosclerosis which may cause, for example, a central retinal artery thrombosis. At the optic disc it divides into four main branches which are technically arterioles, each of which is an end vessel with no anastomosis. These arterioles have a media of smooth muscle 7-8 cells thick. While these vessels can undergo arteriolar sclerosis or hypertensive changes they are not involved in atherosclerosis and the relatively sparse amount of elastic tissue in them may account for their protection from giant cell arteritis. The major arterial branches run in the nerve fibre layer below the internal limiting membrane, and where they cross the accompanying veins there is a common adventitial sheath. Cilioretinal arteries are seen in about 20% of patients and can account for the major macular supply in a minority.

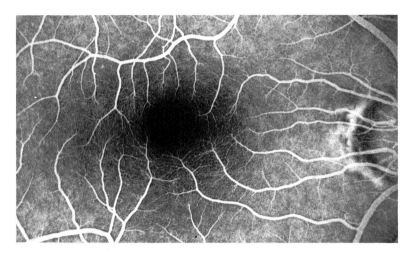

Fig. 13.11 There is a capillary-free zone around the retinal arteries of 200 μm and across the foveola of about 400 μm diameter. The foveola, therefore, is unencumbered by blood vessels which would otherwise obscure the visual acuity; like the rest of the photoreceptors, this area receives its blood supply from the choroid. In the posterior pole, there are superficial (nerve fibre layer) and deep (outer plexiform layer) capillary plexuses which fuse to become a single layer in the peripheral retina.

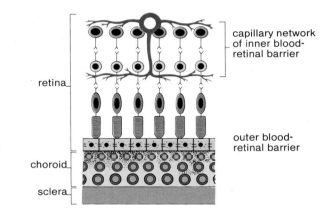

Fig. 13.12 A relatively large branch retinal artery and vein are seen (top) lying under the internal limiting membrane. The retinal arteries have a thicker media than the veins and at an arterio-venous crossing both share the same adventitial sheath (top centre). A van Gieson's for elastic tissue shows this to be absent in the retinal vessels (bottom centre) but a pronounced internal elastic lamina can be seen in the choroid of the same eye (bottom).

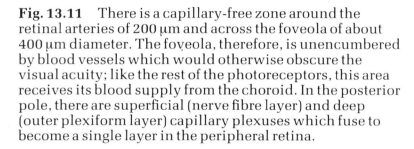

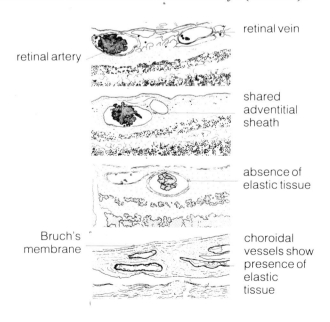

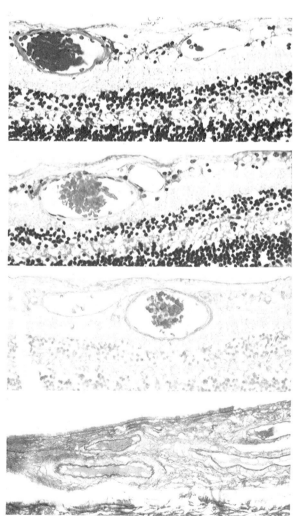

Fig. 13.13 The retinal capillaries consist of endothelial cells with tight intercellular junctions, a basement membrane and mural pericytes. The tight junctions formed by the endothelial cells of the retinal capillaries limit extracellular diffusion and metabolites can only reach the neural retina by active transport processes. This physical barrier, together with the selective active transport processes, is known as the blood-retinal barrier. The retina, therefore, has two protective barrier systems; that formed by the capillary endothelial cells known as the inner blood-retinal barrier and that formed by the RPE, the outer blood-retinal barrier. The retinal environment is also controlled through the blood-aqueous barrier. This photograph of normal rat retina, together with a freeze dried preparation taken after an injection of fluorescein, demonstrate the way in which dye is contained by the endothelial cells within the retinal circulation, but leaks from the choriocapillaris into the choroidal extravascular space to stain the sclera. It is, however, prevented from entering the retina by the RPE.

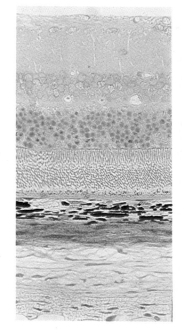
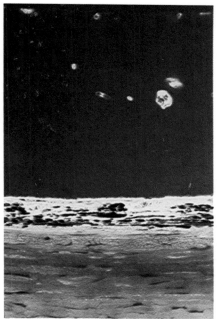

FLUORESCEIN ANGIOGRAPHY

Over the last 20 years fluorescein angiography has greatly advanced the ophthalmoscopic interpretation of retinal disease. Following an intravenous injection of sodium fluorescein, the dye is carried in the blood in its free form and also bound to albumen. Dilute solutions absorb light with a peak wavelength of 480 nm (blue) and emit it with a peak wavelength of 530 nm (yellow green). By using appropriate filters, exciting light can be separated from the emitted light and this forms the basis of fluorescein angiography.

The normal fluorescein angiogram demonstrates two distinct circulations; the retinal and choroidal. The choroidal circulation fills a few seconds before the retinal and the choroidal blood flow is high so that filling is rapidly completed. The choroidal capillaries have holes or fenestrations at the junctions of the endothelial cells and plasma containing fluorescein readily diffuses out of these vessels and fills the extravascular space. This lake of plasma is prevented from leaking into the retina by the tight junctions of the RPE cells (outer blood-retinal barrier) whose pigment also tends to 'mask' the choroidal fluorescence. In contrast the retinal circulation has tight junctions between the capillary endothelial cells which lack fenestrations (inner blood-retinal barrier) so that the fluorescein is confined to the intravascular space. In the angiogram the vessels are, therefore, viewed as the discrete retinal circulation separated from the diffused choroidal circulation by the retinal pigment epithelium.

Fluorescein angiography may be considered as a dynamic study allowing the visualization of the passage of dye from the arterial to the venous systems in the two ocular circulations. Apart from demonstrating the vascular anatomy and its variants, pathological changes within the vessel are demonstrated by their effect on the vascular circulation and breakdown of the inner or outer barriers. Points of particular interest are delay or lack of filling of blood vessels and areas of hypo or hyperfluorescence.

Hypofluorescence can be produced by either a vascular filling defect in the circulation or blocking (masking) of the normal retinal or choroidal fluorescent pattern by, for example, blood or pigment. Hyperfluorescence may result from leakage from retinal vessels (i.e. breakdown of the normal inner blood-retinal barrier), atrophy of the RPE allowing the choroidal fluorescence to be seen more prominently (window defect) or breakdown of the RPE cell barrier in which case fluorescein is seen as pooling and staining in the subretinal space. Neovascular tissue is demonstrated dramatically by fluorescein angiography. All new vessels have loose capillary endothelial cell junctions and therefore leak fluorescein; they fill in the earliest phases of the angiogram and leak intensively as it progresses.

Fig. 13.14 5 ml of 10-20% fluorescein solution is injected intravenously through a butterfly cannula. (Severe anaphylactic reactions can occur and, although rare, full resuscitation equipment must be available). Following a period of 15-20 seconds the dye appears in the eye and can be made to fluoresce with intense blue light of the correct wavelength. The transit of dye through the choroidal and retinal arteries to the veins is observed through appropriate filters and photographed for later study.

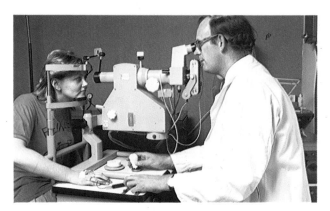

The Normal Fluorescein Angiogram

Fig. 13.15 Colour photographs are taken prior to angiography for later comparison. A small cilioretinal artery can be seen on this optic disc.

In the earliest choroidal phase there is patchy filling of the choriocapillaris, due to its lobular supply, and the deep optic disc capillaries. As the cilioretinal artery derives from the posterior ciliary circulation it also fills in the choroidal phase. Dye is starting to appear in the retinal arteries but the veins are empty and appear black against the background of the choroidal fluorescence.

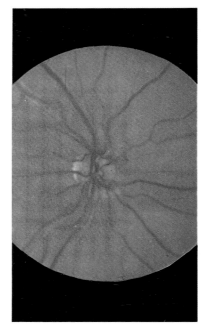
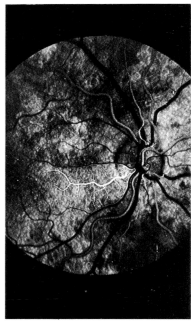

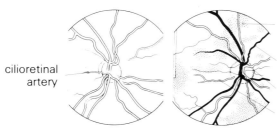

cilioretinal artery

patchy filling of choriocapillaris lobules

empty retinal veins

early retinal artery filling

filled cilioretinal artery

Fig. 13.16 A second or two later choroidal filling is complete so that the retinal circulation is viewed against a uniform choroidal glow, masked in the macula area by both the luteal pigment and the denser pigment in the RPE cells. Retinal arteries are well filled with dye.

The early arterio-venous phase shows complete choroidal and retinal arterial filling and laminar flow in the major retinal veins. This is due to the presence of dye in the plasma adjacent to the vessel wall, the central blood stream being filled by a non-fluorescent core of red blood cells.

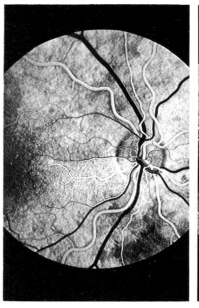
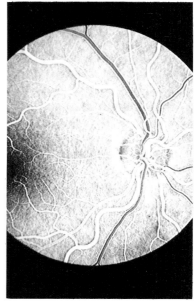

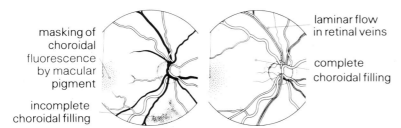

masking of choroidal fluorescence by macular pigment

incomplete choroidal filling

laminar flow in retinal veins

complete choroidal filling

Fig. 13.17 A later photograph shows complete filling of the various systems; laminar flow appears in the retinal arteries as they empty. The vertical fixation pointer is easily seen against the background fluorescence and allows the fovea to be identified precisely.

A late phase photograph shows emptying of the retinal and choroidal circulations and some peripheral hyperfluorescence around the rim of the optic disc from staining of the scleral rim. The fading choroidal fluorescence is masked in the macular area. Some of the larger choroidal vessels are seen as filling defects in the choroidal vascular bed.

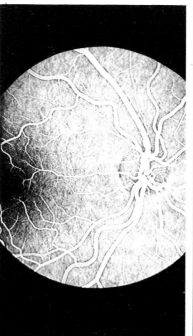
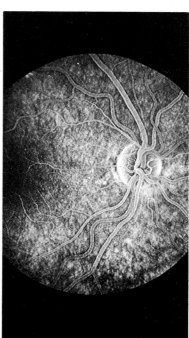

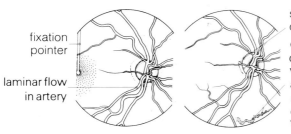

fixation pointer

laminar flow in artery

scleral staining of disc rim

empty choroidal blood vessel seen against background of extravascular fluorescence

PHYSICAL SIGNS OF RETINAL DISEASE

The retina can react in only limited ways to disease and can only exhibit a limited range of physical signs so that similar fundus appearances may be produced by a number of different disease processes. The interpretation of the commoner ophthalmoscopic signs of retinal disease aided by fluorescein angiography is demonstrated here.

Cotton Wool Spots

Cotton wool spots (sometimes incorrectly called soft exudates) lie in the nerve fibre layer of the retina and represent the ophthalmoscopic appearances of the edge of a micro infarct; their presence, therefore, implies an ischaemic microvascular disease. The spots appear initially as white fluffy patches, most commonly in the posterior pole, as this is where the retinal nerve fibre layer is thickest. They become smaller and more circumscribed with time, absorbing completely over 6-8 weeks; although they may persist longer in diabetic retinopathy. At this time, a nerve fibre defect can be seen as a groove in the retina, corresponding to the bundle of infarcted and destroyed axons and producing a corresponding arcuate field defect.

All neurones transport organelles intracellularly between the nucleus and the synapse; this process is known as axoplasmic transport. Pathologically, a cotton wool spot results from accumulation of organelles due to an interruption of axoplasmic transport. This may occur between the retinal ganglion cell and its synapse in the lateral geniculate body (orthograde transport) or vice versa (retrograde transport). Orthograde transport is the more prominent component and consists largely of mitochondria. Electron microscopy and histopathology show that the axonal stumps at the edges of a microinfarct are packed with mitochondria which produces the white appearance. (Papilloedema is produced by the identical mechanism of ischaemia and hold up of axoplasmic flow at the lamina cribrosa). Cotton wool spots are most commonly associated with diseases causing microvascular ischaemia such as hypertension, diabetes, systemic lupus erythematosus and venous infarcts.

Fig. 13.18 These fresh, fluffy cotton wool spots are seen around the optic disc a few days after a transient central retinal artery occlusion. The localisation to the superficial retina can be seen by the way they overlay the retinal vessels. At this acute stage the nerve fibre layer appears intact. Grooves in this layer, which can be observed ophthalmoscopically, take about 6 weeks to appear.

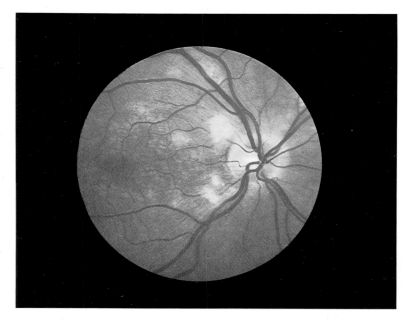

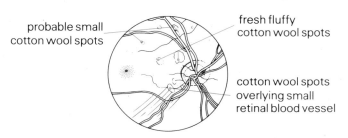

probable small cotton wool spots

fresh fluffy cotton wool spots

cotton wool spots overlying small retinal blood vessel

Fig. 13.19 The fluorescein angiogram shows that the cotton wool spots correspond exactly to small areas of hypofluorescence in the retinal capillary network. These persist throughout the angiogram and are not associated with extravascular leakage, confirming their aetiology as microvascular infarcts.

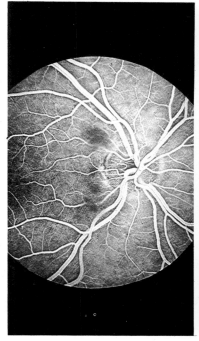
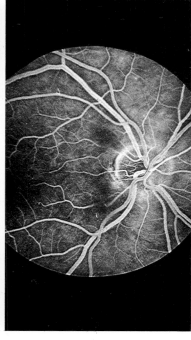

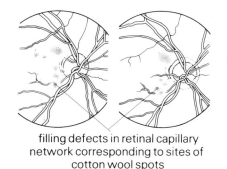

filling defects in retinal capillary network corresponding to sites of cotton wool spots

13.11

Fig. 13.20 Early and late photographs from another patient with an inflammatory arteritis. The early picture (left) shows a fluffy cotton wool spot with some haemorrhage in the acute stage. Note also the arteritic changes of focal sheathing in the upper temporal artery. Six weeks later (right), the soft exudate is absorbing and remains only as small, well-circumscribed spots. The arteritic changes are less prominent and a nerve fibre defect has appeared.

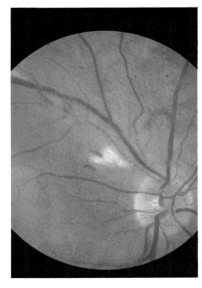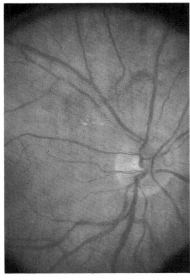

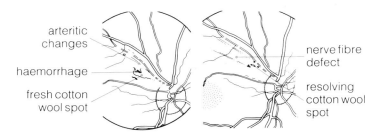

Fig. 13.21 The distinction between complete retinal infarction and axonal infarction is shown by this patient with a recent lower temporal branch artery occlusion. The retina supplied by the obstructed artery appears pale due to cloudy swelling of the infarcted neuroretinal layers which are supplied by the retinal circulation to the depth of the outer plexiform layer. A patch of viable retina

remains in this territory, however, supplied by a cilioretinal artery. These retinal ganglion cells are still able to generate axoplasmic flow which passes along the axon until it reaches the area of ischaemia where it becomes held up as a thin white frill of axoplasma corresponding to a cotton wool spot. (See also arterial occlusions, Chapter 14).

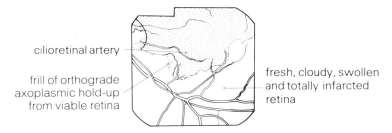

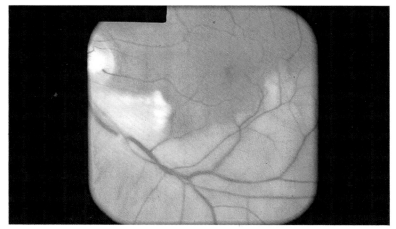

Fig. 13.22 Light microscopy of a cotton wool spot shows the distended and disrupted axons in the nerve fibre layer. Eosinophilic inclusions are seen in the axons and resemble a cell nucleus giving rise to the old-fashioned term 'cytoid body'.

The true nature of 'cytoid bodies' as swollen axonal stumps is clearly demonstrated in silver preparations. In this case the axons have been damaged as they pass over an area of photocoagulated retina. The large swellings occur on the axon segment remote from their cell body and adjacent to the head of the optic nerve.

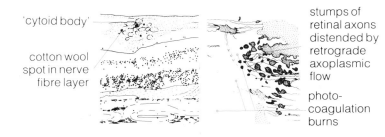

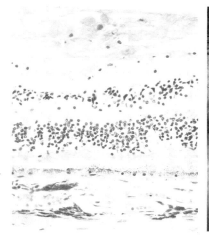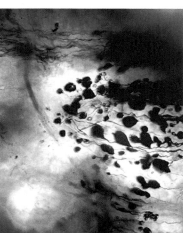

Fig. 13.23 Electron microscopy demonstrates that the 'cytoid bodies' are crammed full of mitochondria and degenerating membrane systems resulting from an interruption in axonal flow. This stump is due to an interruption in retrograde flow and such stumps usually show more marked pathological changes than those resulting from an interruption of orthograde transport. This probably occurs because, unlike the axonal component which is attached to the cell body, active repair mechanisms cannot take place and swelling and degeneration continue unchecked in this isolated axonal segment.

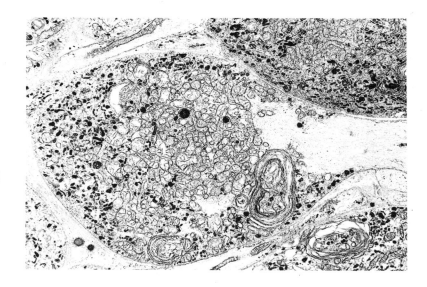

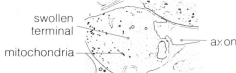

Hard exudates

Hard exudates are formed by the deposition of lipid and lipo-proteins and are a sign of abnormal vascular permeability in either retinal vessels or abnormal subretinal vessels. Such deposits may also be accompanied by macrophages. Lipid deposition does not invariably follow vascular leakage; leakage is an almost universal finding in posterior uveitis and yet hard exudates are rare in this instance. Within the retina a hard exudate is seen as a yellowish, well circumscribed accumulation, deep to the retinal vessels in the outer plexiform nerve fibre layer. Hard exudates occur in two types of distribution in the retina; either a circinate pattern (a complete or partial circle separated from the leaking vessel by a clear zone) or as a macular star, in which case the lipid accumulates in the fibre layer of Henlé

surrounding the macula. Macular stars may result from a leaking vascular focus adjacent to the macula, in the peripheral retina or in the underlying RPE. They may also result from optic disc leakage when they tend to be more prominent on the nasal side of the macula. These are particularly common in the resolving phases of optic disc infarction. Further lipid deposition in a circinate exudate or macular star will progress to form a plaque of exudate.

Choroidal neovascularization with penetration of Bruch's membrane is frequently associated with subretinal deposition of lipid (for example, disciform macula degeneration Chapter 16). Really gross examples of subretinal lipid deposition with serous detachment of the retina are seen with Coats' disease and this can superficially resemble a retinoblastoma (see Chapter 15).

Fig. 13.24 Circinate exudates are seen surrounding the macula. They have a circumscribed yellowish appearance, deep to the retinal vessels. In the macular area they adopt a more linear pattern from deposition within Henlè's layer. Fluorescein angiography demonstrates that the leakage originates from a previous macula branch vein occlusion.

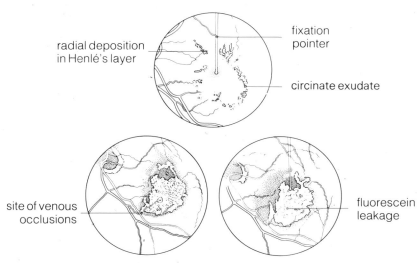

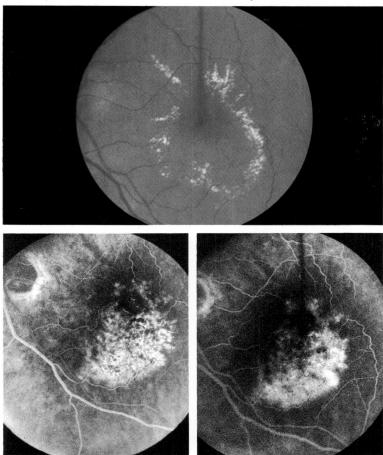

13.13

Fig. 13.25 A photograph taken soon after argon laser treatment to the leaking area of retina shows that the exudates are beginning to break up and absorb, especially inferiorly where the photocoagulation is heaviest.

The angiogram demonstrates scarring of the retinal pigment epithelium from the laser and less pronounced vascular leakage.

Several months later, the hard exudation has completely absorbed leaving RPE scars in the affected area.

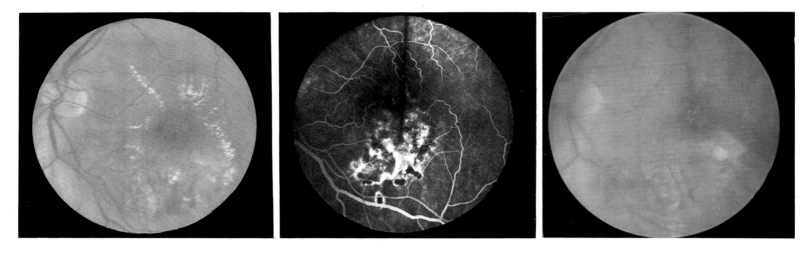

Fig. 13.26 A partial macular star and circumpapillary subretinal hard exudate is seen in a patient with a pale, swollen and infarcted optic disc. Note the linear radial deposition in the fibre layer of Henlé on the nasal side of the macula indicating the optic disc to be the site of leakage.

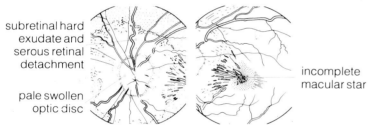

subretinal hard exudate and serous retinal detachment

incomplete macular star

pale swollen optic disc

Fig. 13.27 Histology of a hard exudate shows amorphous deposition of lipid in the outer plexiform layer. Müller cells probably limit the lateral spread of the exudate.

lipid of hard exudate

lipid in outer plexiform layer

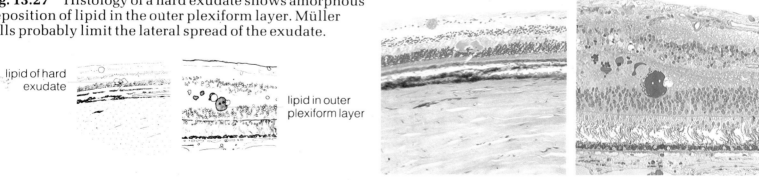

Retinal Haemorrhages
Retinal haemorrhages are always of pathological significance. Their ophthalmoscopic appearance indicates the anatomical location and this has implications for the aetiology and the clinical sequelae.

Fig. 13.28 Haemorrhage may be found in the vitreous gel (intragel haemorrhage), between the posterior hyaloid membrane and retinal surface (preretinal, subhyaloid or retrogel), in the nerve fibre layer (flame-shaped haemorrhages), in the deeper retina (blot haemorrhages), under the photoreceptors or under the retinal pigment epithelium. All types of haemorrhages mask the choroidal fluorescence on angiography.

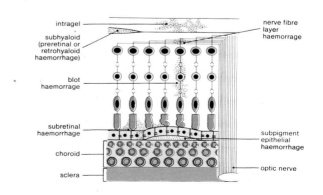

intragel

subhyaloid (preretinal or retrohyaloid haemorrhage)

nerve fibre layer haemorrhage

blot haemorrage

subretinal haemorrhage

choroid

sclera

subpigment epithelial haemorrhage

optic nerve

Fig. 13.29   Preretinal haemorrhages result from bleeding into the subhyaloid space between the internal limiting membrane of the retina and the posterior vitreous face. Sometimes a haemorrhage causes a localised detachment of the vitreous gel and then settles with gravity forming a horizontal fluid level. Preretinal haemorrhage is due to bleeding from retinal tears, superficial retinal neovascularization or from bleeding within the retina, rupturing the internal limiting membrane as in this example.

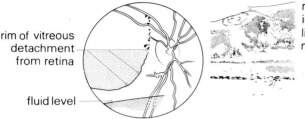

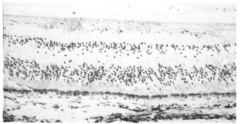

Fig. 13.30   Nerve fibre layer haemorrhages tend to be seen in the posterior pole where the nerve fibre layer is at its thickest. They have a linear, flame-shaped appearance caused by tracking along the retinal axons, and usually absorb with relatively little damage.

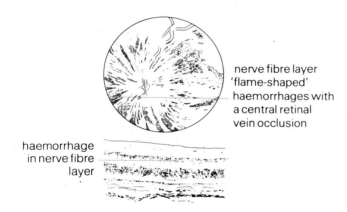

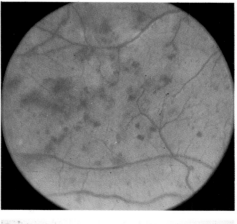

Fig. 13.31   Blotchy haemorrhages lie deeper in the retina in the plexiform or inner nuclear layers, or are seen in the peripheral retina where the nerve fibres are thin. In these regions the vertical arrangement of the Müller fibres and neurones limits lateral spread.

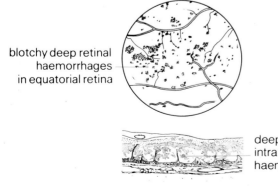

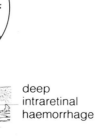

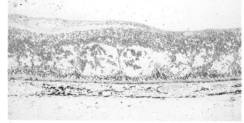

13.15

Fig. 13.32 Dark blot haemorrhages are seen with full-thickness retinal haemorrhage. This is usually a feature of venous occlusions or diabetic retinopathy and is a sign of severe retinal ischaemia with retinal capillary closure, indicating a high risk of subsequent retinal neovascularization.

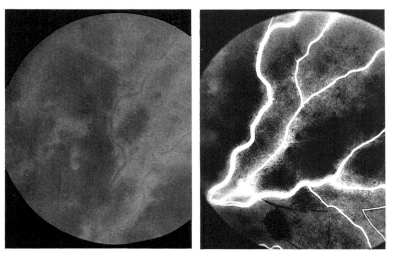

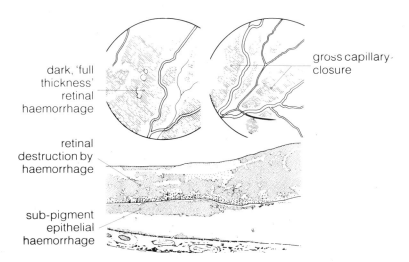

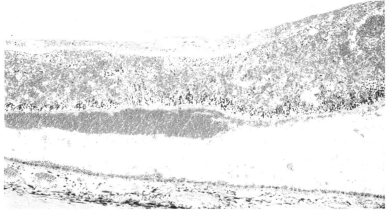

Fig. 13.33 Deep retinal or subretinal haemorrhage appears as a blotchy red area (left), with the retina often elevated by the blood. In the macula, these haemorrhages are frequently associated with choroidal subretinal neovascularization but, in the absence of this, can also occur with trauma. As the haemorrhage absorbs over a period of weeks it can become depigmented with a whitish-yellow appearance (right). Visual recovery depends on the amount of concomitant macular destruction which varies enormously.

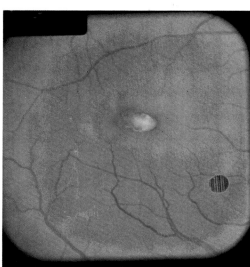

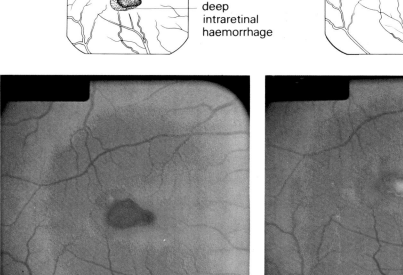

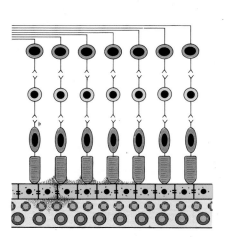

Fig. 13.34 The retinal pigment epithelium masks the redness of subpigment epithelial haemorrhages which consequently appear as a dark, greenish brown, as in this patient with a disciform macular degeneration. Large subpigment epithelial haemorrhages can even be mistaken for a malignant melanoma.

The site of the underlying neovascular membrane can often be seen ophthalmoscopically as a deep palish patch within the haemorrhage. Fluorescein angiography will demonstrate the underlying disciform membrane but the density and extent of the haemorrhage can mask the neovascular membrane and, if treatment is to be considered, the patient must be observed until the haemorrhage clears sufficiently to allow precise localization. In a case such as demonstrated, this might take 2 or 3 weeks.

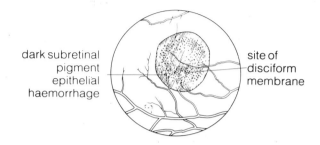

dark subretinal pigment epithelial haemorrhage

site of disciform membrane

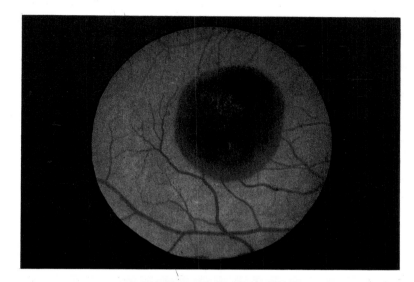

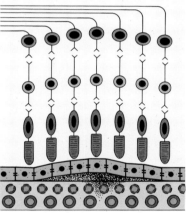

Roth's Spots

Fig. 13.35 These are haemorrhages with a white center corresponding to a cotton wool spot (haemorrhagic infarcts) or a collection of polymorphs. Often thought of as a manifestation of subacute bacterial endocarditis, they are a non-specific sign although they tend to be seen more frequently in patients who are anaemic and who usually have other haematological diseases.

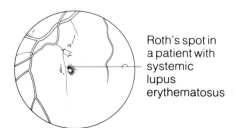

Roth's spot in a patient with systemic lupus erythematosus

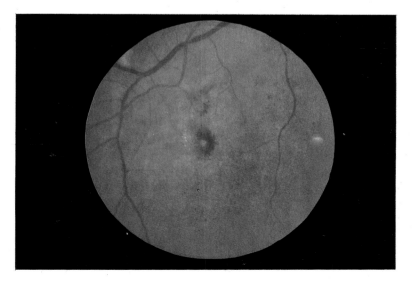

Macular Oedema

The macula and the fibre layer of Henlé are particularly susceptible to the accumulation of fluid and lipid from leaking vessels lying adjacent to the macula, in the optic disc or in the peripheral retina. Macular oedema is a common feature of posterior segment inflammation, retinal ischaemia or retinal vascular leakage with hard exudation.

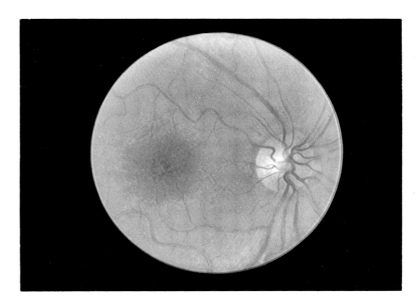

Fig. 13.36 Macular oedema is difficult to diagnose by direct ophthalmoscopy and can only be satisfactorily studied with either a Hruby or fundus contact lens (Chapter 1). It occurs in either a diffuse pattern where the macula appears generally thickened with a dull light reflex, or, in more severe cases, as cystoid oedema where cystic accumulations of fluid surround the macula in a petaloid appearance, as in this patient with posterior uveitis.

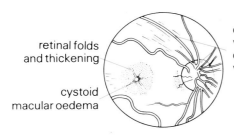

retinal folds and thickening

optic disc and retinal vessels partially obscured by vitreous debris

cystoid macular oedema

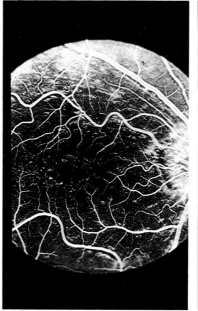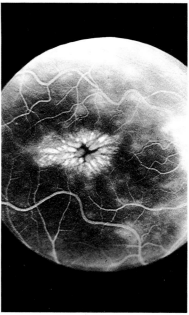

Fig. 13.37 Early and late phases of the fluorescein angiogram demonstrate a large amount of leakage from the veins and capillaries of the retina and optic disc with the later pictures showing pooling of the fluorescein in the extravascular tissue space corresponding to the clinical picture. Macular oedema is usually, but by no means always, associated with reduced visual acuity. It may persist for prolonged periods of time and with resolution it can leave a relatively normal macular appearance. The visual acuity depends on the degree of associated retinal damage.

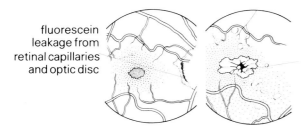

fluorescein leakage from retinal capillaries and optic disc

late phase angiogram showing petaloid cystoid macular oedema

Fig. 13.38 Histology of cystoid macular oedema shows pooling of fluid within the inner retinal layers. Note the trapping of fluid between the outer plexiform and ganglion cell layers and the almost complete loss of intermediary neurones. Lateral spread of fluid is limited by the survival of glial elements of the Müllers fibres.

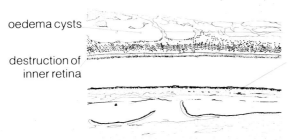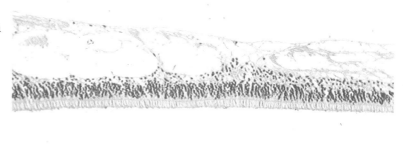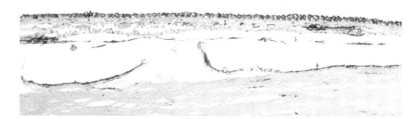

oedema cysts

destruction of inner retina

Müller fibres limit lateral spread RPE

Retinal Pigment Epithelial Disturbances

The retinal pigment epithelium normally partially masks the background choroidal fluorescence during angiography so, therefore, increased pigmentation will hide the choroidal fluorescence further (causing a 'masking' or 'transmission' defect), whereas atrophy allows the choroidal fluorescence to show more prominantly ('window' defect). Atrophy of the retinal pigment epithelium from any cause is usually accompanied by adjacent areas of pigment hypertrophy. Frequently RPE atrophy is not very obvious ophthalmoscopically but fluorescein angiography clearly demonstrates the window defect. Large areas of atrophy often appear to have a hyperfluorescent rim adjacent to the normal retina in the later phases of the angiogram which is due to fluorescein leakage from the adjacent intact choriocapillaris diffusing laterally to stain the sclera in the area of RPE and choriocapillaris atrophy.

Leakage of fluorescein through the retinal pigment epithelium occurs as a result of either mechanical or functional breakdown of the RPE cellular barrier or as a result of choroidal neovascularization breaking through Bruch's membrane and the RPE. The angiographic appearance is of increasing fluorescein leakage throughout the angiogram, producing a hyperfluorescent pool in the subretinal space; neovascular tissue being distinguished by the greater intensity of such leakage.

Fig. 13.39 Benign pigment epithelial hypertrophy is a common finding in Caucasian fundi and is a good example of a lesion which produces masking of the choroidal fluorescence. The flat, black lesion is avascular and well circumscribed. It results from hypertrophy of RPE cells and is totally benign and easily distinguishable from a choroidal naevus or melanoma. With time, the central pigmentation can atrophy leaving a depigmented centre with surrounding pigment known as a 'sunburst'.

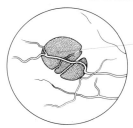

benign pigment epithilial hyperplasia

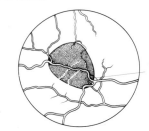

dense masking of choroidal fluorescence

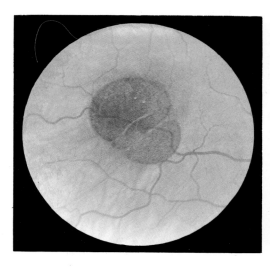

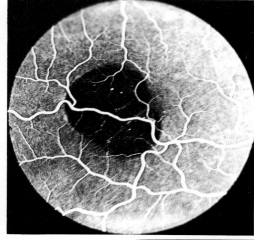

Fig. 13.40 RPE hypertrophy can take a variety of patterns collectively known as 'grouped pigmentation', or, more colloquially, as 'bear tracks' from their morphological appearance. RPE hypertrophy must be distinguished from intraretinal pigmentation which is always pathological and is usually seen in various patterns as a sign of retinal dystrophies, degeneration or inflammation. In the late stages of retinitis pigmentosa areas of black spidery 'bone corpuscular' pigmentation are characteristically seen in the retina, frequently adjacent to blood vessels. Concomitant atrophy of the RPE is always present as the 'bone corpuscular' pigment is formed by the migration of RPE cells into the neural retina, (see Chapter 16 retinitis pigmentosa).

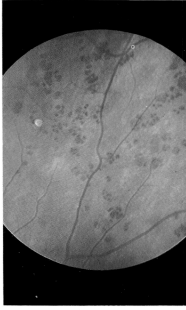

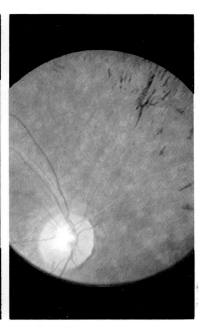

Fig. 13.41 This patient has angioid streaks and shows atrophy of the RPE with some associated pigmentary hypertrophy. Whilst this is not very noticeable in colour photographs, fluorescein angiography clearly demonstrates the fracture of Bruch's membrane and the RPE atrophy as a window defect. Adjacent areas of RPE hypertrophy mask the background choroidal fluorescence.

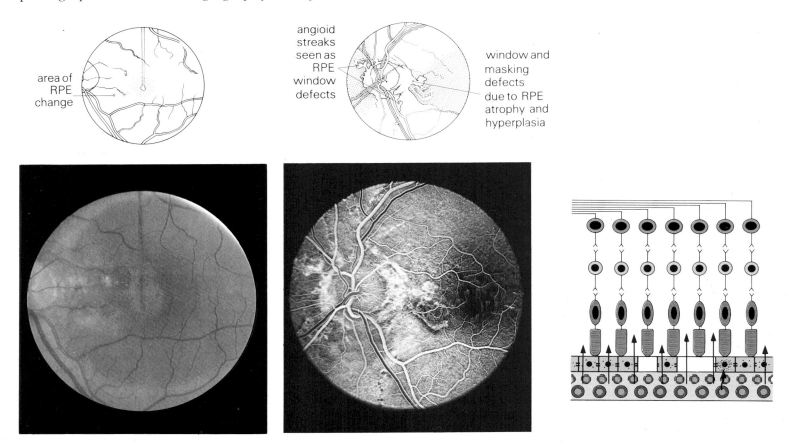

Fig. 13.42 All neovascular tissue within the eye, whether initially derived from the retinal or choroidal circulation, lacks tight endothelial cell junctions and therefore leaks fluorescein intensively. It is also fragile and tends to bleed with subsequent fibrosis, exudation and retinal destruction. Re-examination of the patient seen in Fig. 13.41 some months later shows signs of choroidal neovascularization in the area of the angioid streak. Colour photography shows fresh subretinal haemorrhage and oedema with the RPE disturbances. Early phase angiograms show the neovascular complex which leaked intensively as the angiogram progressed, staining the adjacent tissue. The haemorrhage masks some areas of underlying hyperfluorescence.

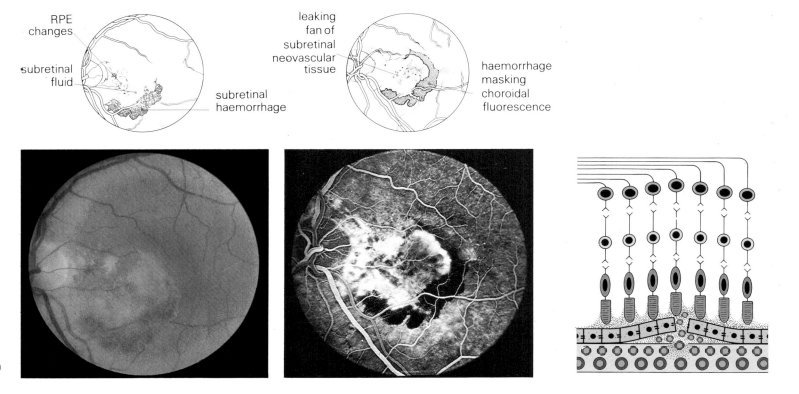

Fig. 13.43   Mechanical breakdown of the RPE is illustrated by this patient with central serous retinopathy. A blister of subretinal fluid has accumulated between the RPE and outer segments of the photoreceptors, thus elevating the macula. Angiography demonstrates a focal leak in the RPE through which this fluid has been derived. Although this stains with increasing intensity as more fluorescein leaks out during the angiogram it lacks the early and sharply increasing intensity of a neovascular leakage.

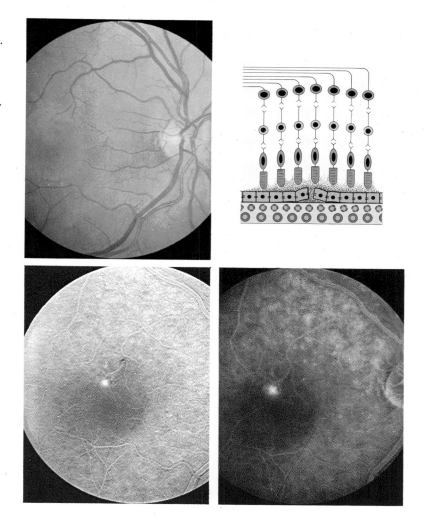

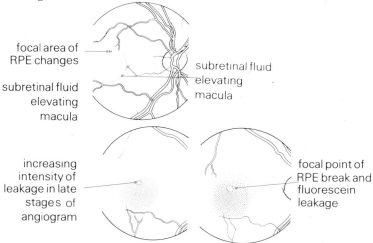

Ageing Changes in the Retina

Drusen (or colloid bodies) are a common senile change in the middle-aged or elderly Caucasian eye (they are uncommon in black patients) and represent accumulations of lipofuscin and other debris from the metabolism and phagocytosis of the photoreceptor outer segments by the RPE cells. Under normal circumstances, this material appears to be voided from the RPE cell through Bruch's membrane to the choriocapillaris. With age, however, there is progressive thickening of Bruch's membrane and, in some people, this presumably restricts the ability of the RPE to void waste products, leading to the formation of drusen. These lie on the retinal aspect of Bruch's membrane and may increase in size aggressively such that they displace overlying RPE cells. There is often associated RPE atrophy with a substantial risk of subsequent neovascularization from the choroid if the macular area is involved. (See Chapter 16 for further discussion of the disciform response).

Fig. 13.44   Drusen are commonly found in the macular area but may be found anywhere in the posterior pole. They are yellowish circumscribed areas of varying size in the retinal pigment epithelium varying in appearance from fine granular deposits to large, juicy confluent areas or hard, glistening calcific lesions, (see Chapter 16). Associated atrophy and hypertrophy of the RPE is common with more pronounced disease. Drusen are sometimes confused with hard exudates but they are easily distinguished by their deeper, less-defined appearance, their topographical location and the absence of concomitant vascular leakage.

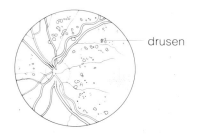

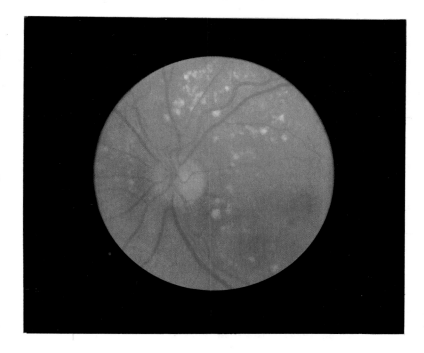

13.21

Fig. 13.45 During fluorescein angiography drusen usually take up dye with a low intensity staining which fades towards the later phases of the angiogram. If more intense leakage occurs it is usually a sign of early choroidal neovascularization.

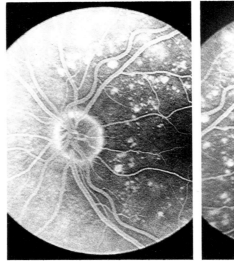
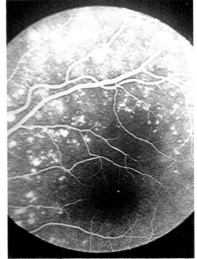

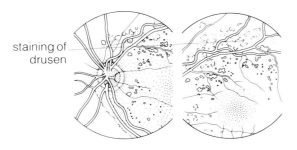

staining of drusen

Fig. 13.46 Light microscopy of drusen confirms the clinical impression that they have two major forms; a discrete rounded form which causes a small focal displacement of RPE cells, or a larger more diffuse form which produces large areas of RPE disturbance. The latter form is illustrated as this is the type that seems to cause focal changes that predispose to the penetration of Bruch's membrane by neovascular tissue, as shown in the lower half of the slide.

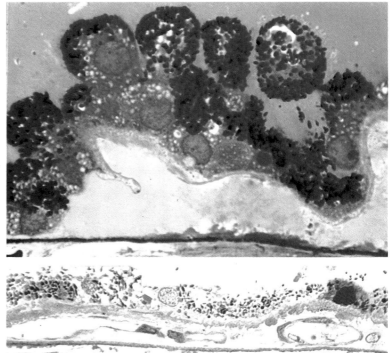

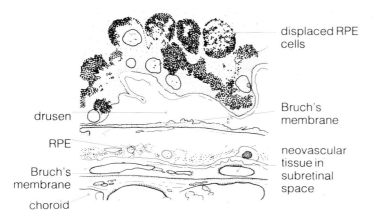

displaced RPE cells

drusen

RPE

Bruch's membrane

choroid

Bruch's membrane

neovascular tissue in subretinal space

The Neovascular Response

New blood vessel formation (neovascularization) within the eye from retinal disease is associated with a variety of diseases such as diabetes, retinal vein occlusions, retrolental fibroplasia or Eales' disease. The common factor between these widely varying conditions appears to be retinal hypoxia which is usually manifested clinically by areas of closure and loss of the retinal capillary bed. The precise reason for retinal capillary closure in the eye is as yet unknown. It usually occurs at the time of the initial vascular insult, for example with a venous occlusion, but the area of capillary closure can extend to some extent subsequently. It has been postulated that retinal hypoxia stimulates the formation of a protein or polypeptide factor from the affected retina which in turn stimulates new blood vessel formation from the surrounding healthy retina. There is now both good circumstantial clinical evidence and some experimental evidence to support this. The release of this unknown substance and its diffusion

can stimulate new blood vessel formation on the retina, optic disc or from the choroid, depending on the particular circumstances. In the presence of retinal or optic disc neovascularization it is postulated that further diffusion through the vitreous gel and aqueous humour results in neovascularization on the iris and in the angle of the anterior chamber. Corneal neovascularization is probably also caused by similar neovascular factors and there is good evidence of such factors in relation to the induction of pathological vascularization by tumours elsewhere in the body.

Within the eye, all new blood vessels lack barrier properties. They will leak rapidly and intensively during fluorescein angiography and this is a useful demonstration if their clinical recognition is in doubt. Neovascularization is always of serious importance. The blinding sequelae result from the fragility of these neovascular vessels, and their tendency to haemorrhage with obscuration of the ocular media, subsequent fibrosis and traction detachment of the retina. Deposition of hard exudate is a less common feature with optic disc or retinal neovascularization, but is common with subretinal neovascularization.

In the case of optic disc or retinal neovascularization, it is seen initially as a flat area of fine blood vessels. Vitreous detachment from the retina is induced at an early stage and this drags the new vessels forward allowing them to proliferate on the posterior hyaloid face ('forward new vessels'). Invasion of the vitreous gel itself is exceptionally uncommon possibly due to inhibitory factors within the gel. In the clinical assessment of neovascularization it is important to assess whether it is localized to either the retina or optic disc, or both, and whether it is flat or pulled forwards from the retina. The attachment of forward new vessels to the posterior vitreous face makes them all the more vulnerable to minor trauma and haemorrhage from movement and traction by the vitreous gel. The neovascular response and its managements are further discussed in relation to diabetic retinopathy Chapter 15, retinal vein occlusion Chapter 14 and the disciform response Chapter 16.

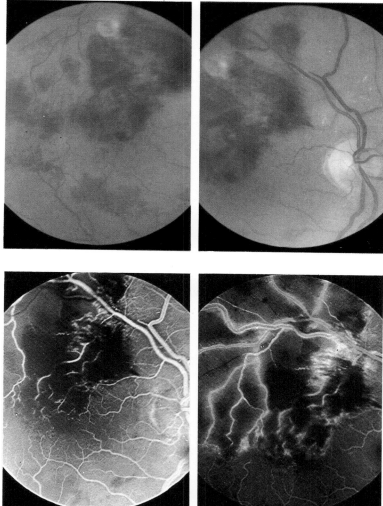

Fig. 13.47   Retinal capillary closure is almost always seen as a precursor of retinal neovascularization, no matter what the primary cause. In this patient, with a superior temporal branch vein occlusion, the presence of capillary closure and retinal hypoxia can be inferred from the dense dark, full-thickness retinal haemorrhage and the presence of cotton wool spots.

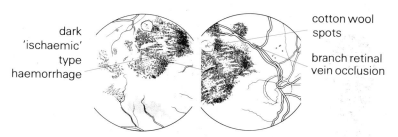

Fig. 13.48   Fluorescein angiography at this acute stage demonstrates massive capillary closure in the affected area with some leakage and staining of major vessel walls in the hypoxic area in the later phases.

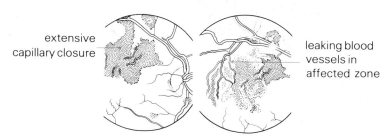

Fig. 13.49   Fluorescein angiography is not invariably needed to show capillary non-perfusion and closure because this can often be inferred by the type of retinal haemorrhage or the slightly darker appearance and different light reflex of the non-perfused retina, as in this diabetic. Sometimes, major vessels terminate at the junction of perfusion and closure, or become sclerosed as they pass through the affected area (see Chapter 14).

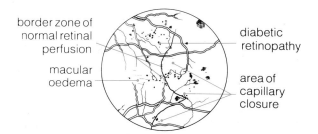

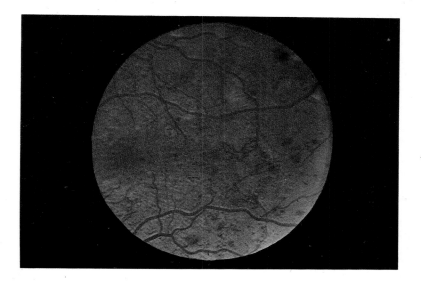

13.23

Fig. 13.50 Following a venous occlusion neovascular tissue begins to appear on the retina or optic disc 2-3 months after the induction of hypoxia. In this patient there is early neovascularization on the optic disc and retina following a superior temporal branch vein occlusion several weeks previously. Note the intense leakage of fluorescein from the new vessels. This eye has a substantial risk of developing vitreous haemorrhage, and possibly fibrosis with traction retinal detachment.

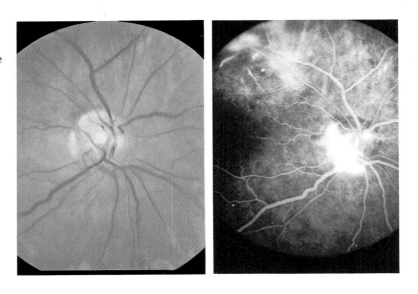

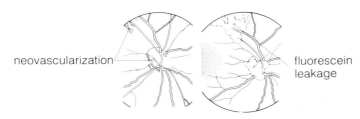

neovascularization — fluorescein leakage

Fig. 13.51 Neovascularization can occur on the retina or optic disc as in the previous example, subretinally from the choroid as seen in Fig. 13.43 or intraretinally. This example shows the development of fine, stunted, intraretinal new vessels and vascular remodelling over a period of several months following a branch retinal vein occlusion. These intraretinal new vessels are a common phenomenon adjacent to areas of retinal ischaemia but they remain stunted and do not grow progressively. They do not cause any ocular morbidity nor do they have the blinding sequelae of superficial neovascularization and are often thought of as an abortive attempt at revascularization of the ischaemic retina.

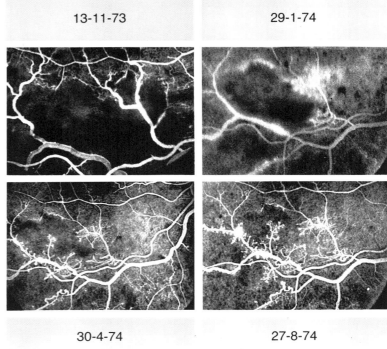

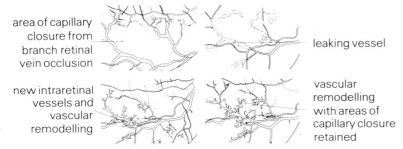

area of capillary closure from branch retinal vein occlusion

leaking vessel

new intraretinal vessels and vascular remodelling

vascular remodelling with areas of capillary closure retained

Fig. 13.52 Capillary closure can occur in discrete topographical areas such as in venous occlusions, or diffusely over the whole retina, as is usually the case in diabetic retinopathy, or in the peripheral retina, as in some haemaglobinopathies, retrolental fibroplasia or retinal vascular inflammatory diseases. This photograph shows the equatorial retina of a patient with Hb SC disease. With retinal disease, neovascularization usually occurs at the junction of the normal and hypoxic tissue and in this patient fronds of neovascularization, with some associated fibrosis, are seen at the junction of vascularized and non-vascularized retina; distal to this the large retinal vessels are occluded and are seen as thin white lines.

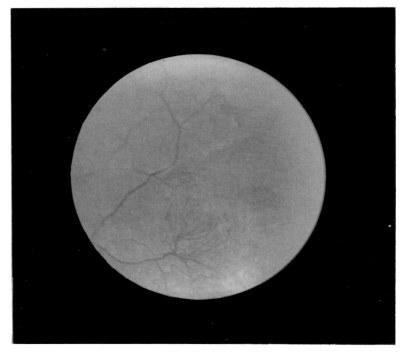

border of retinal perfusion

normally perfused retina

white sclerosed vein

elevated neovascular fronds

peripheral capillary closure

Fig. 13.53 Early and late-phase angiograms show the area of non-perfusion and capillary closure with abnormal shunt vessels between major arteries and veins with gross fluorescein leakage from the neovascular frond in the later stages. Not all ocular neovascularization carries a devastating prognosis; in some types such as Hb SC disease with peripheral vascular closure, vitreous haemorrhage and blinding sequelae from the neovascularization are relatively uncommon.

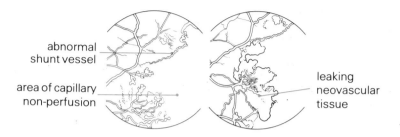

abnormal shunt vessel

area of capillary non-perfusion

leaking neovascular tissue

Fig. 13.54 The optic disc is particularly prone to developing new vessels, possibly because it is itself a site of junctional blood supply. When this occurs it tends to carry a poorer visual prognosis than retinal neovascularization and this is probably due to vitreous attachment to the optic disc with traction on ocular movement.

This diabetic patient shows the development of optic disc neovascularization over a two year period of observation from a few minute changes, only recognisable with the help of fluorescein angiography, to an extensive complex and further retinal ischaemia which requires treatment by photocoagulation (cf. Chapter 15).

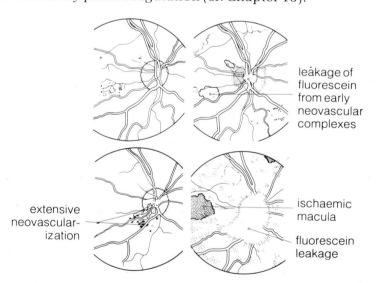

leakage of fluorescein from early neovascular complexes

extensive neovascular-ization

ischaemic macula

fluorescein leakage

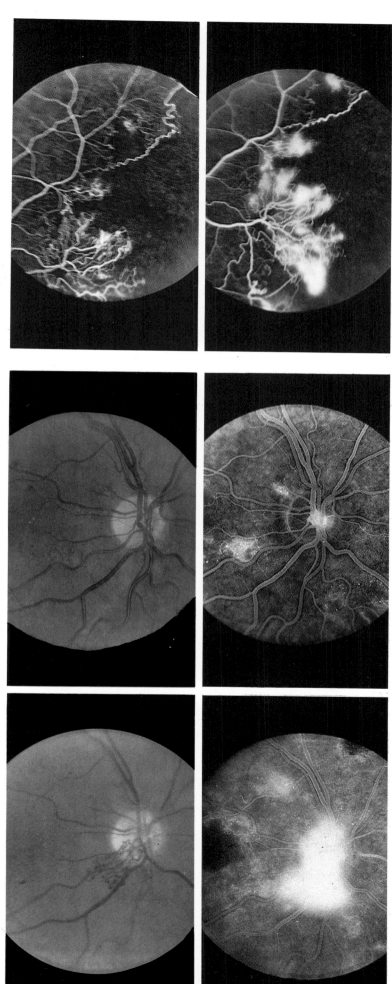

Fig. 13.55 A more marked example of optic disc neovascularization is seen in this diabetic with gross neovascular changes on the disc and surrounding retina. At this stage some early fibrosis, as indicated by the associated white tissue, is already present. A few development of retinal traction, distortion and loss of vision. The combination of neovascularization and fibrosis is known as retinitis proliferans. Contraction of the fibrous tissue leads to traction retinal detachment.

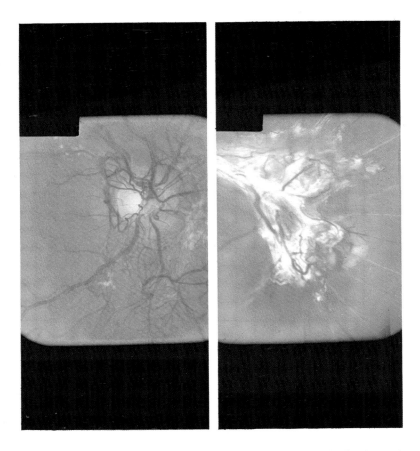

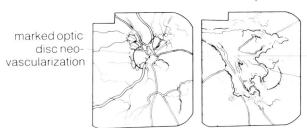

marked optic
disc neo-
vascularization

fibrosis and
traction
retinal
detachment

Fig. 13.56 A photograph of this macrodissection shows a fibrovascular membrane extending across the surface of the optic disc. The neovascular elements within this complex, seen in the histology, have fenestrated endothelial cells and therefore leak profusely.

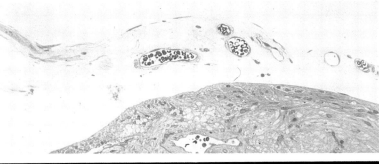

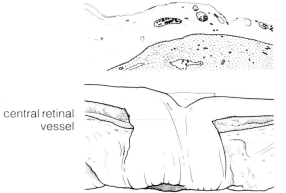

blood vessels
in neovascular
membrane

retinal nerve
fibres entering
optic disc

neovascular
membrane

central retinal
vessel

posterior
ciliary vessel

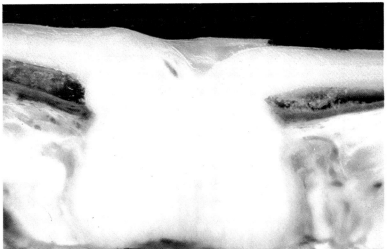

Epiretinal Membranes

Membrane formation on the retinal surface at the vitreo-retinal interface is associated with a wide variety of causes such as vascular occlusive retinopathies, heavy photocoagulation or cryotherapy, or posterior uveitis but many patients present with epiretinal membranes with no other apparent ocular disease. In these cases, senile posterior vitreous detachment appears to be the underlying cause. It appears that the common feature linking these diverse conditions is a physical disruption of the internal limiting membrane allowing glial cells to spread from the retina on to its surface and to proliferative with subsequent traction and distortion. In the idiopathic variety patients usually present in their 50's and 60's with moderately blurred vision and metamorphopsia. Once formed, epiretinal membranes are usually stable and do not progress to more severe distortion over the years.

Fig. 13.57 Cellophane maculopathy is the mildest form of epiretinal membrane formation and usually presents as slight blurring of acuity. In this patient there are the typical appearances of undulating shallow folds in the internal limiting membrane around the macula and the tortuosity of the surrounding small vessels is more prominent than usual.

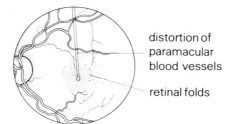

distortion of
paramacular
blood vessels

retinal folds

Fig. 13.58 This patient shows a more severe membrane with an epicentre on the superior temporal vessels. There are prominent retinal folds with traction and distortion of the macula producing metamorphopsia.

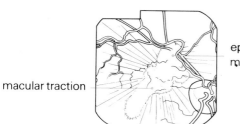

epicentre of epiretinal
membrane

macular traction

Fig. 13.59 Some epiretinal membranes can simulate macular oedema or a senile macular hole. In this patient the vascular anatomy is distorted and pulled into the membrane overlying the macula which is demonstrated by the angiogram. It is not unusual to see associated vascular leakage and macular oedema caused by traction and distortion of the retinal vessels in the affected area. Epiretinal membranes may occasionally peel off the retina spontaneously with visual improvement. In severe cases with marked visual loss, surgical removal by vitrectomy has been tried but visual results can be variable, sometimes with reformation of membrane a few months later after apparently successful surgery.

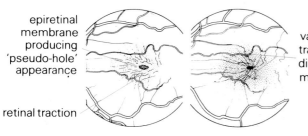

epiretinal
membrane
producing
'pseudo-hole'
appearance

vascular
traction and
distortion from
membrane

retinal traction

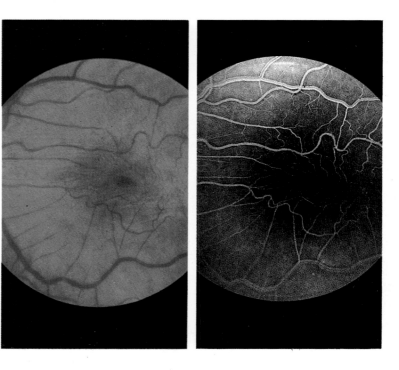

Fig. 13.60 Photomicrograph of an epiretinal membrane on the surface of a diabetic retina. Glial cells migrate through dehiscences in the inner limiting membrane of the retina and then proliferate along its vitreal aspect. Once a cellular membrane is established, the cells may contract and do so between sites of anchorage at the dehiscences in the limiting membrane. In this way the underlying retina is drawn up into a series of corrugations between points of anchorage.

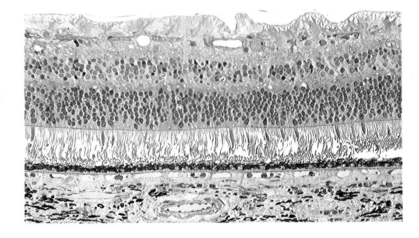

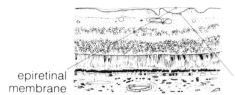

epiretinal membrane

distortion of internal limiting membrane

14. The Retina: Vascular Disease I

D. J. Spalton
J. S. Shilling
T. J. ffytche

Introduction

Retinal vascular occlusions are a common cause of visual loss particularly in the elderly, the hypertensive, diabetic or arteriosclerotic patient. They present with sudden, unilateral visual loss but this might only be noticed coincidentally some time after the initial event, particularly in elderly people. All patients need a careful assessment of their cardiovascular system for associated underlying systemic hypertension, diabetes or other atherogenic diseases, together with an assessment of their cardiac and cerebral vascular circulations for subclinical disease in case prophylactic medical or surgical treatment might be indicated to prevent further infarction.

ARTERIAL OCCLUSIONS
Central Retinal Artery Occlusion

This is usually a disease of the elderly and is most commonly caused either by thrombosis of the part of the central retinal artery which lies in the optic nerve, or by blockage of the artery by an embolus, usually originating in the heart or carotid artery. All patients should be screened for hypertension, diabetes and cardiac or carotid atheromatous disease. In younger patients, the underlying

aetiology is occasionally found to be an inflammatory arteritis of which polyarteritis nodosa, systemic lupus erythematosus or syphilis are, perhaps, the most common causes. Temporal arteritis occasionally presents as a central retinal artery occlusion although an anterior ischaemic optic neuropathy is a much more common sign (see Optic Disc, Chapter 17). Spasm of the central retinal artery is an ill-defined and controversial phenomenon which only occurs in exceptional circumstances such as drug toxicity with quinine or ergot overdosage, or possibly with pre-eclamptic toxaemia of pregnancy.

Occasionally, in some eyes with central retinal artery occlusion there is some visual recovery, and this is probably due to fragmentation and dispersion of an embolus. If a patient is seen within a few hours of the initial loss of vision it is worthwhile to presume that it is embolic in nature. Working with this hypothesis, attempts should be made to dislodge the embolus by massage of the globe to fluctuate intraocular pressure and intravenous acetazolamide or paracentesis of the anterior chamber to lower intraocular pressure. However, visual recovery is rare and the prognosis is generally very poor.

Fig. 14.1 The fundus of a recent central retinal artery occlusion shows a cloudy, opaque and swollen infarcted retina, particularly noticeable in the posterior pole where the retina is thickest. As the foveal area is the thinnest area of the posterior retina there is little tissue here to infarct, and the underlying redness of the choroid contrasts with the whiteness of the surrounding infarcted retina to give the classical 'cherry red spot' appearance. Within a few hours mild swelling of the optic disc often appears due to

accumulation of retrograde axoplasmic transport in the optic nerve head. In the acute stage blood in the retinal arteries is dark from stagnation and the arteries themselves are often attenuated. These acute appearances subside over a period of 2-4 weeks leaving the eye blind, or with vague perception of light, and a pale optic disc with no other signs; the retinal arteries usually regain their normal appearance.

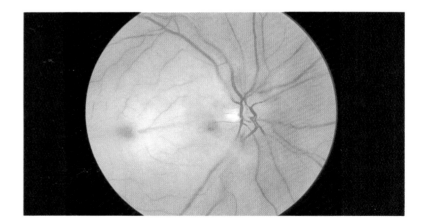

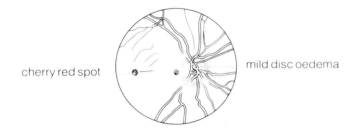

cherry red spot mild disc oedema

Fig. 14.2 Fluorescein angiography is not usually performed but, if it is done in the acute stages, there is a considerable delay in filling of the central retinal artery circulation following injection of dye; this is seen as black against the normal background fluorescence which, of course, is unaffected by the occlusion. The artery fills eventually, either directly, or by retrograde flow from the venous circulation. The central vessels in the posterior pole fill poorly, possibly due to the retinal oedema increasing external tissue pressure.

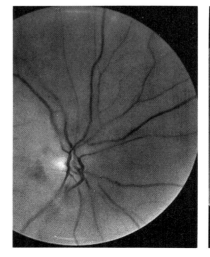
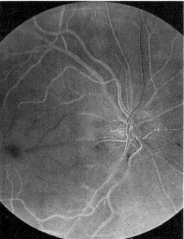

Fig. 14.3   The optic disc one year after occlusion of the central retinal artery. Note the ischaemic damage to both disc and nerve fibres and the extensive glial repair around the disc vessels.

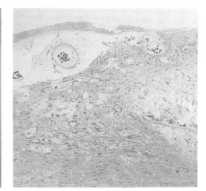
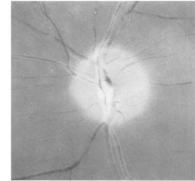

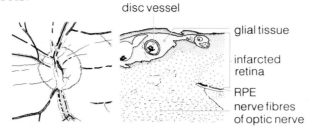

Cilioretinal Arterial Sparing and Occlusion

Fig. 14.4   Cilioretinal arteries of varying size are found in about 20% of eyes. These are part of the posterior ciliary circulation and are, therefore, spared in a central retinal artery occlusion leaving a patch of viable retina, which, if the patient is fortunate, may supply the macula.

A small cilioretinal vessel is seen clearly in this patient, supplying an area of retina temporal to the optic disc. Minute emboli can be seen in the inferior and superior temporal arteries and also in a small branch artery adjacent to the macula, indicating the aetiology of the occlusion.

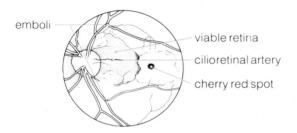

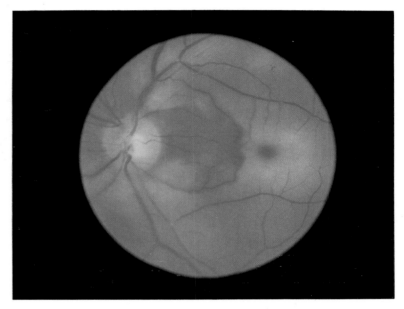

Fig. 14.5   Fluorescein angiography demonstrates the slow rate of filling of the retinal circulation (left), and the normal filling of the cilioretinal artery and choroid (right).

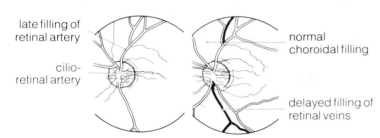

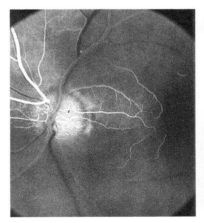
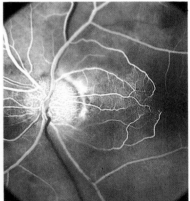

Fig. 14.6   Another example of cilioretinal sparing in the presence of a central retinal artery occlusion in a negro eye demonstrates clumping of the blood column in the artery. This characteristic sign of a stagnant retinal circulation is known as 'cattle trucking'.

A clinical estimation of ophthalmic artery pressure can be made by applying digital pressure to the eye during ophthalmoscopy and observing the onset of pulsation of the central retinal artery and then of complete closure which correspond to systolic and diastolic pressures respectively.

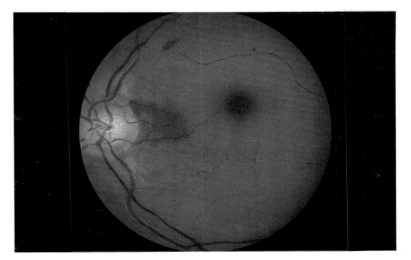

Fig. 14.7 Cilioretinal infarction with central retinal artery sparing is the converse situation to that shown in Fig. 14.6. Here, a small cilioretinal branch is occluded, thus infarcting the retina temporal to the optic disc. A frill of axoplasmic material from the viable retina is seen surrounding the cilioretinal infarct. Cilioretinal infarcts have a similar aetiology to anterior ischaemic optic neuropathy and, although temporal arteritis usually presents as more extensive infarction of the optic disc, it must be excluded as a potential cause.

Cilioretinal infarction is sometimes seen with a central retinal vein occlusion and this is thought to be due to compromise of a small cilioretinal artery by increased external tissue pressure within the optic nerve head.

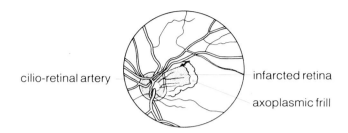

cilio-retinal artery — infarcted retina

axoplasmic frill

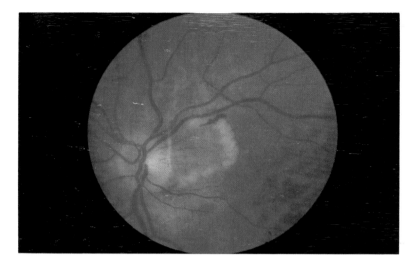

Retinal Emboli

Embolisation of the retinal circulation usually occurs with cholesterol or fibrin and platelet emboli from the carotid arteries, or calcific fragments from a stenosed aortic valve. Occasionally more exotic material such as talc in drug addicts or fat emboli in patients with multiple fractures can be seen. Emboli may produce permanent or transient visual loss, and cholesterol emboli are also frequently seen coincidentally on routine examination of an asymptomatic eye. Transient uniocular visual loss is known as amaurosis fugax and is virtually always due to embolisation whether or not emboli are actually seen on examination. Patients typically notice uniocular visual loss starting as a concentric peripheral dimming of vision or a horizontal curtain coming over the eye, depending on whether the central retinal artery or a branch retinal artery is affected. The attack lasts for periods from a few minutes to 2-3 hours before vision quite rapidly returns to normal. Attacks may happen singly or in groups sometimes occurring in clusters or showers during a day. Patients with retinal embolisation have a substantial risk of developing a permanent stroke over the next few months, particularly if the amaurosis fugax is accompanied by signs of transient cerebral ischaemia. The appreciation of this in recent years has meant that the ophthalmologist plays an important role in the management of these patients by referring them for prophylactic medical or surgical treatment to forestall the development of permanent neurological sequelae.

Fig. 14.8 Cholesterol crystals are seen frequently as a coincidental finding in elderly patients and are a sign of atheromatous disease, usually in the carotid artery at the bifurcation of the internal and external carotid arteries. They are flat crystals which glint and reflect light as the ophthalmoscope is tilted to examine the fundus, and are most commonly found at bifurcations of the retinal arteries. Because of the planar shape of the crystal, blood flow may not be disturbed and the patient does not complain of any symptoms. Cholesterol emboli are also known as 'Hollenhorst plaques'.

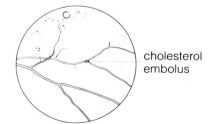

cholesterol embolus

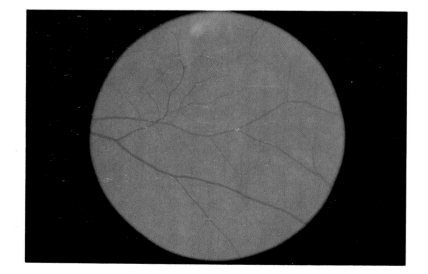

Fig. 14.9 A carotid angiogram of the common carotid artery at its bifurcation to form the internal and external branches shows a large atheromatous plaque with gross stenosis of the vessel. Other methods of diagnosis of carotid artery atheroma are the signs of a bruit, Doppler ultrasonography or digital substraction angiography; ophthalmodynamometry is generally considered to be unsatisfactory. Such an atheromatous lesion is suitable for surgical removal if the patient is otherwise well, if not, low dose aspirin therapy is probably the treatment of choice.

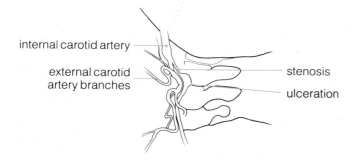

internal carotid artery

external carotid artery branches

stenosis

ulceration

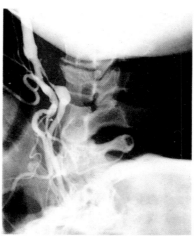

Fig. 14.10 Occlusion of a branch retinal artery is almost always the result of embolisation. In this patient with an inferior temporal artery occlusion and partial 'cherry red spot' at the macula a small embolus can be seen in the artery on the disc. The inferior rim of the disc is slightly swollen due to a halt in retrograde axoplasmic transport and a frill of axoplasm lies inferiorly, probably from an area of retina preserved by a small unidentifiable cilioretinal artery.

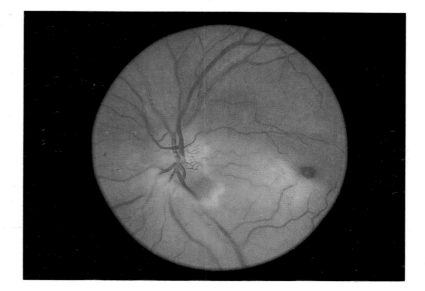

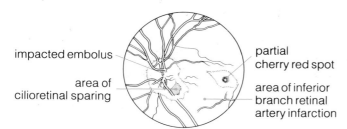

impacted embolus

area of cilioretinal sparing

partial cherry red spot

area of inferior branch retinal artery infarction

Fig. 14.11 Lipid deposition may be seen in the retinal arterial wall following vascular endothelial cell damage after embolisation. In this patient there is marked yellowish white sheathing at the origin of the superior temporal artery and, peripheral to this, the vessel is thin, attentuated and fibrosed. Collateral vessels can be seen on the retina and the optic disc has sectorial pallor; the patient had a large inferior nasal arcuate scotoma. Sometimes the lipid deposition occurs at a bifurcation of a major retinal arteriole giving a 'trouser leg' pattern of sheathing to the vessel.

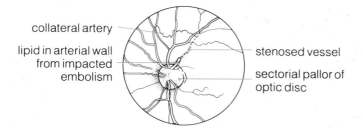

collateral artery

lipid in arterial wall from impacted embolism

stenosed vessel

sectorial pallor of optic disc

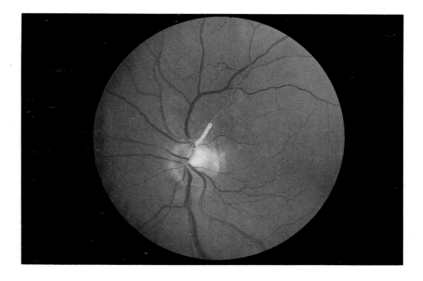

14.5

Fig. 14.12   Platelet and fibrin emboli originate from an ulcerating atheromatous plaque and look like soft porridgey material in the vessel. They produce amaurosis fugax and can sometimes be observed moving slowly through the retinal arterial circulation as the attack evolves.

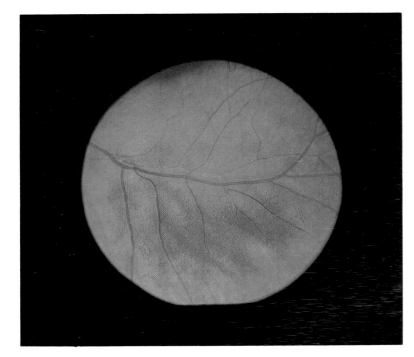

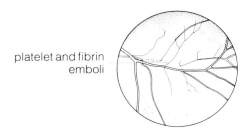

platelet and fibrin emboli

Fig. 14.13   Red free photography shows the emboli to better advantage in the same patient. Carotid angiography confirmed the presence of an ulcerating plaque at the bifurcation of the carotid artery which was removed surgically. The patient was also advised to stop smoking.

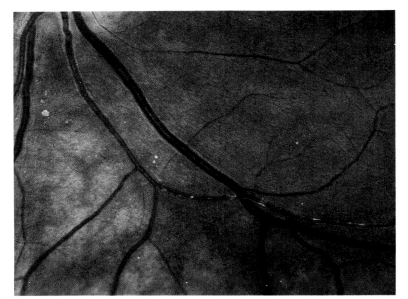

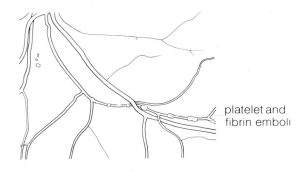

platelet and fibrin emboli

Fig. 14.14   Fragments of a calcific aortic valve are seen occasionally; they have a characteristic appearance which differs from that of other types of emboli and enables their exact source to be identified. They tend to be larger and globular, with a pearly white appearance, and lodge in the larger arteries at the optic disc. Echocardiography confirms the diagnosis.

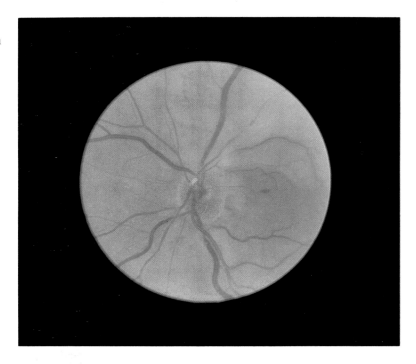

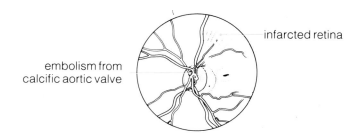

infarcted retina

embolism from calcific aortic valve

RETINAL MACROANEURYSMS

Macroaneurysms of the retinal arterioles are usually seen in elderly patients with systemic hypertension; they are similar in pathology to the Charcot-Bouchard aneurysms of the cerebral circulation which are thought to originate from embolisation with damage to the arterial wall. Retinal macroaneurysms may be found either coincidentally or because they cause visual disability due to haemorrhage or leakage of lipid with macular oedema.

Studies have shown that the haemorrhagic complications resolve spontaneously and do not require specific treatment, but that the exudative response should be treated by photocoagulation since permanent visual loss may result from damage to the fovea. Retinal macroaneurysms must be distinguished from Leber's miliary aneurysms (see Chapter 15) or vascular anomalies due to venous occlusions or diabetes.

Fig. 14.15   This eye shows an area of gross preretinal and subretinal haemorrhage from a macroaneurysm.

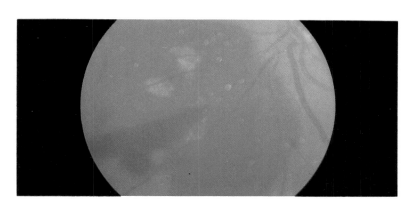

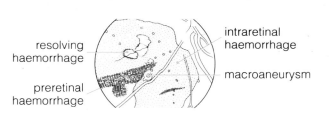

Fig. 14.16   A macroaneurysm is often difficult to identify by ophthalmoscopy but is readily demonstrated by fluorescein angiography. The haemorrhage masks the background choroidal fluorescence and the aneurysm is seen as a hyperfluorescent saccular dilatation of the artery.

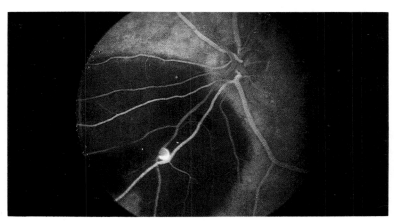

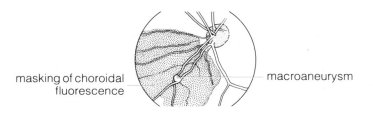

Fig. 14.17   This patient shows a macroaneurysm on the superior temporal artery with a macular star producing visual loss. Fluorescein angiography demonstrates the hyperfluorescent aneurysm, together with leakage in the macular area.

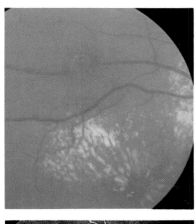

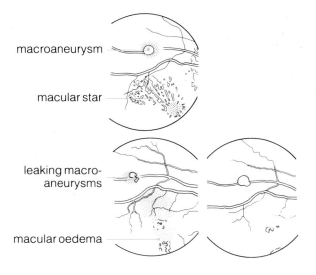

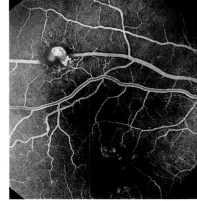

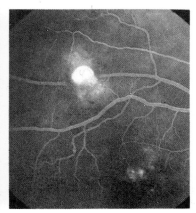

Fig. 14.18 Following laser photocoagulation in the same patient some weeks later retinal pigment epithelial atrophy is seen around the lesion and the hard exudate is absorbing.

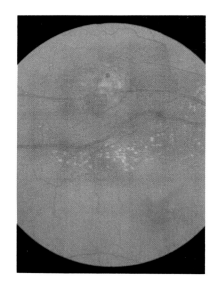

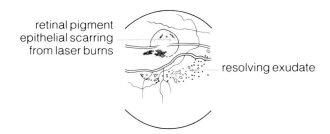

retinal pigment epithelial scarring from laser burns

resolving exudate

RETINAL VENOUS OCCLUSIONS

Retinal vein occlusions may be divided according to whether the central retinal vein or its tributaries are affected. The typical signs in the early stages are haemorrhage in the part of the retina supplied by the vein, dilatation of the affected veins, retinal oedema and varying amounts of ischaemia with cotton wool spots. Venous occlusions vary considerably in their severity and the visual disability will depend on the area of retina affected, the severity of the occlusion and the amount of retinal ischaemia. Mild venous occlusions cause visual disability from haemorrhage or vascular leakage and macular oedema, whereas the more severe lesions also produce ischaemia, retinal capillary closure and the risk of neovascularization.

Central Retinal Vein Occlusion

Mild central retinal vein occlusions can be asymptomatic but more severe occlusions typically present with loss of vision varying from minor to severe blurring, with a haemorrhagic fundus, dilatation of the retinal veins, retinal oedema and variable amounts of ischaemia. Signs of severity vary from a grossly haemorrhagic fundus with optic disc oedema, to partial forms with only a few fundus haemorrhages and mild vascular changes. This range of appearances is reflected by the initial visual symptoms and the subsequent clinical sequelae.

The aetiology is often difficult to elucidate. There is a higher incidence of the disease in diabetic and

hypertensive patients and those with other vascular diseases. The role of associated arterial disease in the pathogenesis remains controversial, but the condition is more common in arteriosclerotic individuals and it is possible that as the central retinal artery and vein share a common fascial sheath in the optic nerve, thickening and hypertrophy of the artery compromises the venous diameter, leading to obstruction. Patients often notice that the symptons are present on waking, vision having been normal the previous night and it has been postulated that these patients might have a particularly labile vascular response to posture and blood pressure. Hyperviscosity states produce a similar picture to central vein occlusion from venous stasis but the retinopathy is bilateral and is usually less severe in that the ischaemic and haemorrhagic types are not usually seen.

Inflammatory phlebitis has been shown to cause central retinal vein occlusion, for example, in sarcoidosis and some authorities believe that central retinal vein occlusion in younger patients is a form of vasculitis and should be investigated and treated accordingly. However, there is usually no evidence of either intraocular or systemic inflammation in most of these patients and such a diagnosis is usually difficult to substantiate.

Chronic glaucoma is an important association of central retinal vein occlusion in both the affected and the fellow eye and is frequently overlooked.

Fig. 14.19 Central retinal vein occlusion may produce gross optic disc swelling; in contrast to papilloedema, the haemorrhgagic fundus changes spread into the equatorial retina. This patient shows marked optic disc oedema, gross retinal haemorrhages, venous dilatation and cotton wool spots. Deep haemorrhages are seen in the peripheral retina.

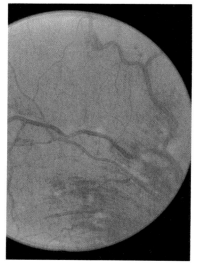

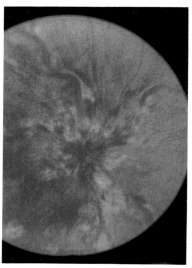

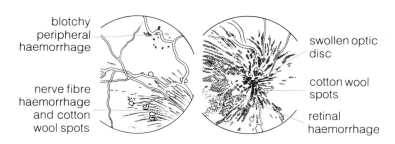

blotchy peripheral haemorrhage

nerve fibre haemorrhage and cotton wool spots

swollen optic disc

cotton wool spots

retinal haemorrhage

Fig. 14.20   A mild central vein occlusion shows venous engorgement, retinal haemorrhage and an optico-ciliary venous collateral vessel on the optic disc indicating that blood is being shunted from the retinal circulation to the lower pressure choroidal circulation to leave the eye by the vortex veins. Optico-ciliary shunts are derived by dilatation of normal vascular channels on the optic disc and their appearance indicates that obstruction has probably been present for some time.

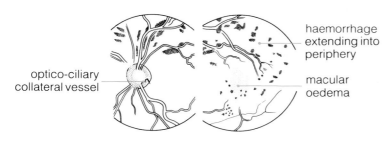

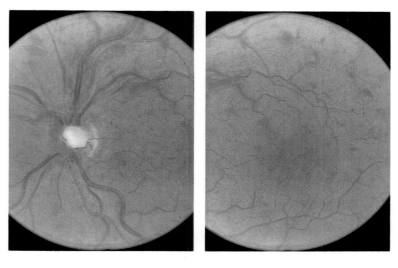

Fig. 14.21   Fluorescein angiography shows venous and capillary leakage on the optic disc and in the retina with macular oedema. Retinal haemorrhages mask the choroidal fluorescence.

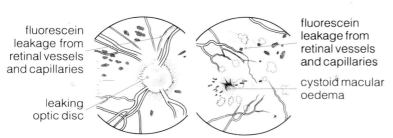

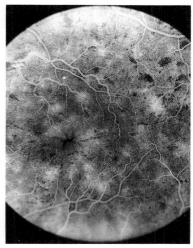

Fig. 14.22   Such patients present with blurring of vision which tends to improve over 2-3 months as the central retinal vein recanalises or collateral vessels develop on the optic disc with the choroidal circulation. At this stage the visual acuity may improve and the retinal haemorrhages absorb and fluorescein angiography shows only minimal vascular leakage. The collateral vessels do not leak fluorescein, in contrast to neovascularization, because they are derived from normal vascular channels with tight junctions between the endothelial cells. In this patient the optico-ciiliary collateral vessels are well developed on the optic disc and there are possible signs of early glaucomatous cupping. In more severe cases the macular oedema may persist with consequent visual loss.

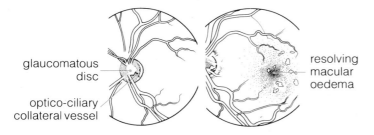

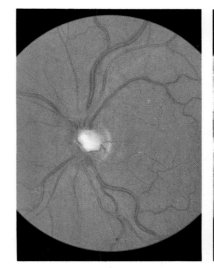

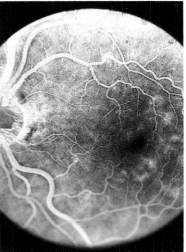

Fig. 14.23 Cotton wool spots and dense, dark, blotchy retinal haemorrhages are a sign of severe retinal ischaemia with capillary closure. This is a common but poorly understood phenomenon that is usually observed soon after the initial occlusion, although it may progress in extent over the following few months.

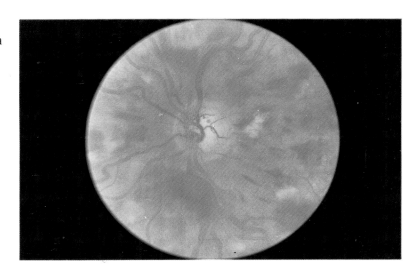

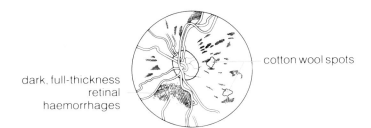

Fig. 14.24 Fluorescein angiography of the same patient shows that the major retinal vessels fill with dye but that the capillary bed is grossly abnormal with large areas of absent capillary perfusion and islands of dilated sparse coarse capillaries remaining. Retinal haemorrhage masks the background choroidal fluorescence. In the later stages there is gross leakage of dye from the major retinal vessels and the optic disc, especially in the ischaemic areas. Surprisingly, marked capillary closure in the posterior pole can be compatible with reasonable preservation of visual acuity, although the majority of such eyes have extremely poor vision.

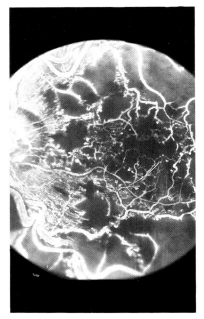

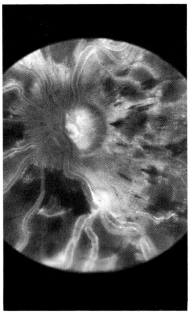

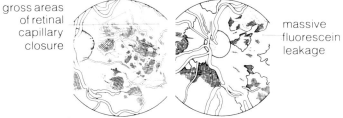

Fig. 14.25 In the presence of gross capillary closure, between 30-50% of eyes will develop rubeosis iridis and progress to thrombotic glaucoma. Most of these eyes can be made comfortable by topical steroid and mydriatic therapy, but a proportion of these eyes will eventually have to be enucleated as blind painful eyes. Rubeosis iridis classically appears about 3 months after the vein occlusion. In the earliest stages a fine neovascular network is seen around the pupil or in the angle of the anterior chamber. This is followed by development of ectropion uveae from contraction of the neovascular membrane, further vascular proliferation, glaucoma and corneal oedema (see Glaucoma, Chapter 8). This sequence of events can be forestalled by early panretinal photocoagulation. Following this, the rubeotic iris vessels will atrophy to leave the patient with an eye that has poor vision but is, at least, comfortable. For some reason, retinal or optic disc neovascularisation is extremely uncommon after a central retinal vein occlusion.

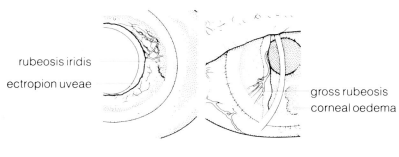

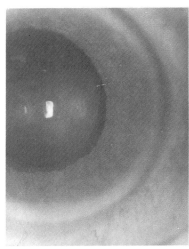

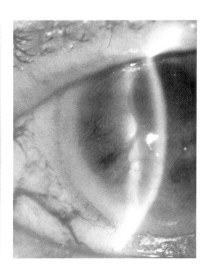

Fig. 14.26   Collateral vessels often persist on the optic disc after other signs of venous occlusion have resolved and occasionally can be confused with neovascularisation. However, they are easily distinguished by fluorescein angiography and do not produce ocular morbidity. Coarseness of the capillary pattern in this posterior pole is also due to previous venous disturbance.

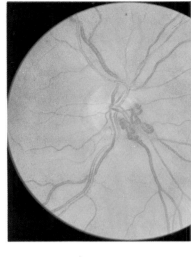
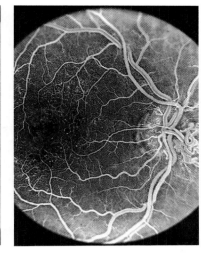

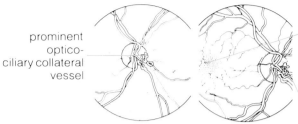

prominent optico-ciliary collateral vessel

capillary changes from previous central retinal vein occlusion

no fluorescein leakage from collateral vessels

Fig. 14.27   The optic nerve of a patient whose eye was enucleated for thrombotic glaucoma shows gliosis and atrophy of the nerve (compare with the normal nerve, Chapter 17). The common fascial sheath of the central retinal artery and vein is demonstrated; the artery is identified by its muscular wall. A thrombus containing cholesterol crystals is lodged in the arterial lumen, the vein is pushed to one side and there is recanalisation with multiple channels.

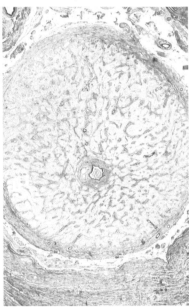
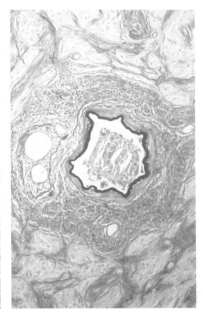

atrophic optic nerve

central retinal vessels

subarachnoid space

gliosis of optic nerve axons

recanalized central retinal vein

central retinal artery

thrombosis with cholesterol clefts

Branch Retinal Vein Occlusion

Occlusion of branches of the central retinal vein produces a similar fundus picture to that of central vein occlusion but is limited, as would be expected, to the affected area. Most branch vein occlusions occur in the temporal retina at arteriovenous crossings in patients with systemic hypertension or arteriosclerosis. Thickening of the artery leads to compression of the underlying vein within the shared fascial sheath (The Retina, Chapter 13). Branch vein occlusions at other sites may occur with an

inflammatory phlebitis (Inflammatory Eye Disease, Chapter 10), with diabetes or, occasionally, at the rim of a deeply cupped glaucomatous optic disc where the vein bends over the rim. Occasionally, there may be a congenital anomaly of venous drainage with late fusion of the upper and lower retinal branch veins in the optic nerve head so that a hemisphere vein occlusion may be produced in a way analogous to a central retinal vein occlusion.

Fig. 14.28   This patient shows haemorrhages in the nerve fibre layer from a superior temporal vein occlusion occuring at an arteriovenous crossing on the margin of the optic disc. Most of the haemorrhage is superficial without cotton wool spot formation, which suggests that little deep retinal ischaemia and capillary closure has occurred and that the prognosis for vision will be good.

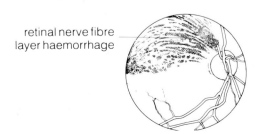

retinal nerve fibre layer haemorrhage

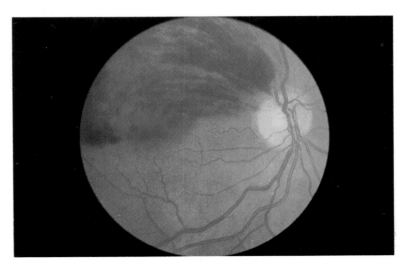

Fig. 14.29 The fluorescein angiogram demonstrates masking of background choroidal fluorescence by the retinal haemorrhage but an absence of any marked degree of capillary closure. There is some leakage of dye from the large retinal vessels and capillaries in the affected area.

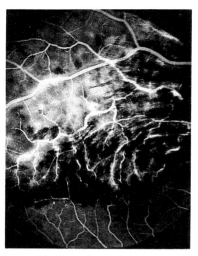

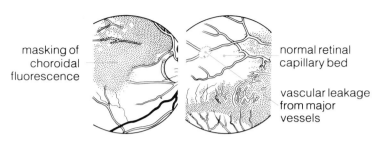

masking of choroidal fluorescence

normal retinal capillary bed

vascular leakage from major vessels

Fig. 14.30 A small macular branch vein occlusion is seen in a hypertensive patient who presented with blurred vision. Fluorescein angiography shows the site of occlusion at an arteriovenous crossing with retinal vascular leakage, haemorrhage and oedema in the affected area. Some weeks later, the haemorrhage can be seen to be resolving with corresponding improvement in vision.

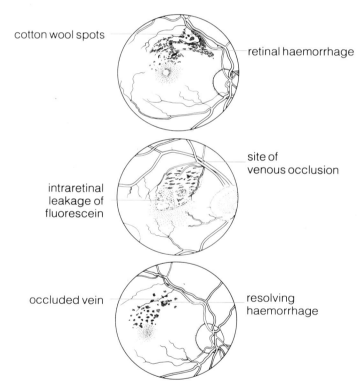

cotton wool spots

retinal haemorrhage

site of venous occlusion

intraretinal leakage of fluorescein

occluded vein

resolving haemorrhage

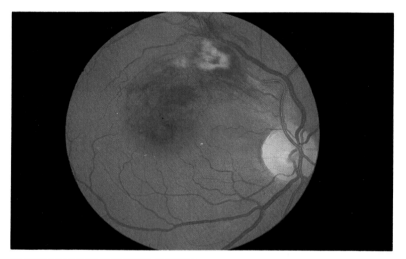

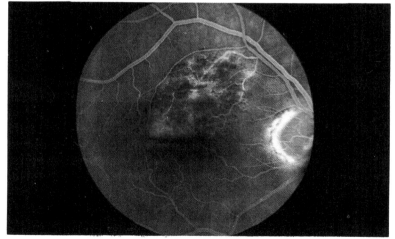

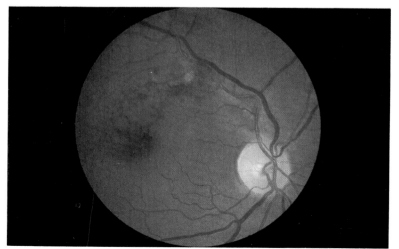

Sequelae of Branch Retinal Vein Occlusion

Fig. 14.31   Following a hemisphere branch occlusion, collaterals may develop across the horizontal meridian from the affected to the normal venous return. These vessels resemble venous collaterals on the optic disc in that they are "mature" and do not leak fluorescein or produce ocular morbidity.

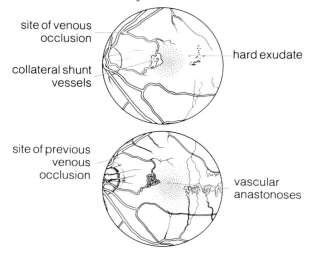

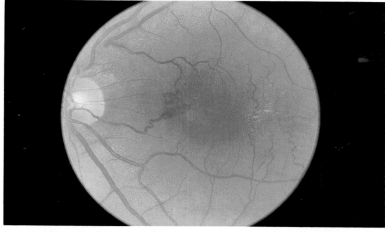

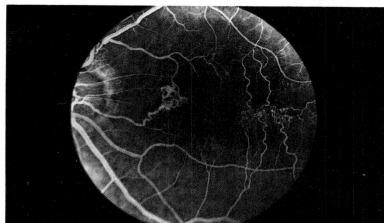

Fig. 14.32   Major retinal arteries or veins that pass through an ischaemic retina may become white and sheathed with fibrosis and lipid deposition in the vascular walls. These photographs show a recent superior temporal vein occlusion with cotton wool spots indicating retinal ischaemia.

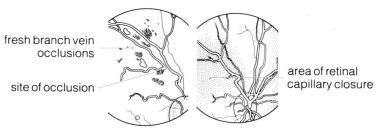

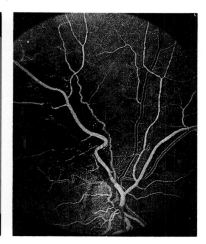

Fig. 14.33   Some months later, in the same patient, the artery and vein within the ischaemic retina are white and sheathed. Angiography shows the artery is still patent although attenuated. There is vascular remodelling of the venous return and, in the later phases, the vein fills by retrograde flow from collaterals. Such sheathing must be distinguished from the whiter, ill-defined and fluffy appearance of a vasculitis.

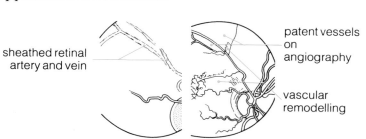

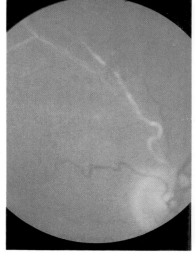

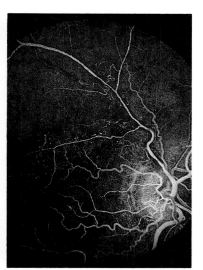

14.13

Fig. 14.34 Visual loss in the acute stages is due to involvement of the macula by haemorrhage or oedema. Vision may improve as these changes resolve over weeks or months and if the capillary arcade surrounding the macula is left intact the visual prognosis is comparatively good. Persistent visual loss may be caused by ischaemic macular damage, epiretinal membrane formation or chronic macular oedema. Whilst photocoagulation has been tried for the latter, it has not proved effective. Lipid exudate sometimes occurs some months after the initial occlusion and produces further loss of visual acuity, as in this patient where there is a plaque of hard exudate overlying the macula in the viable and functioning retina. Angiography demonstrates marked capillary dilatation and leakage in the area of the previous occlusion. If this area is photocoagulated, the lipid will slowly absorb and further visual loss will be prevented.

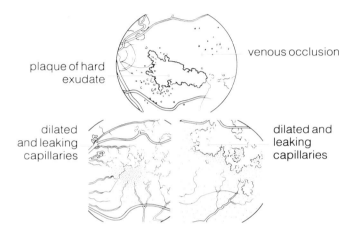

Fig. 14.35 Severe branch vein occlusion with capillary closure may be followed by neovascularization in a similar way to that seen in diabetes (cf. Chapters 13 and 15). This patient shows cotton wool spots and retinal haemorrhages in the affected area (top left) and fluorescein angiography demonstrates extensive capillary closure (top right). Several weeks later, a fan of neovascular-ization has developed at the junction of the ischaemic and normal retina (bottom left) which leaks fluorescein profusely (bottom right). The patient has a substantial risk of developing a vitreous haemorrhage and requires photocoagulation to the ischaemic area.

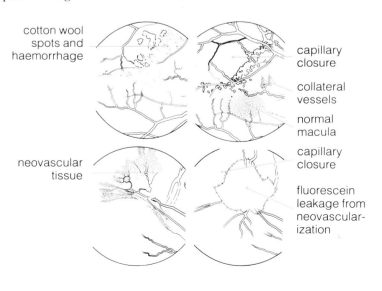

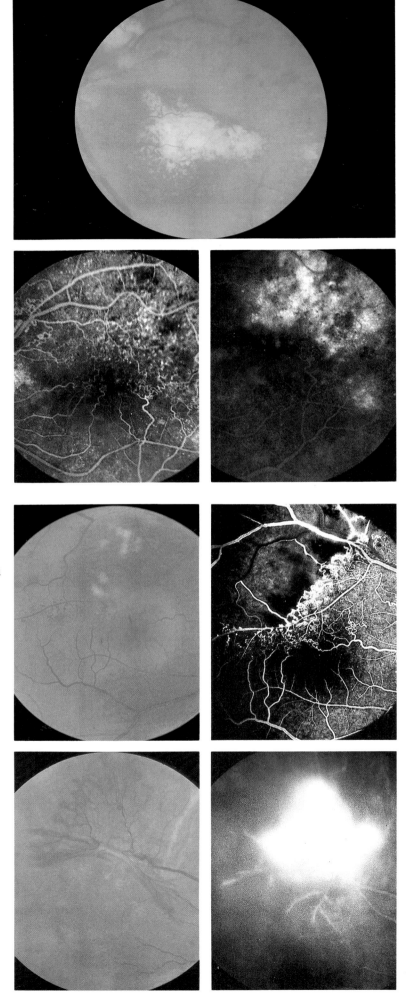

Fig. 14.36 Following a branch vein occlusion with capillary closure, neovascularisation can occur on the retina, usually adjacent to the ischaemic area, or on the optic disc. This patient shows a patch of fine, thready neovascularization on the optic disc. This is a serious complication which carries a poorer prognosis than peripheral neovascularization, especially if the vessels are pulled forwards to the posterior hyaloid face. These vessels readily regress following panretinal photocoagulation of the area of ischaemic retina and this therapy is indicated, especially if the patient has already suffered a vitreous haemmorhage. Rubeosis iridis is comparatively uncommon and, if it does occur, it hardly ever progresses to thrombotic glaucoma.

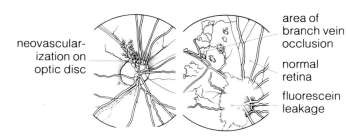

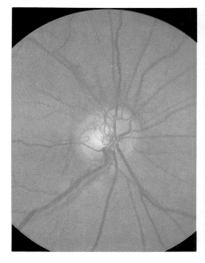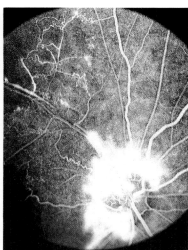

HYPERTENSIVE RETINOPATHY

Systemic hypertension produces changes in the choroidal, retinal and optic disc circulations and these changes depend on the severity, rapidity of onset and duration of the hypertension and on the age of the patient. The branch retinal 'arteries' are, in fact, arterioles by histological criteria. The pathological sequence of events in these vessels, in response to a rise in blood pressure, has been described as an initial arteriolar constriction of the ocular vessels due to autoregulation. This is followed by necrosis of the smooth muscle in the media from ischaemia, subsequent vascular dilatation and leakage of plasma into the vessel's wall producing fibrinoid necrosis. Occlusion, haemorrhage and infarction follow.

The eye is the only site in the body where blood vessels can be directly observed and there have been several attempts to classify and grade the effect of hypertension on these vessels. However, it is impossible to differentiate adequately between the early changes of hypertension and the normal ageing changes of arteriolar sclerosis which will also produce changes in the reflex of the arteriolar wall (silver wiring, copper wiring) and arteriovenous crossing changes. Apart from the presence of a frank retinopathy, perhaps the most reliable sign of systemic hypertension is focal areas of attenuation in arteriolar calibre and most ophthalmologists place little emphasis on the light reflex from the vessel wall seen ophthalmoscopically. Severe systemic hypertension of sudden onset produces a microvascular retinopathy with comparatively little change in the major arterioles; the converse is true where the rise in blood pressure has been more gradual and prolonged, allowing time for compensatory sclerotic changes to take place in the major retinal arteries.

Fig. 14.37 This figure illustrates the fundus appearance of a black patient of 40 years of age with systemic hypertension of relatively short duration. The inferior temporal artery has an irregular calibre and light reflex from the vessel wall, and there is pronounced arteriovenous nipping where the vessels cross. Whilst these changes are pathological in a young patient, it would be more difficult to say with certainty that they were so in an elderly patient.

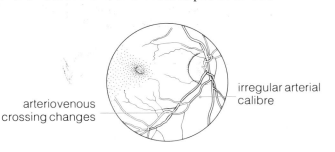

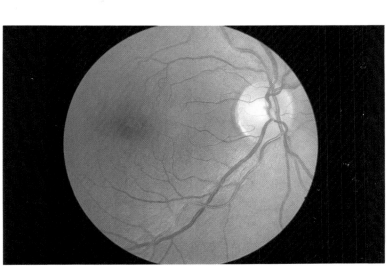

Fig. 14.38 This patient has acute hypertension of rapid onset and shows a more severe retinopathy. Both eyes show cotton wool spots and haemorrhages but the main retinal arteries are comparatively spared, indicating the acuteness and severity of the hypertension.

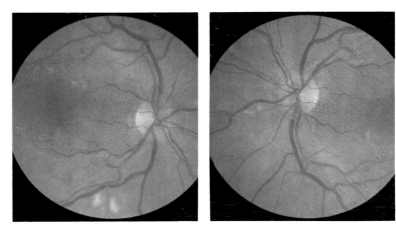

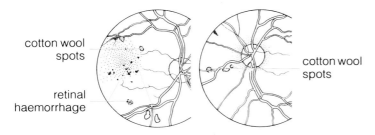

Fig. 14.39 This patient shows cotton wool spots, retinal haemorrhages and marked focal areas of constriction in the retinal arteries, indicating severe and more prolonged systemic hypertension.

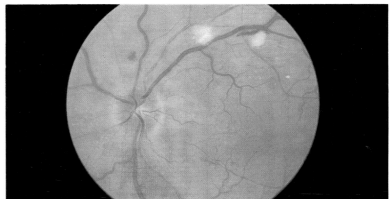

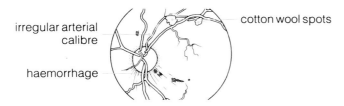

Fig. 14.40 Bilateral optic disc swelling or the sudden appearance of cotton wool spots with hypertensive retinopathy is known as accelerated hypertension. This condition carries a very poor prognosis if the blood pressure is not rapidly controlled, patients being at risk from cardiac failure and hypertensive encephalopathy. Whilst the blood pressure requires urgent control, this

must be done carefully and gradually as a sudden drop in tissue perfusion pressure can result in infarction in the optic disc, or elsewhere. Swelling of the optic disc with accelerated hypertension probably results from local tissue ischaemia rather than raised intracranial pressure which is usually said to be normal. Visual acuity remains normal in the absence of macular changes.

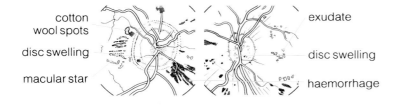
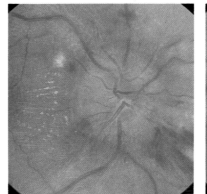
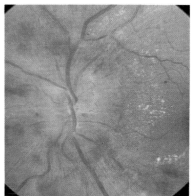

Fig. 14.41 Fluorescein angiography demonstrates the optic disc changes generally seen in optic disc oedema of any cause. Macular stars are common as the optic disc oedema resolves and, indeed, their presence often suggests ischaemia as the cause of the disc swelling (see also anterior ischaemic optic neuropathy, Chapter 17). In this patient, choroidal infarcts are seen in the posterior pole and there are widespread segments of focal attenuation in the retinal arterioles indicating severe hypertension of some duration.

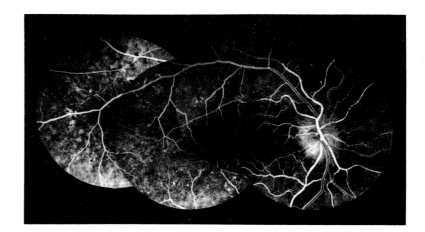

Fig. 14.42 Changes in the choroidal vasculature with hypertensive retinopathy do not usually affect vision. Bullous serous retinal detachments can be seen with acute systemic hypertension, probably as a result of infarction of the choriocapillaris and breakdown of the retinal pigment epithelial cell barrier. Elschnig's spots represent foci of infarction of the choriocapillaris in the posterior pole with overlying changes in the retinal pigment epithelium (cf. Fig. 14.41).

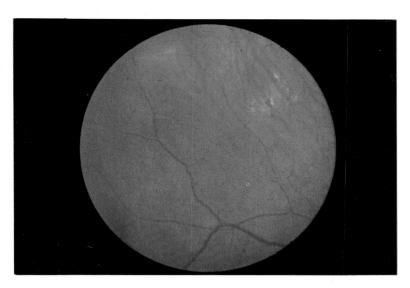

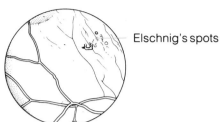

Elschnig's spots

Fig. 14.43 Siegrist streaks are linear areas of infarction, sometimes seen in the peripheral retina. These patterns of choroidal infarction are further support for the concept of a lobular supply to the choroid (Uveal Tract, Chapter 9).

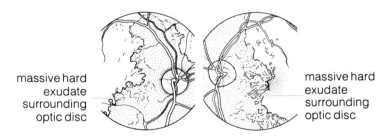

wedge shaped 'Siegrist streak'

Fig. 14.44 Hypertension with renal failure can produce a much more exudative pattern of retinopathy with less evidence of retinal ischaemia.

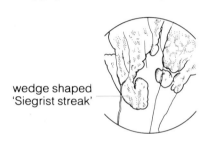

massive hard exudate surrounding optic disc

massive hard exudate surrounding optic disc

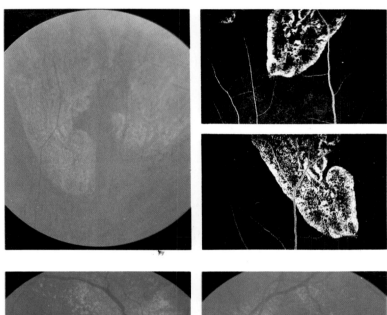

Fig. 14.45 Following control of blood pressure and renal dialysis in the same patient, retinal exudate absorbed over several months and visual acuity returned to normal. Minor focal attentuations can be seen in the arteries.

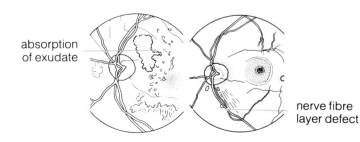

absorption of exudate

nerve fibre layer defect

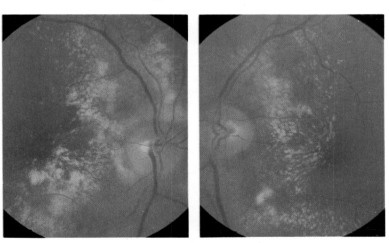

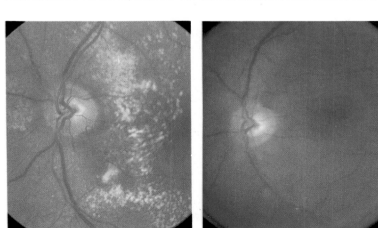

14.17

HYPERVISCOSITY SYNDROMES AND SLOW FLOW RETINOPATHY

Blood viscosity can be raised by polycythaemia, plasma protein macroglobulinaemia, high fibrinogen levels or, exceptionally, by massive leucocytosis with leukaemia. The retinopathy produced is similar in appearance to that from slow flow with carotid artery occlusion or central retinal vein obstruction, except that both eyes are affected in hyperviscoscosity syndromes. In the hyperviscosity syndromes the fundus appearance depends on the degree and duration of venous stasis. Initial changes are seen in the retinal veins which become dilated, haemorrhage into the nerve fibre layer and deeper retina follows, and varying amounts of optic disc oedema or retinal ischaemia are seen. More severe ocular involvement is rare but patients can develop capillary closure and ocular neovascularisation.

Waldenström's macroglobulinaemia

Hyperviscosity results from a myeloma producing large quantities of the IgM class of immunoglobulin, the largest immunoprotein. The initial manifestation is bilateral venous dilatation progressing to retinal haemorrhage and cotton wool spot formation simulating central retinal vein obstruction. Patients also have weight loss, malaise, a tendency to bleed, hepatosplenomegaly and progressive neurological signs from the hyperviscosity.

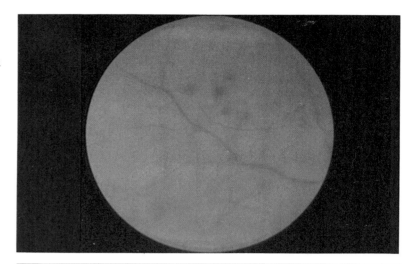

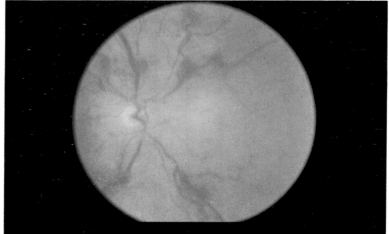

Fig. 14.46 The peripheral retina of both eyes of this 70-year-old man with Waldenströms macroglobulinaemia of some three years duration showed blot haemorrhgages compatible with his anaemia (Hb 7.2gm) but, in spite of an IgM level of 27 gm/l and an elevated plasma viscosity, there was no retinal venous dilation. The right eye of another patient with more marked retinopathy shows dilated retinal veins, retinal oedema and superficial retinal haemorrhages.

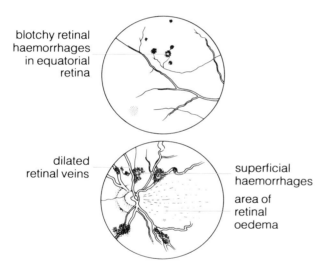

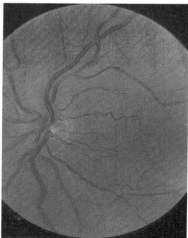

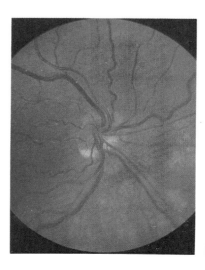

Fig. 14.47 This patient with primary polycythaemia rubra vera shows dilatation of the retinal vessels without other signs of retinal ischaemia. The haemoglobin concentration was 23 g/l. The patient complained of mild blurring of vision which rapidly improved following venesection.

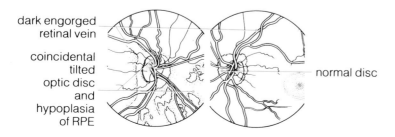

14.18

RETINOPATHY OF PREMATURITY

This disease is becoming more common again due to the advances in neonatal ventilation which allow lower birth weight and very premature babies to survive. The foetal retina vascularises from the optic disc to the periphery and, until vascularisation is complete, the retinal arteries are susceptable to high oxygen concentrations in the retina. Vascularisation is completed on the nasal side first (as this is the shortest distance from the optic disc), but development continues in the temporal retina until about the time of normal birth. This delay in vascularisation is likely to be the reason for the temporal retina being the most severely affected area by retinopathy of prematurity.

The disease can be divided into an active proliferative phase with a subsequent cicatrical phase and either phase can be aborted before it becomes fully developed. Mature retinal vessels are insensitive to high oxygen tensions but immature vessels are sensitive and initially become vasoconstricted and subsequently obliterated (stage 1).

This is followed by a ridge of neovascular budding along the line of retinal ischaemia which penetrates the inner limiting membrane and extends into the vitreous gel (stage 2). Vitreous haemorrhage, fibrosis and retinal traction follow (stages 3 & 4), leading to retinal detachment (stage 5). Retinal changes are seen after a few hours of high oxygen exposure and progress but the process can abort at any stage to be followed by the cicatrical phase. This is also graded from 1–5, but these do not necessarily correspond to the end result of each proliferative phase. In the mildest cases there is myopia with scarring in the temporal periphery (stage 1) progressing to retinal vascular traction (stage 2), macular ectopia and distortion (stage 3), retinal detachment (stage 4), and a retrolental fibrovascular mass (stage 5). The use of vitamin E as a prophylatic antioxidant in infants at risk and the role of cryotherapy to destroy the active neovascular tissue are currently being evaluated.

Fig. 14.48 The retinal changes are best seen in the temporal periphery and may be asymmetrical in each eye. Initially, arterial constriction is followed by a greyish avascular line of peripheral vascular closure; the picture on the left shows peripheral vascular closure and early neovascular budding with collateral vessel formation (stage 2). The picture on the right shows vitreous haemorrhage in a more advanced case (stage 3).

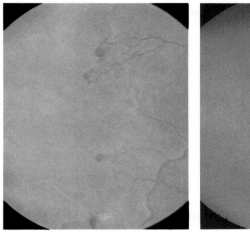
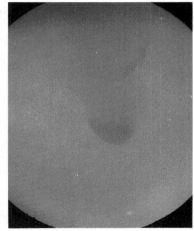

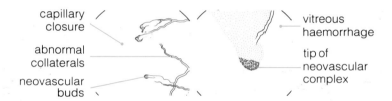

Fig. 14.49 On the left can be seen the mildest degree of temporal scarring, with mild traction on the optic disc (stage 1, cicatrical phase). More severe scarring and traction, as seen in the middle picture produces visual loss from macular distortion (stage 3). The photograph on the right shows the typical appearance of a 'dragged' optic disc.

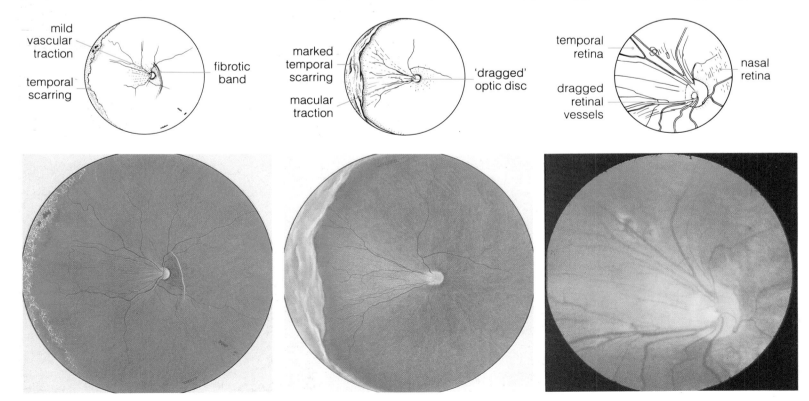

Fig. 14.50 The picture on the left shows scarring and traction, producing a retinal fold (stage 3). Note the flat retinal hole superiorly. (Rhegmatogenous retinal attachment is not uncommon in young adults with cicatrical retinopathy.) Severe folding of the retina destroying the macula can be seen on the left (stage 4).

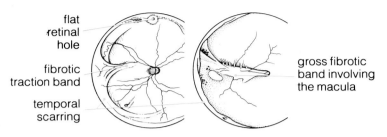

flat retinal hole
fibrotic traction band
temporal scarring
gross fibrotic band involving the macula

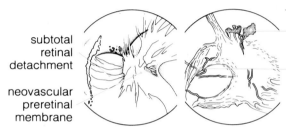

Fig. 14.51 A subtotal retinal detachment from extensive proliferative disease can be seen on the left (Cicatrical stage 4), and on the right similar changes can be seen while still in the active vasoproliferative phase.

subtotal retinal detachment
neovascular preretinal membrane
active neovascular tissue
fibrosis and gross traction

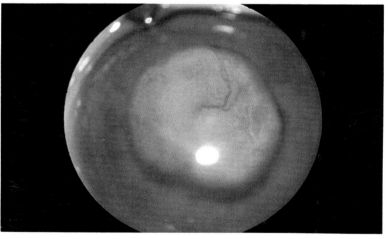

Fig. 14.52 Increasing fibrosis leads to total retinal detachment and organisation which is seen as a white retrolental mass; this must be differentiated from the other causes of leucocoria in an infant (for example, congenital cataract, persistent hyperplastic primary vitreous, endophthalmitis, coloboma, retinal dysplasia, folds or detachment, retinoblastoma).

vascularized white retrolental membrane
retrolental fibrotic mass
cone of fibrotic retina
optic disc

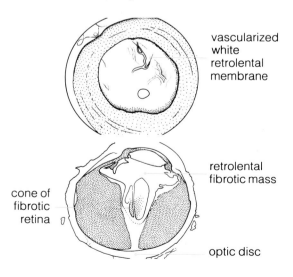

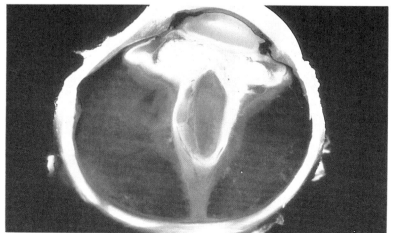

TRAUMATIC RETINOPATHY

Fig. 14.53 Retinal oedema is a common finding following a blunt injury to the eye (Commotio retinae, Berlin's oedema). Any part of the fundus can be affected and appears pale and silvery due to intraretinal oedema of the outer retina. This usually resolves over a few days without sequelae, although a careful examination of the retinal periphery for a dialysis must be made (see Chapter 12). The possibility of traumatic anterior chamber angle recession and future cataract must not be overlooked. More severe trauma may produce a 'choroidal' rupture (cf. Chapter 16).

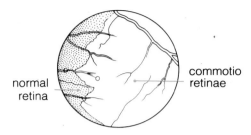

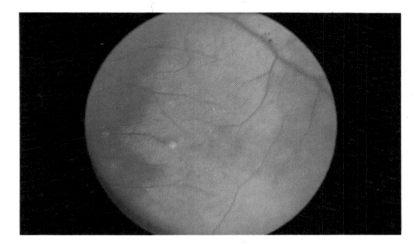

Fig. 14.54 Purtscher's retinopathy is a rare condition seen following compressive chest injuries, multiple trauma or acute pancreatitis. Cotton wool spots, retinal oedema and haemorrhages are found in the posterior pole of each eye. The aetiology is probably a combination of sudden increased venous pressure, fat embolisation and disseminated intravenous coagulation.

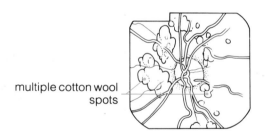

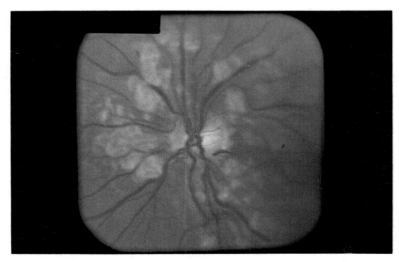

RETINAL INFECTIONS

The retina is an unusual site for infection. Toxoplasmosis is the most common cause of retinochoroiditis and has been discussed in Chapter 10. Less common causes are fungal and neurotropic viral infections which usually present as a posterior uveitis with areas of retinal infiltration. Bacterial infection is usually seen in the context of endophthalmitis and is rare as an isolated retinal septic lesion.

Fig. 14.55 Cytomegalic virus (CMV) retinitis is most commonly seen in immunocompromised individuals, affecting one or both eyes, and has been described as a feature of AIDS (Acquired Immunodeficiency Syndrome, originally seen in promiscuous homosexuals). Patients with CMV present with visual loss and on examination show widespread areas of retinitis and haemorrhage – the 'tomato sauce and salad dressing' fundus. Diagnosis is made by culturing the virus from the eye or warm urine.

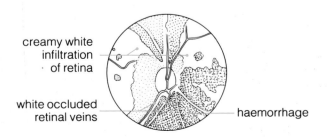

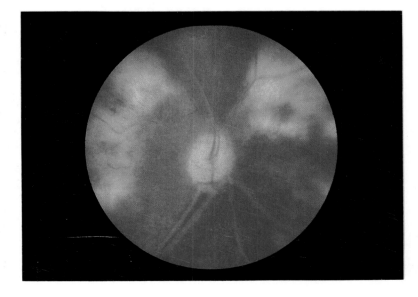

Fig. 14.56 *Candida albicans* retinitis is seen in immunocompromised individuals, drug addicts or patients with longstanding intravenous catheters. The initial lesion is a focus of embolic yeast infection in the retina which bursts through into the vitreous gel and replicates there. Other signs of systemic candiasis may or may not be present. Patients present with a posterior uveitis. They may also show evidence of a focus of retinitis or snowballs joined by threads in the vitreous, the 'string of pearls' sign. Diagnosis is made by culture of the organism from the vitreous gel and the disease responds to antifungal drugs and vitrectomy.

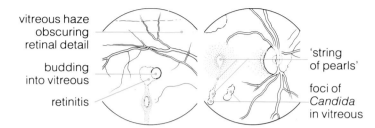

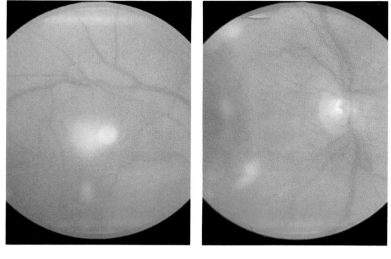

Fig. 14.57 Rubella retinopathy is part of the congenital rubella infection syndrome and patients usually have other signs such as deafness, mental retardation, cardiac defects, cataracts etc. (see Chapter 11). The retinopathy is seen as a pigmentary disturbance of the outer retina which does not result in visual loss except that patients have a risk of developing presenile disciform degeneration in the 30-40 year age group.

This child was referred for ophthalmic assessment because of congenital deafness from rubella. Visual activities were normal and there was no cataract. Retinal examination showed areas of diffuse disturbance of retinal pigment epithelium in the posterior pole with more obvious and better demarcated atrophic changes in the periphery.

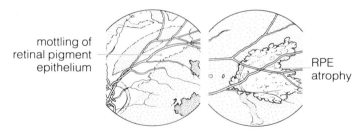

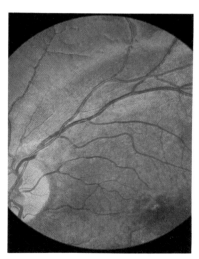
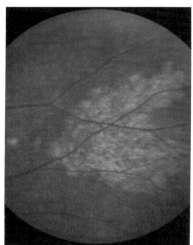

Fig. 14.58 Bilateral acute retinal necrosis (BARN syndrome) is a rare acute necrotic retinitis which affects the peripheral fundus producing confluent scalloped lesions; these progress to gross retinal hole formation and untreatable retinal detachment. There is some evidence that herpes zoster retinitis is the underlying aetiology.

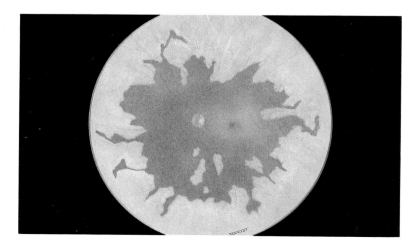

15. The Retina: Vascular Disease II

J. S. Shilling
D. J. Spalton
T. J. ffytche

Introduction

Diabetic retinopathy is the commonest cause of blindness in the working population but with present techniques of blood sugar control and photocoagulation much of this blindness should, in future, be preventable. Diabetes predominantly affects the microvascular ocular circulation and, apart from some minor dilatation of the retinal arterioles and venules, no changes are seen in the major vessels in the early stages. Vitreous fluorophotometry suggests that breakdown of the blood-retina barrier occurs before any ophthalmoscopic evidence of ocular disease. This is followed by increased arteriolar dilatation and retinal blood flow, possibly as an autoregulatory response to tissue hypoxia.

The precise pathological sequence of events which produces a retinopathy is still unknown but the earliest changes appear to start in the retinal capillaries with thickening of the capillary basement membrane and loss of their mural pericytes. Microaneurysms are formed in the capillary circulation, perhaps as a result of a weakness in the capillary wall due to loss of pericytes, or possibly because of an abortive attempt at neovascularization of surrounding hypoxic retina. Basement membrane hypertrophy is produced by the endothelial cells which may initially proliferate but are eventually lost. Capillary closure may result from occlusion by basement membrane hypertrophy, loss of endothelial cells, vascular shunting or changes in the blood, of which hormonal changes or defects in platelet metabolism may play a part. The microvascular abnormalities develop with concomitant leakage of plasma or haemorrhage and, in some cases, the onset of neovascularization. The biochemical stimulus for these structural changes is unknown but there are various theories which centre around the likelihood of some circulating abnormality in the blood, possibly hormonal, secondary metabolic changes due to glucosaemia or interference in the clotting-fibrinolysis pathways. The latter might be mediated through platelet malfunction.

Diabetic retinopathy can be divided into various subtypes. Background retinopathy occurs when microaneurysms, small haemorrhages, cotton wool spots, hard exudates and small areas of capillary closure are seen in the presence of normal visual acuity. Disruption of the blood-retina barrier may progress according to one of two courses. It may lead to a maculopathy, where visual acuity is lost due to macular changes such as oedema, exudation or ischaemia. Alternatively it may give rise to a proliferative neovascular retinopathy where retinal hypoxia and neovascularization predominate and vision is lost due to vitreous haemorrhage or traction retinal detachment. However, these are broad groups and clinically there is a considerable overlap between them.

Retinopathy normally develops many years after the onset of the diabetes but in some adults it will present as the first sign of the disease. Good evidence is accumulating that meticulous control of blood sugar retards the onset of retinopathy. About 25% of juvenile diabetics exhibit retinopathy after ten years of disease duration but adult-onset diabetics seem to develop retinopathy more quickly, occurring in about 50% after ten years of disease. About 90% of visual loss from diabetes is due to maculopathy and, in common with other macular disorders, these patients lose central vision but retain navigating sight. Proliferative retinopathy carries a very much worse visual prognosis with about 70% of untreated eyes being totally blind five years after the onset of neovascularization. The influence of initiating meticulous blood sugar control once a retinopathy is established seems to vary. Early background retinopathy sometimes improves whereas proliferative retinopathy can deteriorate dramatically. Other factors such as pregnancy, systemic hypertension and renal failure appear to lead to deterioration of the retinopathy, whereas myopia of over −5D, optic atrophy, glaucoma, central retinal artery occlusion or carotid artery stenosis appear to offer some protection, possibly from reduction of the metabolic demands in the eye.

Fig. 15.1   A flow diagram illustrates the concept of initial background retinopathy progressing to visual loss from maculopathy or proliferative retinopathy.

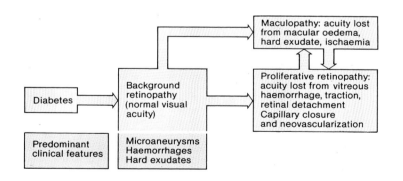

Fig. 15.2   Diabetic retinopathy. The blood vessels are outlined with colloidal carbon injected via the central retinal vein and show both tortuosity and microaneurysm formation at the margin of a small avascular zone. A similarly prepared specimen, on the right, is viewed by phase microscopy to show a focus of capillary closure.

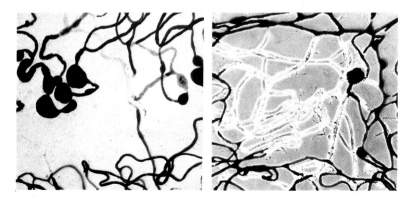

DIABETIC RETINOPATHY
Background Retinopathy

This is the commonest form of diabetic retinopathy. Breakdown of the blood-retinal barrier has already occurred by the time ophthalmoscopic changes are visible, either as a result of changes in the barriers of the retinal circulation or the retinal pigment epithelium. Microaneurysms, small deep blotchy haemorrhages, cotton wool spots and hard exudates are seen in the posterior pole. Microaneurysms are the pathognomic lesions of the diabetic eye. They can be found in other vascular retinopathies, but not in the numbers or to the extent found in diabetic retinopathy. At first, background retinopathy is normally most prominent in the retina temporal to the macula, probably because this is a watershed area in the retinal circulation. Focal areas of closure in the capillary bed are common and may result from occlusion of the feeding precapillary arteriole together with a contribution from external compression due to tissue hypoxia and retinal swelling or intravascular factors in the capillary itself. By definition visual acuity remains normal.

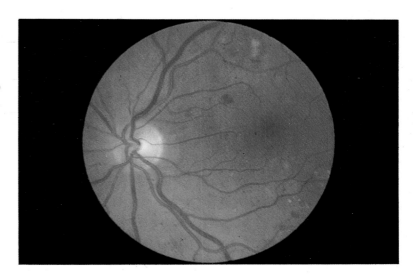

Fig. 15.3   This patient shows the typical changes of early background retinopathy with scattered microaneurysms, blot haemorrhages and hard exudates, and cotton wool spots in the posterior pole. The macula appears normal and the severity of the condition can fluctuate according to the success of the diabetic control. Visual acuity is normal.

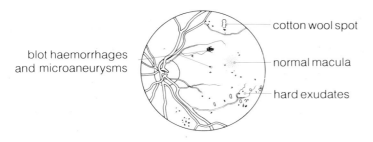

Fig. 15.4   Fluorescein angiography of the same patient demonstrates extensive microvascular changes throughout the posterior pole with scattered microaneurysms and minimal vascular leakage. Many more microanaeurysms are visible than can be seen clinically. Although in some areas capillary patterns around the macula are irregular and show minor areas of capillary closure they are, in the main, complete.

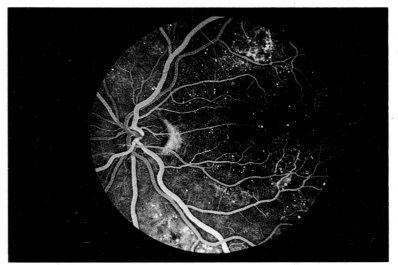

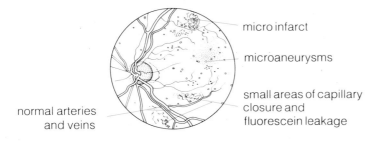

Fig. 15.5   With early retinopathy, the retina temporal to the macula is often susceptible to earlier and more pronounced changes; elsewhere in the posterior pole of this patient, retinopathy is comparatively sparse.

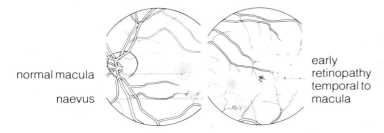

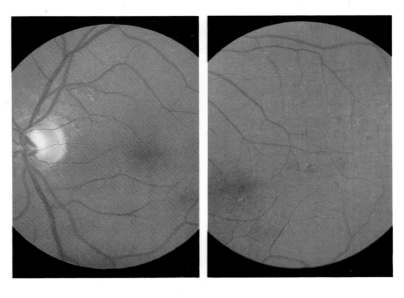

Fig. 15.6 Colour photographs of another patient show a more advanced background retinopathy with some paramacular accumulation of hard exudate.

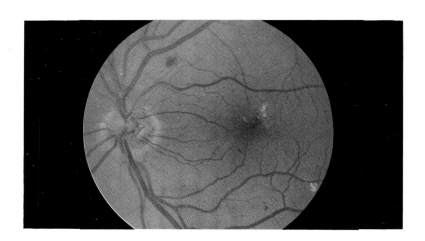

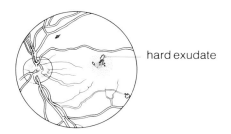

hard exudate

Fig. 15.7 Early and late phases of the fluorescein angiogram of the same patient demonstrate increasing disruption of the blood-retinal barrier. The microaneurysms show increasing leakage of dye from the capillary circulation of both the optic disc and retina. Such a patient is at risk of developing visual loss from a maculopathy.

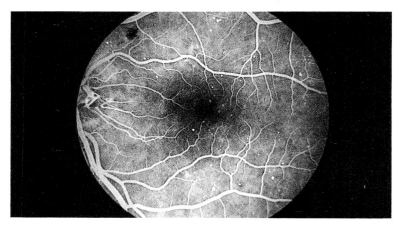

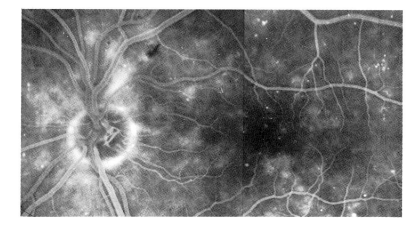

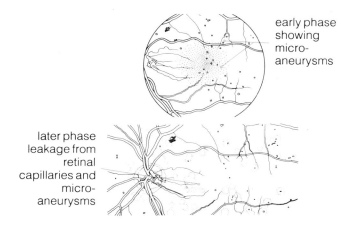

early phase showing micro-aneurysms

later phase leakage from retinal capillaries and micro-aneurysms

Maculopathy

Involvement of the macula is the commonest cause of legal blindness from diabetic retinopathy and occurs in three basic patterns: lipid exudation, diffuse macular oedema or macular ischaemia, all of which are readily diagnosed by fluorescein angiography. Patients retain their peripheral field of vision.

Fig. 15.8 In the exudative type of maculopathy, circinate areas of hard exudate form around foci of leaking microvascular damage and visual acuity is lost from concomitant macular oedema and lipid deposition. This type of maculopathy responds most readily to laser photocoagulation (see Treatment).

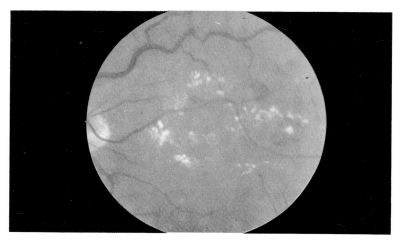

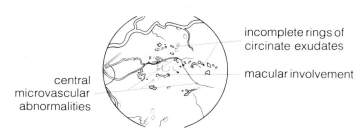

incomplete rings of circinate exudates

macular involvement

central microvascular abnormalities

Fig. 15.9 Fluorescein angiography of the patient seen in Fig. 15.8 demonstrates the areas of capillary abnormality with leakage and oedema in the macular area. From comparison with the colour photograph it can be seen that the centre of the circinate hard exudate contains the microvascular abnormality.

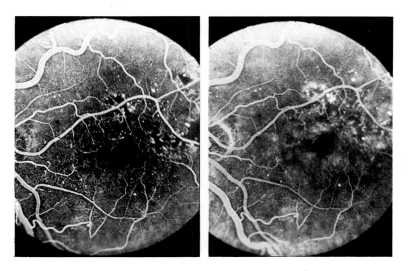

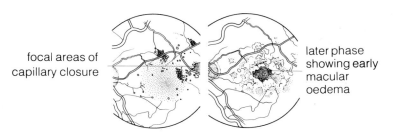

focal areas of capillary closure

later phase showing early macular oedema

Fig. 15.10 The oedematous type of maculopathy is less common. Vascular changes produce macular oedema with relatively little haemorrhage or exudation. These maculas have a thickened, rather amorphous appearance and cystoid spaces are sometimes visible on biomicroscopy. Visual impairment is usually severe.

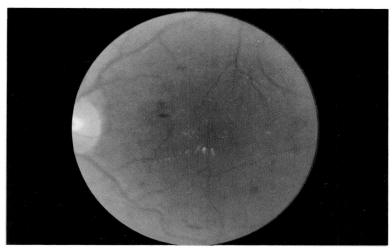

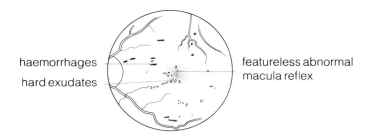

haemorrhages

hard exudates

featureless abnormal macula reflex

Fig. 15.11 Characteristically these individuals show diffuse capillary dilatation over the whole posterior pole with relatively few focal changes. Later phases show massive vascular leakage. These patients do not respond well to photocoagulation.

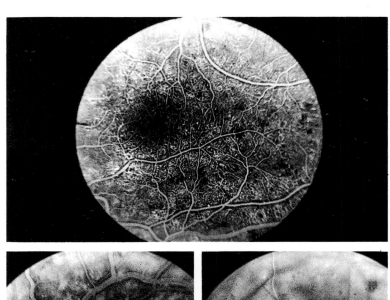

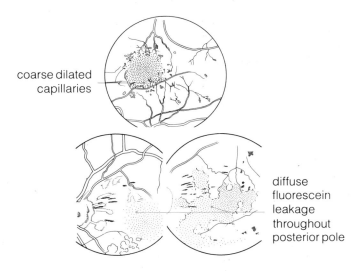

coarse dilated capillaries

diffuse fluorescein leakage throughout posterior pole

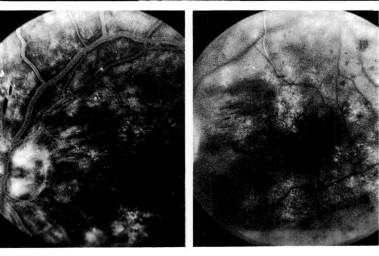

15.5

Fig. 15.12 In the ischaemic type of retinopathy, extensive capillary closure produces deep intraretinal haemorrhage, oedema and ischaemia. Exudates are comparatively sparse but may surround the central disturbance.

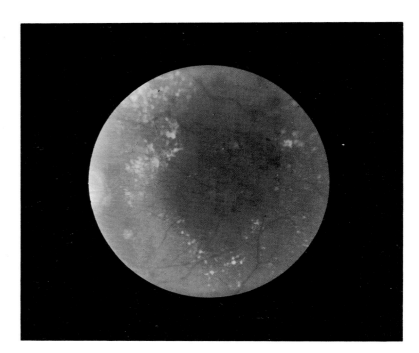

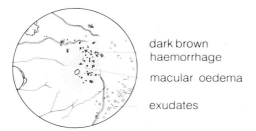

dark brown haemorrhage

macular oedema

exudates

Fig. 15.13 Large areas of capillary closure are seen in the angiogram. Surprisingly, the degree of capillary closure does not correlate with visual acuity; occasionally patients are seen with extensive areas of capillary closure involving the macula and yet retain reasonable vision. Photocoagulation does not help the visual prognosis.

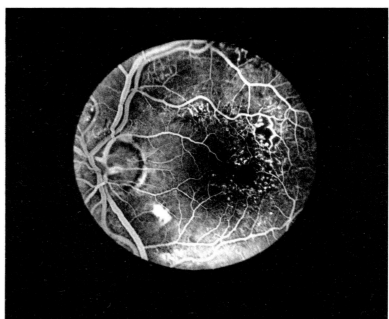

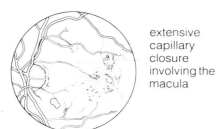

extensive capillary closure involving the macula

Fig. 15.14 Advanced exudative maculopathy results from prolonged and untreated deposition of lipid within the macula. Circinate exudates coalesce to produce massive plaques and, although these will absorb if the sources of vascular leakage are destroyed by photocoagulation, neuronal destruction has occurred to such an extent that vision rarely improves.

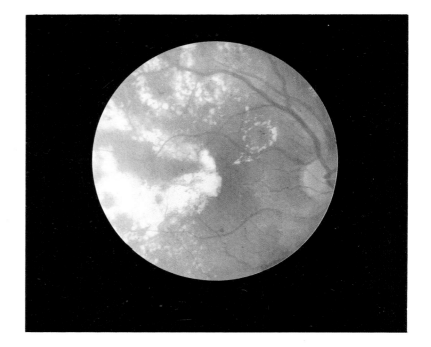

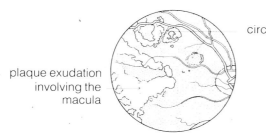

circinate exudates

plaque exudation involving the macula

Proliferative Diabetic Retinopathy

This condition tends to occur in diabetics who have evidence of severe involvement of other systems and these patients generally carry a poorer prognosis for life. A life expectancy, on average, of less than 6 years after the onset of the retinal neovascularization is often quoted but this is improving with better medical treatment, and in good centres these figures for patient survival are now probably pessimistic.

The stimulus for neovascularization, as in other neovascular retinopathies, appears to be gross retinal hypoxia from extensive areas of retinal capillary closure. These changes lead to a reduction of the increased retinal blood flow, which is a feature of background retinopathy, to normal or below normal levels. At this stage, neovascularization starts to appear from the capillaries on the venous side of the circulation and this occurs in two sites, either on the optic disc or on the retina, usually at the junction of normal and hypoxic retina. At first, the neovascular tissue lies flat on the retinal surface under the internal limiting membrane, but induced changes in the vitreous gel cause the gel to collapse and detach from the retina. If the new vessels have penetrated the internal limiting membrane they are dragged forwards with it and their adhesion to its surface acts as a scaffold for their further proliferation on the posterior hyaloid surface. The

neovascular tissue proliferates on the posterior hyaloid face but does not penetrate the vitreous gel, possibly because the gel contains a neovascular inhibitory factor. In common with neovascularization elsewhere in the eye, these vessels have fenestrated endothelial cell junctions which accounts for their tendency to leak, and minor trauma causes them to tear and bleed clouding the ocular media. Subsequent formation of fibrous tissue leads to traction bands forming on the retina and between the retina and the posterior vitreous face, eventually causing contraction and detachment of the retina. This combination of neovascularization and fibrosis is known as retinitis proliferans.

Although proliferative diabetic retinopathy may eventually burn out in a minority of cases leaving inactive fibrosis and scar tissue, untreated proliferative retinopathy carries a very poor visual prognosis in the majority of cases; about 70-80% of patients with optic disc neovascularization progress to no perception of light within 5 years because of vitreous haemorrhage and traction retinal detachment. Peripheral neovascularization carries a rather better prognosis but both types are a firm indication for treatment by panretinal photocoagulation.

Fig. 15.15 Marked cotton wool spot formation, areas of capillary closure or beading of retinal veins are signs of pronounced retinal hypoxia which indicates a significant risk of progression to neovascularization. This is sometimes known as 'pre-proliferative retinopathy'. Whilst these patients do not require treatment at this stage this is a useful description which indicates that the patient requires close supervision.

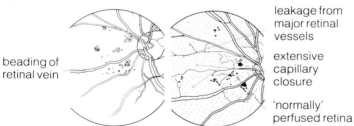

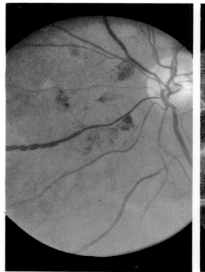

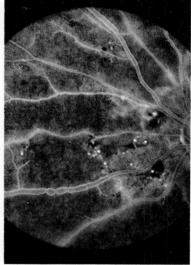

Fig. 15.16 This patient shows very early peripheral retinal neovascularization. Superficially the retinopathy does not look too severe but beading of the retinal veins can be seen in the posterior pole. Fluorescein angiography shows gross areas of capillary closure; the colour photograph can be used to identify hyperfluorescent areas which correspond to new vessels just visible as a fine thready network.

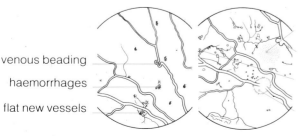

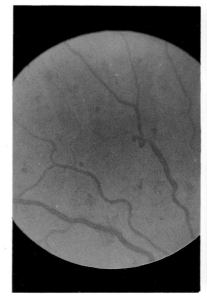

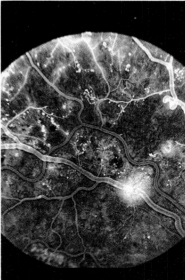

Fig. 15.17 Another patient shows peripheral neovascular tissue with accompanying fibrosis producing a white appearance. Fluorescein angiography shows gross leakage from this tissue which lies at the junction of normal retina and the area of marked capillary closure.

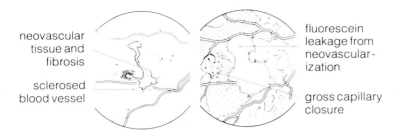

neovascular tissue and fibrosis

sclerosed blood vessel

fluorescein leakage from neovascular- ization

gross capillary closure

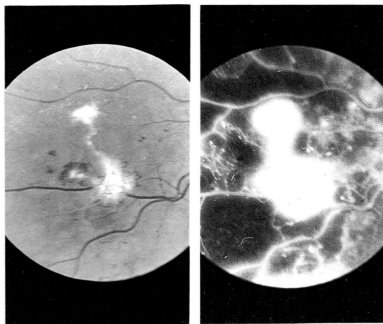

Fig. 15.18 Neovascularization on the optic disc carries a more sinister visual prognosis than peripheral new vessel formation. It develops initially with flat dilated capillaries that give the disc the appearance of having more prominent and more numerous capillaries than are normally seen. Fluorescein angiography shows a dilated and coarse capillary network on the optic disc and surrounding retina with areas of capillary closure. The neovascular tissue fills early and shows gross leakage of fluorescein in the later stages of the angiogram.

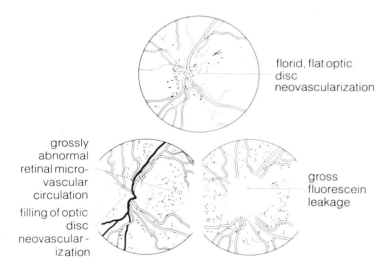

florid, flat optic disc neovascularization

grossly abnormal retinal micro- vascular circulation

filling of optic disc neovascular- ization

gross fluorescein leakage

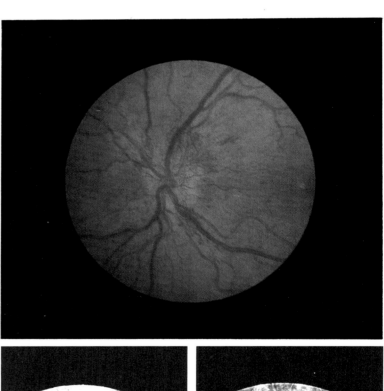

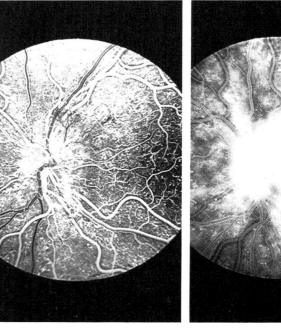

Fig. 15.19 This optic disc shows a more prominent neovascular fan which has been pulled forwards by the detached vitreous gel; the vessels can be seen multiplying on the retrohyaloid face.

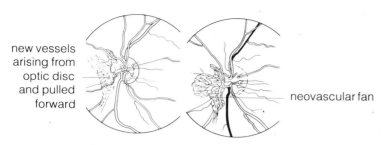

new vessels arising from optic disc and pulled forward

neovascular fan

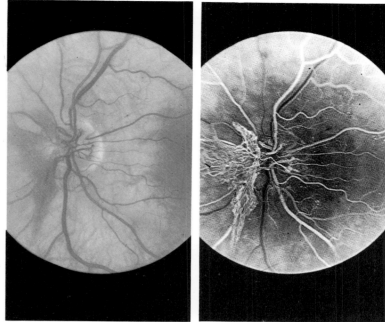

Fig. 15.20 Vitreous haemorrhage is an important complication of neovascularization both on the optic disc and in the peripheral retina. If gross enough it will cause acute loss of vision and lead to secondary fibrotic changes. This eye shows florid neovascularization on the disc and adjacent retina with subretinal haemorrhage. The whitish grey area overlying the haemorrhage is early fibrosis.

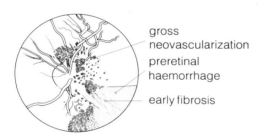

gross neovascularization

preretinal haemorrhage

early fibrosis

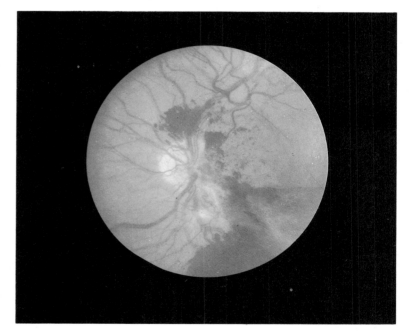

Fig. 15.21 The combination of neovascularization and fibrous traction of the retina is known as retinitis proliferans. This patient shows the early stages with marked neovascularization on the optic disc and inferior temporal arcade. (Vitreo-retinal adhesions along the temporal vascular arcades are very common in diabetes, see Chapter 12). Localised fibrotic changes have produced traction on the retina and distortion of the macula. The natural history would be further fibrotic tissue formation and traction progressing to localised or general traction detachment of the retina.

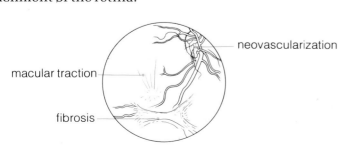

neovascularization

macular traction

fibrosis

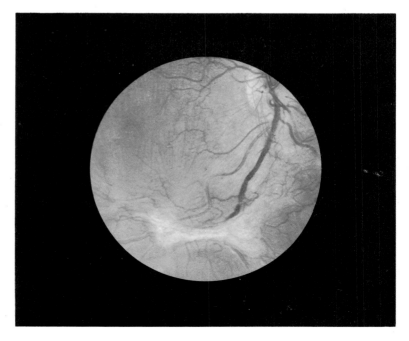

Fig. 15.22 In advanced cases vision is lost as a result of a combination of vitreous haemorrhage and traction detachment. In a few patients, the retinopathy seems to 'burn out' before this final stage. This is probably due to the progression from retinal hypoxia to ischaemia which removes the biochemical stimulus to further proliferation and leaves inactive fibrotic tissue in the area of retinitis proliferans with a varying degree of distortion of the retinal architecture. This patient was left with visual acuities of hand movements and 6/18.

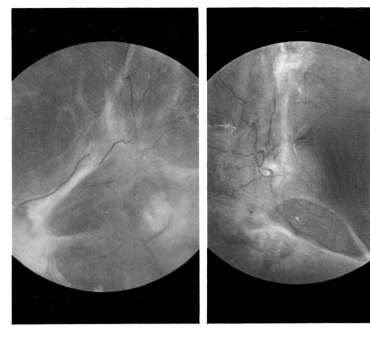

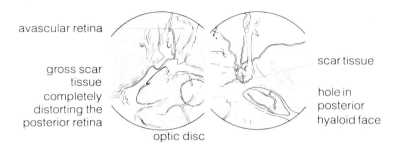

avascular retina

gross scar tissue completely distorting the posterior retina

optic disc

scar tissue

hole in posterior hyaloid face

Treatment of Diabetic Retinopathy

Clinical trials have shown that photocoagulation improves the visual prognosis of neovascular diabetic retinopathy and prevents deterioration of visual acuity in exudative maculopathies. It does not ameliorate visual loss due to macular oedema or ischaemia. While various types of light source can be used, the argon laser offers the most precise and convenient system for both the surgeon and patient. The green light energy is absorbed by both the retinal pigment epithelium and haemoglobin to produce a thermal injury. Adjustment to the laser allows the burn size, intensity and duration of the light burst to be varied as necessary.

Exudative maculopathy can be controlled and its progression halted by photocoagulating the microaneurysms and vascular malformations at the centre of the circinate rings which are responsible for the leakage of plasma and lipid into the retina. The burns should be of low intensity so that the energy is taken up by blood, retinal pigment epithelium and photoreceptors; if the overlying nerve fibre layer is destroyed it results in a small arcuate field defect. The retinal exudates may take several weeks or months to absorb after treatment, depending on their density. In early exudative maculopathies visual

acuity may be improved but in more advanced cases, even though the exudates absorb satisfactorily, the retinal damage is permanent. Clinical trials indicate that to get a good visual outcome the retinopathy must be treated before the visual acuity has fallen below 6/9–6/12. The results of treatment of diabetic cystoid macular oedema or ischaemia maculopathy are poor and vision is generally not improved by photocoagulation.

While maculopathy is treated by focal photocoagulation to the specific vascular abnormalities that create the leakage, control of neovascularization relies on the technique of panretinal photocoagulation and the success of this type of therapy is further evidence for the hypothesis of a neovascular substance produced by the hypoxic retina.

Scattered photocoagulation burns to the retina, outside the temporal vascular arcades, reduce the metabolic requirements of the retina by destroying the retinal pigment epithelium and photoreceptors of the outer retina and reducing retinal thickness, possibly allowing the choroid to supply more of the inner retina. Hypoxic retina is also destroyed, potentially reducing the formation of the vasoactive factor.

Fig. 15.23 The histology of a laser burn shows that there is atrophy of the retinal pigment epithelium and photoreceptors in the area of the burn. The energy is taken up in the retinal pigment epithelium and, providing the amount of energy is restricted, the thermal injury is localized and the inner nerve fibre layer spared. Damage to this layer would result in small arcuate field defects.

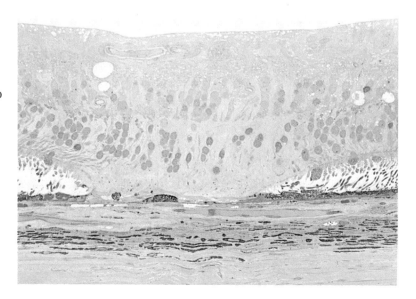

Fig. 15.24 The aim of treatment in exudative maculopathy is to obliterate the leaking microvascular abnormalities in the center of the circinate exudates. These can usually be identified clinically without the need for routine fluorescein angiography. It may be necessary to repeat treatment on several successive occasions; absorption of hard exudates over a period of weeks is a sign of successful treatment.

Fig. 15.25 The photograph shows the fundus appearances pre- and post- laser photocoagulation; some weeks after treatment the exudates have completely absorbed. Faint scars in the retinal pigment epithelium can be seen in the areas of focal photocoagulation.

Fig. 15.26 This patient shows a less gross example of exudative maculopathy. Prior to treatment, early deposition of hard exudate can be seen in the macular area. Eight weeks after treatment the exudate is in the process of being absorbed, and one month later it has disappeared and the scars in the retinal pigment epithelium from the photocoagulation can be seen. Such treatment does not produce any visual impairment so long as the burns are outside the foveal avascular zone and of sufficiently low intensity to protect the overlying retinal nerve fibres.

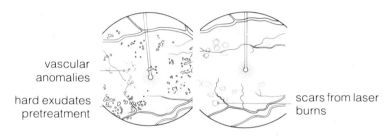

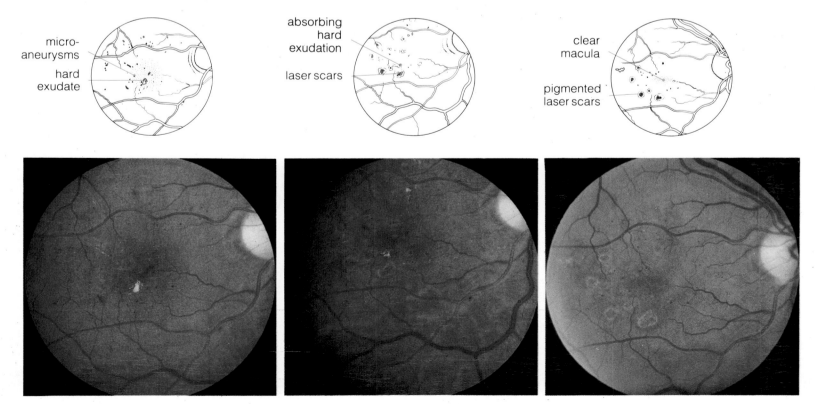

Fig. 15.27 Proliferative retinopathy requires treatment by panretinal photocoagulation. By sparing the macula area, panretinal photocoagulation should not affect visual acuity. 1000 to 2000 burns are usually given to the equatorial retina, normally in one or two treatments, to produce regression of optic disc neovascularization. A few patients require much more treatment and all patients need to be followed up carefully with further treatment if neovascularization reappears. Following panretinal photocoagulation, visual disability is surprisingly slight. Preservation of the inner nerve fibre layer avoids the production of arcuate field loss and patients normally only notice marginal constriction of their visual field and sometimes a reduction in their visual performance in the dark. A similar strategy is used to ablate peripheral retina in the treatment of rubeosis iridis following central retinal vein occlusion (see Chapter 14).

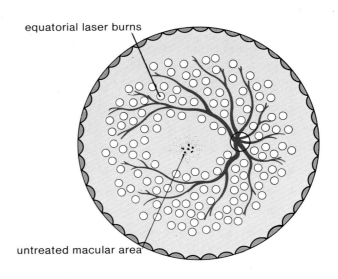

equatorial laser burns

untreated macular area

Fig. 15.28 In practice, the burns must be of sufficient intensity to produce a soft white reaction in the retinal pigment epithelium; a dense white reaction indicates damage to the inner retina. Within a few days the burns become pigmented atrophic scars.

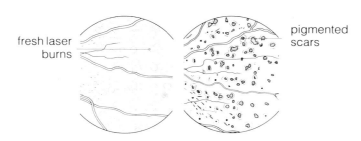

fresh laser burns

pigmented scars

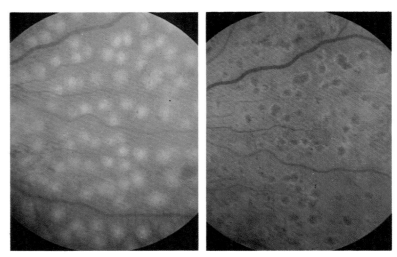

Fig. 15.29 The efficiency of panretinal photocoagulation is demonstrated by this patient who participated in a controlled trial of the effects of panretinal photocoagulation in the early 1970's. At the start of the trial these photographs show normal optic discs, some background retinopathy and normal fluorescein angiograms of the optic discs.

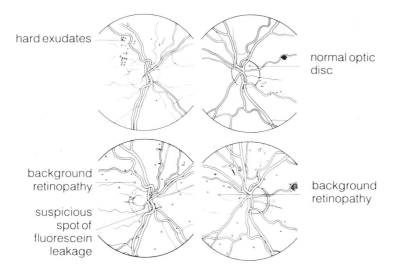

hard exudates

normal optic disc

background retinopathy

background retinopathy

suspicious spot of fluorescein leakage

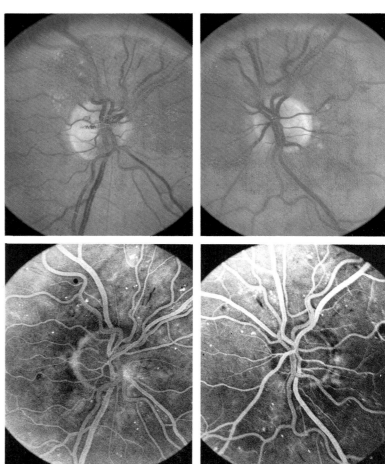

Fig. 15.30 Nine months later, early neovascularization is seen on each optic disc, confirmed by the presence of leakage of the fluorescein angiogram. With informed consent, the right eye was treated with xenon arc photocoagulation, and the left remained untreated as a 'control' eye.

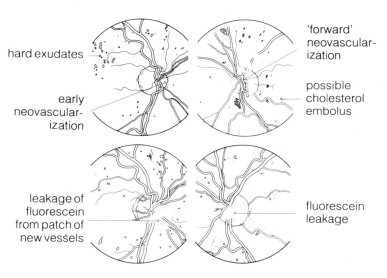

hard exudates

early neovascularization

leakage of fluorescein from patch of new vessels

'forward' neovascularization

possible cholesterol embolus

fluorescein leakage

Fig. 15.31 Fifteen months after panretinal photocoagulation to the right eye, the new vessels on the optic disc have regressed, confirmed by fluorescein angiography and marked chorioretinal scars can be seen from the photocoagulation. Visual acuity remained normal in this eye, with slight loss of visual field and some mild night blindness. In contrast the left has deteriorated to perception of light; there is a marked neovascular membrane arising from the optic disc with total traction retinal detachment. This eye has a substantial risk of developing rubiotic glaucoma.

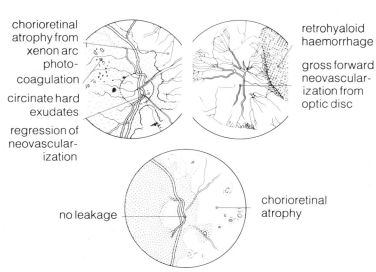

chorioretinal atrophy from xenon arc photocoagulation

circinate hard exudates

regression of neovascularization

retrohyaloid haemorrhage

gross forward neovascularization from optic disc

no leakage

chorioretinal atrophy

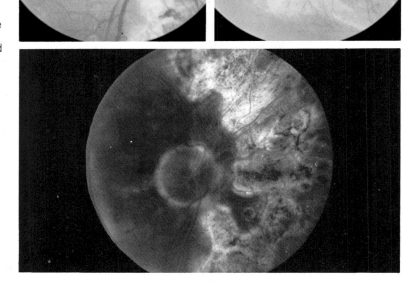

SICKLE CELL RETINOPATHY

A retinopathy which predominantly affects the peripheral retina is a feature of the sickle cell diseases (HbSS, HbSC, sickle thalassaemia). Retinal changes are most commonly seen with HbSC disease, probably because these patients are less anaemic and consequently have a higher blood viscosity than that seen in the other diseases and may, therefore, have a greater tendency to sickling with the formation of thrombotic arteriolar occlusions which appear to be the basic pathological lesion. These occur in the equatorial retina, possibly as a result of the combination of decreasing blood vessel diameter and decreasing pO2 levels. Retinal haemorrhages and capillary closure follow the occlusions, sometimes with subsequent peripheral neovascularization. Vitreous haemorrhage and traction retinal detachment are comparatively uncommon, especially when expressed as a percentage of the total number of affected patients.

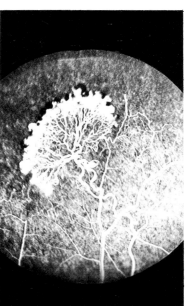

Fig. 15.32 Vascular occlusions can produce retinal haemorrhages (salmon patches) which are red or yellowish and about one disc in diameter. They are seen in the equatorial retina adjacent to the occluded arteriole and are a sign of recent infarction. Black sunbursts are localised disturbances of the pigment epithelium thought to be associated with underlying infarction of choriocapillaries from sickling.

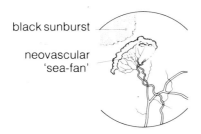

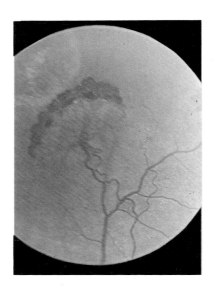
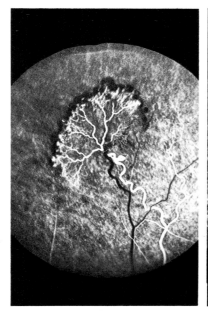

Fig. 15.33 Fluorescein angiography in the same patient demonstrates peripheral capillary closure, leakage from the neovascular frond and the vascular shunt vessels. If necessary, the peripheral hypoxic retina can be treated with photocoagulation, but while this destroys neovascular tissue it can lead to chorio-retinal anastomoses and fresh neovascularization appearing in the previously normal retina making the disease move centripetally. Present clinical trials suggest that photocoagulation does not improve the natural history of the disease.

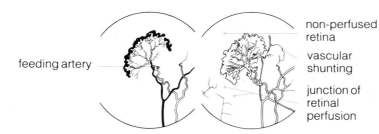

Fig. 15.34 Another example shows peripheral neovascular fronds at the junction of normal retina with peripheral capillary closure. Note the abnormal arterio-venous shunting between the major peripheral blood vessels and the sclerosed blood vessel in the periphery.

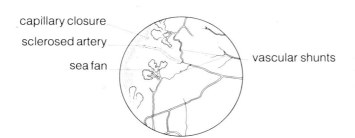

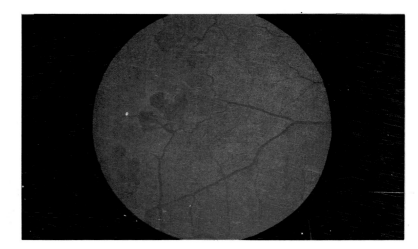

SYSTEMIC LUPUS ERYTHEMATOSIS (SLE)

Retinopathy from SLE is a combination of microvascular ischaemia from the disease itself, with the added effects of secondary systemic hypertension and anaemia. The predominant features are cotton wool spots in the absence of hypertensive vascular changes; arteriolar occlusions may occur on rare occasions. Anaemic patients tend to have retinal haemorrhages and sometimes Roth spots as well. Anterior or posterior uveitis is not a feature.

Fig. 15.35   A cotton wool spot, retinal haemorrhage and arterio-venous crossing changes are seen in a 20-year-old woman with severe SLE.

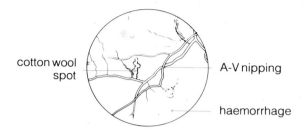

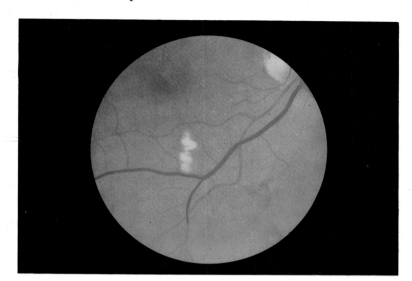

Fig. 15.36   This negro patient with severe SLE shows the more uncommon sign of arteriolar occlusion. Such patients usually have very high levels of circulating immune complexes and it is possible that deposition of these may cause the obstruction.

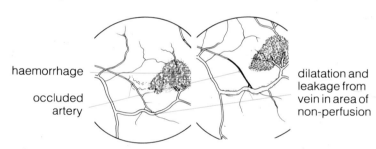

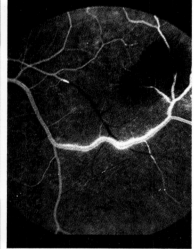

Fig. 15.37   Ocular pathology from a patient with similar retinal signs to those seen in Fig. 15.36 shows a blocked retinal arteriole, with little inflammatory reaction, and hypertrophic choroidal vessels from systemic hypertension. In the choroid there is a marked lymphocytic inflammatory infiltrate.

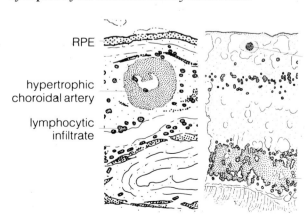

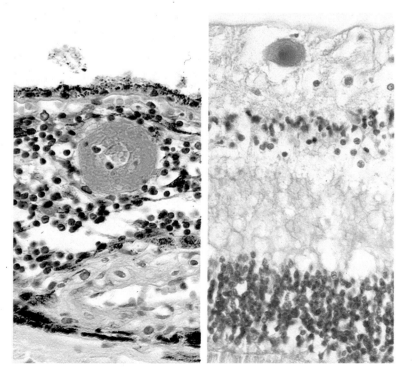

15.15

RETINAL VASCULAR ANOMALIES

There are a number of retinal vascular abnormalities, thought to be developmental in origin, which can affect any component of the retinal vascular system. Occasionally they are associated with intracranial angiomas (Wyburn-Mason syndrome) or cutaneous angiomas (Klippel-Trenaunay-Weber syndrome) and some produce visual loss from vascular leakage and accumulation of hard exudate. Vitreous haemorrhage is rare.

Racemose Malformations

Fig. 15.38 Small localised vascular abnormalities may be discovered as an incidental finding on routine examination. This patient has a small arteriovenous malformation adjacent to the optic disc.

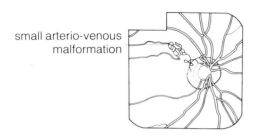

small arterio-venous malformation

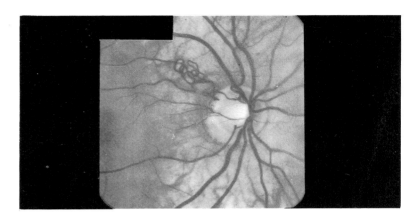

Fig. 15.39 Large arteriovenous malformations have a dramatic fundal appearance. They are normally totally static but visual acuity will be affected if the macula is involved, as is the case in this patient. Angiomas such as these may occasionally be associated with an intracranial angioma and this rare combination is known as the Wyburn-Mason syndrome.

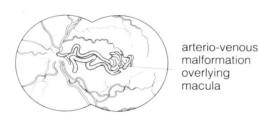

arterio-venous malformation overlying macula

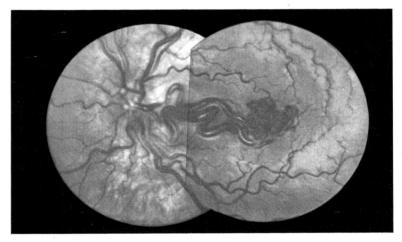

Cavernous Hemangioma

Fig. 15.40 Cavernous hemangioma of the retina is a rare benign lesion. It consists of multiple aneurysmal dilatations localised along a retinal vessel with a fibrous matrix. These lesions do not progress or generally cause symptoms and are not associated with any other vascular disease. Well documented cases have been shown to remain unchanged over many years. The fluorescein angiogram shows that the individual aneurysms fill with dye in the late venous phase, often with a fluid level from the stagnant circulation (fluorescein on top of the stagnant red blood cells), but with no vascular leakage.

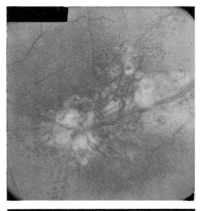

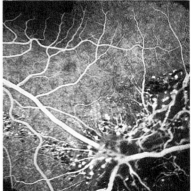

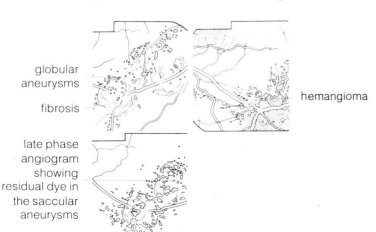

globular aneurysms

fibrosis

hemangioma

late phase angiogram showing residual dye in the saccular aneurysms

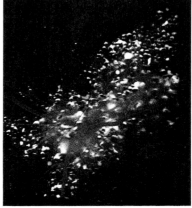

Von Hippel-Lindau Disease

The von Hippel-Lindau syndrome is a dominantly inherited disease with variable penetrance in which characteristic retinal angiomas are associated with haemangioblastomas of the cerebellum and occasionally with renal anomalies and polycythaemia. These angiomas have a progressive course of enlargement, leakage or rupture to produce lipid exudation or vitreous haemorrhage. In view of the complications, these angiomas should be treated with photocoagulation or cryotherapy and the patient must be constantly observed as, with time, new lesions can develop in the eye. CT scanning is indicated to detect intracranial lesions but cerebral angiography is only performed when surgery might be indicated. Genetic counselling of affected families is important.

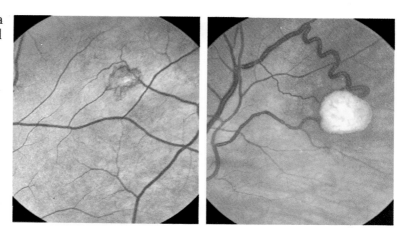

Fig. 15.41 Early tumours are seen in the peripheral retina as red or yellowish bulbous vascular lesions with enlarged feeder vessels.

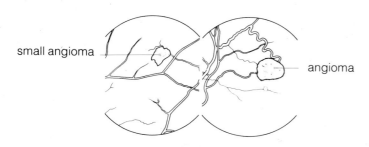

small angioma — angioma

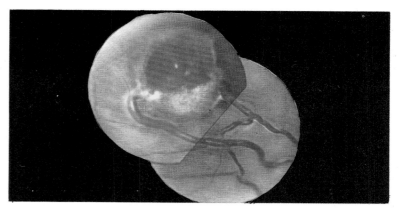

Fig. 15.42 These tumours can eventually reach quite dramatic proportions.

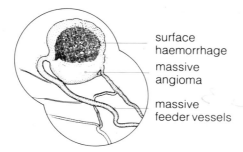

surface haemorrhage
massive angioma
massive feeder vessels

Fig. 15.43 Fluorescein angiography demonstrates the feeder vessels and the large leaking angioma. A shallow retinal serous detachment may occur around the tumour and there are often associated capillary anomalies.

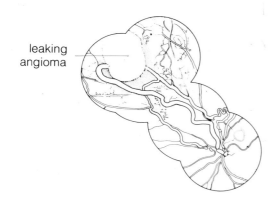

leaking angioma

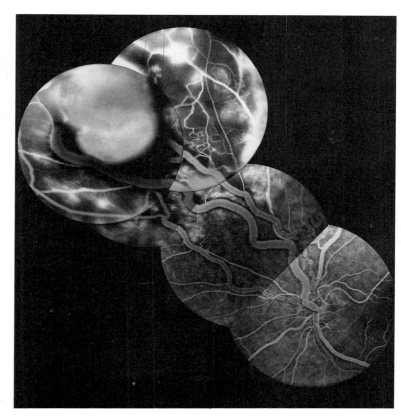

15.17

Leber's Miliary Aneurysms and Coats' Disease

Many authors consider Coats' disease, Leber's miliary aneurysms and paramacular telangiectasia to be part of the same disease spectrum, appearing in different age ranges.

Coats' disease usually presents in young males at the end of the first decade as a uniocular disease in which saccular aneurysmal malformations produce massive subretinal exudation and visual loss. Similar vascular lesions are described as Leber's miliary aneurysms when they present in young adults, usually with less telangiectasia, retinal exudation and destruction. Finally paramacular telangiectasia presents as macular oedema or exudate in middle age. Careful examination of the retinal periphery of these patients may show vascular anomalies.

Fig. 15.44 Massive subretinal lipid exudate and serous retinal detachment in a young boy with Coats' disease can simulate a retinoblastoma. Apart from the difference in age of presentation, the differential diagnosis is aided by demonstrating the vascular anomalies and the yellowish green lipid exudate in contrast to the white or pink fleshy appearance of retinoblastoma.

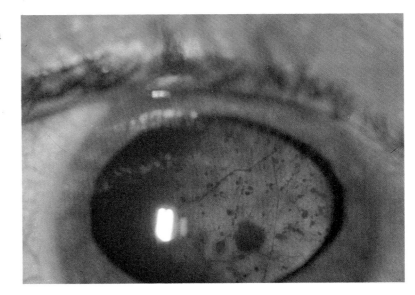

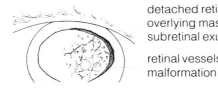

detached retina overlying massive subretinal exudation

retinal vessels and malformation

Fig. 15.45 Massive exudate in the subretinal space extending into the macula is seen in the right eye of a 9-year-old boy. Overlying vascular abnormalities are seen in the retina. It is important to examine the peripheral retina carefully for vascular malformation in any case of undiagnosed macular exudation.

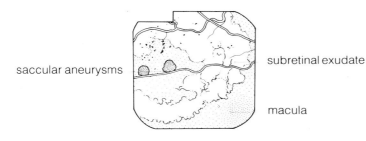

saccular aneurysms

subretinal exudate

macula

Fig. 15.46 Fluorescein angiography demonstrates the saccular vascular dilatations accompanied by coarseness and closure of the capillary bed. Massive leakage of dye occurs in the late phases. Although capillary closure occurs, retinal neovascularization is not seen, in contrast to the usual situation with other retinal vascular disease.

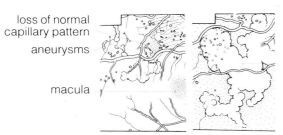

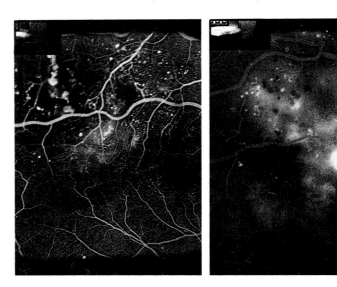

loss of normal capillary pattern

aneurysms

macula

massive leakage of dye

Fig. 15.47   Peripheral vascular abnormalities in a slightly older patient who presented with visual loss from macular exudation, are compatible with Leber's miliary aneurysms.

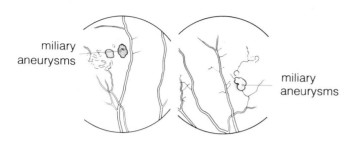

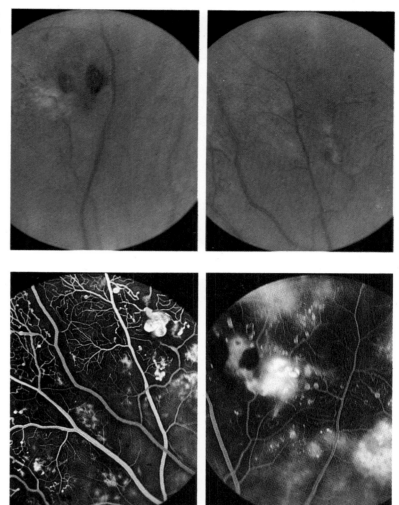

Fig. 15.48   Fluorescein angiography demonstrates the typical changes. Following destruction of the peripheral vascular changes by cryotherapy, the macular exudate absorbed over several months and vision improved.

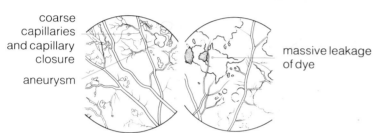

Fig. 15.49   Macular oedema and serous retinal detachment is seen in a middle aged patient who presented with visual blurring in the right eye.

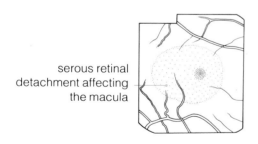

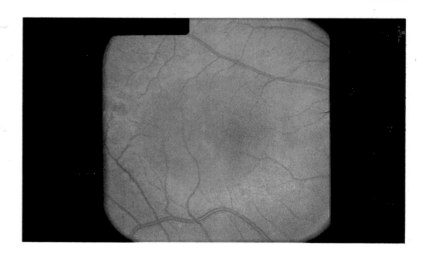

Fig. 15.50   Fluorescein angiography, in the early phases, demonstrates dilated telangiectatic capillaries adjacent to the macula which leak progressively as the angiogram progresses. There were no peripheral retinal lesions but it is important that these are searched for carefully. Such patients can be helped by photocoagulation to the abnormal vascular tissue.

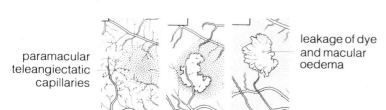

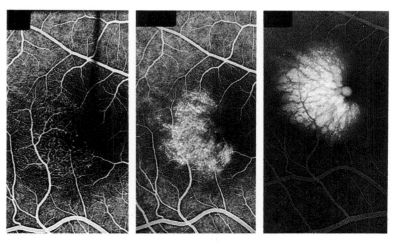

15.19

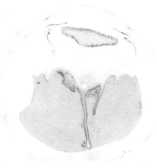
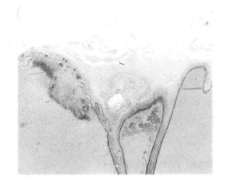

Fig. 15.51   Coat's Disease. In the picture on the left, there is a funnel-shaped detachment of the retina associated with serous subretinal exudation from telangiectatic vessels in the retina. Higher magnification (right) shows serohaemorrhagic exudation from a group of abnormally dilated blood vessels in the retina.

RETINOBLASTOMA

After choroidal malignant melanoma or metastasis, retinoblastoma is the most frequent ocular malignancy and, although rare, is one of the most common malignancies of childhood, (together with leukaemias and neuroblastoma). About 1% of childhood deaths from cancer are due to retinoblastoma.

The tumour occurs either as a dominantly inherited condition with poor penetrance or sporadically or as a new genetic mutation. One or both eyes can be affected. In about 35% of patients both eyes are affected and bilateral involvement is always due to genetically inherited disease. Uniocular cases may be either sporadic (in which case there is no risk to siblings or the next generation), a new genetic mutation in which case the patient's future children may be affected, or as unilateral disease in an affected family. The poor penetrance of the gene makes it mandatory to examine parents and siblings of any patient and to give the patient and family genetic counselling. In the future, it is likely that recombinant DNA technology will be used to identify a specific genetic defect, which will simplify counselling. The incidence of retinoblastoma is given as 1:15,000 to 50,000 live births, but with increasing survival of patients retinoblastoma genes are becoming more common in the general population. It is one of the few tumours that occasionally undergo spontaneous regression and, with treatment and the increasing long term survival of patients, a high incidence of second primary tumours such as osteogenic sarcoma is being seen in the same patients. Genetically determined retinoblastoma appears to be related to deletion on chromosome 13 and conditions such as trisomy 13 (Patou's Syndrome) also have retinal dysplasia as part of their manifestation. Retinoblastoma can be present at birth but most tumours are diagnosed at about 18 months of age and 90% have presented by three years of age. Presentation with increasing age gets increasingly uncommon and after two years of age is rare. Patients present with leucocoria, squint, visual loss and less commonly with hypopyon, hyphema, uveitis, buphthalmos or metastases.

Fig. 15.52   Retinoblastoma must be differentiated from the other common causes of a white pupillary reflex in childhood.

Common Causes Of Leucocoria

Congenital cataract

Persistant hyperplasic primary vitreous

Retrolental fibroplasia

Tumours – retinoblastoma
            medulloblastoma (diktyoma)

Retinal dysplasia e.g. Norrie's disease

Coats' disease

Large chorioretinal coloboma

Long-standing retinal detachment

Intraocular inflammation
e.g. *Toxocara*, metastatic endophthalmitis

Fig. 15.53   Genetic counselling is mandatory and requires a thorough examination of both parents and all siblings. The poor penetrance of dominantly inherited disease means that a firm answer cannot be given as to whether or not an isolated unilateral case is of sporadic or genetic origin. The parents can be given the statistical risk of further siblings being affected, an affected child transmitting the gene to the next generation or the chances of an unaffected sibling being an asymptomatic carrier.

GENETIC COUNSELLING IN RETINOBLASTOMA

Type of Case	% Risk			
	Bilateral Familial	Unilateral Familial	Bilateral Sporadic	Unilateral Sporadic
Further siblings having affected eyes	40	40	5.7	0.6
Unaffected siblings being carriers	10	10	very low	very low
Unaffected carriers, children being affected	7	7	very low	very low
Affected patients, children being affected	40	40	40	8

Fig. 15.54 Bilateral leucocoria is seen in a one-year-old child with gross ocular involvement. A convergent squint is also present.

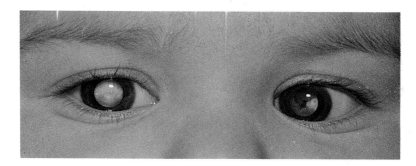

Fig. 15.55. In common with any other blinding disease of childhood, affected children poke and rub their eyes, probably to get some visual sensation from the production of phosphenes by manual stimulation.

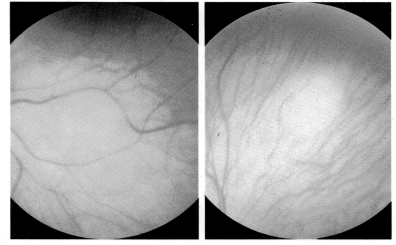

Fig. 15.56 Small retinoblastomas appear as raised white or pink lesions, best identified with the indirect ophthalmoscope. The tumour is multifocal and fresh tumours may develop during follow-up. These early, slightly raised lesions obscure the background pattern of the choroid.

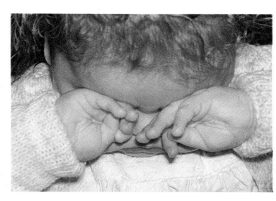

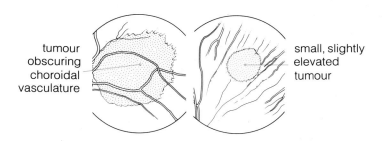

tumour obscuring choroidal vasculature

small, slightly elevated tumour

Fig. 15.57 A larger lesion can be seen bursting into the vitreous gel (left). Growth into the gel is known as endophytic tumour whereas subretinal spread is known as exophytic tumour; rarely, tumours may spread diffusely in the retina. Calcification is common occurring in areas of necrosis within the tumour and this is a helpful diagnostic sign which can be confirmed by ultrasonograpy or CT scanning. Raised levels of lactic dehydrogenase occur in the aqueous humour and help to make a diagnosis; whilst this can be easily measured by paracentesis the procedure carries a risk of spreading the tumour outside the eye. This tumour (right) shows seeding into the vitreous gel, a common finding with endophytic tumours.

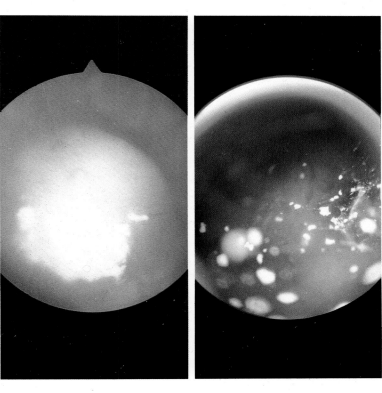

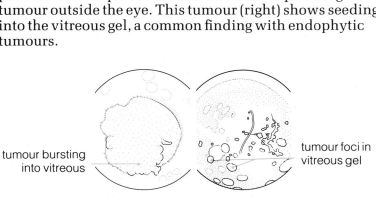

tumour bursting into vitreous

tumour foci in vitreous gel

15.21

Pathology and Treatment

The tumour is derived from malignant change in the photoreceptors. At a cellular level, the degree of differentiation ranges from anaplasia to the formation of rosette-shaped structures which are a primitive attempt at differentiation into photoreceptors. Necrosis and calcification are common findings. Extraocular extension occurs by infiltration of either the choroid or the optic nerve, and it is essential at enucleation to remove as much optic nerve as is feasible. Patients are best managed by those with experience of the disease. Extraocular spread systemically, or to the orbit or brain, carries a very poor prognosis. Small intraocular tumours can be treated conservatively to preserve vision by localised photocoagulation, cryotherapy or radiotheraphy but large tumours or those with optic nerve involvement require enucleation. All patients need prolonged follow-up to detect new lesions. Parents of affected children should be examined for signs of asymptomatic regressed disease as evidence of this helps to establish a genetically inherited tumour and all siblings of any affected child must be examined periodically for asymptomatic lesions.

Fig. 15.58 Retinoblastoma. Posterior part of the globe showing complete filling of the vitreal cavity by tumour with extension into the optic nerve.

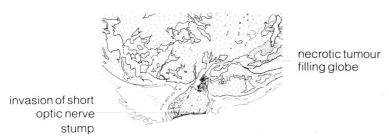

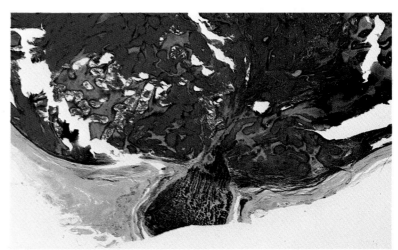

invasion of short optic nerve stump

necrotic tumour filling globe

Fig. 15.59 This tumour consists of small cells with round, hyperchromatic nuclei arranged in well-developed Flexner-Wintersteiner rosettes which are interpreted as a primitive attempt at photoreceptor differentiation.

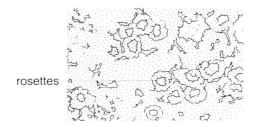

rosettes

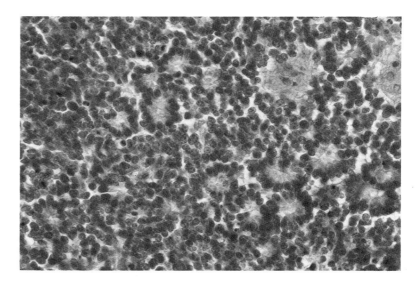

Fig. 15.60 In cross section the optic nerve shows invasion by tumour cells adjacent to the central blood vessels.

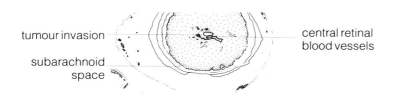

tumour invasion

central retinal blood vessels

subarachnoid space

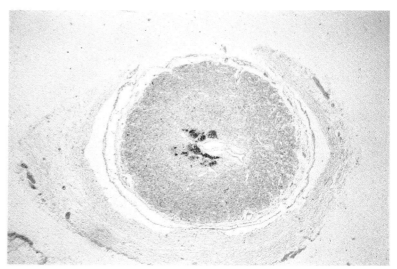

16. The Retina: Macular Diseases and Retinal Dystrophies

T. J. ffytche
D. J. Spalton
J. S. Shilling

INTRODUCTION

This volume deals with the commoner types of degeneration and inherited dystrophies of the macula and retina. Proper functioning of the macula is essential for normal visual acuity and many patients with retinal disease only present when the macula is involved and central vision is disturbed. Central distortion of the visual image (metamorphopsia) or minification (micropsia) are pathognomonic for macular disease. Closer questioning may reveal symptoms of photophobia, glare or dazzle, poor colour perception and a central or paracentral scotoma. Clinically, it is useful in the differential diagnosis and classification of macular lesions to localise the primary defect to the correct anatomical layer; it may be situated in the choriocapillaris, Bruch's membrane, the retinal pigment epithelial cell/photoreceptor complex or the neuroretina. This is not always easy as dystrophies and degenerations of the outer retina produce parallel changes in the photoreceptors, the retinal pigment epithelium and choriocapillaris and it is difficult in the majority of these diseases to localise precisely where the initial defect has occurred, although examination and investigation can provide good circumstantial evidence.

Investigation of macular disease requires careful refraction and assessment of acuity for distance and near vision. Stereoscopic examination of the macula through a dilated pupil using a Hruby or fundus lens is essential, and fundus photography with fluorescein angiography is of enormous value in the diagnosis and documentation of the lesion. Macular lesions are small and although they produce a scotoma in the visual field this can be difficult to demonstrate by standard methods of perimetry; it is most easily shown by using the Amsler grid chart, static perimetry or a Bjerrum screen with a red target.

Occasionally, the differentiation of visual loss from macula or optic nerve disease can be difficult as both produce poor acuity, colour loss and a central scotoma. Retinal lesions produce a 'positive' scotoma which the patient notices as a dark and missing area of field whereas 'negative' scotomas (which are a sign of optic nerve or neuro-ophthalmic lesions), are only noticed as field loss: we are not positively aware of the negative scotoma in our visual field from our own optic discs. Another useful and easily performed clinical test is the photostress test. Macular lesions produce a delayed recovery in visual acuity after dazzle with a bright light, whereas visual acuity recovers quickly and normally with optic nerve lesions. Careful colour vision testing can be helpful too, but is time-consuming and not routinely available. Macular disease produces a blue-yellow pattern of colour blindness whereas optic nerve lesions produce a red-green pattern. The use of electrodiagnostic tests in the investigation of retinal disease is expensive and time-consuming and is only indicated for the diagnosis and documentation of inherited retinal disease.

Apart from the use of low visual aids, no treatment is available for the vast majority of retinal dystrophies and degenerations. In the management of the patient, perhaps the most important factor is to be able to give a diagnosis, visual prognosis and genetic and occupational counselling where required. It is unusual for any degenerative macular disease to progress to total blindness and very reassuring for the patient to know this; most patients have a central scotoma with good peripheral vision and can lead independent lives.

MACULAR DEGENERATIONS
Macular Holes

These originate from a variety of causes all of which have a different natural history. Full-thickness macular holes with vitreo-retinal traction are a rare cause of rhegmatogenous retinal detachment, normally occurring in high myopes (see Chapter 12 Vitreous and Vitreo-retinal Disorders). Solar burns are seen as minute central macular pits in the inner retina in patients with a history of sun gazing. Senile macular holes are an ageing change of unknown aetiology; these produce large, partial-thickness macular holes seen predominantly in elderly females as uniocular lesions which virtually never progress to retinal detachment. Cystoid macular oedema from any cause may rupture through the neuroretina to leave a partial-thickness hole.

Fig.16.1. Solar burns from sun gazing are seen in the macula of this drug addict. Such small lesions are usually associated with quite good acuities in the region of 6/18; they are found as a parafoveal pit in the neuroretina. Fluorescein angiography is normal. Occasionally identical lesions are seen in patients without a history of solar exposure.

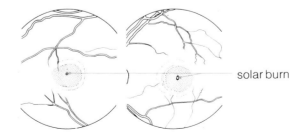

solar burn

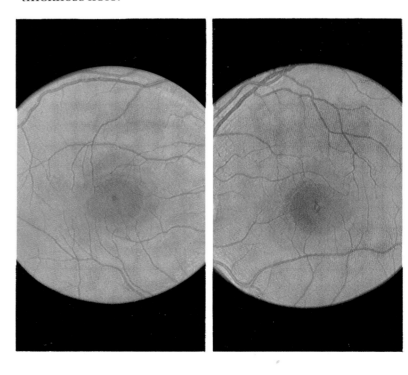

Fig.16.2. Senile macular holes are much larger and reduce the visual acuity to the region of 6/60 to counting fingers. They are most commonly seen in elderly females. Bilateral involvement is unusual (less than 10% of patients). Typically the retina surrounding the hole is thickened with some oedema and small yellowish excrescences can be seen on the surface of the exposed retinal pigment epithelium. Fluorescein angiography will show a mildly hyperfluorescent area corresponding to the diameter of the hole. The lesion does not progress in size or visual disability after its appearance.

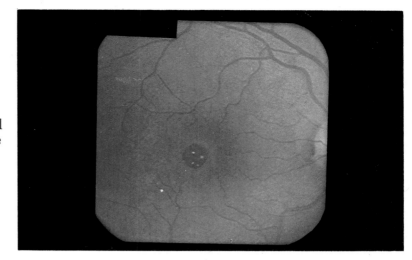

Fig.16.3. The development of the hole is associated with age-related cystoid degeneration of the retina at the macular. Some haemorrhage is also visible.

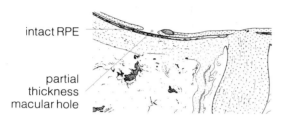

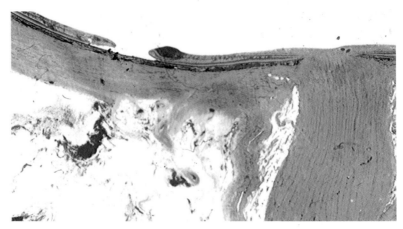

Central Serous Retinopathy

This condition is most commonly seen in patients between the ages of 20 and 40, in a male to female ratio of 8:1. The aetiology is unknown. A serous detachment develops under the macula; it is associated with a focal area of leakage through the retinal pigment epithelium which is usually sited above the horizontal meridian and outside the avascular central zone. The leaking point breaks down the retinal pigment epithelial cell barrier to allow fluid to pass freely from the choriocapillaris and accumulate in the subretinal space between the

photoreceptors and retinal pigment epithelium.

Patients present with micropsia and slightly blurred vision, typically improved by a +ID lens. The photostress test is positive. The condition usually has a self-limiting course of several months but recovery can be accelerated by laser photocoagulation of the leak although the final visual result is unchanged. This treatment prevents further leakage of fluid into the subretinal space and allows the existing fluid to absorb spontaneously.

Fig.16.4. The typical appearance is of a thin translucent blister underlying the macula which can be difficult to see by direct ophthalmoscopy but is more readily seen by using an indirect ophthalmoscope or biomicroscopy. A diagram illustrates the small break in the retinal pigment epithelium and the serous retinal detachment elevating the macula.

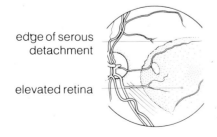

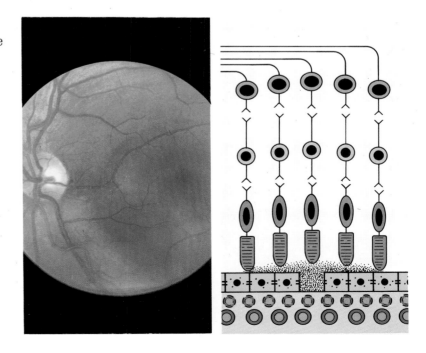

16.3

Fig.16.5. Fluorescein angiography of central serous retinopathy in the early stages of the disease shows a focal defect in the RPE with a typical "smoke-stack" pattern of leakage. The fluorescein leakage appears as a small hyperfluorescent spot at the site of the breech in the retinal pigment epithelium and flows upwards in a column influenced, presumably, by local changes in temperature and viscosity. When the dye reaches the upper margin of the detachment it spreads laterally along the circumference and eventually fills the whole detachment.

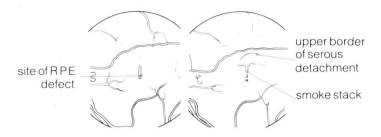

Fig.16.6. In the established case the area of retinal pigment epithelial defect can often be seen as a pale spot. Red-free photography shows the elevated retina more clearly.

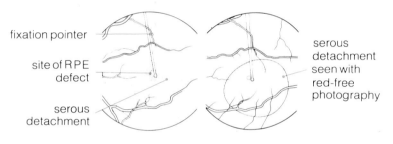

Fig.16.7. With time the leaking point loses its "smoke-stack" appearance and shows as a localised diffusion of dye from the central leaking point, known as an ink blot. This may be due to increasing viscosity of the subretinal fluid limiting diffusion of the dye.

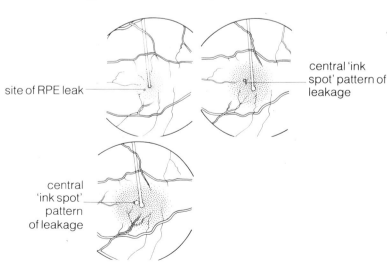

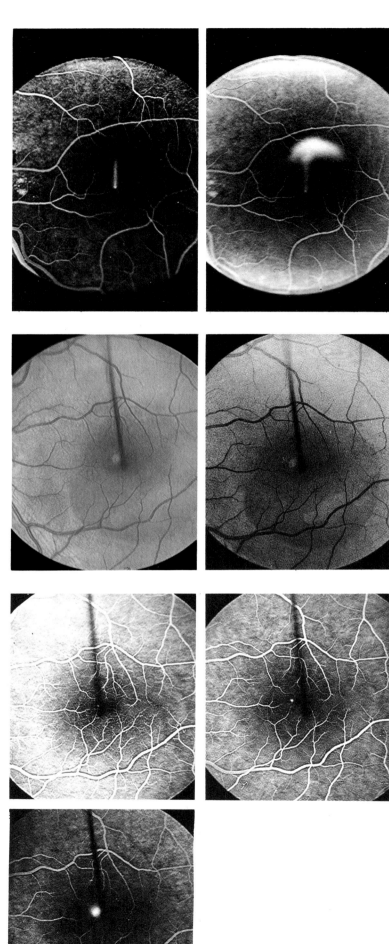

Retinal Pigment Epithelial Detachment

Fluid may collect beneath the retinal pigment epithelium and Bruch's membrane to form a localised pigment epithelial detachment. This condition occurs at the posterior pole in both sexes in either the 20-40 years age group, where it may be a variation of central serous retinopathy, or in the elderly as part of the degenerative macular disease process. A retinal pigment epithelial detachment is seen as a well demarcated localised elevation in the macular area that can be distinguished from central serous retinopathy by its rather more solid and better defined appearance. Pigment epithelial detachments vary in size from ¼ to 2 or 3 disc diameters. Fluorescein angiography confirms the diagnosis by showing a steadily increasing diffuse, even pattern of leakage, without any focal area of hyperfluorescence,

which in this situation might be an indication of associated subretinal neovascularization. Intense, well-defined leakage is seen in the later stages.

In the younger group of patients the visual prognosis is relatively good and no treatment is indicated; the detachment may persist for many years without significant alteration of vision. In elderly patients controlled trials have not shown any marked benefit from laser photocoagulation and, therefore, the condition is best left untreated in all patients. Visual acuity may be suddenly lost in some patients by a tearing of the detached retinal pigment epithelium which may flap back under itself, sometimes with a simultaneous haemorrhage. This pathological event is known as a pigment epithelial tear (or 'rip-off' syndrome).

Fig.16.8. A colour photograph shows the well-circumscribed elevation of the macula which has a more prominent and thicker appearance than that seen with central serous retinopathy. In elderly patients other signs of macular degeneration such as drusen, pigmentation and atrophy are frequently seen. A drawing demonstrates the position of the lesion beneath an intact retinal pigment epithelium.

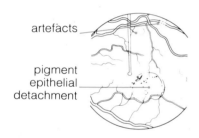

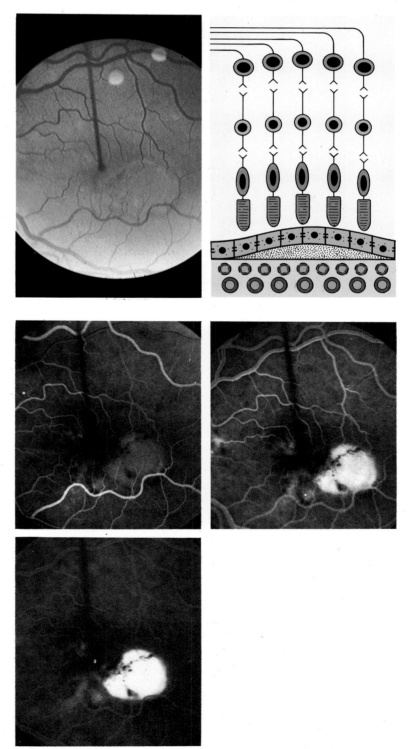

Fig.16.9. The fluorescein angiogram shows the early diffuse leakage which increases in intensity as the run progresses, but remains localised to the area of the lesion. Other degenerative changes in the retinal pigment epithelium are often seen, and in the elderly group some patients may have an underlying neovascular membrane and thus represent part of the spectrum of disciform macular degeneration.

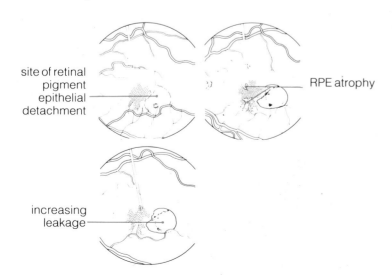

SENILE MACULAR DEGENERATION

This is the commonest cause of legal blindness in the elderly Caucasian population, but is comparatively rare in other races. The primary lesion appears to occur at the level of Bruch's membrane and the retinal pigment epithelium (RPE) where there is a progressive thickening of the former with increasing age. This is associated with localised deposition of lipofuscinoid material, both in the membrane itself and the adjacent RPE cells, which is seen clinically as drusen (see Chapter 13). One can speculate that the progressive, age-related thickening of Bruch's membrane increasingly interferes with the high metabolic activity of the photoreceptor-RPE cell complex leading to the deposition of metabolites and their accumulation as drusen. Subsequent atrophy of the overlying RPE cells, photoreceptors and the underlying choriocapillaris are probably due to secondary metabolic changes.

Drusen usually start to appear in middle age and slowly and progressively increase in number and size over a period of many years. They are associated with increasing macular destruction which is seen clinically as spots of atrophy and pigmentation in the macular area. Eventually, central vision will be lost in a substantial number of patients, although the disease is very haphazard in its extent, severity and progression. Both eyes are usually affected, although the funduscopic appearances and visual symptoms may be very asymmetrical. In the most severely affected patients, acuity falls to levels of counting fingers, with a large central scotoma extending up to 20° from fixation. At this stage further deterioration ceases and peripheral vision remains unaffected so that the patient retains peripheral vision and can lead an independent life.

Established senile macular degeneration follows two main forms: in the "dry" or atrophic type, RPE atrophy predominates, whereas in the "wet" or disciform type, subretinal neovascularization occurs. Apart from laser photocoagulation for certain types of subretinal neovascular membrane, no specific treatment has been shown to be of any use, but supportive help with low visual aids can be very worthwhile.

Atrophic Macular Degeneration

Drusen occur in three types: as small, isolated, discrete yellowish subretinal bodies, usually in the macular area; as confluent yellowish masses at the macula; or as hard glinting, calcific lesions.

Fig.16.10. This patient shows discrete drusen well confined to the macular area with relatively little evidence of RPE atrophy, although this is difficult to assess without fluorescein angiography. At this stage one would expect relatively good visual acuity but the long term visual prognosis is uncertain. Both eyes are normally affected although often asymmetrically. Drusen and senile macula degenerations are rare in negro and heavily pigmented eyes.

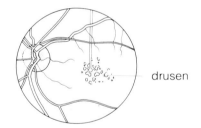

drusen

Fig.16.11. This patient shows large areas of confluent drusen under the macula. Such patients are at considerable risk from developing a disciform lesion and should be advised accordingly. Fluorescein angiography shows the staining of the drusen and window defects from RPE atrophy, but the absence of an intense focal leak shows that there is no evidence of neovascularization of the main confluent mass. The small hyperfluorescent area between the macula and optic disc is probably either a small pigment epithelial detachment or an early neovascular membrane and needs to be watched carefully.

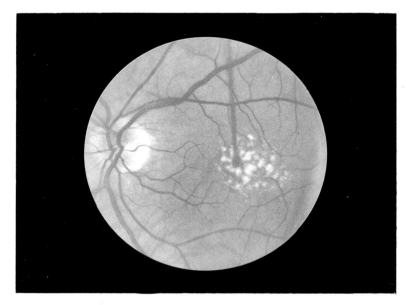

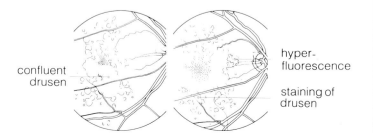

confluent drusen

hyper-fluorescence

staining of drusen

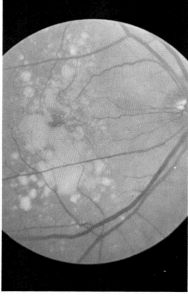

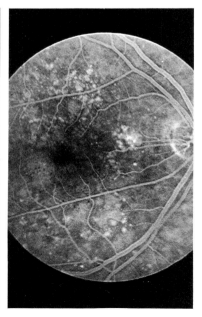

Fig.16.12. Calcification is common in longstanding, rather indolent drusen and gives them a flat, glinting and refractile appearance. In a more gross example with very extensive calcific drusen, widespread paramacular RPE atrophy is apparent showing the prominence of the underlying choroidal vasculature; in spite of these gross changes visual acuity remained at 6/12 as the foveal area was relatively well preserved.

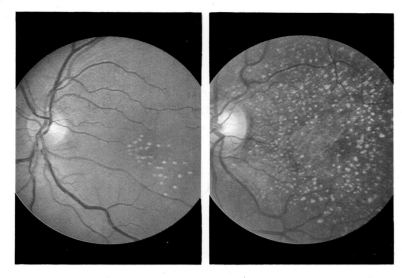

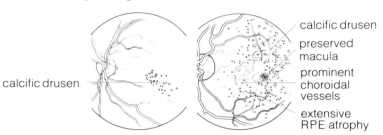

Fig.16.13. Drusen usually occur sporadically, but occasionally, in some families, they appear to be inherited as a dominant trait. Affected members, unlike those with the senile form, may lose central vision in middle age from disciform degeneration. In these patients the drusen are more widespread and are distinguished by their presence in the retina nasal to the optic disc. The arcuate regions along the temporal vessels are also usually affected and the drusen can have the appearance of a fine subretinal meshwork of plaque.

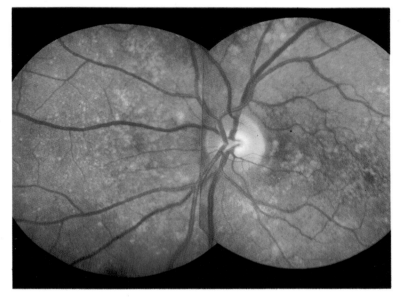

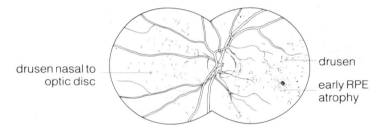

Fig.16.14. These two eyes show established atrophic dry senile macular degeneration. Multiple drusen with pigmentation and atrophy can be seen on the left. The picture on the right shows calcific drusen and extensive RPE atrophy which is only apparent on fluorescein angiography.

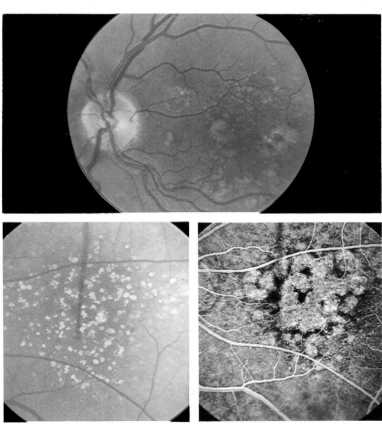

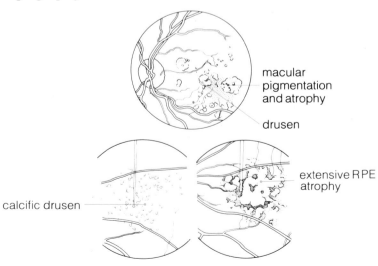

16.7

Fig.16.15. Central areolar choroidal sclerosis is usually seen as a variant of senile macular degeneration but on rare occasions it may occur in younger people as a familial dominant macular dystrophy. There is a sharp demarcation between the normal and abnormal retina, and the condition is characterized by this well-circumscribed atrophy of the RPE, photoreceptors and choriocapillaris in the macula area, revealing the large, underlying choroidal blood vessels. This patient shows advanced atrophic macular changes with loss of central vision. The larger choroidal vessels are easily seen and often appear white although pathological specimens show no evidence of sclerosis.

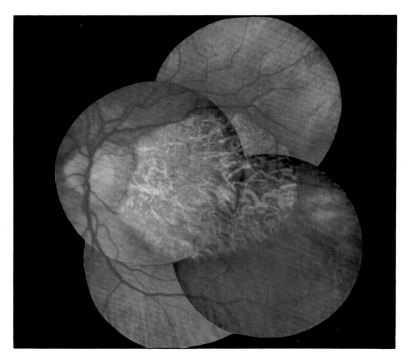

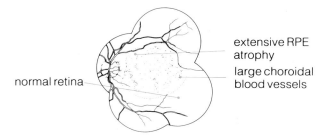

Fig.16.16. The fluorescein angiogram of the same patient shows the large window defect due to loss of the retinal pigment epithelium and choriocapillaris. Note the underlying large choroidal blood vessels, which fill normally, and the sharp junction between normal and abnormal retina.

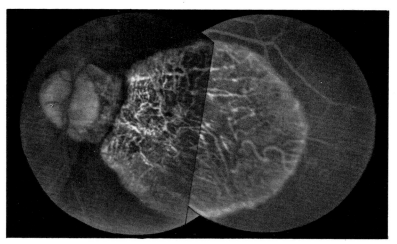

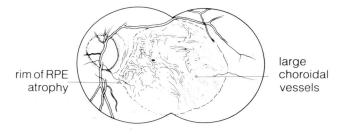

Fig.16.17. Pathology of early senile macular degeneration shows that the retinal pigment epithelium is slightly disorganised where it is separated from Bruch's membrane by a layer of acellular, hyaline material (basal linear deposit) and there are early atrophic changes in the photoreceptor outer segments.

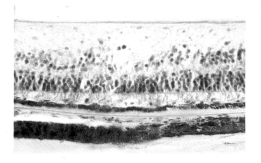

Fig.16.18. Other examples show thickening of Bruch's membrane and irregular RPE hyperplasia (top), and patchy loss of the RPE with some photoreceptor loss and degeneration (centre). In the bottom picture, the RPE is preserved on the left-hand side, but on the right, part of the RPE is absent and the choriocapillaris is lost, similar to the clinical appearances seen in central areolar sclerosis.

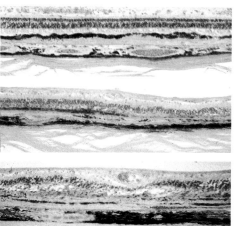

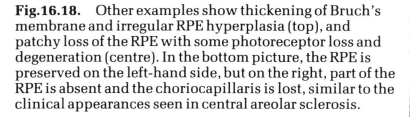

The Disciform Response

Disciform degeneration of the macula is an old name derived from the raised elevated mass of fibrosis and exudate which is seen replacing the macula in the terminal stages of the disease. The earliest pathological changes are rupture of Bruch's membrane with penetration of a neovascular membrane derived from the choriocapillaris. This invades drusen material and the subpigment epithelial and subretinal spaces. The process occurs in the posterior pole of the eye either under the macula, in the paramacular area, or occasionally adjacent to the optic disc. Similar lesions in the equatorial or peripheral retina do not appear to occur. In common with neovascular tissue elsewhere, these vessels bleed and leak producing subretinal exudate and fibrosis with consequent disruption of the macular anatomy and destruction of central vision. While the disciform response is usually associated with senile macular degeneration it can be the end result of a number of other diverse pathological conditions which affect the posterior pole of the eye and which appear to have in common the ability to damage Bruch's membrane. The exact stimulus for this neovascular process is unknown but it might be speculated that the changes in Bruch's membrane lead to local cellular hypoxia with release of some neovascular factor, in a way analogous to that seen in retinal disease. Serial sections of eyes with drusen have shown that neovascularization of drusen in the posterior pole is not uncommon but that only a minority of these lesions progress to a clinically apparent disciform lesion.

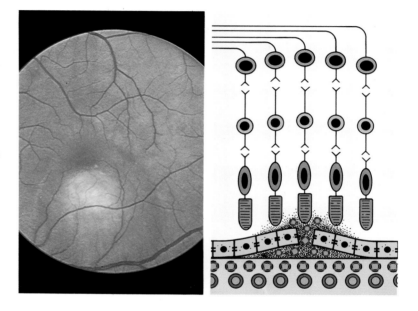

Fig.16.19. The typical disciform lesion, no matter what the aetiology, consists of subretinal elevation either beneath or adjacent to the fovea, surrounded by an area of serous retinal detachment. Recent lesions often have a pale, raised appearance with variable amounts of lipid or haemorrhage. A subretinal haemorrhage in the macular area should always be considered neovascular in origin unless shown otherwise. Presenting symptoms are either metamorphopsia or blurring of vision, depending on the size and the site of the lesion. A drawing demonstrates the anatomical relationships of the neovascular tissue.

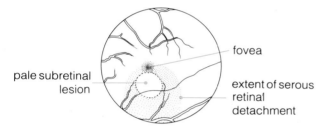

pale subretinal lesion

fovea

extent of serous retinal detachment

Fig.16.20. Early phase fluorescein angiography of the same lesion shows the classical appearance of a neovascular complex lying beneath the retina which, since it is derived from the choroid, fills early in the angiogram. Individual vessels in the neovascular membrane may be identified and the lesion is often surrounded by a thin hypofluorescent margin delineating the extent of the serous retinal detachment. In common with other neovascular tissue, the capillaries in the neovascular membrane have loose cell junctions, and in late stages the membrane shows intense leakage into the adjacent retina.

neovascular membrane — limit of serous retinal detachment

— fixation pointer

intensive leakage in later phases

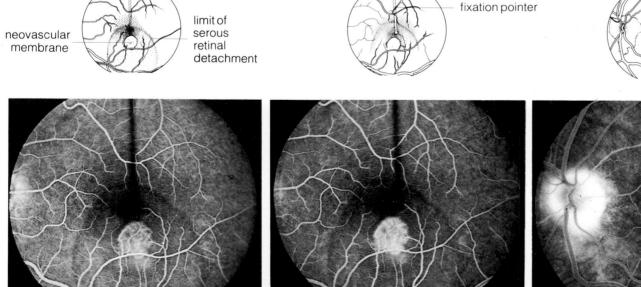

Fig.16.21. Disciform degeneration is often associated with subretinal haemorrhage and this haemorrhage from the membrane may be responsible for the sudden drop in central visual acuity which brings the patient to the ophthalmologist. In this patient the membrane is seen as a pale area at the lower margin of the haemorrhage. Hard exudates are beginning to form inferiorly and there is extensive serous retinal detachment.

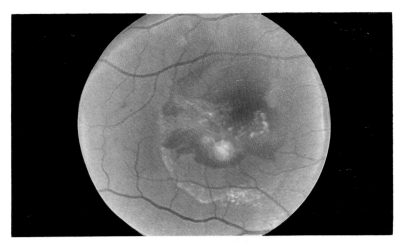

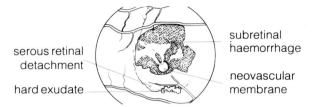

serous retinal detachment

hard exudate

subretinal haemorrhage

neovascular membrane

Fig.16.22. Fluorescein angiography identifies the site of leakage but the haemorrhage masks the underlying choroidal fluorescence and in these circumstances it can be difficult to show the true extent of the neovascular membrane.

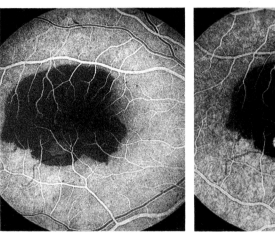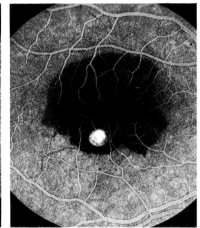

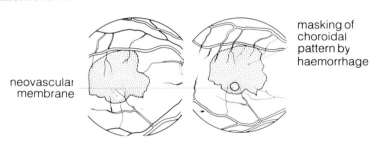

neovascular membrane

masking of choroidal pattern by haemorrhage

Fig.16.23. An exudative reaction may occur around a disciform lesion producing a circinate subretinal exudate with central subretinal neovascularization. In some patients exudates form the major aspect of the fundus appearance.

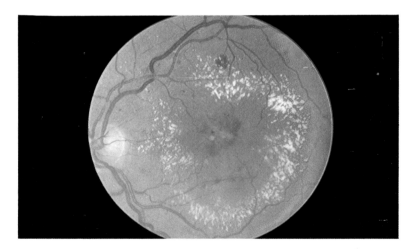

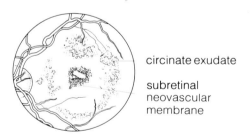

circinate exudate

subretinal neovascular membrane

Fig.16.24. Massive exudation and subsequent retinal fibrosis are the late signs of advanced disciform lesions. Collateral vascularization from the retinal circulation can occur. An extensive serous detachment may initially accompany these late changes, but eventually subsides leaving a burnt out lesion characterised by a white, elevated, subretinal fibrous scar which can occasionally be mistaken for an amelanotic malignant melanoma.

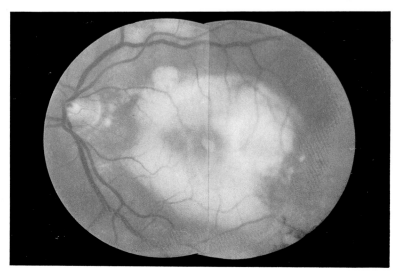

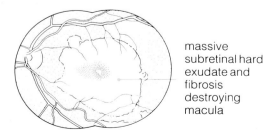

massive subretinal hard exudate and fibrosis destroying macula

Fig.16.25. Pathology of an advanced case (top) shows that the RPE is separated from Bruch's membrane by a layer of hyaline material. In front of the disrupted RPE, a layer of vascularized fibrous tissue replaces the photoreceptors. In another gross example (bottom) the RPE layer is completely disrupted and the neuroretina is replaced by an elevated mass of fibrovascular tissue.

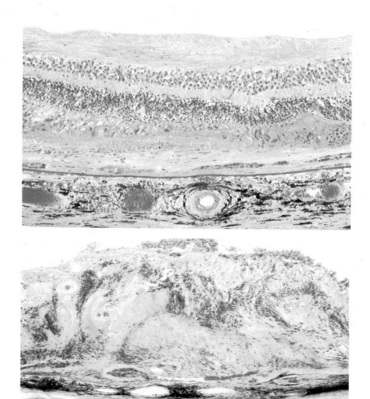

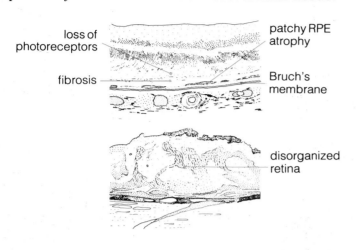

OTHER CAUSES OF DISCIFORM MACULAR DEGENERATION
Juxta-papillary Disciform Degeneration
Fig.16.26. Subretinal neovascularization may develop adjacent to the optic disc either spontaneously or in association with disc abnormalities such as tilting or chronic pathological disc swelling. Lesions extending into the papillomacular region cause a profound loss in central vision but if the membrane lies away from this, vision is not necessarily affected.

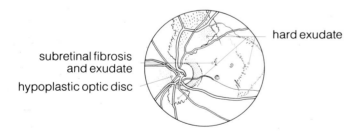

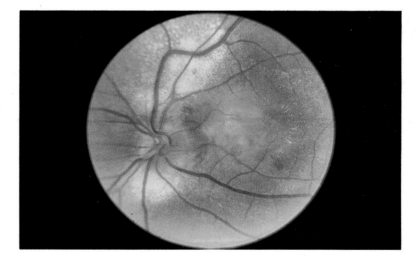

Fig.16.27. The early stages of fluorescein angiography demonstrate the subretinal neovascular complex filling and extending from the disc margin, leading to leakage in the later stages.

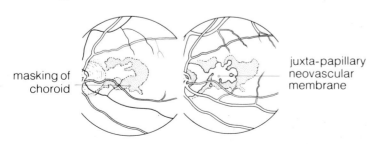

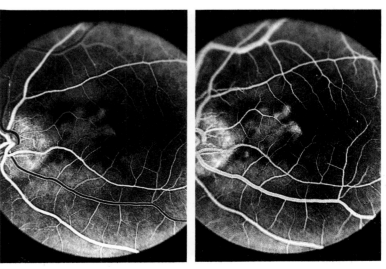

16.11

Myopic Disciform Degeneration

Fig.16.28. High myopes have an increased risk of developing a disciform lesion as young adults. In contrast to other forms of the disease it usually presents as a rather small localised haemmorhage with overlying pigment deposits (Forster-Fuchs' spot) and does not give rise to extensive exudate or serious detachment. Visual recovery is much better than is other types.

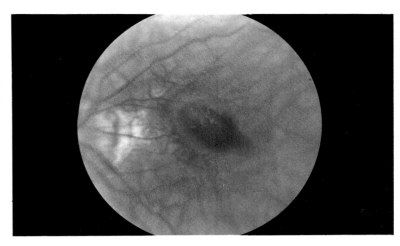

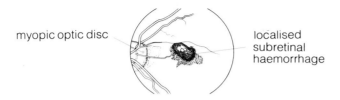

Fig.16.29. Fluorescein angiography in myopic disciform degeneration shows the subretinal neovascular membrane associated with haemorrhage. Myopic degenerative changes can also be seen around the optic disc and in the retinal pigment epithelium of the posterior pole.

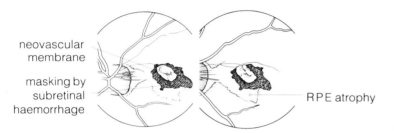

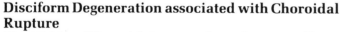

Disciform Degeneration associated with Choroidal Rupture

Fig.16.30. 'Choroidal rupture' may be caused by a severe blunt injury to the eye but the appearance is, in fact, due to a rupture of Bruch's membrane. If the rupture extends into the macular area it can be associated with subretinal neovascularization, which usually occurs some years later. In this patient the rupture is seen as a typical chorioretinal scar concentric with the optic disc in which the neovascular membrane underlies fixation.

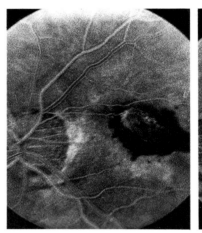

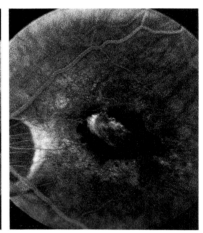

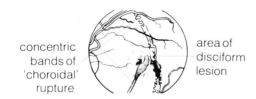

Fig.16.31. Fluorescein angiography demonstrates the extent of the RPE and choriocapillaris atrophy from the initial trauma and the subretinal neovascular membrane underlying the macula.

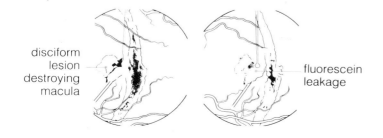

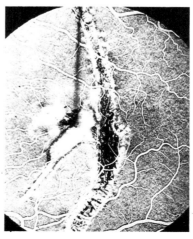

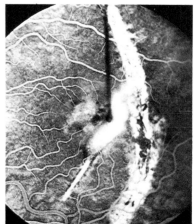

Disciform Degeneration in the Presumed Ocular Histoplasmosis Syndrome

Fig.16.32. The presumed ocular histoplasmosis syndrome describes a pattern of fundus abnormalities which are related to *Histoplasmosis capsulatum* infection which is endemic in the Midwest states of North America. An identical fundus picture is seen in patients without histoplasmosis and the aetiology of these cases is unknown, (see Chapter 10 Intraocular Inflammation). The typical picture consists of the triad of atrophic changes around the optic disc, localised punched-out areas of pigment epithelial atrophy in the posterior pole, atrophic RPE lesions in the equatorial retina which often have a linear pattern and a disciform macular degeneration. When the atrophic areas are in the region of the macula there is a substantial risk of a disciform lesion developing later, typically in early middle age.

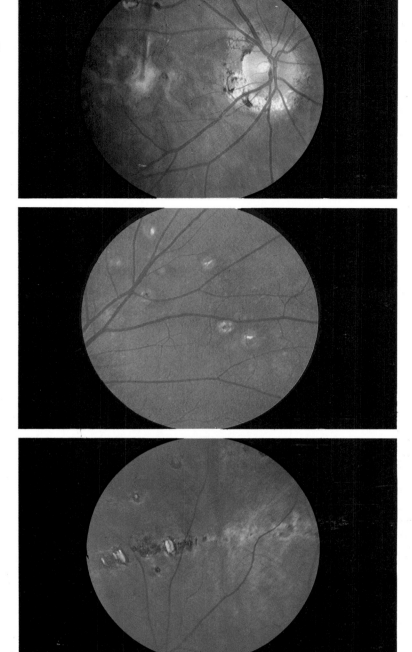

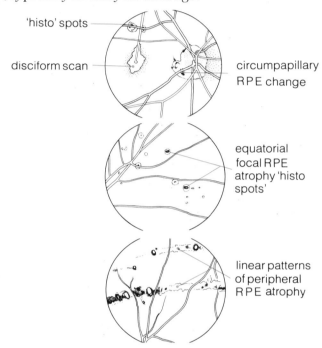

Disciform Degeneration Associated With Angioid Streaks

Angioid streaks are splits in Bruch's membrane. They appear as linear fractures which arise from the optic disc and ramify towards the periphery, mimicking retinal blood vessels. They are usually reddish brown in colour but may show degenerative pigmentary changes. Subretinal neovascularization is a frequent complication occurring in the papillomacular region or alongside the optic disc. Angioid streaks can occur as an isolated ocular finding or with systemic associations which include elastic tissue disorders such as pseudoxanthoma elasticum and Ehlers-Danlos syndrome. Angioid streaks have also been described in sickle cell anaemia and Paget's disease; fragility of Bruch's membrane is the underlying common factor.

Fig.16.33. Patients with pseudoxanthoma elasticum show typical changes in the skin of the neck and flexure creases producing the texture of 'chicken' skin.

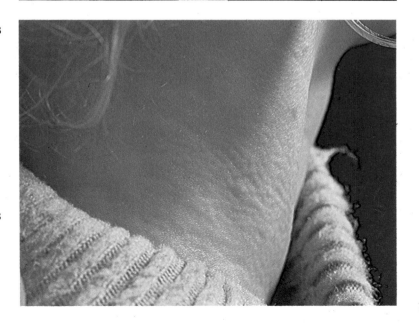

Fig.16.34. This patient shows remarkably conspicuous angioid streaks radiating from the optic discs which are deformed by optic disc drusen, a well-recorded association. Juxta-papillary and subretinal fibrosis can be seen in each eye from burnt out disciform subretinal changes.

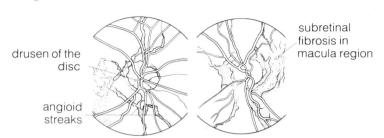

Fig.16.35. The appearance of angioid streaks on fluorescein angiography depends on the degree of associated RPE pigmentation and choriocapillaris atrophy; the majority of streaks show hyperfluorescence but in the early stages they may mask the underlying choroidal fluorescence. In this patient, widespread changes in the RPE are demonstrated together with the areas of subretinal neovascularization already mentioned.

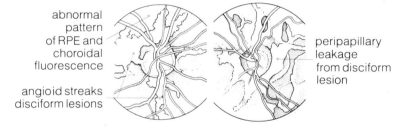

Fig.16.36. Patients with pseudoxanthoma elasticum may also show an alteration in Bruch's membrane and the retinal pigment epithelium of the posterior pole which gives the fundus a slightly mottled refractile yellowish appearance known as 'peau d'orange'. This is most noticeable temporal to the macula and contrasts with the normal, more peripheral, retinal appearances.

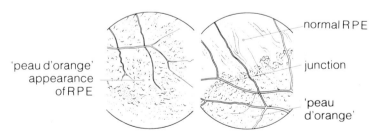

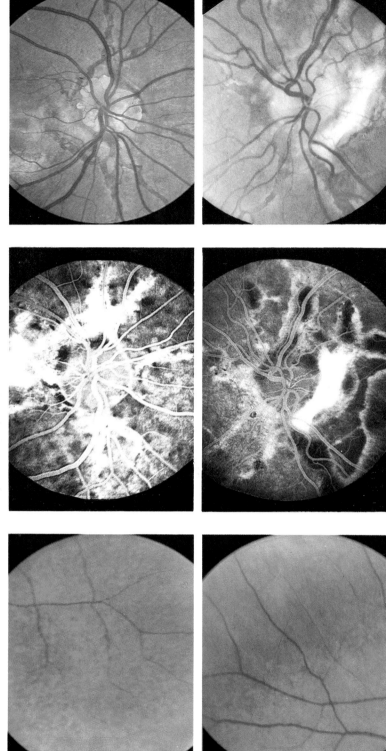

Treatment of Disciform Degeneration

A thermal burn produced by the argon or krypton laser provides a means by which subretinal neovascular tissue may be directly destroyed in an attempt to limit further retinal destruction and visual loss. Energy from the argon laser is taken up by the retinal pigment epithelium (RPE) and blood, and that from the krypton laser by the RPE and choroidal pigment. To achieve success the destruction of a membrane must be total; partial treatment will only cause a recurrence or even provoke a more rapid extension of the residual neovascular tissue. The criteria for treatment with photocoagulation vary according to the type of laser used and also depend on the proximity of the subretinal membrane to fixation and whether or not it underlies the luteal pigment in the ganglion cells of the macular area. Subretinal neovascular membranes that lie outside the central avascular zone are amenable to treatment with the argon laser, although the scar produced will be larger than the area treated. The macular luteal pigment will also absorb argon laser energy, in which case the burn will extend into the inner retina destroying the nerve fibre layer with extension of the scotoma. This limits the use of the argon laser in the region of the fovea; it may be that the krypton laser has advantages in the treatment of lesions in this area and this is currently being investigated in clinical trials. At present, lesions can be treated to within 200μ of fixation but treatment any closer than this incurs a risk of damaging the fovea. In practice this means that patients who present with visual acuities in the region of better than 6/24 may have treatable lesions whereas those with poorer levels of acuity at presentation are usually untreatable.

Fig.16.37. This patient has a fresh parafoveal disciform lesion with serous detachment extending into the fovea and an acuity of 6/12. Fluorescein angiography is essential prior to treatment to assess the full extent of the membrane. The most important pictures are taken in the earliest arterial phases of the angiogram before leakage of dye into the retina obscures the fine vascular detail.

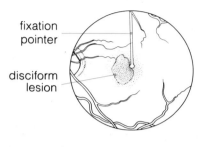

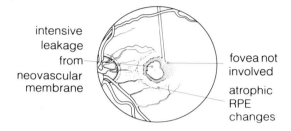

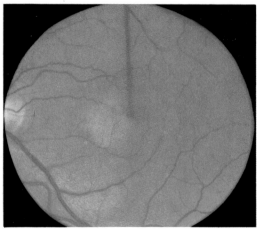

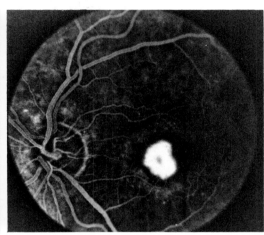

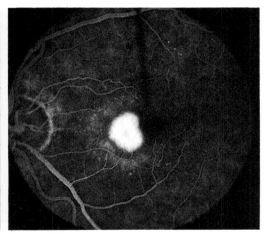

Fig.16.38. Immediately following treatment with the argon laser, the opaque white reaction in the deep outer retina can be seen. The more intense burn in the parafoveal region is the result of absorption of energy by the luteal pigment. Visual acuity fell to 6/24 immediately after treatment.

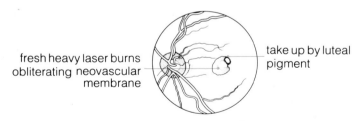

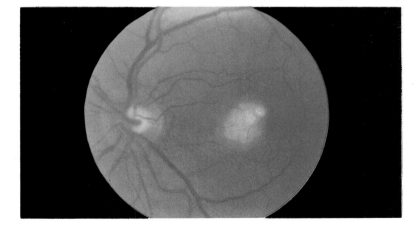

Fig.16.39. Four weeks later a pigmented scar has formed in the region of the burns. Fluorescein angiography shows complete destruction of the membrane. Visual acuity improved to 6/9 with a small paramacular scotoma which was easily ignored by the patient.

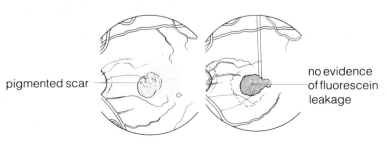

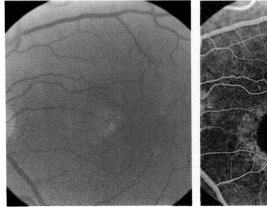

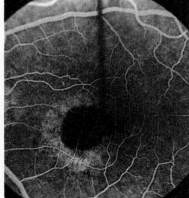

MYOPIC MACULAR DEGENERATION

Myopes of over −10D carry a very high risk of developing atrophic macular degeneration (as well as glaucoma, cataracts and retinal detachment). Advanced macular changes are seen as well-circumscribed areas of widespread chorioretinal atrophy centred on the macula, often in association with a posterior staphyloma. Myopic disciform degeneration may also occur (see Fig.16.30). Less severe cases show generalised thinning of the RPE with more pronounced patches of pigment atrophy and splits in Bruch's membrane known as 'lacquer' cracks.

Fig.16.40. This patient shows a large myopic crescent on the temporal side of the optic disc. Retinal vessels are pulled straight as they enter the enlarged posterior pole. In the macula there is patchy pigmentary disturbance and fine cracks in Bruch's membrane.

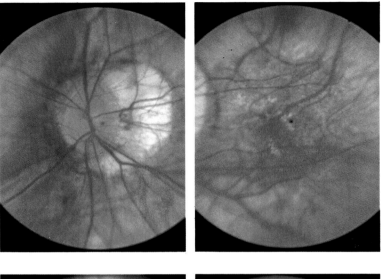

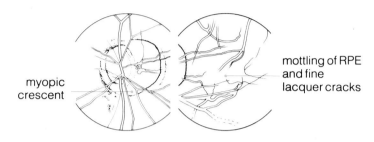

Fig.16.41. A more severe case shows gross chorioretinal atrophy of the macula in the right eye with exposed bare sclera. In the left eye the atrophy is less extensive but a small disciform degeneration is present.

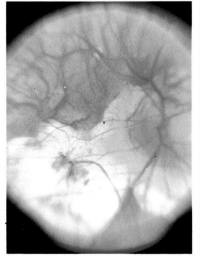
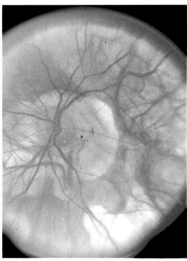

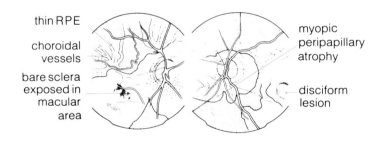

RETINAL DYSTROPHIES

There are a large number of inherited retinal dystrophies but many of these are excessively rare. Their manifestations can be purely ocular or associated with systemic disease, although this is comparatively unusual. In most cases the underlying metabolic defect is unknown but inherited retinal disease can be classified genetically by its mode of inheritance and anatomically by the site of the cellular lesion within the eye; the latter is not known with certainty for many of these diseases since little pathological material of early cases is available for study. It has already been seen with degenerative macular disease that destruction of one cellular constituent of the retina can be followed by secondary atrophy of its neighbours. In many types of retinitis pigmentosa (RP) it is not possible to say whether the primary lesion occurs in the photoreceptor, retinal pigment epithelium or perhaps even the choriocapillaris. However, with the aid of fluorescein angiography and electrodiagnostic tests, this information can be inferred in the majority of cases. These tests are also useful in documenting the progression of the disease and the selective involvement of various cellular retinal components. Morphological fundus appearances have to be interpreted with caution as a wide variety of inherited retinal diseases can produce a similar fundus appearance. To use the example of retinitis pigmentosa again, some experts suggest that the fundus appearance of RP will eventually be shown to reflect up to 30 or 40 different retinal metabolic defects.

Apart from one or two rare examples, no specific treatment is available for inherited retinal dystrophies but genetic counselling, a visual prognosis and occupational advice are important for the patient. In order to do this, thorough family studies and a wide clinical experience are essential. The widespread variations in the disease morphology within a family and its visual effects can make it difficult to link isolated patients into a specific diagnostic category. It is important to recognise that superficially comparable families may not necessarily have the same disease and therefore may not have the same visual outcome. Myopia and cataracts are common associates of many retinal dystrophies.

Classification of Inherited Retinal Disease

Clinically, patients are often described as having a primary rod or cone dystrophy but, whilst this might be true of early cases, advanced cases show a combined effect on both types of cell so that patients with a rod dystrophy also lose cone function with time and vice versa. Combined rod-cone dystrophies (mixed receptor dystrophies) are also seen as a specific entity from the earliest stages and these patients usually have severe visual loss with early onset.

Fig. 16.42. Dystrophies other than those of the photoreceptors appear to start in the retinal pigment epithelium, the choriocapillaris, the Müller cells or the neuroretina.

Presumed anatomical classification of retinal dystrophies	
Layer	**Type**
1. Neuroretina	x-linked retino schisis (congenital stationery night blindness, Oguchi's disease)
2. Photoreceptor	colour deficiencies, achromatism
3. Photoreceptor – retinal pigment epithelial cell complex	retinitis pigmentosa fundus albipunctatus cone dystrophies mixed receptor dystrophies
4. Retinal pigment epithelium – Bruch's membrane	Stargardt's disease Best's disease (and butterfly dystrophy) Sjögren's reticular dystrophy dominant drusen central areolar sclerosis
5. Choroid	choroideraemia gyrate atrophy high myopia

Retinitis Pigmentosa

This name is given to a group of diseases which have the triad of night blindness, visual field constriction and a typical fundus appearance. Most of these diseases are purely ocular in their manifestation but a few rare types have important systemic associations. The diseases appear to have a factor in common, in that they affect the photoreceptor-RPE cell metabolic complex and, although in most types the precise biochemical lesion is not known, it appears that in a substantial number the defect may be located in the photoreceptor. The initial involvement of the equatorial and peripheral retina suggests that the disease affects rod metabolism primarily but increasing evidence of cone malfunction is seen clinically, electrophysiologically and pathologically with time.

The fundus morphology is non-specific and cannot be used to differentiate between genetically inherited patterns. The earliest changes are seen in the equatorial retina as areas of atrophy and hypertrophy of the retinal pigment epithelium producing a dappled appearance; this is readily apparent on fluorescein angiography as widespread spotty atrophy and masking of the RPE. The typical intraretinal bone corpuscular pigmentation which is such a hallmark of the disease is a comparatively late sign probably only seen after the disease has been present for several years. Other characteristic fundus changes are a pale 'waxy' optic disc pallor and attenuation of the retinal arterioles. The macula is spared until comparatively late in the disease.

Patients present with night blindness or symptoms from their peripheral visual field loss, which is usually so insidious that it is not noticed until there is extreme constriction of the field. Photophobia and glare are important secondary symptoms. The electro-oculogram is lost early in the disease, sometimes before fundus changes are noticeable; the electro-retinogram can be used to follow progressive rod and cone deterioration. Retinitis pigmentosa (RP) must be differentiated from pseudo-retinitis pigmentosa in which the fundus morphology is mimicked, for example, by trauma, infection or previous retinal detachment.

Purely ocular retinitis pigmentosa has a definite family history in about 50% of cases and can be inherited in recessive, dominant or X-linked patterns, each varying in their age of onset, severity and rate of progression. RP affects both eyes, although sometimes asymmetrically, and true uniocular disease is not seen. Sectorial retinitis pigmentosa is a variant of the disease in which the appearances are limited to one area of the retina in each eye. The presence of the typical RPE changes without the normal intraretinal pigmentation is sometimes called 'retinitis pigmentosa sine pigmente' and this is probably due to early disease. Systemic disease is associated with retinitis pigmentosa in a group of rare syndromes in which deafness and neurological or renal problems are often other features. Some of these, such as Refsum's disease (RP, hypertrophic peripheral neuropathy, deafness, cardiomyopathy and icthyosis with deposition of phytanic acid) and abetalipoproteinaemia are important as they are examples of known biochemical defects. Early treatment has been shown to improve the visual prognosis of abetalipoproteinaemia. Recently there has been considerable interest in whether light may have a toxic effect on a dystrophic retina, enhancing the rate of degeneration.

Other well known syndromes are Usher's syndrome in which congenital sensineural deafness is associated with RP appearing in childhood and the Laurence-Moon syndrome (polydactyly, mental retardation, truncal obesity, hypogonadism and RP). Leber's amaurosis presents in an infant as congenital blindness with a normal fundus appearance and is distinguished from cortical blindness by the absence of the ERG; patients usually develop the fundus appearances of retinitis pigmentosa many years later. A pigmentary retinopathy is sometimes seen as a feature of chronic progressive external ophthalmoplegia, dystrophia myotonica, Hallgren's syndrome, Alport's syndrome and others.

Fig.16.43. This patient, a 17-year-old male, has advanced presumed autosomal recessive retinitis pigmentosa and severe visual disability although acuities remain at 6/12 and 6/18. Both optic discs are pale and the retinal arteries grossly attenuated. The macula has a glassy sheen to it from associated preretinal membrane formation and is relatively spared, but the retinal pigment epithelium appears progressively more mottled and grossly abnormal towards the equatorial retina. Visual fields were constricted to the central 10°.

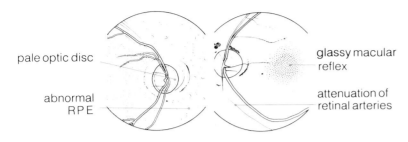

pale optic disc

abnormal RPE

glassy macular reflex

attenuation of retinal arteries

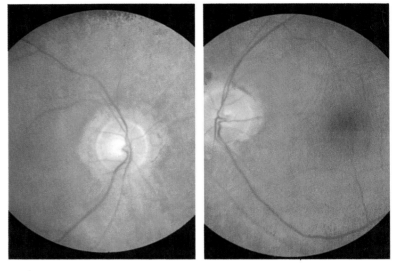

Fig.16.44. Peripheral photographs of the same patient show heavy intraretinal bone corpuscular pigmentation spreading outwards in the equatorial retina. This pigmentation is heavier and more marked than is frequently seen and reflects the severity and duration of the disease in this patient.

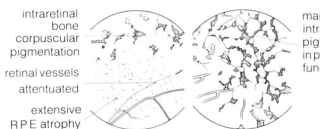

intraretinal bone corpuscular pigmentation

retinal vessels attentuated

extensive RPE atrophy

marked intraretinal pigmentation in peripheral fundus

Fig.16.45. This patient shows the typical features of the Laurence-Moon syndrome with a fat moon-shaped face, truncal obesity and polydactyly, which is seen more clearly in the photograph of another patient. Extra digits are often removed at birth leaving scars as the only evidence in later life of their presence.

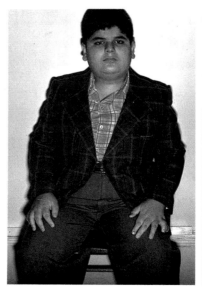
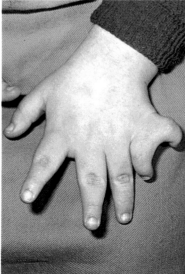

Cone Dystrophies

Cone dystrophies are less common than rod dystrophies. Dominant inheritance of these conditions is the most common pattern but recessive cases do occur. Patients normally present as young adults with poor acuity, photophobia and, occasionally, with nystagmus or poor colour vision. The typical appearance is of a 'bull's eye' maculopathy in which there is an area of hyperpigmentation surrounded by concentric rings of hypopigmentation and hyperpigmentation. Other patients may show a picture of diffuse central amorphous pigmentary atrophy and both patterns can be seen in the affected members of the same family. Rarely, central areolar sclerosis can be a manifestation of a cone dystrophy, although senile macular degeneration is a much more common cause.

Early cases of cone dystrophy show a severe loss of cone functions in the ERG with moderate loss of rod function and a subnormal EOG. As the disease progresses visual acuity falls to levels of 6/60, or counting fingers, with progressive macular destruction, attenuation of retinal vessels, central field loss and progressive deterioration in the ERG and the EOG, reflecting the increasing area of retinal involvement. In children, a bull's eye maculopathy can be the presenting feature of a fatal neurolipidosis known as juvenile Batten's disease. Severe chloroquine toxicity also produces a similar fundus appearance.

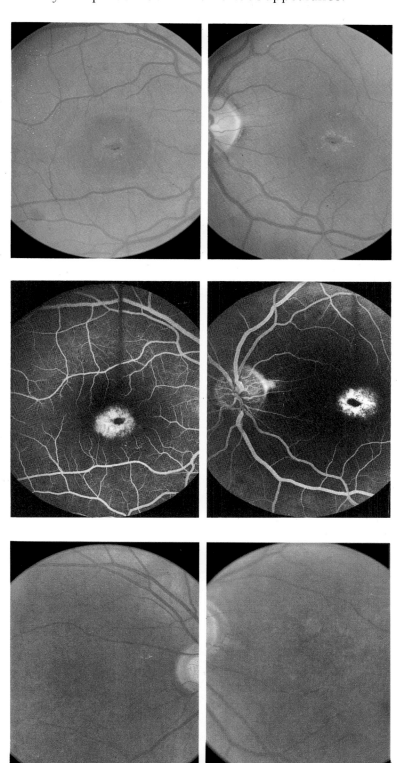

Fig.16.46. Typical bull's eye macular changes are seen in this 18-year-old patient with a dominantly inherited cone dystrophy. Note the central hyperpigmentation of the macula surrounded by atrophy, in contrast with the normal retinal vessels and optic disc.

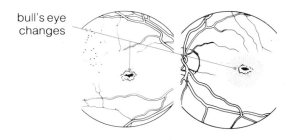

Fig.16.47. Fluorescein angiography demonstrates the retinal pigment epithelial hypertrophy and atrophy confined to the macula.

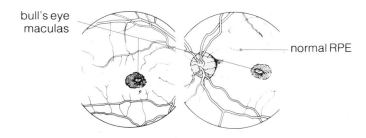

Fig.16.48. This patient shows the diffuse type of atrophy of the macula with no bull's eye appearance on ophthalmoscopy. Visual acuities were 6/12 in each eye with paramacular scotomas. The ERG showed absent cone and reduced rod responses and the EOG was subnormal, reflecting the extent of the retinal disease.

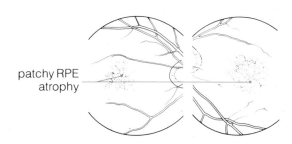

16.19

Fig.16.49. Fluorescein angiography shows the widespread pigmentary disturbance at each macula which has a vague bull's eye pattern. Retinal arteries are attenuated to some degree. The RPE appears normal outside the posterior pole.

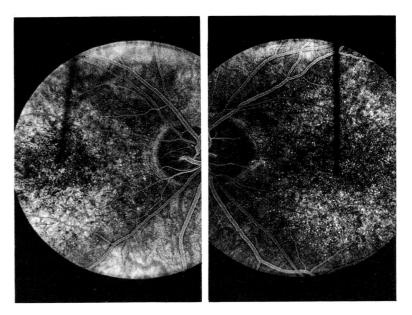

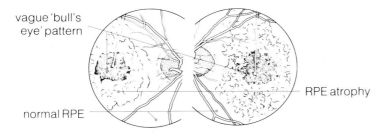

Mixed Receptor Dystrophy

This is relatively rare. Symptoms usually start in childhood and both rod and cone function are affected from the onset and the visual handicap is severe. Patients normally have nystagmus and photophobia. Fundus examination shows both peripheral and central pigmentary changes. Leber's amaurosis might be included as a subtype of this category.

Fig.16.50. This 24-year-old patient shows a pigmentary macular disturbance with surrounding atrophy and a rather thin transparent peripheral retina with widespread retinal pigment epithelial changes on fluorescein angiography. Retinal arteries are attenuated. He had grossly constricted fields, acuities of HM and 6/60, nystagmus and was also mentally subnormal, although this might have been related more to difficulty with his education than to an organic defect.

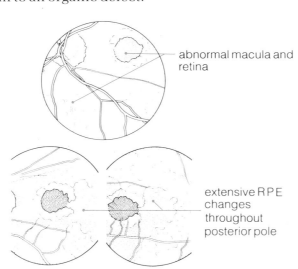

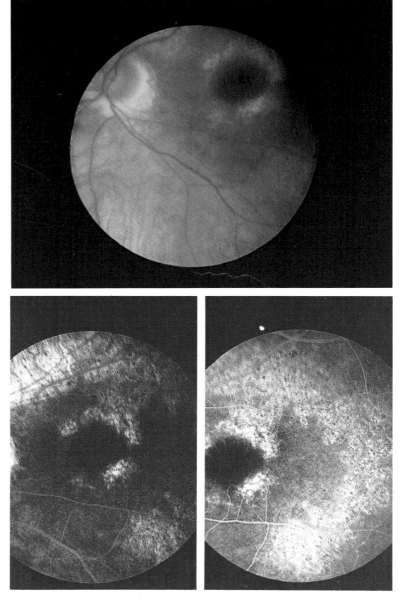

Stargardt's Disease

This disease is usually inherited in an autosomal recessive pattern and presents as visual loss in a teenager or young adult. There are two patterns of fundus appearance. In the most common type the macula is atrophic and surrounded by concentric, whitish flecks at the level of the RPE. These flecks are about the same size as drusen and are yellowish white with a vaguely triangular appearance which has been likened, somewhat dubiously, to a fish tail. They appear initially in the macular region and spread centrifugally with the passage of time, evolving from a well defined lesion to one with soft fluffy borders. Progressive macular atrophy is accompanied by visual acuity falling to levels of counting fingers in middle age. Other patients have the characteristic flecks without macular atrophy. This is known as fundus flavimaculatus and these patients tend to have good acuity until much later in life. Both these fundus appearances can sometimes be found in members of the same family indicating that they are different parts of the same disease spectrum. The EOG is subnormal and mirrors the extent of the RPE change. The ERG shows progressive loss of cone function and, subsequently, rod function. Available pathology seems to indicate a lesion at the level of the RPE.

Fig.16.51. This patient shows comparatively early disease affecting the macula which is atrophic and surrounded by typical whitish subretinal flecks. Fluorescein angiography shows that fresh flecks, which are the most equatorial, do not fluoresce as much as older, more central lesions which are accompanied by RPE atrophy.

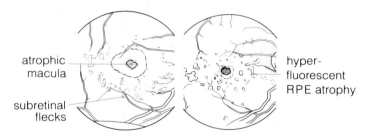

Fig.16.52. This 23-year-old patient shows more extensive disease. The EOG was 175% of the normal level, the cone ERG markedly subnormal but rod functions were relatively well preserved. In the equatorial fundus the flecks are fresh and lie in almost concentric waves. The visual acuity was 6/36 in this eye.

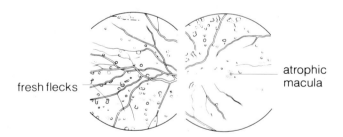

Fig.16.53. Signs of progressive macular atrophy in another patient can be seen in these photographs taken 6 years apart.

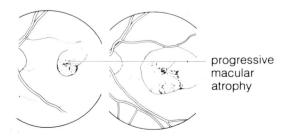

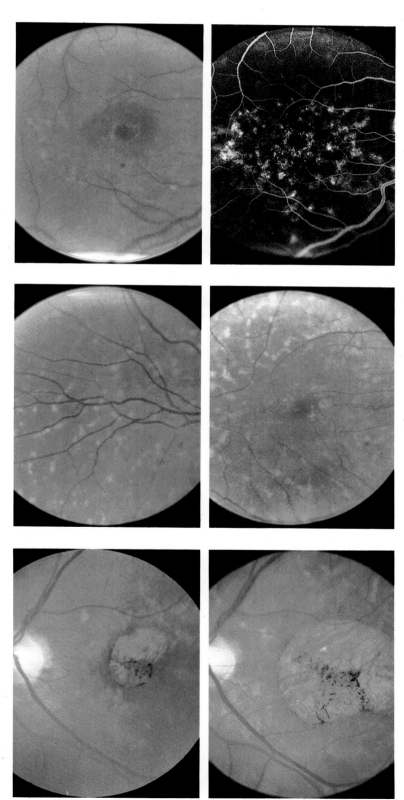

16.21

Vitelliform Macular Dystrophy (Best's Disease)

This is a dominantly inherited disorder with variable penetrance in which the basic defect appears to occur at the level of the retinal pigment epithelium. The EOG is reduced in the presence of a normal ERG and this appears to be a consistent finding whether or not the patients show the characteristic fundus morphology and is, therefore, of great diagnostic help in genetic counselling.

Fig.16.54. The initial lesion is a curious yellowish accumulation of material beneath the macula producing the characteristic 'poached egg' appearance. The overlying retina and vessels are normal. These lesions are submacular and usually single but occasionally may be multiple. They can be seen in early childhood and at this stage do not affect visual acuity. Fluorescein angiography shows that the lesion masks the choroidal pattern but that there is no abnormal leakage.

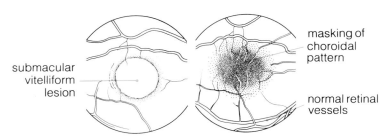

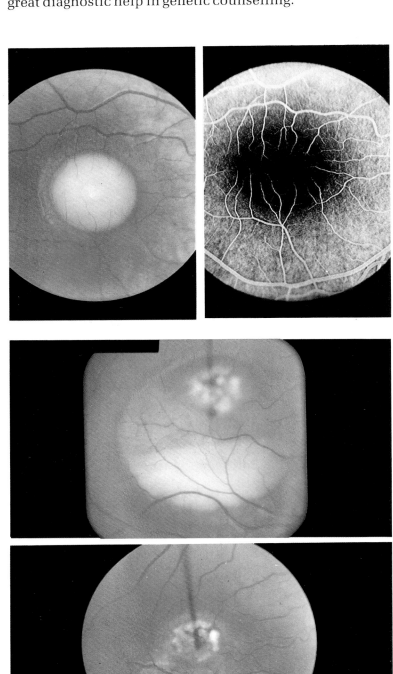

Fig.16.55. Patients usually present in the second decade with some decrease in acuity when the lesion ruptures. The material absorbs but may be left (or reform) as a subretinal fluid level known as a pseudohypopyon. Complete absorption leaves mottled changes at the level of the RPE sometimes described as the 'scrambled egg' stage.

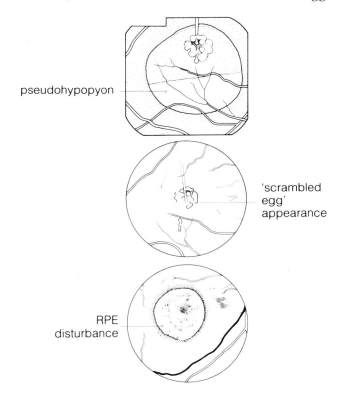

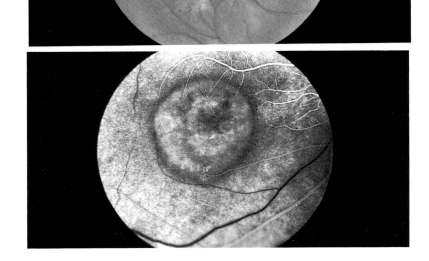

Fig.16.56. Patients may retain reasonable levels of central vision until middle age when there is a high risk of developing disciform macular degeneration which destroys the remaining central vision.

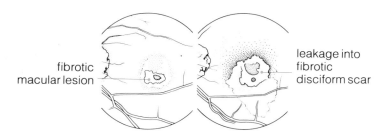

fibrotic macular lesion

leakage into fibrotic disciform scar

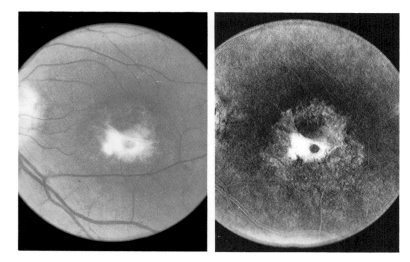

Juvenile X-Linked Schisis

This is a rare macular dystrophy inherited in an X-linked manner which presents as poor visual acuity in boys. Female carriers of the gene cannot be identified. The lesion seems to be related to a defect in the Müller cells and on ERG a selective defect is seen in the B wave. The characteristic findings are of a fine reticular microcystic disturbance in the inner retina overlying the fovea; it is difficult to see without using stereoscopic biomicroscopy, but appears as radial lines, rather like the pattern of a cartwheel. Fluorescein angiography is normal. With time the macula lesion becomes atrophic, losing its typical appearance. About 50% of patients will have a peripheral retinal schisis.

Fig.16.57. Typical fine striations can be seen radiating from the macula in this boy. Microcystoid changes lie within the macula.

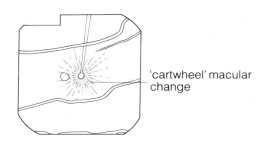

'cartwheel' macular change

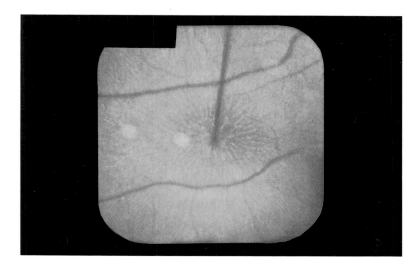

Tay-Sachs Disease

This is a rare, recessively inherited neurolipidosis usually seen in Jewish infants in the first few months of life. Patients present with a progressive neurological deterioration, become spastic and blind and die in the first 2 to 3 years of life. The defect is due to a deficiency of hexosaminidase A leading to storage of ganglioside GM_2 in neurones. This is seen ophthalmoscopically as a whitish ring around the macula, the abnormal material being deposited where the retinal ganglion cells are thickest and contrasting with the redness of the relatively neurone-free macula.

Fig.16.58. This infant with Tay-Sach's disease shows a prominent cherry red spot at the macula. A similar fundus appearance can be seen in teenagers with the excessively rare cherry red spot myoclonus syndrome in which there is a sialidase deficiency.

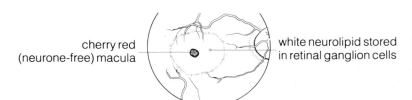

cherry red (neurone-free) macula

white neurolipid stored in retinal ganglion cells

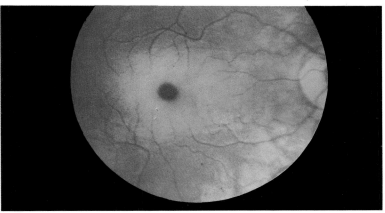

16.23

Choroideraemia

Fig.16.59. This is an X-linked retinal dystrophy in which males in their second decade present with night blindness; visual acuity remains fairly good until 40-50 years of age. Initial changes appear in the equatorial retina with patchy, ill-defined atrophy of the choroid and overlying retina which progresses so that in the affected areas only the sclera remains. The macula is spared until late in the course of the disease. In contrast to retinitis pigmentosa, the retinal vessels and optic disc remain comparatively normal and intraretinal pigmentation does not occur (top). Female carriers of the disease can be identified by characteristic mottled changes in the retinal pigment epithelium and some affected females lose vision in later life (bottom).

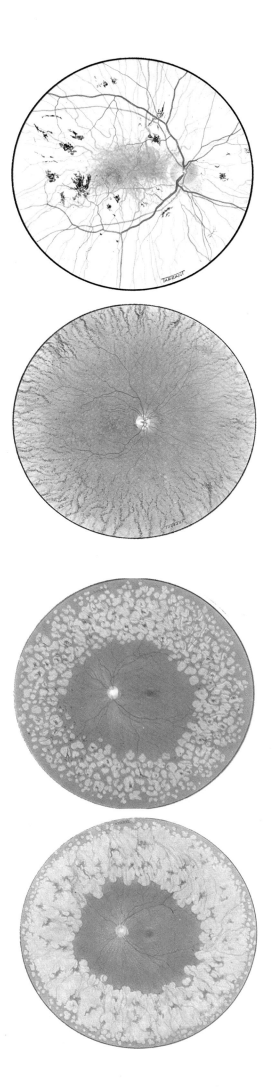

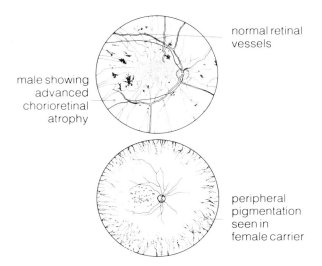

normal retinal vessels

male showing advanced chorioretinal atrophy

peripheral pigmentation seen in female carrier

Gyrate Atrophy

Fig.16. 60. This is an excessively rare, recessively-inherited dystrophy, but is important because there is a known defect in the metabolism of the amino acid ornithine, high levels being found in the blood and urine. Patients present with poor night vision in their 20's and 30's. Fundus examination of the equatorial retina shows scalloped and well-circumscribed areas of chorioretinal atrophy surrounded by normal retina. The affected areas expand centrally and peripherally with severe loss of vision. Retinal blood vessels and optic discs remain normal. These paintings show the fundus appearance of two siblings with the disease.

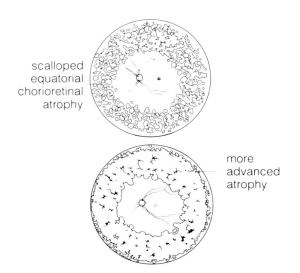

scalloped equatorial chorioretinal atrophy

more advanced atrophy

17. The Optic Disc

D. J. Spalton

M. D. Sanders

THE NORMAL OPTIC DISC

The normal optic disc is about 1.5mm. in diameter and lies between 10 and 15 degrees from fixation in the nasal retina and usually slightly above the horizontal meridian. Each optic nerve contains about 1.2 million afferent nerve fibres which originate in the retinal ganglion cells and synapse at the lateral geniculate body. In addition, there are probably a few efferent fibres in each optic nerve with vasomotor functions, although the presence of these has not been conclusively demonstrated in man. About twenty-five percent of the sensory input to the brain is visual.

The scleral opening is rigid and non-expansible. Behind the cribriform plate, the axons, which have a diameter of about one micron, acquire a myelin sheath, and the optic nerve enlarges to a diameter of 3-4mm. The nerve fibres are topographically arranged in both the retina and the optic nerve. The optic nerve sheath is a continuation of the meninges and the axons in the nerve are divided into approximately one thousand bundles by fibrous septa (derived from the pia mater) which also carry centripetal blood vessels. The subarachnoid space communicates intracranially so that the nerves are surrounded by the cerebrospinal fluid (CSF) which transmits the intracranial pressure.

Two posterior ciliary arteries leave the ophthalmic artery posteriorly in the orbit and divide to form about fifteen or twenty short posterior ciliary arteries which pierce the sclera radially, adjacent to the optic nerve, and anastomose to form an incomplete circle of Zinn. These branches supply the scleral and choroidal lamina of the disc and peripapillary choroid. The blood supply of the optic disc is derived entirely from the short posterior ciliary arteries, either by direct branches or indirectly from the choroidal circulation. Centripetal vessels pass directly into the disc from the adjacent choroidal circulation but the exact proportion of blood that the optic disc receives from either of these sources is still unknown. The central retinal artery penetrates the optic nerve about 12mm. posterior to the cribriform plate and supplies the nerve by means of centrifugal branches but does not contribute to the supply of the disc itself, apart from some supply to the most superficial nerve fibre layer.

Fig. 17.1 Schematic diagram illustrating the blood supply of the optic disc and distal optic nerve by the posterior ciliary artery circulation.

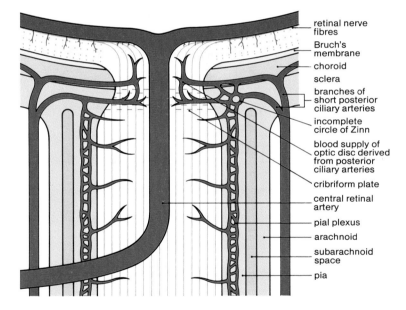

retinal nerve fibres
Bruch's membrane
choroid
sclera
branches of short posterior ciliary arteries
incomplete circle of Zinn
blood supply of optic disc derived from posterior ciliary arteries
cribriform plate
central retinal artery
pial plexus
arachnoid
subarachnoid space
pia

Fig. 17.2 Low-power micrograph showing a longitudinal section of the distal part of the optic nerve with the optic nerve head and the retina. There is a considerable increase in the transverse diameter of the optic nerve after it has passed through the scleral canal. This increase is due to myelination.

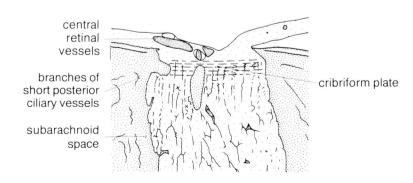

central retinal vessels

branches of short posterior ciliary vessels

cribriform plate

subarachnoid space

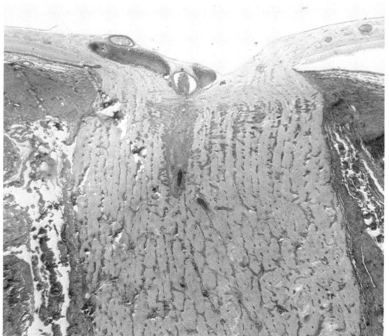

Fig. 17.3   Transverse section of optic nerve showing the meninges and subarachnoid space and the division of nerve fibres into bundles by fibrous septae derived from the pia mater.

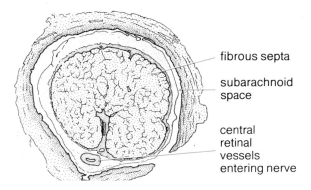

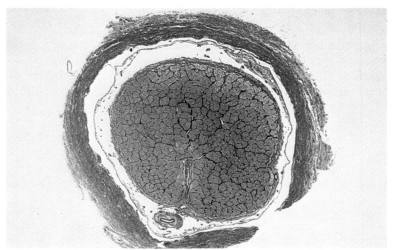

fibrous septa

subarachnoid space

central retinal vessels entering nerve

CONGENITAL ANOMALIES AND PSEUDOPAPILLOEDEMA

Normal optic discs can vary in size, shape, and contour and the accurate appreciation of this is extremely important. Anomalies of the disc can reflect defects in closure of the foetal fissure, degeneration of the hyaloid vascular system, the shape of the globe (which is usually indicated by the refractive state), or developmental anomalies of the anterior visual pathways.

Anomalous discs can appear swollen because of the

distortion of the normal nerve fibre pattern but careful scrutiny of the disc with white and 'red-free' light will usually reveal whether or not a disc is pathologically swollen. When doubt remains fluorescein angiography and careful observation (together with photography) over a period of time resolve the question. Congenitally anomalous discs can be associated with visual function varying from gross visual loss to complete normality.

Fig. 17.4   Glial remnants are thought to be derived either from hyaloid artery remnants or vitreous condensations. Depending on their form and distribution they can simulate swelling or tumours of the disc.

Occasionally, fibrous remnants of the hyaloid artery can be seen in the vitreous, sometimes attached to the posterior lens pole. Remnants of the tunica vasculosa lentis are sometimes seen more peripherally as a Mittendorf dot.

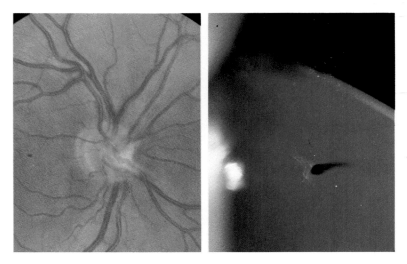

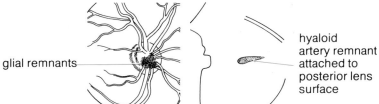

glial remnants

hyaloid artery remnant attached to posterior lens surface

Colobomas of the Disc

A coloboma is a congenital defect resulting from a malclosure of the foetal cleft. They vary in size and shape but usually occur inferiorly with varying involvement of

the retina and uveal tracts. Colobomas are occasionally inherited in an autosomal dominant fashion.

Fig. 17.5   The foetal fissure of the optic cup lies inferiorly and normally closes (starting at the middle and spreading anteriorly and posteriorly) at about 5-7 weeks of gestation. Defects in this process produce a coloboma. These can occur in many shapes and sizes and typically involve the inferior temporal area of the disc, retina and choroid.

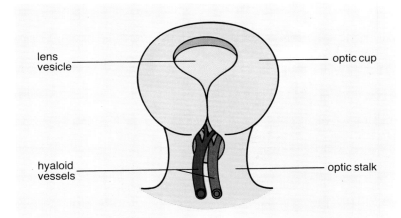

lens vesicle

optic cup

hyaloid vessels

optic stalk

Fig. 17.6   A small coloboma of the disc associated with sectorial hypoplasia of the inferior pigment epithelium in a pigmented eye. The disc appears slightly smaller vertically, and wider horizontally than normal. Choroidal vessels can be seen more easily through the thinned pigment epithelium. There might be reduced sensitivity of the superior temporal visual field.

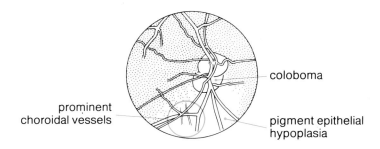

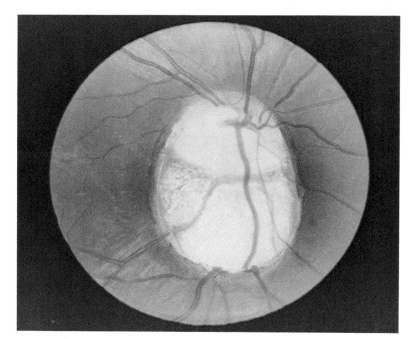

Fig. 17.7   A large coloboma of the disc. There may also be associated colobomas of the retina and choroid, lens or iris. (cf. The Uveal Tract and The Lens — Volumes 9 and 11). A field defect is common and acuity may be poor if macula fibres are affected.

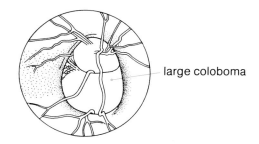

Fig. 17.8   A variant of coloboma is the morning glory disc. This rare congenital deformity of the disc is characterized by a mass of central glial tissue with radiating blood vessels, peripapillary atrophy, and pigmentation. It is sometimes called a central coloboma of the disc. The vision in the affected eye is poor and there may be associated midline intracranial anomalies such as basal encephalocoeles. This is especially true if there are signs of malclosure of the foetal facial clefts such as palatal deformity, accessory facial nodules, or telecanthus.

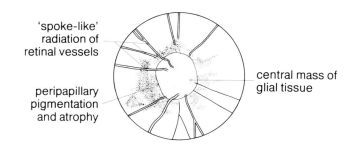

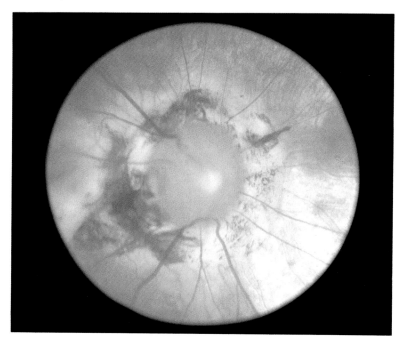

Fig. 17.9 Typically, a pit of the optic disc has a greyish appearance and lies on the temporal border of the disc (which is of normal or slightly larger diameter), penetrating deeply into its substance: the aetiology is uncertain. Those pits centred on the maculo-papular bundle are frequently associated with a serous detachment of the macula with corresponding visual loss, as in this patient, and usually present in early adulthood. A late-stage fluorescein angiogram demonstrates leakage from the pit with masking of background fluorescence in the region of the serous macular detachment. The origin of the subretinal fluid is unknown but it has been suggested that it might be derived from communication with either the orbit or the subarachnoid space, through the disc substance, or the vitreous, via defective vitreous attachments over the pit, which seems more likely. Treatment with photocoagulation is unhelpful.

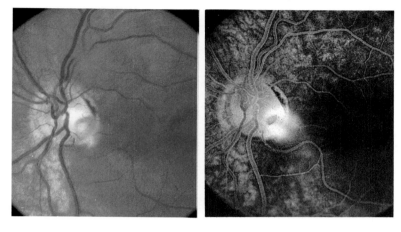

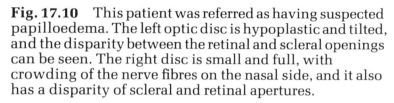

Hypoplastic Discs

Partial optic disc hypoplasia (small discs) occurs in varying degrees of severity and can be either unilateral or bilateral. Visual acuity can vary from normal to severely defective. Poor acuity and strabismus are common and the discs can look swollen in the more severe forms. Characteristically, there is a disparity between the diameter of the retinal opening and the smaller scleral diameter of the disc.

Fig. 17.10 This patient was referred as having suspected papilloedema. The left optic disc is hypoplastic and tilted, and the disparity between the retinal and scleral openings can be seen. The right disc is small and full, with crowding of the nerve fibres on the nasal side, and it also has a disparity of scleral and retinal apertures.

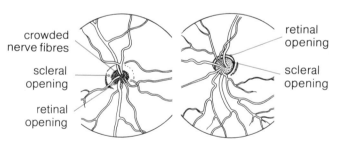

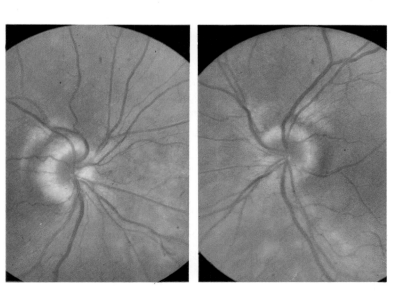

Fig. 17.11 Tilted or asymmetrical discs are frequently associated with a high astigmatic correction, but not necessarily in the axis of the tilt. Most commonly there is a deficiency on the nasal aspect of the disc suggesting an anomaly of development.

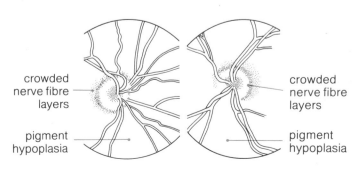

Fig. 17.12 Fewer fibres than normal enter a tilted disc on the defective side and this can produce field defects that simulate a bitemporal loss due to chiasmal compression. Careful perimetry shows that these defects cross the vertical meridian, a feature never seen in chiasmal compression, allowing the patient to be reassured and spared neuroradiological studies.

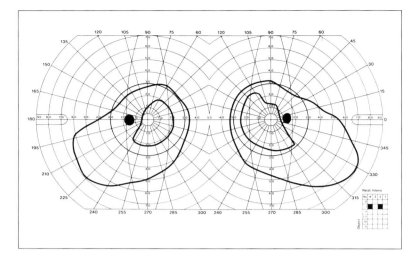

Fig. 17.13 Optic nerve hypoplasia is seen in its most severe form as part of the rare syndrome of septo-optic dysplasia of de Morsier. These children have very poor vision and associated midline intracranial anomalies of which an absent septum pellucidum is typical. Abnormalities of pituitary hormonal function, especially of growth hormone, are common. These optic discs show a grossly hypoplastic right disc although some nerve fibres are present: the left contains virtually no nerve fibres at all. The child had short stature due to deficient growth hormone function.

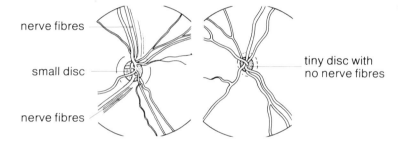

nerve fibres

small disc

nerve fibres

tiny disc with no nerve fibres

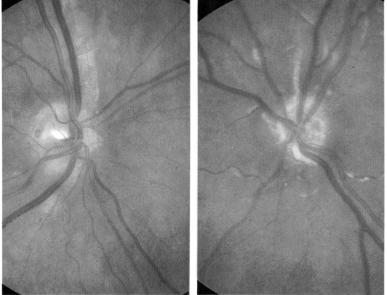

Fig. 17.14 CT scan of the same patient shows an absence of the septum pellucidum so that both lateral ventricles are united into a single cavity.

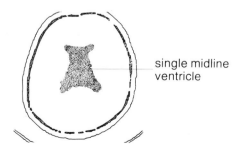

single midline ventricle

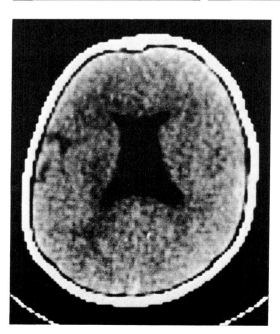

Miscellaneous Anomalies

Fig. 17.15 Optic nerve myelination is usually completed by about nine months of gestation. Myelinated fibres sometimes spread onto the surface of the disc or surrounding retina in feathery white patches which can simulate disc swelling or retinal oedema in a wide variety of patterns. The presence of myelinated nerve fibres is usually inconsequential but has been reported to be more common with neurofibromatosis.

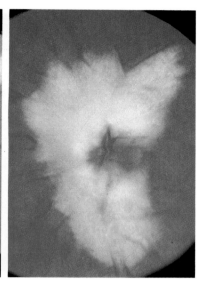

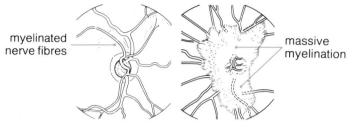

Fig. 17.16 Drusen of the disc. These opalescent excrescences are seen on the surface of the disc and/or buried in its substance and are thought to be derived from axonal debris. Typically, the retinal vessels exit centrally and branch anomalously and the disc has a swollen or full appearance with no physiological pit. These signs can be mistaken for papilloedema. Arcuate nerve fibre defects and subretinal peripapillary haemorrhages are common. In some families, drusen of the disc are inherited in an autosomal dominant manner (they have no relationship to colloid bodies of the retina). There are increased associations between drusen of the disc and both retinitis pigmentosa and angioid streaks.

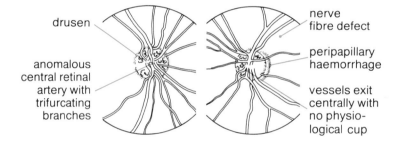

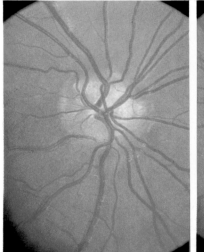
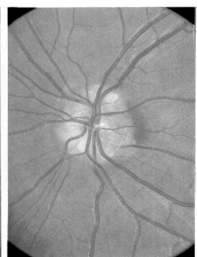

Fig. 17.17 When viewed through a fundus camera prior to fluorescein angiography, exposed drusen of the disc will autofluoresce and this can be a useful diagnostic aid. Additional information can be gained from axial CT scans through the optic nerve head which will show calcification within the drusen.

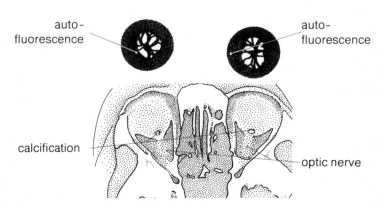

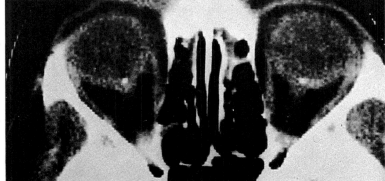

17.7

Fig. 17.18 Congenitally anomalous discs are often mistakenly thought to be pathologically swollen. The discs are of normal size with no physiological cup and the vessels exit centrally in an anomalous pattern. On the retina there is congenital tortuosity, largely affecting retinal veins, with typical reverse loops pointing backwards towards the disc, a sign of their congenital aetiology.

The retinal nerve fibres are not swollen and do not cover the vessels: furthermore, the superficial vascular plexus on the disc is not dilated.

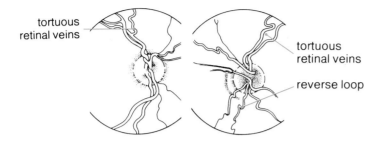

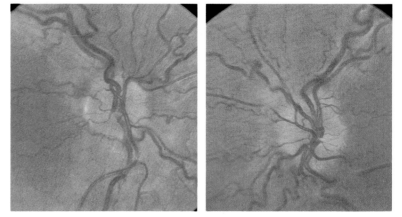

REFRACTIVE ANOMALIES

The axial length and size of the eye will also influence the size and shape of the optic disc. Hypermetropic eyes are smaller in size than normal and consequently, optic discs are frequently smaller and have a crowded or 'full' appearance that can suggest swelling.

Myopic discs are large and surrounded by a white crescent of bare sclera on the temporal side, occasionally with some pigmentation along the border. The physiological pit is normally broad and shallow and the disc tends to be paler than in emmetropic eyes. These findings can mask glaucomatous changes from the unwary. The physiological pit in hypermetropia is usually small or absent but there are no haemorrhages or dilated capillaries on the disc and retinoscopy gives the clue to the underlying aetiology. Fluorescein angiography can be confusing as these discs sometimes show mild hyperfluorescence.

Fig. 17.19 The appearance of the optic discs in a patient with + 6D of hypermetropia in each eye. The discs are small and full with a crowded nerve fibre pattern.

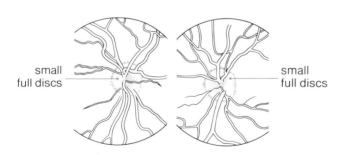

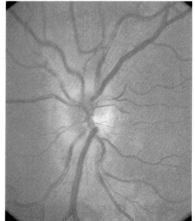

Fig. 17.20 A myopic disc. There is associated peripapillary atrophy and a temporal crescent. Because of the larger intraocular surface area, the retinal pigment epithelium and choroid appear to be thinned and pale and sometimes the temporal retinal vessels are stretched into a posterior pole staphyloma.

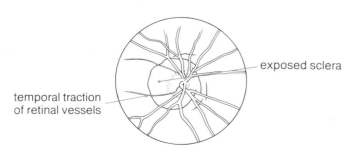

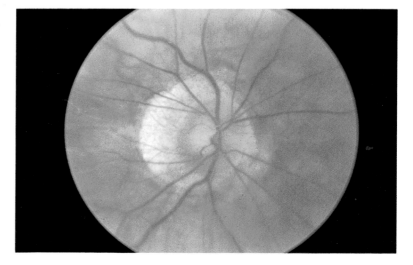

Fig. 17.21 Histology shows that the retinal aperture is larger than the scleral aperture of the optic disc with a deficiency of retina and choroid on the temporal side revealing the bare sclera. There is temporal traction of the blood vessels caused by the stretching or pulling of the retina into the expanded posterior pole of the eye.

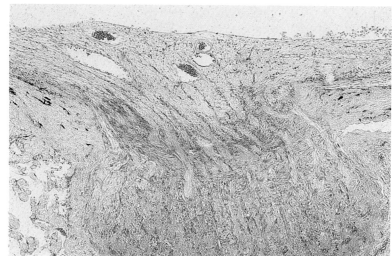

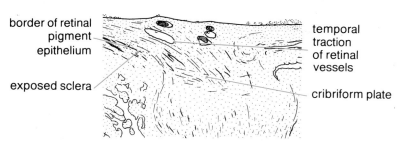

border of retinal pigment epithelium

exposed sclera

temporal traction of retinal vessels

cribriform plate

THE PATHOLOGICALLY SWOLLEN OPTIC DISC

PAPILLOEDEMA

It is almost always impossible to determine the aetiology of pathological optic disc swelling merely from the appearance of the disc. Accurate diagnosis depends upon eliciting the concurrent history and physical signs. Any patient with suspected optic disc swelling needs a careful history and examination of visual acuity, refraction, colour vision, pupillary responses, ocular movements, and visual fields of both eyes before making a diagnosis. Today, the term papilloedema implies optic disc swelling due to raised intracranial pressure and, while CT scanning has made many of the more dangerous neuroradiological investigations unnecessary, the diagnosis still retains serious implications. Early papilloedema is difficult to diagnose and the optic disc should be carefully scrutinized with white and 'red-free' light (which shows vascular and nerve fibre detail more easily) to look for swelling of the retinal nerve fibres at the disc, dilatation of the superficial capillary plexus, and the presence of haemorrhages in the surrounding nerve fibre layer. The presence of retinal folds, (Paton's folds), choroidal folds, venous dilatation and shunts, absence of venous pulsation, and the size of the optic disc itself are all important features in distinguishing pathological swelling from pseudopapilloedema.

Papilloedema itself does not produce visual symptoms other than transient obscurations of vision until very late in its course. Obscurations are episodes of unilateral or bilateral visual loss lasting a few seconds during which the patient notices a greying out of vision which rapidly returns to normal. They are sometimes related to bending, straining or a Valsalva manoeuvre. Prolonged papilloedema leads to nerve fibre destruction and field loss but visual acuity is not usually affected until the terminal stages. At this point, relief of CSF pressure sometimes seems to hasten visual loss. Papilloedema may be subdivided on descriptive grounds into early, acute decompensated, chronic or terminal.

Early Papilloedema

Fig. 17.22 The earliest histological feature seen in any swollen disc is axonal dilatation following hold-up of orthograde axoplasmic transport in the retinal neurones as they pass through the cribriform plate. Axoplasmic transport is a complex traffic of intracellular organelles from the cell nucleus to the synapse (orthograde) or vice-versa (retrograde) transport.

Vascular engorgement and oedema add to the swelling but the initial changes are found in the nerve fibres. The precise mechanism causing these changes is not fully understood but probably consists of a mixture of hypoxic, mechanical, and vascular factors (stained with Masson Blue).

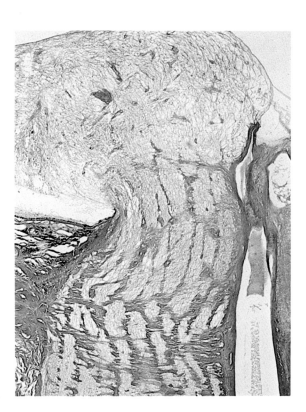

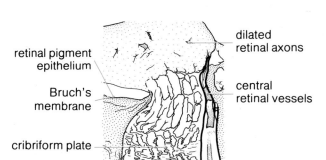

retinal pigment epithelium

Bruch's membrane

cribriform plate

dilated retinal axons

central retinal vessels

Fig. 17.23 This patient illustrates the earliest changes seen in papilloedema as the nerve fibre detail is clearly seen against the background of the negroid fundus. There is an apparent dilatation of the retinal axons in each eye (more so in the right), retinal folds (Paton's folds) adjacent to the right disc, and a tiny haemorrhage into the nerve

fibre layer of the right eye. Papilloedema usually affects both optic discs, although not always to the same extent. When visible venous pulsation is present on the disc, this suggests that the CSF pressure is not raised above 200mm Hg but this is by no means a conclusive physical sign.

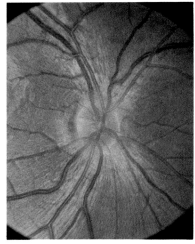
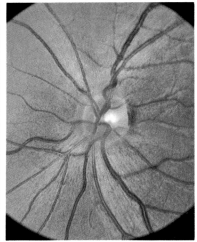

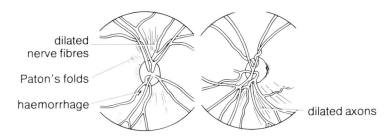

Fig. 17.24 The details of the right optic disc of this patient are seen more clearly by viewing the disc with a green or 'red-free' light which enhances the vascular and nerve fibre changes, (magnification x 2). There is some loss in clarity of the nasal disc margin but at this stage nerve fibre dilatation does not mask the larger retinal vessels. While these nerve fibre changes might be missed

or thought to be within the normal limits, the presence of tiny haemorrhages indicates a pathological process. Fluorescein angiography of the right optic disc in the early stages of the run showed the dilated capillary network on the surface of the disc. The haemorrhage masks background fluorescence. Late-phase angiograms showed mild hyper-fluorescence of the disc.

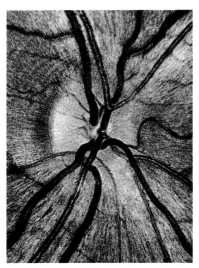
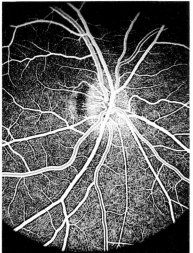

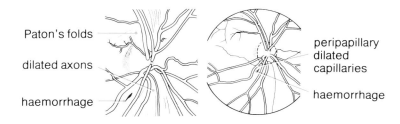

Fig. 17.25 CT scan of the same patient revealed a large enhancing pinealoma with dilatation of the third and lateral ventricles (the patient also had signs of Parinaud's syndrome). This patient had a marked disparity between the optic disc appearances and the extent of the intracranial pathology. The degree of papilloedema is influenced by the severity, rate of increase, and duration of the CSF pressure rise as well as local factors at the optic disc itself.

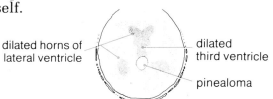

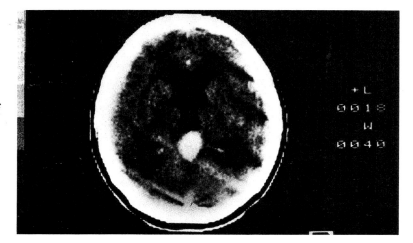

Fig. 17.26 The early changes of papilloedema are more obvious here. Dilatation of the nerve fibre bundles is clearly seen together with superficial haemorrhages and some masking of the retinal vessels. The discs are hyperaemic with blurred margins.

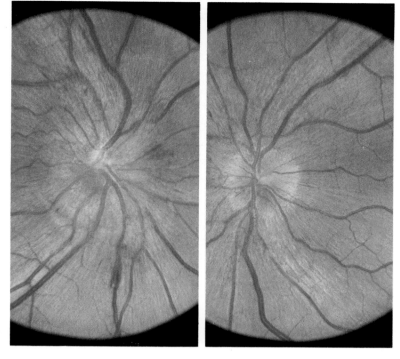

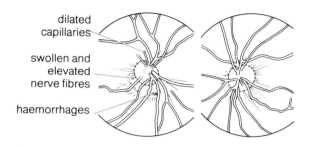

Acute Decompensated Papilloedema

Fig. 17.27 Both discs are grossly swollen with dilated nerve fibres masking the blood vessels at the disc borders. This patient had a posterior fossa tumour. There are haemorrhages into the nerve fibre layer around the disc and cotton-wool spots on the disc surface. These are signs that the patient has suffered a rapid rise in intracranial pressure. The optic cup is still preserved.

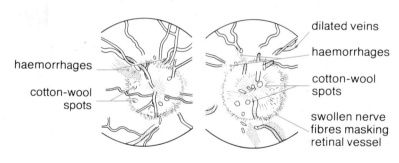

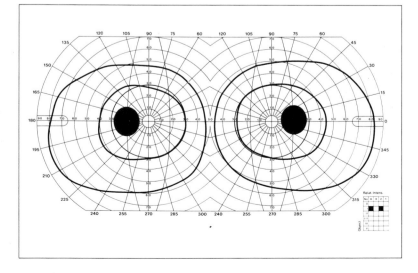

Fig. 17.28 Acute papilloedema is associated with a full visual field and normal visual acuities and colour vision. The blind spots are enlarged probably as a result of crowding and masking of photoreceptors by swollen nerve fibres. This is of no diagnostic importance, however, as it correlates with the visual appearances of the disc.

17.11

Chronic Papilloedema

Fig. 17.29 A more insidious onset of raised intracranial pressure produced grossly swollen discs in this patient who had benign intracranial hypertension of many months duration prior to diagnosis. There are fewer haemorrhages and cotton-wool spots as the retinal vasculature had had time to compensate.

The physiological cups are still preserved. Papilloedema never extends to involve the macula.

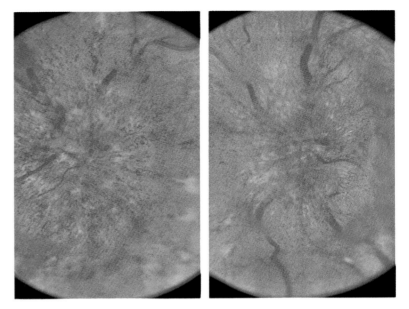

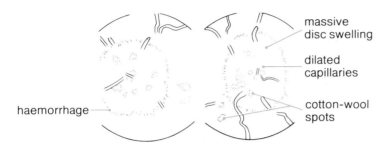

Fig. 17.30 Fluorescein angiography demonstrates the dilated capillary plexus on the surface of the right optic disc together with extensive deep leakage in the late stages of the angiogram spreading into the adjacent arcuate regions just off the disc.

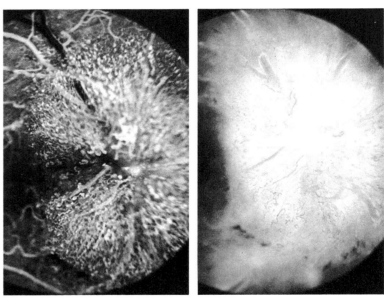

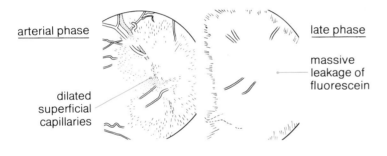

Fig. 17.31 Prolonged increased CSF pressure dilates the subarachnoid space and expands the optic nerve sheath. The axial and coronal orbital scans of this patient show the optic nerve sheath to be enlarged in diameter and more tortuous than normal. High resolution CT scanning following injection of metrisamide (a water-soluble contrast medium) will show that the enlargement in nerve diameter is due to a dilatation of the subarachnoid space.

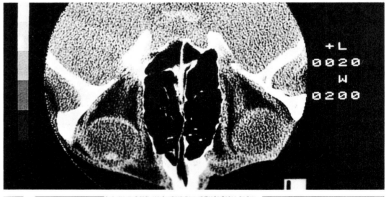

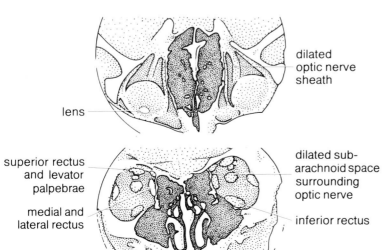

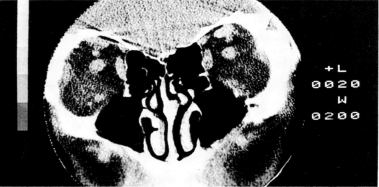

Fig. 17.32 The patient's intracranial pressure remained elevated for several months despite treatment. The disc swelling began to subside; the cotton-wool spots and haemorrhages absorbed and signs of optic atrophy appeared. There are signs of chronic papilloedema, such as choroidal folds, and relative pallor of the right optic disc has appeared indicating nerve fibre loss. There is also some attenuation of the retinal arteries which is often seen after prolonged papilloedema.

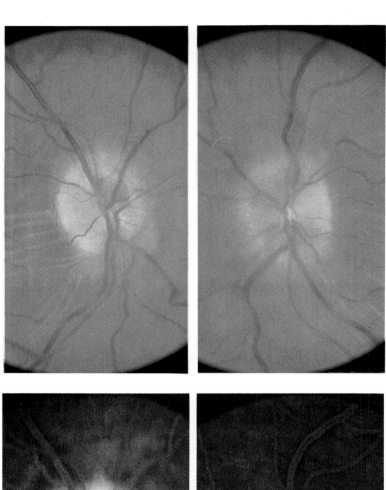

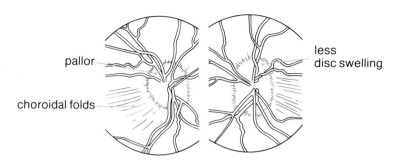

Fig. 17.33 Fluorescein angiography now shows less leakage of dye in each disc than Fig. 17.30.
The hypofluorescent choroidal folds are easily seen in the left eye, a sign of prolonged papilloedema. In the right eye there is a disturbance of the pigment epithelium surrounding the disc, possibly due to previously present subretinal fluid associated with the massive swelling.

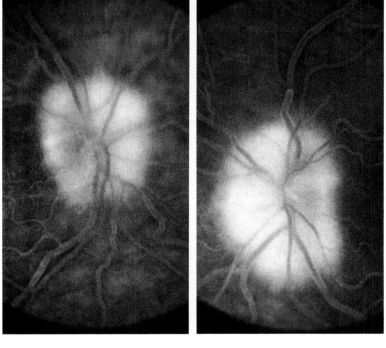

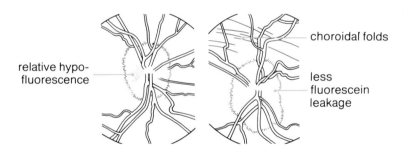

Fig. 17.34 At this stage, the left eye still retains a full field of vision but the blind spot is less enlarged, corresponding to the reduced disc swelling. The right visual field shows changes characteristic of chronic papilloedema with an enlarged blind spot, arcuate nerve fibre defects, and peripheral constriction correlating with the disc pallor and destruction of nerve fibres: the patient's visual acuities were normal. With further uncontrolled CSF pressure, the arcuate fibre defects and peripheral constriction would coalesce to constrict the visual field to tunnel vision.

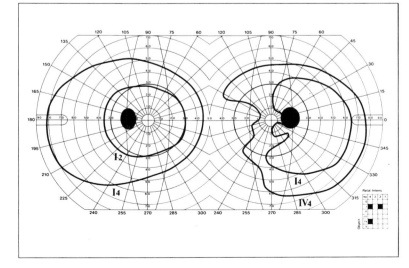

17.13

Fig. 17.35 Sustained intracranial pressure over a prolonged period eventually leads to pallid swollen discs with tiny opalescent excrescences on the disc surface. Nerve fibre damage can now be seen and the opalescent areas probably represent debris from axonal destruction. These discs sometimes have a superficial appearance similar to drusen of the disc.

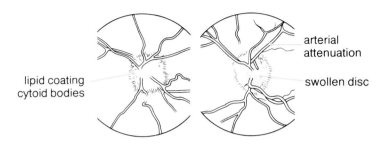

lipid coating
cytoid bodies

arterial attenuation

swollen disc

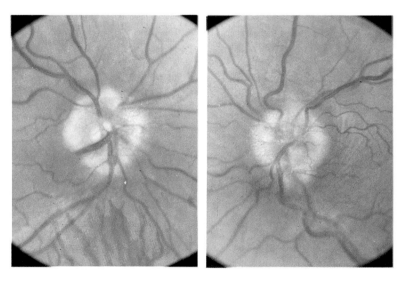

Optociliary venous shunts are present (a sign that there has been chronic swelling of the disc), removing blood from the retinal circulation to lower pressure in the choroidal circulation, leaving the eye by the vortex veins. The visual fields will be grossly and irreversibly constricted with poor visual acuity. The visual prognosis is hopeless regardless of treatment.

Fig. 17.36 Terminal atrophic papilloedema results from prolonged raised CSF pressure. Nerve fibres are eventually destroyed and the optic disc, without viable nerve fibres, does not swell. (If there are no axons left, there can be no hold-up of axoplasmic transport). This mentally retarded patient had long-standing benign intracranial hypertension. The discs are pale, slightly swollen, and there is some arterial attenuation.

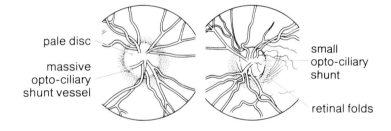

pale disc

massive opto-ciliary shunt vessel

small opto-ciliary shunt

retinal folds

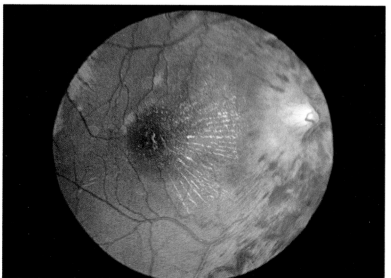

Fig. 17.37 Papilloedema with a macular star. This is one of the few occasions when papilloedema is accompanied by decreased visual acuity. Macular stars are the result of leakage of plasma lipids from a swollen optic disc and are sometimes seen with either chronic papilloedema or resolving disc swelling following treatment. The lipid exudate lies within the radiating nerve fibres of Henle surrounding the macula and is usually more marked on the nasal side.

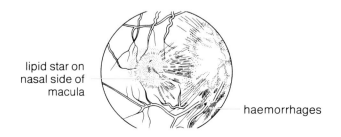

lipid star on nasal side of macula

haemorrhages

PAPILLITIS

This condition describes swelling of the optic disc caused by local inflammation of the optic nerve head. It is accompanied by signs of optic nerve damage — reduced visual acuity, colour desaturation, an afferent pupillary defect, and a central scotoma in the visual field. Disc swelling resulting from papillitis cannot be distinguished by its appearance from that due to other causes although it is usually less florid.

Papillitis is usually acute, unilateral and is most commonly seen in young adults and children. In the acute stages it is associated with retrobulbar pain, tenderness, and pain on ocular movement although these symptoms are usually less dramatic than when seen with acute retrobulbar neuritis. Papillitis occasionally follows viral respiratory infections or the exanthemata: these tend to recover and have a benign visual and neurological prognosis. There are many other causes of the disease but in young adults multiple sclerosis is probably the most common. Retrobulbar neuritis, in which the plaque of demyelination lies within the optic nerve and the optic disc is initially normal, is a more common presentation of this disease.

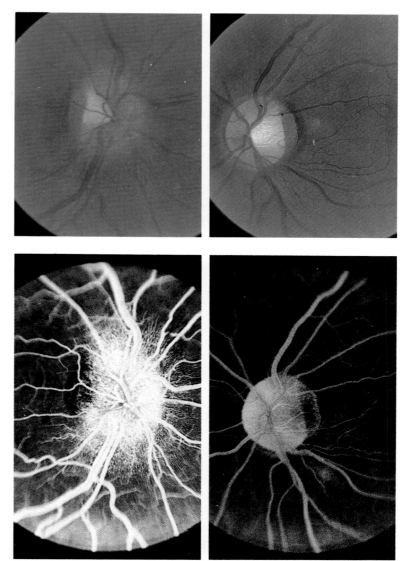

Fig. 17.38 This twenty-five-year-old girl has a normal left optic disc and swelling of the right with haemorrhages into the nerve fibre layer. In the right eye, acuity was reduced to counting fingers, colour vision was lost, and there was some pain and tenderness on ocular movement.

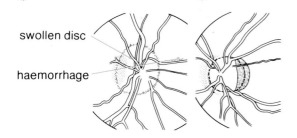

Fig. 17.39 The disc swelling is demonstrated by fluorescein angiography. Although the swelling is usually not severe, it is impossible to distinguish between papillitis and papilloedema by either fluorescein angiography or ophthalmoscopy and the differentiation is made by finding signs of optic nerve damage. Papillitis occasionally produces a mild inflammatory vitreous infiltrate. Sheathing of retinal equatorial veins has been reported in a minority of cases of acute retrobulbar neuritis; these are known as Rucker's lines.

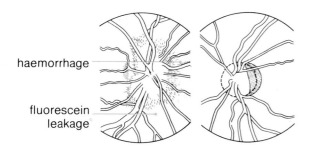

Fig. 17.40 The left visual field is normal, the right has a large central scotoma. This can be easily demonstrated at the bedside by using a red target and a confrontation visual field to show central desaturation. The visual evoked response will show a slight reduction in amplitude with considerable delay of the waveform.

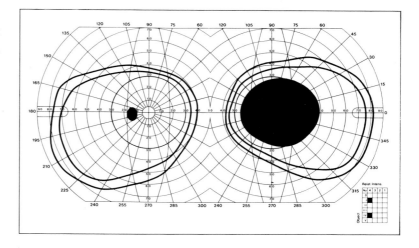

Fig. 17.41 The swelling of the right optic disc subsided over a period of several weeks. The vision improved to 6/6 with colour perception and the afferent pupillary defect returned almost to normal. Two years later, the patient developed papillitis in the left eye in addition to signs of multiple sclerosis in the spinal pathways. The majority of patients with retrobulbar neuritis eventually develop other signs of multiple sclerosis with varying degrees of severity.

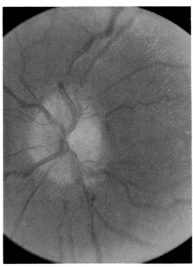
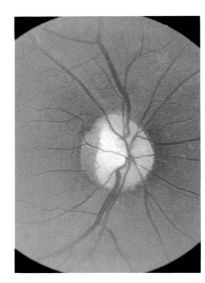

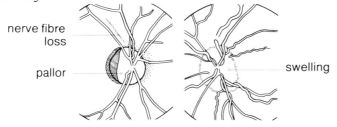

Fig. 17.42 The appearance of the optic disc and the presence of disc oedema depend upon the location of the plaque of demyelination and inflammation in the optic nerve. Plaques of demyelination proximal to the disc will not cause disc oedema and are known as retrobulbar optic neuritis. This patient had chronic multiple sclerosis and the chiasm and posterior parts of the optic nerves are involved with gross plaques of demyelination. (PTA stain for glia, paler areas are demyelinated.)

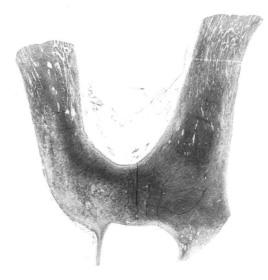

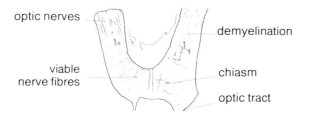

ISCHAEMIC PAPILLOPATHY

The optic disc receives its blood supply from the short posterior ciliary arteries. Acute obstruction of these arteries will produce a unilateral infarcted disc which is pale and swollen with surrounding nerve fibre haemorrhages. For some unknown reason this tends to occur segmentally with the superior hemisphere of the disc being most commonly affected. The inferior hemisphere of the disc can be compromised by the adjacent infarct and its oedema and sometimes appears to have more hyperaemia and more florid swelling. This produces asymmetrical disc swelling where the

orthograde axoplasmic flow is arrested. The aetiology of ischaemic papillopathy is unknown but it seems to be more common in atherosclerotic or hypertensive individuals. Occasionally, however, vasculitis or migraine can be the underlying factor. Patients typically present in late middle-age with sudden painless loss of vision in one eye. If macula fibres are damaged, acuity is lost as well. The vision sometimes deteriorates further over a few days as a result of oedematous compression of the remaining viable nerve fibres. There is no effective treatment.

Fig. 17.43 The left optic disc of this sixty-five year old man shows asymmetrical pallid swelling with more hyperaemia and oedema inferiorly where the viable nerve fibres are compromised. The fluorescein angiogram demonstrates the relative avascularity of the superior hemisphere of the disc.

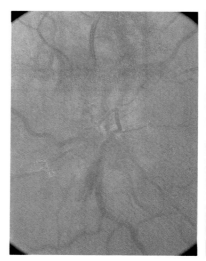
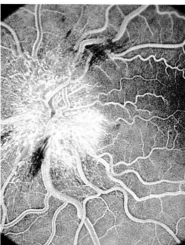

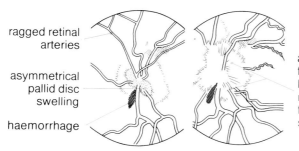

Fig. 17.44 Ischaemic papillopathy produces a characteristic inferior altitudinal field defect which can be most helpful in making the diagnosis. Acuity will be lost if macula fibres are involved.

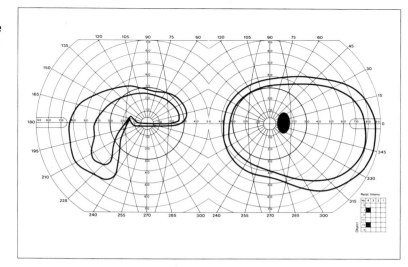

Fig. 17.45 The disc swelling of this patient subsided over a few weeks leaving asymmetrical disc pallor. The field defect remained unchanged. Macular stars are frequently seen in the resolving stage and the fluorescein angiogram clearly demonstrates segmental filling defects in the disc circulation. Changes in the arteriole calibre are also evident. There is a substantial risk of the fellow eye being affected subsequently.

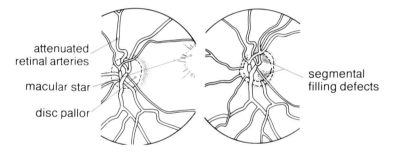

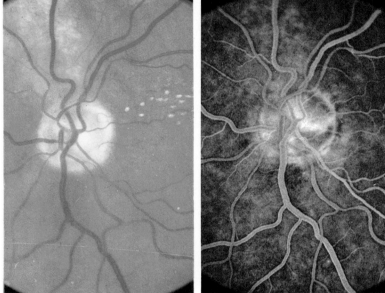

Ischaemic Papillopathy due to Temporal Arteritis

Temporal arteritis must be considered in any person over fifty-five years of age who presents with sudden loss of vision and the clinical appearances of ischaemic papillopathy.

Fig. 17.46 The temporal arteries of this lady were tender, inflamed, and non pulsatile, but frequently the signs are more subtle. The diagnosis is suggested by finding a high erythrocyte sedimentation rate (ESR) and confirmed by temporal artery biopsy. Prompt treatment with steroids is required as there is a grave risk of involvement of the fellow eye or development of a cerebral stroke.

In making this diagnosis, it is helpful to search for a history of characteristic temporal headaches, neckache or stiffness, jaw claudication, malaise, or weight loss in addition to polymyalgia.

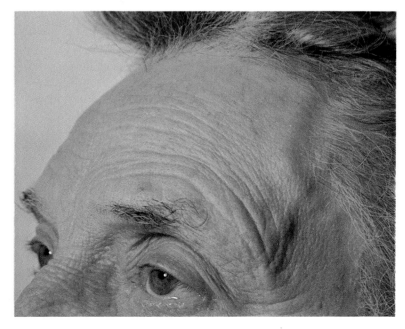

17.17

Fig. 17.47 The optic disc of this elderly lady who suddenly lost vision in the right eye, is completely infarcted, pale, and slightly swollen. The fluorescein angiogram in the venous phase shows delayed filling of the optic disc and peripapillary circulations due to involvement of the short posterior ciliary arteries with some leakage of dye into the optic disc. Central retinal artery occlusion does occur but is uncommon in temporal arteritis.

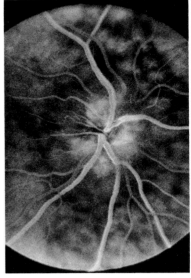

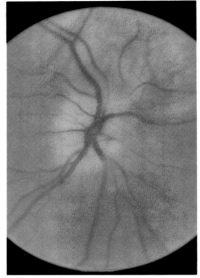

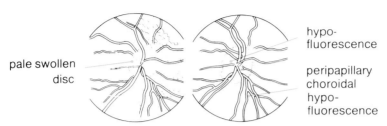

Fig. 17.48 Temporal artery biopsy within the first forty-eight hours following presentation is essential to confirm the diagnosis as the histological picture may be difficult to interpret following steroid therapy. These elderly patients may need prolonged steroid therapy to control the arteritis and side effects of treatment are common.
The biopsy of this patient shows inflammatory changes throughout the entire arterial wall but these are mainly concentrated in the media with fragmentation of the internal elastic lamina, multinucleated giant cells, and occlusion of the lumen. Skip lesions can occur and it is necessary to examine sections over several millimetres of the vessel to exclude this possibility. It is important to take the surgical specimen with care since rough handling can make pathological interpretation difficult. If the biopsy is negative in suspicious circumstances, an additional biopsy of the other temporal artery may sometimes be positive.

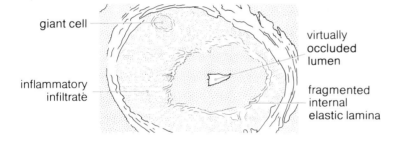

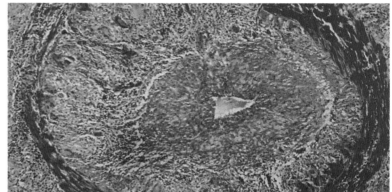

JUXTAPAPILLARY CHOROIDITIS
The aetiology of juxtapapillary choroiditis is the same as that of choroiditis elsewhere in the eye. Congenital toxoplasmosis is by far the most common cause especially if there is evidence of previous chorioretinal scarring.

Fig. 17.49 This optic disc appears swollen from a combination of inflammatory chorioretinal exudate, oedema, and axoplasmic stasis inferiorly. The patient presented with poor vision, a superior arcuate field defect, and a marked cellular vitreous infiltrate in this eye.
The fluorescein angiogram demonstrates leakage of dye from the disc spreading along the retinal vessels — a sign of intraocular inflammation.

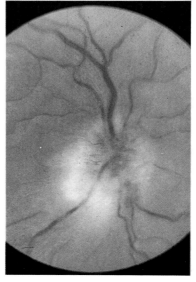

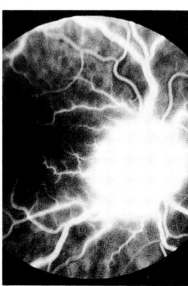

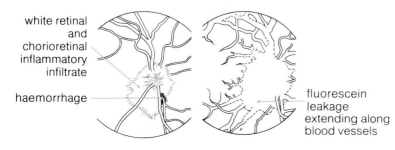

OPTIC DISC INFILTRATION

The optic disc occasionally becomes infiltrated by a lymphoma, metastasis or granuloma. With disc swelling of obscure aetiology it is important to search for a vitreous cellular infiltration or peripheral vasculitic lesions in the retina. Visual acuity and field loss can vary but the usual pattern is one of poor acuity with a central scotoma.

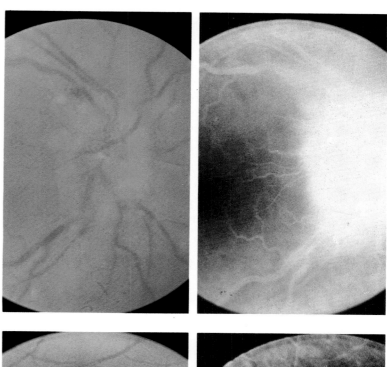

Fig. 17.50 This patient with sarcoidosis has a swollen disc which appears blurred due to vitreous cellular infiltration. The fluorescein angiogram shows disc leakage and periphlebitis, consistent with intraocular inflammation. Macular oedema may be present although it is not apparent in this example.

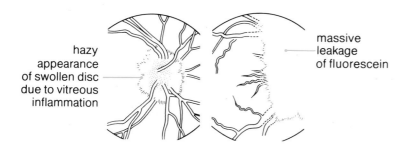

hazy appearance of swollen disc due to vitreous inflammation

massive leakage of fluorescein

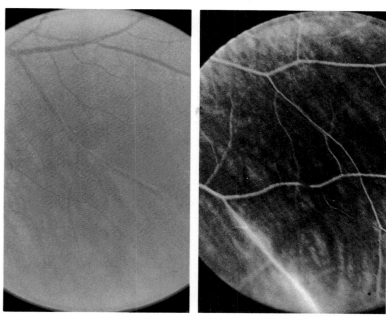

Fig. 17.51 The same patient has peripheral equatorial periphlebitis, confirming the inflammatory origin of the optic disc swelling and suggesting investigations for systemic causes of retinal vasculitis such as sarcoid, Behcet's disease, systemic lupus erythematosis, or multiple sclerosis.

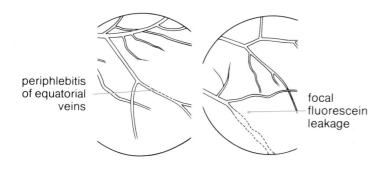

periphlebitis of equatorial veins

focal fluorescein leakage

Fig. 17.52 A large sarcoid granuloma is seen lying within the optic nerve head. Optic disc swelling with posterior uveitis is not uncommon and is due to local infiltration or oedema and vascular engorgement, which will resolve as the inflammation regresses sometimes with signs of optic atrophy. On rare occasions, the disc swelling can be marked and the inflammatory signs mild, so that papilloedema is mistakenly diagnosed.

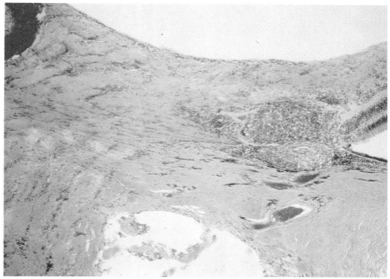

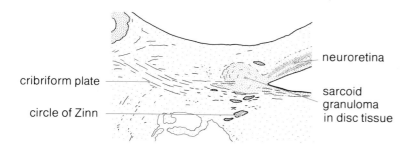

cribriform plate

circle of Zinn

neuroretina

sarcoid granuloma in disc tissue

ACUTE LEBER'S OPTIC ATROPHY

This fascinating and rare condition affects young men and, occasionally, elderly females in a familial fashion, without conforming to a recognised pattern of inheritance. Affected individuals do not appear to transmit the condition to their children and this has raised the question of a cytoplasmic mode of inheritance. Patients present with uniocular visual loss of rapid onset and signs of an optic nerve lesion. The fellow eye follows the same course soon afterwards.

Fig. 17.53 Potential carriers of the disease can often be diagnosed by their anomalous optic discs which appear to be full and slightly swollen with telangiectatic capillaries that characteristically do not leak fluorescein, and retinal arteries which are often more tortuous than usual. Some unknown factor seems to precipitate acute decompensation and further swelling.

In this patient, disc swelling subsided and six weeks later the disc is becoming pale. There is loss of nerve fibres and the vascular dilatation has diminished. Treatment with massive doses of hydroxycobalamin and steroids is controversial. Vision has a tendency to improve slowly many years after the initial attack.

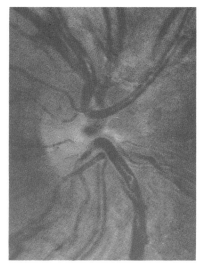
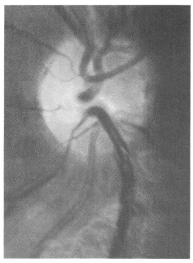

teleangiectatic vessel

hyperaemic disc

prominent nerve fibres

vascular dilation

loss of macula nerve fibres

vessels less dilated

TUMOURS OF THE OPTIC DISC

These are rare and usually benign but can cause diagnostic problems. They are diagnosed on their morphology. Optic disc tumours usually arise locally within the disc itself — a metastasis to the optic disc is extremely rare and patients with carcinomatous optic neuropathy usually have normal or pale discs. Invasion of the optic disc can be seen with a retinoblastoma or choroidal melanoma and is a firm indication to enucleate the eye.

Melanocytoma

Fig. 17.54 Melanocytoma is a densely pigmented benign naevus which is usually situated in the inferior part of the disc and is more commonly found in dark-skinned people. The disc is usually larger than normal. The lesion may increase in size slowly and protrude into the vitreous or spread out onto the retina, in which case differentiation from a malignant melanoma of the choroid can be exceptionally difficult. Field defects can occur although visual acuity is not normally affected. Fluorescein angiography shows no intratumour circulation.

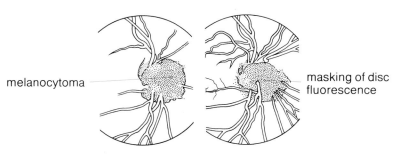

melanocytoma

masking of disc fluorescence

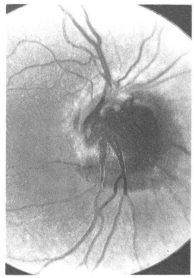
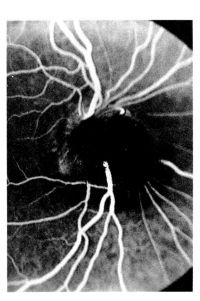

Fig. 17.55 The deeply pigmented cells form a well-circumscribed lesion with no invasion of the disc tissue. The cells are uniform and densely pigmented.

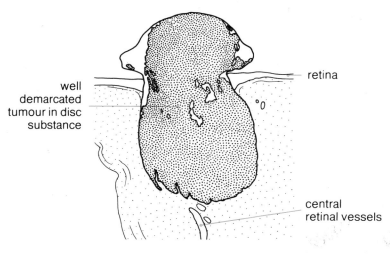

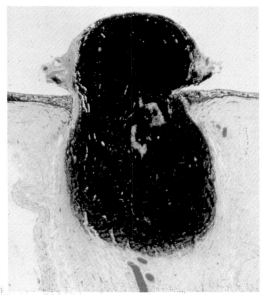

well demarcated tumour in disc substance

retina

central retinal vessels

Astrocytic Hamartoma

While astrocytic hamartomas are often found in patients with tuberous sclerosis, they can also occur independently of the disease. Patients and relatives must be carefully examined for other signs of skin or cerebral involvement of this autosomal dominant condition which has a very variable phenotype.

Fig. 17.56 This is a typical nodular white mulberry tumour arising from the superficial retina. Multiple lesions are not uncommon and can sometimes be mistaken for a retinoblastoma in a child. The tumours can be observed to grow slowly over many years often beginning as a greyish opalescent thickening of the nerve fibre layer which becomes raised and pearly white; intra-tumour calcification is common. The lesions have also been described inappropriately as 'giant drusen'.

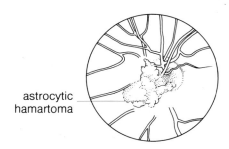

astrocytic hamartoma

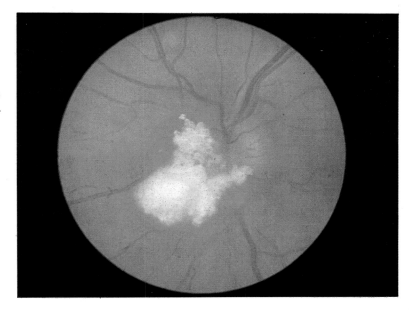

Fig. 17.57 Histology shows this peripapillary tumour to be composed of astrocytes derived from the superficial retina. Areas of bluish calcification can be seen within the tumour.

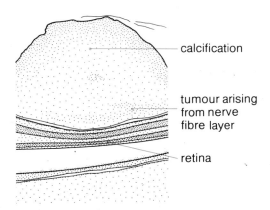

calcification

tumour arising from nerve fibre layer

retina

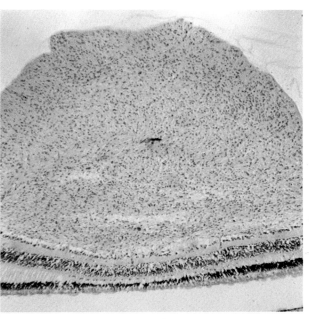

17.21

Pigment Epithelial Hamartoma

Fig. 17.58 Benign pigment epithelial hamartoma is a rare congenital condition in which the optic disc is swollen by mottled pigmented tissue derived from the pigment epithelium. This spreads onto the surrounding retina, sometimes causing traction and retinal folds. There are greyish vitreous condensations on the surface. Patients present as young adults with poor vision; the tumour growth is very slow.

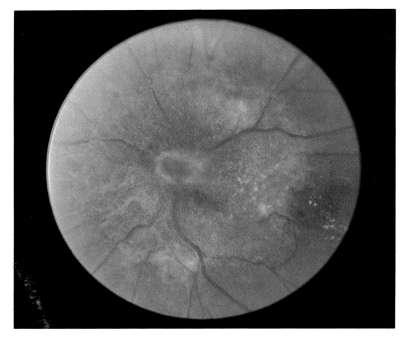

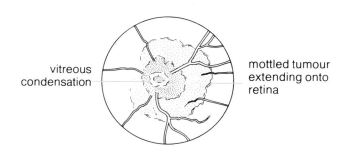

Fig. 17.59 Fluorescein angiography demonstrates the vessels within the tumour substance which leak as the angiogram progresses.

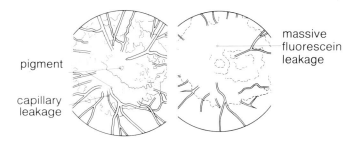

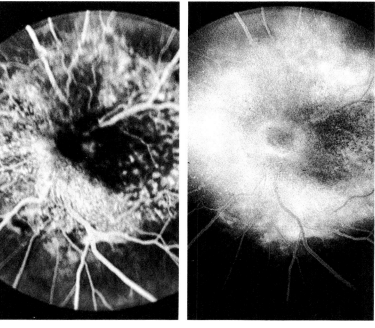

Capillary Angioma

Fig. 17.60 Capillary angioma is another rare benign hamartomous lesion. Slightly elevated pinkish tissue spreads from the disc inferiorly, containing fine blood vessels which leak on the fluorescein angiogram. These lesions can be mistaken for a neoplastic infiltration of the disc.

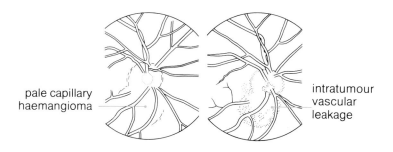

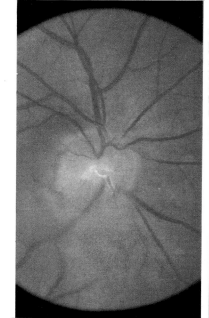

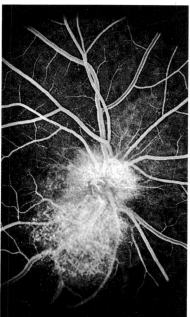

18. Strabismus

P. Fells

J. P. Lee

Introduction

Defects of ocular motility constitute a large proportion of ophthalmic problems. It has been estimated that two percent of the population have a manifest strabismus, four percent have no demonstrable stereoscopic vision (suggesting a primary defect of binocular vision) and the vast majority of children admitted to ophthalmic units have strabismus that requires surgery for functional or cosmetic reasons. Increased awareness of the importance of early diagnosis of strabismus and prompt treatment has greatly helped in the prevention of amblyopia, a defect of visual acuity reversible in the vast majority of cases, but which may cause severe disability in later years if the patient loses the non-amblyopic eye as a result of disease or injury.

In this chapter, a general overview of concomitant strabismus and its variants will be described. Methods of examination and measurement are not discussed in detail but instead, the emphasis has been placed on clinical methods which require the minimum of equipment and give reliable results. Details of surgical techniques are not described and surgical methods are only discussed where they illustrate the principles of management.

DEFINITIONS

Strabismus (squint) is present when the foveas of both eyes are not simultaneously aligned on the object of regard. For distance fixation, this is equivalent to non-parallelism of the visual axes. Strabismus may be classified on the direction of the deviation; if the visual axes converge there is eso-deviation; if they diverge, there is exo-deviation; if the visual axes differ in vertical direction, there is a hyper- or hypo-deviation, depending on whether the eye described is higher or lower than its fellow. The globes may rotate about vertical and horizontal axes and torsional movements are also possible. Torsional strabismus may be categorized as incyclotorsional or excyclotorsional. It will be seen that for cyclovertical deviations it is necessary to define the eye with the deviation, since a right hypertropia is equivalent (under most circumstances) to a left hypotropia.

Strabismus may be concomitant, that is when the angle of deviation remains constant (or nearly so) whatever the position of gaze; or incomitant, when the angle of deviation varies with the gaze direction. Incomitant deviations are generally associated with ocular muscle paresis or mechanical restriction of rotation of the globe.

Strabismus may be manifest; a 'tropia', if the deviation is present with both eyes open – or latent; a 'phoria', when the deviation may only be demonstrable when the eyes are dissociated and the binocular visual reflexes are disrupted.

Associations of Strabismus

Fig. 18.1 A number of circumstances are associated with a higher than expected incidence of strabismus and it is essential to obtain a careful history of these from the parents at the first interview. These factors include difficulties during pregnancy, birth trauma of various types, or a history of squint in other members of the family. Children who have other congenital anomalies, cerebral palsy, mental retardation from any cause, or metabolic diseases all have a high risk of strabismus. Strabismus occurs more commonly in a child with poor health (as in cystic fibrosis, for example), or may be seen first after a particularly severe illness or injury.

Associations of Concomitant Strabismus

problems during pregnancy,
e.g., intrauterine infections, prematurity, dysmaturity

birth trauma,
e.g., forceps, breech delivery, Caesarian section etc.

family history of squint

congenital anomalies, mental retardation, chromosomal defects, cerebral palsy etc.

poor general health, severe intercurrent infections

other ocular defect or disease

Fig. 18.2 In the vast majority of cases, strabismus is not associated with ocular or neurological disease. However, any condition which prevents the formation of a clear retinal image, such as high refractive errors, ptosis, maldevelopment of the eye, or intraocular disease in childhood may cause strabismus. The most serious example of this is shown by this child with strabismus and leucocoria from a retinoblastoma.

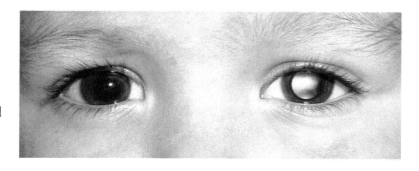

Pseudo-strabismus

Fig. 18.3 'Pseudo-strabismus' may cause diagnostic problems. Causes include epicanthus, wide interpupillary distance, unilateral myopia, exophthalmos, facial asymmetry, and variation in angles alpha or kappa. These conditions are deceptive and strabismus has to be excluded by a carefully performed cover test.

Causes of Pseudostrabismus

epicanthus	facial asymmetry
wide interpupillary distance	variation of angle alpha or kappa
unilateral myopia and exophthalmos	

Fig. 18.4 Epicanthus is by far the most common cause of misdiagnosed convergent strabismus. It is common in both Caucasian and Oriental babies and leads to a false impression of convergence. It should not be forgotten, however, that the presence of epicanthus does not exclude strabismus, as demonstrated in the lower photograph showing esotropia.

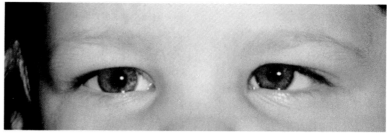

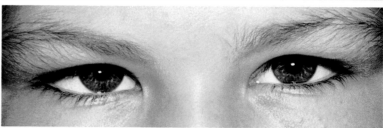

Fig. 18.5 The line which exactly bisects the eye in the antero-posterior direction does not necessarily run through the fovea. In the average eye, the fovea is displaced slightly to the temporal side and the angle between the geometric axis and the visual axis (line of sight) is called angle alpha. An easier angle to estimate clinically is angle kappa, where the line normal to the centre of the cornea intersects the visual axis.

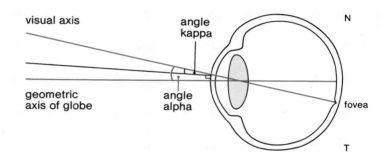

Fig. 18.6 When the fovea lies temporal to the geometric axis the angle alpha is said to be positive, and if the fovea lies nasally the angle is said to be negative. A large positive angle alpha gives an impression of divergent strabismus, as in this child, whereas a negative angle simulates a convergent deviation, despite the fact that in each case, the foveas are used for simultaneous fixation. The only way to distinguish between apparent and real strabismus is by means of the cover test (cf. Fig. 18.10).

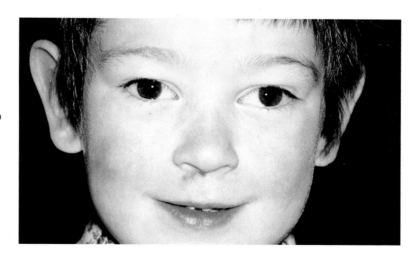

DETECTION OF STRABISMUS
Clues to Diagnosis

Patients with strabismus sometimes exhibit associated signs, the most common of which are various types of abnormal head posture. Not all of these abnormal head postures are adopted for ocular reasons but when they are they frequently enable the patient to achieve a limited area of binocular vision. It is advisable to note the head posture before commenting upon it, as the patient may have learnt to control any abnormality in the interest of his appearance. A child may have been told 'hold your head straight' by its parents and only manifest the diagnostic head posture in the waiting room. In adult patients with symptoms of diplopia and ocular muscle underaction, childhood photographs showing an abnormal head posture can help to establish the diagnosis of decompensation and breakdown of a previously controlled deviation and save much time and effort on wasted neurological investigations.

Fig. 18.7 Causes of abnormal head posture.

Causes of Abnormal Head Posture

Ocular	Nonocular
maintenance of single vision e.g.,paretic squint, A and V patterns, Duane's syndrome	habitual – no detectable cause
to maximise separation of diplopia for ease of discrimination (rare)	to relieve pain
to level the subjective horizon in cyclovertical muscle weakness	skeletal abnormalities in the neck
dampening of intensity of congenital nystagmus	sternomastoid contracture secondary to birth injury
in unilateral or bilateral ptosis (chin elevation to clear visual axis)	unilateral deafness
to compensate for hemianopic field defects	vestibular disease

18.3

Fig. 18.8   When examining for the presence of an abnormal head posture it is important to have the patient standing unsupported, legs and feet together, with trunk straight and fixating on a distant target. Photography is a useful method of recording the head posture, and cover test and stereo tests should be done with and without the head posture to assess its effect. Persistence of abnormal head postures for many years may cause secondary skeletal abnormalities, e.g., scoliosis.

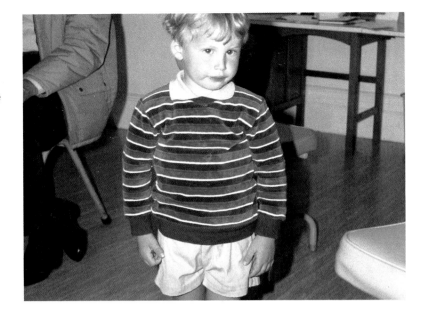

Fig. 18.9   Many patients with intermittent exotropia are seen to close one eye in bright sunlight. The cause is obscure, but family photographs often show the sign.

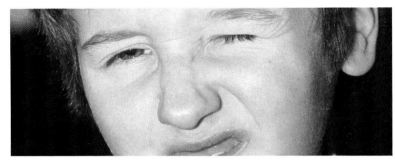

The Cover Test

A variety of methods have been devised to detect strabismus, but the most useful of these are all variants of the cover test. The principle involved in the cover test is that interruption of fixation of one eye will produce an attempt to fixate the object of regard with the other eye (unless acuity is exceptionally poor.) Observation of the fixational movements can elicit a considerable amount of useful data.

In manifest strabismus, covering the fixating eye results in a fixational movement of the fellow eye. In a latent strabismus or phoria (eg. esophoria or exophoria), the binocular fixation reflexes keep the eyes straight, despite a tendency for them to drift apart, so that in normal circumstances the eyes are straight. If the eyes are dissociated and the binocular reflexes interrupted, the eyes will tend to adopt the position of relaxation. A cover-uncover test will cause some dissociation of binocular

reflexes, and a recovery movement to take up fixation will signify a latent deviation. In many patients, however, the habit of binocularity is strong, particularly in exo-deviations, and a simple cover-uncover test will not reveal the deviation or will underestimate it. More prolonged dissociation is required. This may be achieved by the use of dissimilar images, as in the Maddox rod test, or by haploscopic devices such as the Maddox wing, but is best demonstrated by an alternate cover test. (See Fig. 18.12.)

Cover tests should be performed routinely for near and distant fixation, and with and without an associated head posture if this is present. Cover testing in different directions of gaze discloses a degree of incomitance if this is present (eg. A & V patterns) and also allows accurate measurements of the deviation to be made. If spectacles are worn, cover testing with and without them will disclose any accommodative element.

Fig. 18.10   This photograph illustrates a cover-uncover test on a patient with manifest esotropia of the right eye. The fixating eye is covered, forcing the other eye to take up fixation (an accommodative fixation target must be used which is interesting – a light is insufficient). On removing the cover, the right eye will not hold fixation, which snaps

back to the left eye. The inference is that the visual acuity of the left eye is better than that of the right eye. The speed and accuracy of the refixation movement gives information about the difference between the acuities and also shows the direction and degree of strabismus.

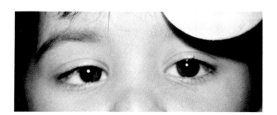
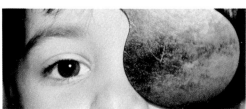
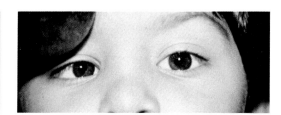

Fig. 18.11 The fixation has changed from the right to the left eye following cover, and this persists after uncover.

This is called alternation and signifies equal or nearly equal acuity in the two eyes.

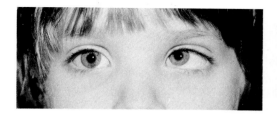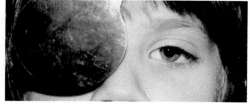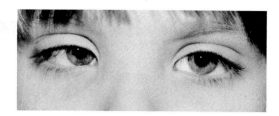

Fig. 18.12 With a latent strabismus, the eyes are normally straight but have a tendency to deviate if the binocular reflexes are interrupted. A very reliable method of detecting latent strabismus is the alternate cover test when the occluder is moved from one eye to the other without permitting binocular fixation during the test. The movement made by the freshly uncovered eye is opposite in direction to the deviation (ie., the inward movement in a latent divergent deviation or exophoria illustrated in this drawing.) Typically, the size of the movement increases during the first few uncovers and then reaches a plateau.

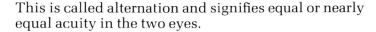

Latent Exophoria

bifoveal fixation   right occlusion

left occlusion   uncover–may be delay

Measurement of Strabismus

Clinically, there is frequently an element of latent strabismus present with a manifest strabismus and in order to measure the total deviation, it is necessary to dissociate the eyes fully and measure the angle between the visual axes. A variety of methods exist to do this, but one of the most reliable is the prism and alternate cover test (prism cover test), where an alternate cover test is performed using a graduated prism before one eye.

Fig. 18.13 In the prism cover test, the strength of the prism is increased until the eye gives no detectable recovery movement on cover testing and this is equal to the deviation which is expressed in prism dioptres or △. The test should be performed at 33 centimetres and 6 metres, and sometimes at 60 metres (for intermittent exo-deviations). If spectacles are normally worn, the test should be performed both with and without them.

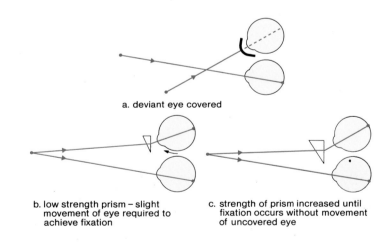

a. deviant eye covered

b. low strength prism – slight movement of eye required to achieve fixation

c. strength of prism increased until fixation occurs without movement of uncovered eye

Fig. 18.14 Some patients, either because of age or other handicap, may not fixate reliably for a prism cover test. Other patients may have a squinting eye of such poor acuity that it will not fixate on the target. Under these circumstances, a fixation light is used and the angle of strabismus can be estimated from the position of the light reflex on the strabismic eye when the reflex on the good eye is central. This is termed the Hirschberg test, and the 'rule of thumb' is that 1 mm≡7°. Therefore, with the light reflex on the limbus, the deviation is approximately 35°.

In order to obtain a more accurate measurement of the deviation in such cases, the light reflex may be centralized on the deviated eye by means of prisms placed before the fixing eye. This is known as the modified Krimsky test.

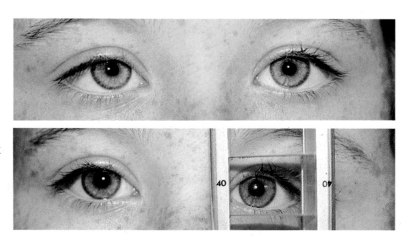

18.5

EXAMINATION OF EYE MOVEMENTS

The range of ocular movements must be tested whenever possible. Binocular conjugate movements are called versions, uniocular movements are ductions. Careful note must be taken of the range of eye movement, any signs of restriction of rotation, retraction of the globe, or abnormal lid movement.

Voluntary gaze movements, saccadic refixational movements, and pursuit movements can also be tested and these are discussed in more detail in Chapter 19 (Neuro-Ophthalmology). Vergence movements will require a suitable accommodative fixation target.

In unconscious patients, or patients with a gaze palsy, saccadic or pursuit movements may be deficient or impossible to elicit. Integrity of the pontine and infra-nuclear pathways may be demonstrated by utilising the vestibulo-ocular reflex, which moves the eyes in the opposite direction to which the head is turned. This is known as the 'doll's head' reflex.

In infants with doubtful vision, a rotational test must be performed in which the baby is briskly rotated and then stopped suddenly. This induces a vestibular input from the semicircular canals which drives the eyes with a nystagmus with a fast phase in the opposite direction to rotation. On ceasing rotation, an infant with normal vision should immediately override this reflex and re-establish fixation: in blind children, the eyes will stay in a deviated position for some seconds, only gradually returning to the central position.

ACCOMMODATION AND STRABISMUS

In a hypermetropic eye, rays of light from a distant object would theoretically be brought to focus behind the macula, but in practice a blurred retinal image is created. By accommodation, the lens refracting power is increased and hypermetropic patients can thus produce a clear retinal image of a distant object (cf. Chapter 11 The Lens); this means that even greater accommodative effort has to be used to view a near object. Infants and children have immense accommodative power (up to +14D) and can compensate for much hypermetropia. However, the close physiological linkage of accommodation to convergence means these patients show a tendency to eso-deviation which may be either latent or break down to become intermittently or completely manifest. Removal of accommodative effort by prescribing spectacles to correct the hypermetropia has a beneficial effect on the eso-deviation.

All patients with strabismus require an accurate refraction with accommodation eliminated. In adults this can be done by using a fogging technique with convex lenses, but in infants and difficult or unreliable patients a topical cycloplegic agent must be used. 1% atropine ointment applied twice daily to both eyes for three days prior to refraction is the most reliable: G. cyclopentolate 1% produces less reliable cycloplegia but is more convenient for follow up refractions. For full hypermetropic correction make allowance for the refraction working distance only (no reduction is made for any cyclopegic used).

Fig. 18.15   Versions are observed as the child follows movement of the target.

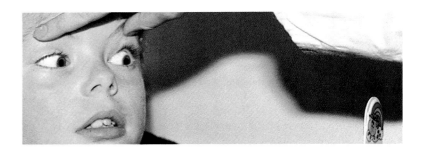

Fig. 18.16   Doll's head movements are demonstrated by turning the patient's head manually while the patient looks at the examiner's face. This test is extremely helpful in uncooperative or unconscious patients.

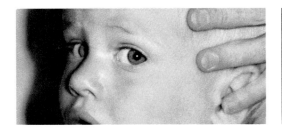
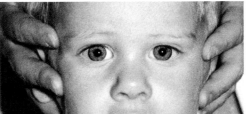
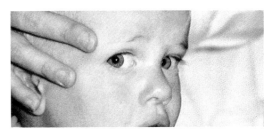

Fig. 18.17   Non-conjugate eye movements are called vergences. They may be simply assessed by asking the patient to fix a target which is moved towards and away from him. The ranges of convergence and divergence may be measured on the synoptophore, with prisms, or the R.A.F. near-point rule, as shown in this photograph. The near-point of convergence is the distance at which diplopia is first appreciated; the range of accommodation is the distance at which the target becomes blurred

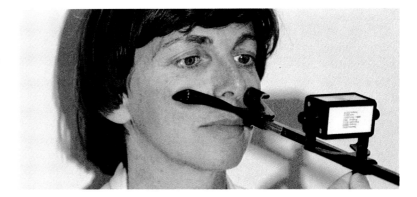

Fig. 18.18 A hypermetropic patient needs to exert accommodation even to see distant objects. This boy is orthophoric on distant fixation but breaks down to a left esotropia for near vision. Spectacles with the full hypermetropic correction abolish the strabismus which is therefore a fully accommodative esotropia.

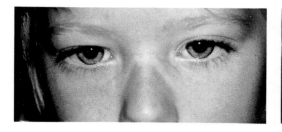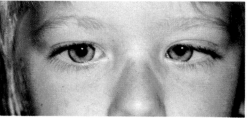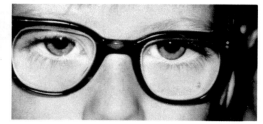

AC/A Ratio

The linkage of accommodation and convergence in the near reflex tends to have a constant relationship in any given patient. This is termed AC/A ratio, where accommodative convergence is expressed in prism dioptres and accommodation in lens dioptres. A commonly used method of measuring this ratio is by performing the prism cover test with and without $-3.0\,D$ spectacle lenses which induce 3 dioptres of accommodation. The ratio is calculated by dividing the change in total deviation by the dioptres of accommodation. Average values are between 3 and 5 prism dioptres of convergence to 1 dioptre of accommodation.

Fig. 18.19 High or low AC/A ratios may be responsible for different types of strabismus. The most common type of strabismus is a convergence excess eso-deviation. In such cases, even after full correction of any hypermetropia, fixation on a near target still induces an inappropriately large amount of convergence which is expressed as an esophoria or tropia.

	Esodeviations	Exodeviations
High AC/A Ratio	convergence excess	divergence excess
	esotropia	exotropia
	eso near > distant	exo distant > near
Low AC/A Ratio	divergence deficiency	convergence deficiency
	esotropia	exotropia
	eso distant > near	exo near > distant

18.20 Accommodative strabismus with convergent excess may be treated with 'executive bifocals' with the segment line at the level of the pupil. Miotics, such as phospholine iodide, may be used as a temporary measure to reduce convergence e.g. following surgery with persistent esotropia.

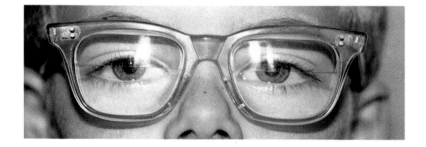

VISUAL ACUITY AND STRABISMUS

All patients with strabismus require regular recording of their visual acuity. This should be measured uniocularly and binocularly, with and without corrective lenses if worn, and with and without an abnormal head posture if this is present. In older, literate patients, the acuity is measured at 6 metres on a Snellen chart, where the 6/6 (20/20) letter subtends 5 minutes of arc and the thickness of each constituent line 1 minute of arc when viewed from 6 meters. In young patients, other methods must be employed. For very small children, the ability to see and pick up tiny sugar cake decorations ('hundreds and thousands') on the examiner's outstretched hand using each eye in turn may show differences of acuity. Resentment of occlusion of the 'good' eye, or searching movements of the 'bad' eye suggest poor vision.

Fig. 18.21 A small child picking up 'hundreds and thousands'.

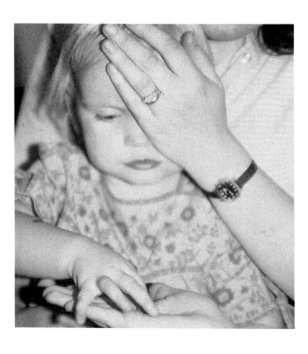

Fig. 18.22 A reliable test for slightly older children is the Sheridan-Gardiner test. This requires recognition rather than identification and is suitable for the child who does not yet know the names of the letters. Cooperative children between two to three years of age can perform the test.

The child has a chart of capital letters before him, and the examiner has a flip-over book with letters of the various Snellen equivalent sizes. The test may be performed at three or six metres distance. The results are reproducible, and as acuities of up to 6/3 (20/10) may be recorded, subtle degrees of amblyopia may be detected. The main disadvantage of this test concerns the phenomenon of 'crowding'. (See caption to Fig. 18.23.)

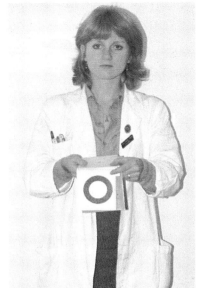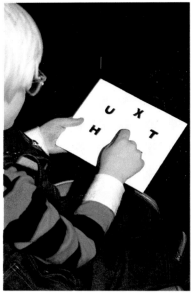

Amblyopia

Amblyopia is a deficiency of visual acuity ('form sense') occurring with otherwise normal field of vision, colour vision, and the ability to detect movement. In addition, no structural abnormality of the fovea can be detected on ophthalmoscopy and no relative afferent pupillary defect is found unless the amblyopia is very dense.

It is conventional to divide amblyopia into functional or organic (where there is a retinal lesion); in clinical practice, however, amblyopia usually refers to the functional type.

Functional amblyopia is reversible in younger children if treated early and this usually implies treatment before the binocular visual reflexes have become mature by about six to seven years of age. Many forms of management have been put forward but the most successful and the mainstay of management is occlusion of the eye with the better visual acuity, in order to stimulate the use of the amblyopic eye and the development of its acuity. In general, the younger the child the speedier the response and the better the prognosis for visual improvement. Occlusion is usually performed on a part-time basis, for a few hours a day, with careful monitoring of the visual acuity since in young children there is a real risk of the occluded eye becoming amblyopic in its turn.

Fig. 18.23 The physiological basis of amblyopia seems to be the lack of a clear and focused retinal image. This is accompanied by maldevelopment of the retinal ganglion cells subserving visual acuity with subsequent changes in the lateral geniculate body and visual cortex. Functional amblyopia can be produced by stimulus deprivation (eg. ptosis or cataract), strabismus or anisometropia.

Many patients with amblyopia show the phenomenon of 'crowding', in which the visual acuity of the affected eye is better when viewing single letters than for rows of letters, and this should be borne in mind when using the Sheridan-Gardiner and other single letter tests.

Classification of Amblyopia

Functional	Organic	Hysterical
stimulus deprivation	e.g. receptor dystrophy	
strabismic	neonatal macular haemorrhage	
anisometropic	early drug toxicity	

Fig. 18.24 Although occlusion may be effective in older children, it should be employed with caution, because of the risk of creating intractable diplopia.

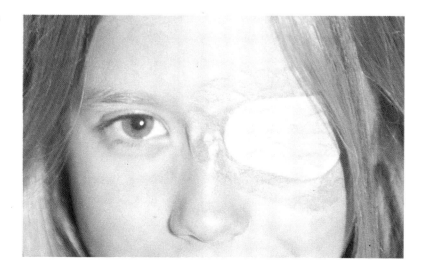

ANATOMY AND MUSCLE ACTIONS

Ocular posture is controlled by the six extraocular muscles, four recti and two obliques. The recti arise at the orbital apex and insert anterior to the equator of the globe. Contraction of the recti therefore produces a movement of the line of sight in the direction of the muscle's line of action. The insertion of the vertical recti nasal to the axis of horizontal rotation of the globe makes them accessory adductors of the globe and also produces torsional effects, the superior rectus intorting and the inferior rectus extorting the globe.

To understand the actions of the oblique muscles one must consider their actions with respect to the horizontal and vertical axes of rotation of the globe. The obliques exert their action from the anterior medial part of the orbit, the inferior oblique arising there, and the superior oblique passing through its trochlea (a small fibrous pulley on the frontal bone). The line of each muscle's action runs temporally and posteriorly, inserting into the superior posterior and inferior posterior temporal sclera respectively. Contraction of the superior oblique therefore causes depression of the visual axis and similarly, the inferior acts as an elevator. In addition, both muscles have an abducting action and the superior oblique intorts the globe, whereas the inferior oblique acts as an extorter.

When the line of sight coincides with the line of action of the vertical ocular muscles they will function as pure elevators or depressors. This occurs with the vertical recti in abduction, and with the obliques in adduction. Therefore, when testing ocular movements and especially in the examination of patients with diplopia, the principal actions of the external ocular muscles will be as illustrated below. The horizontal recti generally function as simple adductors and abductors, and so represent less of a diagnostic problem.

Fig. 18.25 The four recti muscles and their insertions into the right globe.

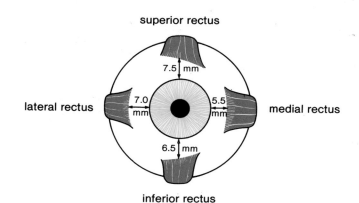

Fig. 18.26 The insertion of the oblique muscles into the right globe.

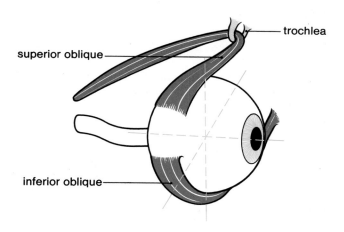

Fig. 18.27 The lines of maximal action of the recti and oblique muscles of the right eye.

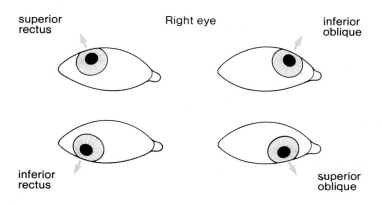

18.9

A AND V PATTERNS

Certain concomitant deviations show a difference in the horizontal angle of deviation on changing from up to downgaze. Cases which are less convergent or more divergent on upgaze are termed 'V' patterns, and cases which are less convergent or more divergent on downgaze are termed 'A' patterns.

It is important to identify such patterns as they may cause a compensatory head posture in binocular patients. In addition, failure to recognise and treat these anomalies may lead to failure of corrective surgery. Minor degrees of 'A' and 'V' phenomena are quite common.

V Patterns

Figs. 18.28 and 18.29 illustrate the 'V' patterns of eso- and exotropia. In many of these patients there is clinically overaction of the inferior oblique muscles, as shown by upshoot of the adducted eye on horizontal versions. The probable cause of these anomalies is thought to be a variation in the lines of insertion of the oblique muscles, causing a greater mechanical advantage in one pair of oblique muscles compared to the other, which is best elicited as a vertical deviation in far lateral gaze. This represents a minor degree of incomitance existing in an otherwise concomitant strabismus.

Fig. 18.28 This girl has a manifest exotropia which increases markedly on upgaze. In addition, on horizontal gaze the adducting eye can be seen to be elevated compared to the abducting eye. This signifies inferior

oblique overaction and may in many cases require bilateral inferior oblique weakening procedures in addition to horizontal rectus surgery to correct the exotropia.

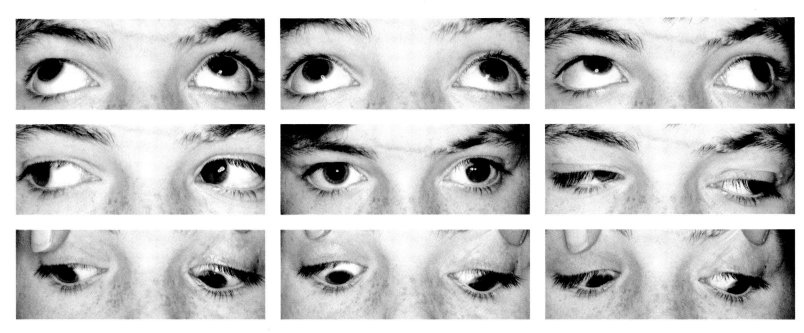

Fig. 18.29 This is probably the commonest type of deviation associated with A and V phenomena. This child has a marked V esotropia with right hypertropia in the primary position. On upgaze, the eyes are almost straight,

but the esotropia increases in downgaze. On horizontal gaze, both inferior oblique muscles overact, the right more than the left. Even where there is asymmetry, it is advisable to weaken both overacting obliques surgically.

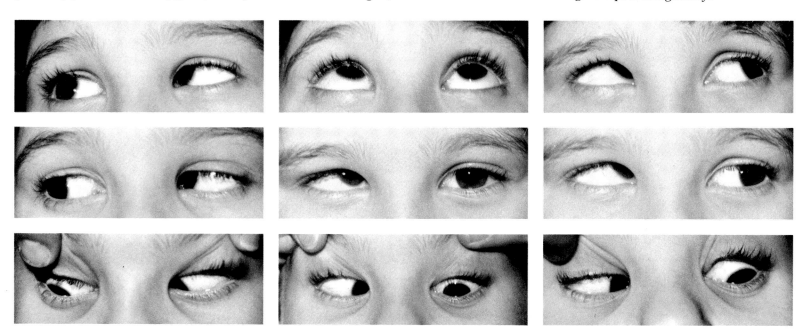

A Patterns

'A' patterns are less common than 'V' patterns and tend to be associated with oblique muscle overactions. Overaction of the superior obliques, for example, will cause a downdrift of the adducted eye on horizontal versions. An 'A' exotropia may present with a chin-down head posture in an attempt to reduce the deviation. A missed 'A' pattern may cause failure of horizontal strabismus surgery.

Oblique muscle dysfunction may be confused with alternating sursumduction (alternating hyperphoria, dissociated vertical divergence). This is a phenomenon of unknown cause in which occlusion of an eye makes it deviate upwards and outwards, often with excyclotorsion of the globe. On removing the cover, the eye makes a rather deliberate recovery movement. The condition is usually bilateral but more marked when the eye with the poorer acuity is occluded. Common associations are a congenital strabismus (usually esotropia) and also latent nystagmus, a condition in which cover of either eye induces nystagmus (with the fast phase towards the uncovered eye), with a proportional drop in visual acuity. With latent nystagmus, binocular visual acuity is characteristically much better than that of either eye alone.

Fig. 18.30 This patient has had previous strabismus surgery, which has left her with an A exotropia. This is best seen in downgaze, where the visual axes are markedly divergent. Overaction of the right superior oblique may be seen in left gaze, but overaction of the left superior oblique is not apparent. In the primary position the appearance is good, and there is no diplopia due to suppression.

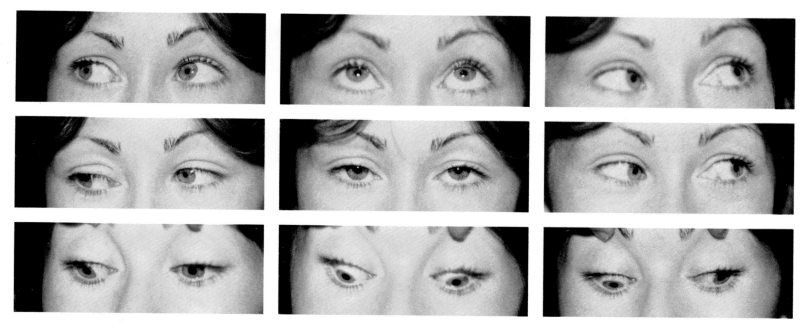

Fig. 18.31 This patient's eyes are straight or marginally divergent in downgaze, with an exotropia in upgaze. There is bilateral superior oblique overaction, best seen by the downdrift of the adducting eye in both right and left depression. The adducting eye may also be seen to be slightly hypotropic on right and left elevation (underaction of the inferior obliques).

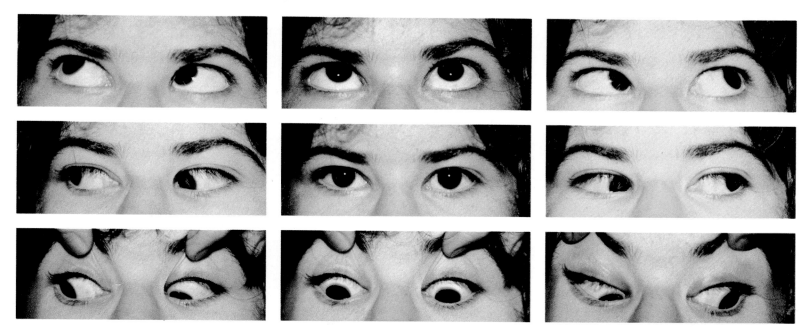

MUSCULO-FASCIAL SYNDROMES
Brown's Syndrome

Brown's syndrome is a congenital condition which may be unilateral or bilateral and in which there is limitation of elevation of one or both eyes in adduction, simulating inferior oblique palsy. Patients present with an abnormal head posture, tilting the head towards the affected side to increase their field of binocular vision. The parents often first note the over elevation of the eye on the unaffected side. On testing ocular movements, there is downdrift of the affected eye in adduction, and, in some cases, a 'click' may be heard or felt in the region of the trochlea of the superior oblique tendon on attempted elevation. Resistance is encountered on passive elevation of the globe with forceps under local or general anaesthetic, especially in the adducted position. Various hypotheses have been advanced to explain the condition, such as anomalous innervation or a congenitally short superior oblique tendon. The most convincing suggestion is the presence of a swelling on the superior oblique tendon preventing free passage through the trochlea and, rarely, acquired tethering will be seen in rheumatoid patients. Some authorities term the condition 'the superior oblique tendon sheath syndrome.' Most cases have normal fusion, and a large proportion tend to improve spontaneously by the age of twelve. Surgery is reserved for cases with a cosmetically unacceptable head posture, or where there is a risk of permanent skeletal changes in the cervical spine.

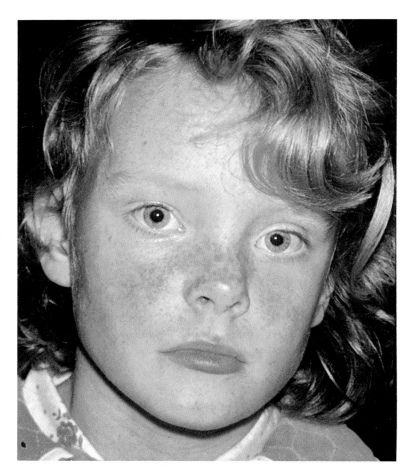

Fig. 18.32 Position of face with head posture. This child has a head posture of tilting to the left, a face turn to the right and chin depression to compenste for a severe left Brown's syndrome.

Fig. 18.33 Observation of the ocular movements demonstrates a remarkable degree of restriction of elevation of the left eye in adduction.

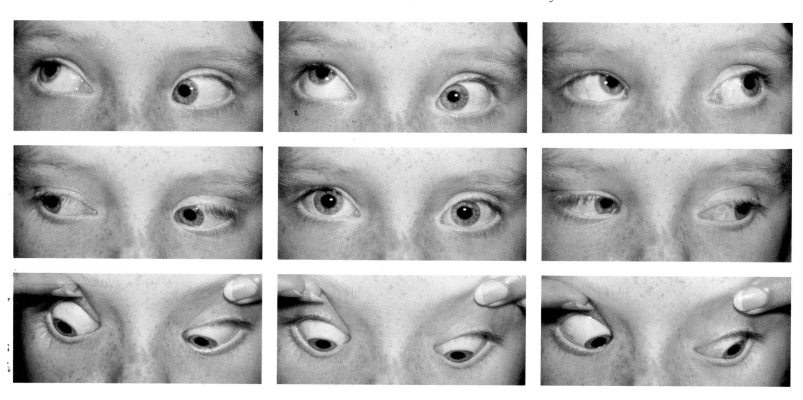

Duane's Syndrome

Duane's retraction syndrome (Stilling-Turk-Duane syndrome) is a congenital condition which is usually unilateral, although bilateral cases occur. Various classifications exist but it is easiest to divide cases into typical and atypical cases. In typical Duane's syndrome, there is a marked deficit of abduction of the affected globe which may be mistaken for a lateral rectus palsy. In addition, there is widening of the palpebral aperture on attempted abduction, and narrowing of the aperture on adduction with retraction of the globe into the orbit.

Adduction may be normal or slightly limited. In the atypical form adduction is more limited than abduction resulting in an exodeviation. Characteristic changes and globe retraction on attempted adduction are still found.

Although various fibro-fascial abnormalities of the orbit have been described, there is good clinical and electromyographic evidence that the condition is due to anomalous co-contraction of the horizontal rectus muscles – in the typical form the lateral rectus is inhibited on attempted abduction, causing limitation of movement, and active on adduction, causing the retraction of the globe. Of interest is the postmortem finding in one patient of absence of the abducens nucleus in the pons with innervation of the lateral rectus by a branch from the oculomotor nerve in the orbit. This fits with the clinical and EMG findings. Changes in the degree of anomalous innervation and the amount of fibrosis in the lateral rectus explain the other variants.

Patients may present with an abnormal head posture of a face turn to the affected side, or with diplopia, or with an esotropia with suppression and amblyopia. Surgery is of value in improving the abnormal head posture and lessening the degree of retraction, but with only a small increase in abduction of the affected eye.

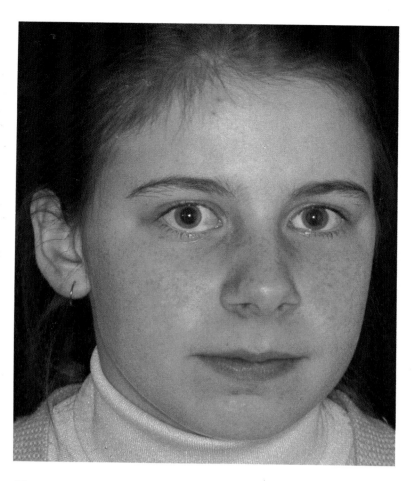

Fig. 18.34 Head posture in a child with typical left Duane's syndrome shows a face turn to the left in order to compensate for the deficient abduction of the left eye.

Fig. 18.35 Ocular movements in left Duane's syndrome demonstrate a limitation of abduction with widening of the palpebral aperture. Left adduction is associated with narrowing of the palpebral aperture and retraction of the globe.

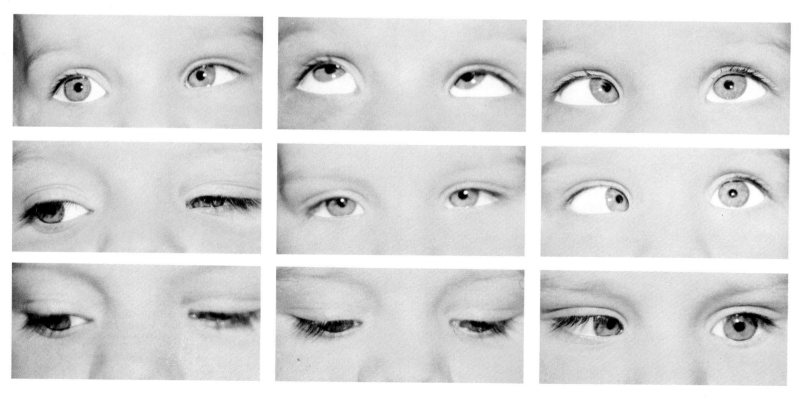

INCOMITANT STRABISMUS

Strabismus is termed incomitant when the angle of deviation between the visual axes varies with the position of gaze. This is usually seen with neurological palsies of the external ocular muscles or mechanical factors restricting free rotation of the globes, but minor degrees of incomitance are also seen in concomitant strabismus with A and V phenomena.

Diplopia

Diplopia is the prime symptom of incomitance and is due to abnormal and non-corresponding retinal projection of the image in the deviant eye. In the presence of an acquired ocular deviation, normal retinal projection still applies and, providing that there was normal binocular vision preceding the onset, two symptoms occur at the same time.

Confusion

Confusion is produced by the foveas being stimulated by two different objects, with the images projected to the same point in space (i.e., straight ahead) and these are seen as either superimposed or alternating images. Confusion is rarely complained of because of foveal suppression. Diplopia is always maximal in the direction of action of the affected muscle. In this position, the image from the eye with the muscle palsy will always be more peripheral because retinal projection is at its most disparate: it will also be less distinct, as the retinal area being stimulated is less sensitive than the fovea. To localize diplopia, it is important to know whether it is horizontal or vertical, the direction of maximum separation, and whether it varies with near or distant vision or can be improved by a change of head posture. Simple questions based on these facts serve to elicit the paretic muscle in most cases. Red and green goggles with a fixation light may also be used.

Several methods are available to study the evolution or resolution of diplopia. Many cases will simply improve while in the others, surgical intervention must be delayed until all improvement has ceased. A simple and useful method of monitoring the patient's progress consists of plotting the field of binocular single vision with the head fixed using an arc perimeter. (Serial charts show whether changes are occurring.)

Fig. 18.36 Common causes of incomitant strabismus classified by pathological process.

Pathological Process	Common Causes
Congenital	nerve palsy, forceps injury, hydrocephalus, agenesis of muscle
Acquired Trauma	orbital fracture, head injury, surgery
Acute Inflammation	orbital cellulitis, cavernous sinus thrombosis, meningitis
Chronic Inflammation	syphilis, orbital pseudotumour, dysthyroid ophthalmopathy, tuberculous meningitis
Tumour	glioma, meningioma, acoustic neuroma, orbital tumour, metastases
Demyelination	multiple sclerosis
Vascular	aneurysm, diabetes mellitus, hypertension, ischaemic cerebral disease, embolism, giant-cell arteritis
Degenerative	progressive external ophthalmoplegia

Fig. 18.37 Common causes of incomitant strabismus classified by the anatomical site of lesion.

Incomitant Strabismus

Site of Lesion	Common Causes
Internuclear Lesions	vascular accident, intracranial tumour, demyelination, etc.
Cranial Nerve Paresis	trauma, aneurysm, vascular (including diabetes), intracranial tumour, raised intracranial pressure
Neuromuscular Junction	myasthenia gravis
Muscular	progressive external ophthalmoplegia, orbital myositis, thyrotoxic myopathy
Orbital	orbital fracture, trochlear damage, multiple adhesions, secondary contracture of antagonist, misdirection-regeneration, 'musculo-fascial' syndromes, e.g., Brown's syndrome, Duane's syndrome

Fig. 18.38 This patient has a left sixth nerve palsy. In the primary position there is a moderate left esotropia. In the left gaze the deviation increases and in right gaze there is no esotropia. The deviation is therefore incomitant.

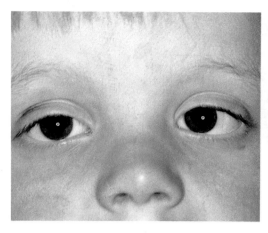
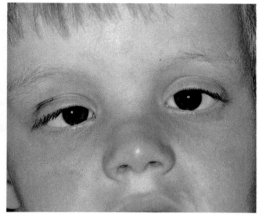
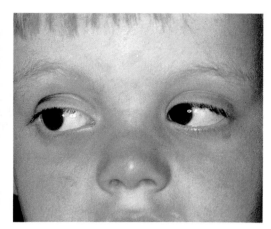

Fig. 18.39 This diagram illustrates how an object 'X' in the temporal field of vision stimulates a retinal element in the nasal retina. Similarly, an object, Y, in the nasal field will stimulate a temporal retinal element. Each retinal element has its own characteristic projection value, that for the fovea being 0^0 or straight ahead. In the right-hand diagram, of a patient with right esotropia objects at (aX_1) and (aY_1) stimulate the foveas and could cause confusion. This is rare and short lived, however, due to foveal suppression. The object at (aX) stimulates the left fovea and is seen as straight ahead. It also stimulates a nasal retinal element in the convergent eye. This projects temporally and the object is seen at (aX_1), causing diplopia.

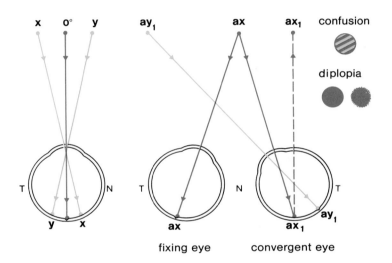

Fig. 18.40 The field of binocular vision can be plotted by using an arc perimeter with the head fixed (left). The chart (right) shows the area of single vision shaded in.

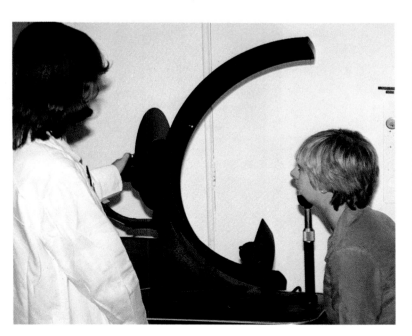
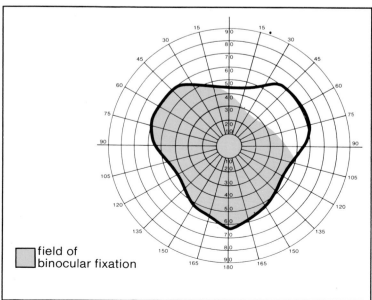

18.15

CRANIAL NERVE PALSIES

Acquired cranial nerve palsies affecting the ocular muscles may be due to a variety of causes including congenital anomalies, trauma or vascular disease (cf. Figs. 18.36 and 18.37).

Fourth Nerve Palsies

Fourth nerve palsies may be unilateral, bilateral, congenital or acquired. Patients with congenital fourth nerve palsies frequently have an abnormal head posture. The superior oblique is a powerful intorter of the globe, in addition to its actions of depression and abduction. If it is weak, the patient tends to adopt a posture where the head is tilted away from the affected side, placing the affected eye in an extorted position.

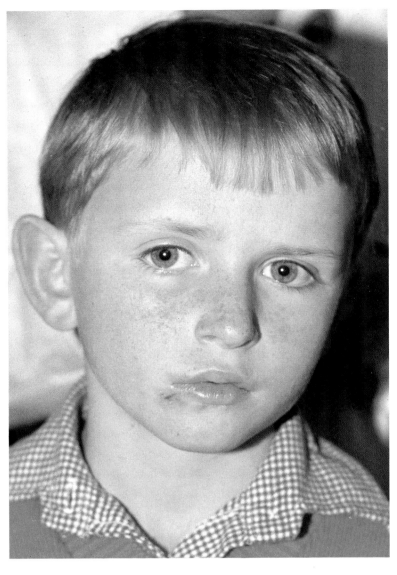

Fig. 18.41 Full-face position of a patient with congenital right fourth nerve palsy. The clues to diagnosis are an unusually high degree of vertical fusion and old photographs showing the head posture. Normal intorsion of the fellow eye facilitates single vision and the patient maintains a larger area of binocular vision than he would otherwise. A face turn to the opposite side and chin depression are less constant features. A congenital fourth palsy that has been compensated by an abnormal head posture in childhood may sometimes decompensate in adult life.

Fig. 18.42 Patient with left fourth nerve palsy. It can be seen that the affected left superior oblique causes underaction of the globe in attempted right depression, with associated overaction of the ipsilateral inferior oblique in right elevation due to unopposed action.

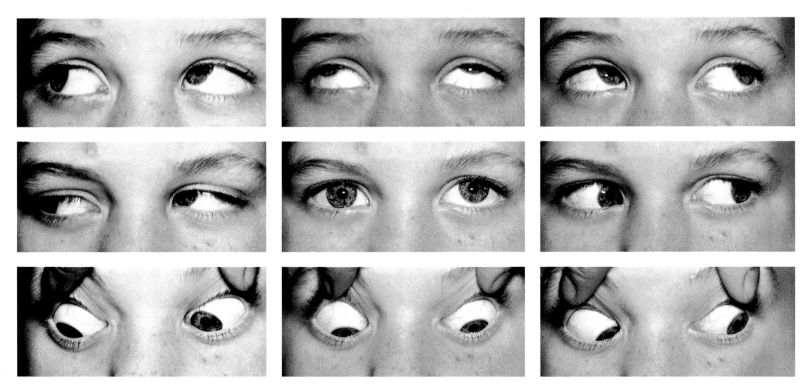

Bilateral Fourth Nerve Palsy

Bilateral fourth nerve palsies are almost invariably due to blunt head trauma which ruptures the nerve rootlets by contusion on the tentorium as they decussate superiorly over the midbrain. There is particular difficulty with reading and close work, as the inferior recti, acting to depress the eyes without the assistance of the superior obliques, cause the eyes to extort on downgaze, producing a torsional diplopia. Symptoms are often severe even in the absence of a gross ocular deviation. Asymmetry is common, and it is advisable to suspect bilateral palsies, especially in traumatic unilateral cases. Patients may gain some relief from chin depression, allowing the eyes to be used in relative elevation.

It may be impossible to demonstrate fusion on orthoptic testing in such cases, but the majority of patients show it when the torsional problem is corrected. Fourth nerve palsies are more often missed than third or sixth nerve palsies, and patients may be erroneously labelled as 'compensation neurosis'. Specific questions for torsional diplopia, using a straight fixation target such as a pen, may be valuable.

In the case of cyclovertical muscle weakness, it may be extremely difficult to decide whether the patient is suffering from a superior oblique palsy of one side, or a superior rectus palsy of the other, on the basis of ocular movements alone. Here the Bielschowsky head tilt test is of value (cf. Fig. 18.45).

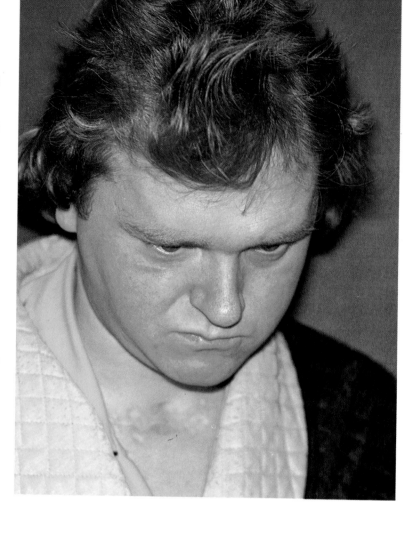

Fig. 18.43 Full-face position of a patient with bilateral fourth nerve palsy showing chin depression to maintain single vision in the reading position.

Fig. 18.44 Ocular motility in a patient with bilateral fourth nerve palsy. Note limited depression in adduction of each eye.

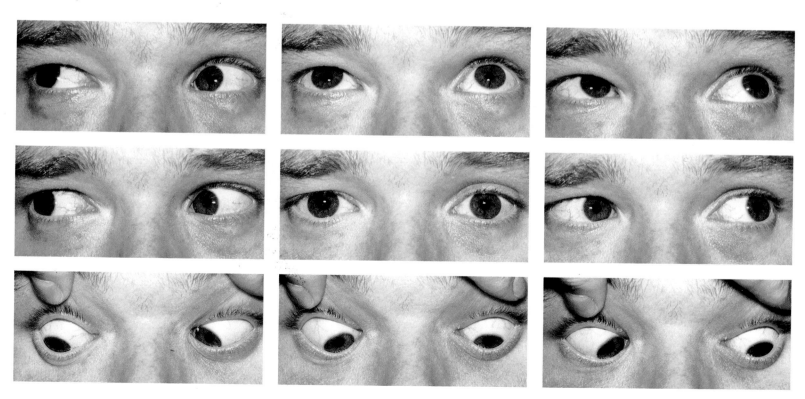

18.17

Fig. 18.45 In the Bielschowsky head tilt test, the patient is asked to fixate on a target and the head is firmly tilted by the examiner towards the higher eye, (i.e., the side with possible superior oblique paresis.) This stimulates intorsion. If the superior oblique is weak – the other intorter of the globe (the superior rectus) is also utilized and its secondary action of elevation will be manifest as a discernable upshoot of the affected eye, as an increase in the vertical separation of the patient's diplopia or increased hyperphoria on cover testing. A positive head tilt test therefore confirms a diagnosis of superior oblique palsy affecting the right eye in this case.

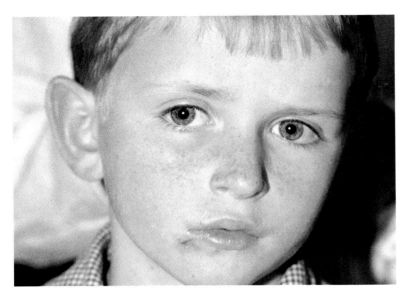

Fig. 18.46 Diagram of mechanism of Bielschowsky test.

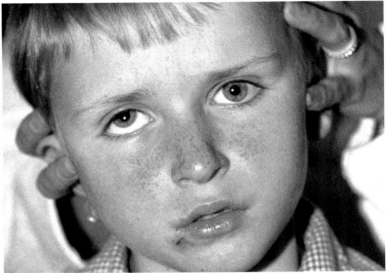

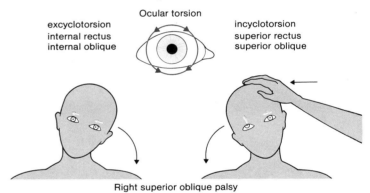

Bielschowsky's Head-Tilt Test

Ocular torsion

excyclotorsion
internal rectus
internal oblique

incyclotorsion
superior rectus
superior oblique

Right superior oblique palsy

head–tilt to left compensates for weak intorter of right eye

forced tilt to right induces intorsion of right globe – unopposed secondary action of right superior rectus causes ocular elevation

Third Nerve Palsy

Third nerve palsy may be congenital or acquired. Common causes include trauma, intracranial aneurysm, and vascular disease. As all but two of the extraocular muscles are supplied by the third nerve, lesions cause gross restriction of ocular movement. With a total palsy there is complete ptosis and internal ophthalmoplegia of the pupil and ciliary muscle with the eye assuming a downward and outward position. The presence of an intact fourth nerve in this situation can be demonstrated by intorsion of the globe on downgaze. Partial third nerve palsy, in which some muscles are more affected than others, is not uncommon and orbital disease may affect either the superior or inferior divisions of the nerve as it divides at the superior orbital fissure.

Examination of the pupils is of particular value in any patient with a third nerve palsy (cf. Neuro-Ophthalmology Chapter 19). Acute presentation of a painful isolated third nerve palsy in an adult is most commonly due to either aneurysmal compression or ischaemic vascular disease. The pupillary fibres lie externally and dorsally in the nerve as it passes through the subarachnoid space, and are almost invariably compressed by a distending aneurysm of the posterior communicating artery. These patients will therefore have a dilated pupil and require carotid angiography prior to surgical ligation of the aneurysm, whereas ischaemic vascular disease spares the pupil and can be treated expectantly. A third nerve palsy accompanied by a small pupil usually indicates involvement of the sympathetic pathways, most frequently by disease in the cavernous sinus.

Surgical management of third nerve palsy is very difficult due to the extensive nature of the paralysis. At best, a small field of binocular single vision may be achieved in the primary position and downgaze. The accompanying ptosis may be invaluable in preventing intractable diplopia. Bilateral third nerve palsy is fortunately very rare but is occasionally seen following pituitary apoplexy.

In some cases of third nerve palsy, particularly those due to trauma and aneurysms, and in some congenital cases, recovery of the palsy may lead to the misdirection – regeneration syndrome ('aberrant regeneration'). In this condition, it is presumed that the regenerating fibres 'lose their way' and terminate in the wrong muscle. This is most

apparent when testing synkinetic reflexes. For instance, in the normal patient lid elevation is induced by upward ocular movement, and miosis of the pupil is associated with convergence in the near reflex. In misdirection-regeneration, the patient's lid may elevate on adduction or downgaze, and miosis may occur on downgaze. Simultaneous contraction of both superior and inferior recti on attempted upgaze may prevent elevation of the globe.

Fig. 18.47 Ocular motility in a patient with left third nerve palsy. The globe is divergent because of the unopposed lateral rectus.

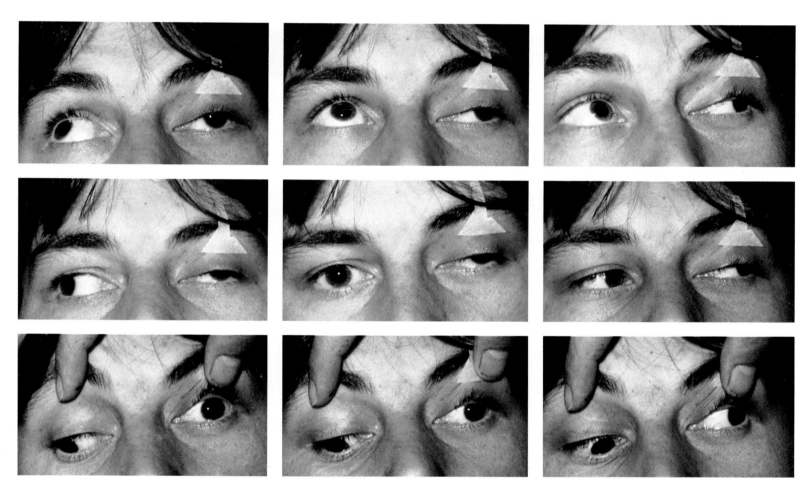

Fig. 18.48 Pupillary involvement with an isolated, painful, third nerve palsy indicates compression by a posterior communicating artery aneurysm. Such patients have a substantial risk of subarachnoid haemorrhage and require carotid angiography.

Isolated pupil sparing third nerve palsy is usually associated with hypertensive or diabetic vascular disease and may be painful. In the absence of other signs, these patients do not need invasive neuroradiological studies and the palsy usually improves over several weeks.

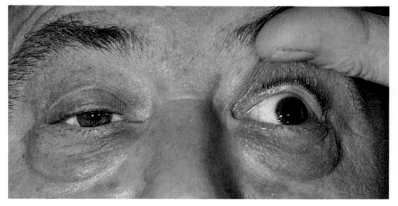
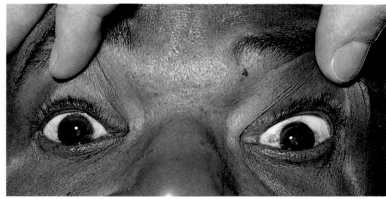

Fig. 18.49 Angiography of the internal carotid artery shows a large aneurysm of the posterior communicating artery compressing the third nerve and producing an oculomotor palsy with pupillary involvement which required neurosurgical management (cf. Chapter 19 Neuro-Ophthalmology).

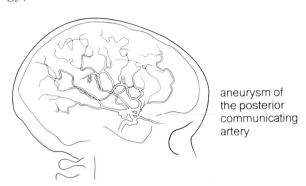

aneurysm of the posterior communicating artery

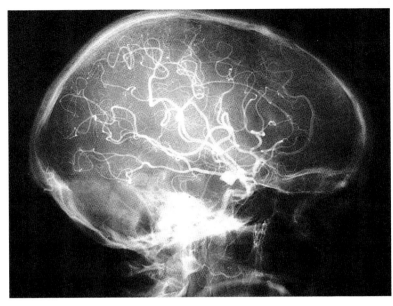

Fig. 18.50 Ocular motility in misdirection-regeneration syndrome. Aberrant regeneration is seen following traumatic and compressive lesions but never after ischaemic lesions. Various patterns of abnormal lid or pupillary constriction can be seen on ocular movement and the direct light reflex may be poor, causing confusion with Adie's myotonic pupil or light-near dissociation. This patient with a right third nerve palsy (whose pupils had been dilated for fundoscopy), shows lid elevation on medial and downgaze.

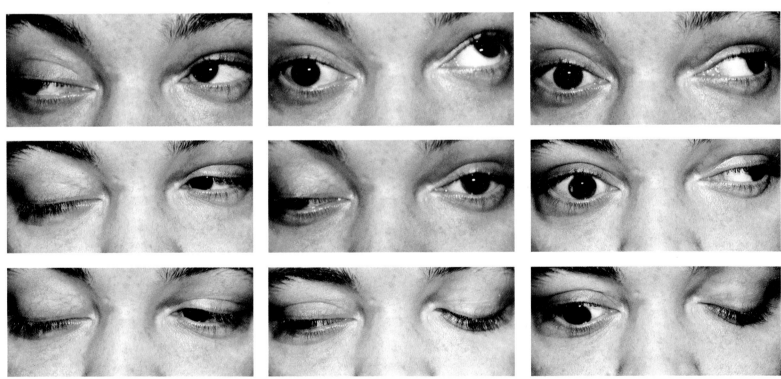

Sixth Nerve Palsy

Sixth nerve palsy is the most common cranial nerve palsy affecting ocular motility. It may be congenital or acquired, unilateral or bilateral. One possible reason for its frequency is the long intracranial course of the sixth cranial nerve, which is nearly vertical in the posterior cranial fossa.

Patients present with horizontal diplopia, which is worse on looking to the affected side, and often a face turn to the affected side. (See Fig. 18.38.)

Sixth nerve palsy may be due to orbital, cavernous sinus, subarachnoid, or pontine lesions. The sixth nerve palsy seen as a false localizing sign with raised intracranial pressure is due to compression of the nerve against the apex of the petrous bone as it turns to enter the cavernous sinus. Patients with isolated sixth nerve palsy require systemic investigation but it is not unusual for no other disease to be found. Isolated sixth nerve palsies in the elderly are usually due to 'vascular' disease: in children they can sometimes follow virus infection. Sixth nerve palsy must be differentiated from Duane's syndrome, myasthenia gravis, thyroid ophthalmopathy, orbital disease and hysterical convergence spasm.

Sixth nerve palsy, unlike third or fourth nerve palsy, is relatively easy to manage with prisms, although surgery may be offered when the deviation ceases to improve spontaneously.

Fig. 18.51 Infants with large congenital esotropias often have poor abduction and use the left eye for the right field and vice versa. This is known as 'cross-fixational esotropia.'

Such patients may be erroneously classified as bilateral sixth nerve palsies. The distinction may be made on rotational or doll's head movement testing, as any movement of the eyes lateral to the midline suggests that no paralysis is present.

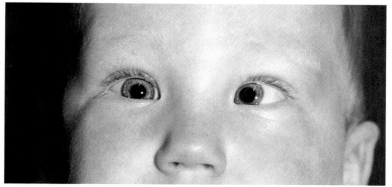
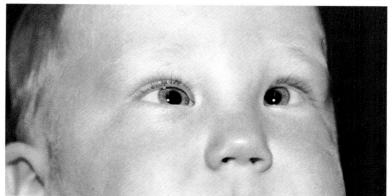

OCULAR RESTRICTION

Incomitant squints, specially vertical ones, are not always due to extraocular muscle palsy. Every ocular rotation requires both muscle contraction and relaxation of its direct antagonist. For example, failure of elevation in dysthyroid eye disease is not due to superior rectus ophthalmoplegia but to inferior rectus fibrosis, which tethers the eye: once the maximal extension of the inferior rectus has been reached further contraction of the superior rectus causes the globe to be retracted into the orbit.

Ophthalmic Graves' Disease

Graves' disease is an auto-immune condition with infiltration by large numbers of chronic inflammatory cells, the deposition of excessive amounts of mucopolysaccharides and increased extracellular fluid volume. The sites affected are the fingertips, the pre-tibial area, the extraocular muscles and orbital tissue, and the thyroid gland.

Simple hyperthyroidism may cause lid retraction. Ophthalmic Graves' disease produces inflammatory changes in extraocular muscles.

The disease is often asymmetrical, with a tendency for the inferior and medial recti to be affected. The orbital tissues are similarly affected, and proptosis may occur, although CT scans have shown that swelling of the extraocular muscles accounts for much of the increased orbital contents. Dangerous complications include corneal exposure from proptosis and optic neuropathy from compression of the optic nerve by the swollen rectus muscles at the orbital apex. These complications may respond to high dose systemic corticosteroids, or may require surgical decompression of the orbit (cf. Chapter 20 The Orbit and Lacrimal System).

Patients can present in hyperthyroid, or hypothyroid states but most are hyperthyroid when first seen.

The extraocular muscles are weaker than normal but, more importantly, are very inelastic and do not relax well to permit ocular rotations. As the disease 'burns out', the inflammation leads to fibrosis, thus worsening the restrictions. Patients present with diplopia, and show variable patterns of restricted upgaze and abduction, simulating superior and lateral rectus palsies.

Fig. 18.52 A patient with longstanding severe ophthalmic Graves' disease. The face shows chronic periorbital oedema, red eyes, and conjunctival chemosis. The fingers show 'clubbing' of the terminal phalanges (thyroid acropachy) and the legs show pretibial myxoedema.

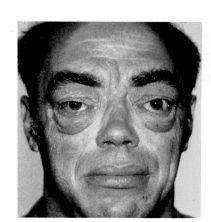
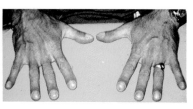
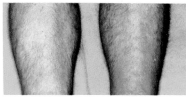

Fig. 18.53 This patient with dysthyroid ophthalmopathy shows asymmetrical restriction of upgaze and abduction. Diplopia is frequently severe and difficult to control with prisms. Surgery is not indicated until the condition stabilizes.

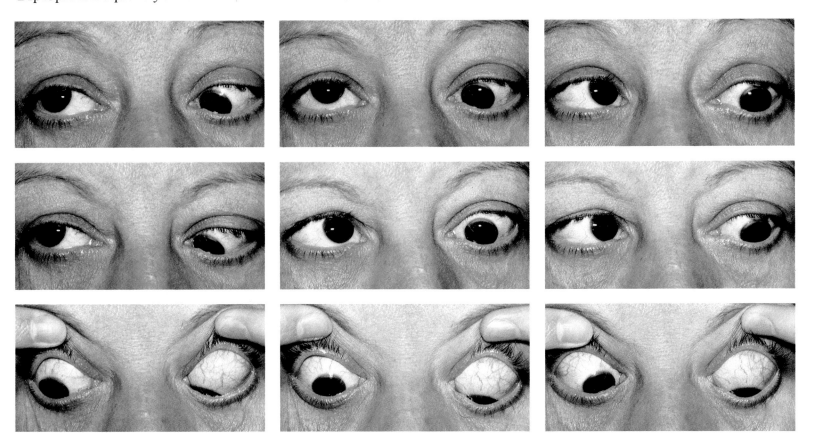

Orbital Fractures

Orbital fractures may involve the orbital margins and/or the orbital walls. A specific type with intact orbital rim is termed a 'blow-out' fracture, and is generally caused by a direct blow to the eye through closed lids. The wave of pressure created is transmitted through the orbital contents to the walls, which tend to fracture where they are thinnest – at the floor nasal to the infraorbital groove, and the medial wall, in the orbital plate of the ethmoid bone. A portion of the orbital tissues may become trapped in the fracture site and, because of this attachment to the extraocular muscles, restrict rotation of the globe. The fracture and prolapsed tissue ('tear drop sign') may be seen in tilted postero-anterior skull x-ray and confirmed on orbital tomography.

Restriction of ocular movements is the main sign of orbital floor fractures causing vertical diplopia on up and downgaze. The restriction of the field of binocular single vision may be severe, and the globe may retract on attempted vertical movements. Although medial wall fractures may cause ocular restriction, symptoms are less prominent due to the vastly greater ability to fuse horizontal rather than vertical disparity. Enophthalmos, due to loss of orbital contents, may be a major cosmetic problem.

Many patients will recover spontaneously within the first two weeks. Severe enophthalmos, large fractures severe retraction on upgaze, and complete lack of improvement by fourteen days are indications for exploration of the orbital floor and the freeing of any trapped tissue.

Fig. 18.54 The normal anatomy of the orbital walls can be compared to that following a 'blow-out' fracture. Pressure from a direct blow to the eye is transmitted through the orbital contents to the walls, which fracture at their thinnest place. A portion of the orbital tissues may become trapped at the fracture site and so restrict rotation of the globe. Air may enter the lids from the surrounding paranasal sinuses, especially on blowing the nose, and cause crepitus on palpatation. In blow-out fractures of the orbital floor, the infraorbital nerve may be contused, causing numbness of the cheek and the incisor area of the upper jaw.

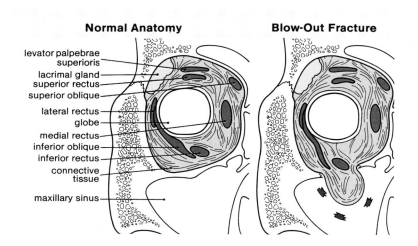

Fig. 18.55 Subconjunctival and lid haematomas following a blunt injury to the orbit should alert one to the possibility of a blow-out fracture. In this patient, blood has accumulated forward from an orbital floor fracture site. Altered infraorbital sensation should be checked for by direct questioning. The presence of crepitus, especially following blowing the nose, strongly suggests an orbital wall fracture.

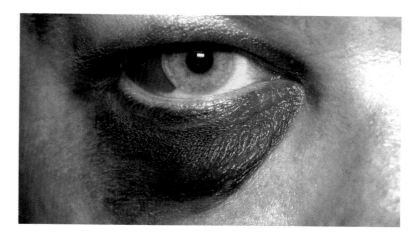

Fig. 18.56 Postero-anterior skull x-ray of blow-out fracture shows right-sided orbital floor fracture with herniation of orbital contents into the maxillary antrum, which is known as the 'teardrop' sign. There is frequently some antral haziness due to haemorrhage from the mucosa. In doubtful cases, tomography or CT scan may help in showing the prolapse. The ethmoidal sinuses along the medial wall should also be inspected for signs of fracture.

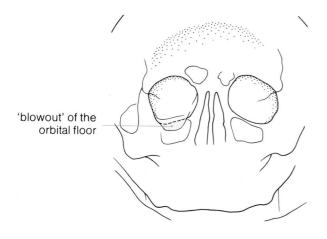

'blowout' of the
orbital floor

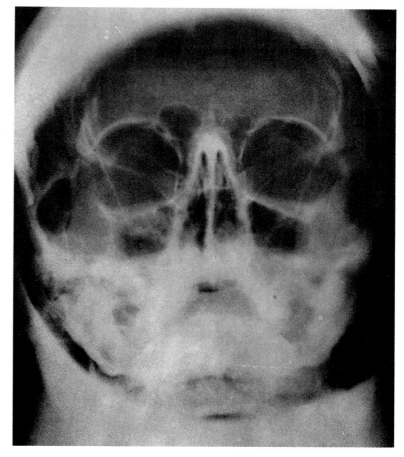

Fig. 18.57 This patient has a right orbital floor blow-out fracture. The right eye is relatively enophthalmic in the primary position. It is restricted in its excursion in both attempted elevation and depression. The cause is not incarceration of the inferior rectus muscle in the fracture site, but fibrous orbital septa connected with the inferior rectus, which are trapped. The patient has vertical diplopia with a small central area of binocular vision.

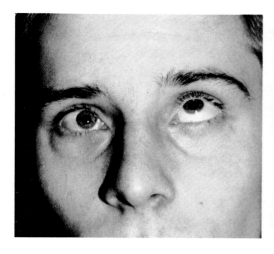

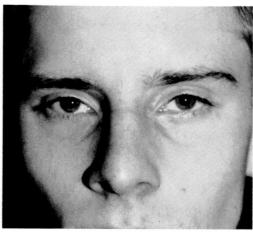

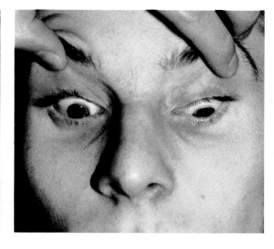

Fig. 18.58 Retraction of globe on upgaze. Retraction is not pathognomonic of orbital fracture, but will occur whenever an agonist muscle attempts to pull against a tight antagonist, causing the globe to be pulled back into the orbit. Other causes include Duane's syndrome, dysthyroid ophthalmoplegia, contracted rectus muscles, etc. The patient is observed from the side in attempted up- and downgaze.

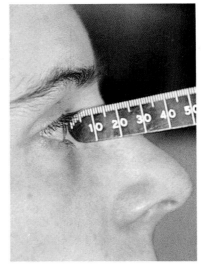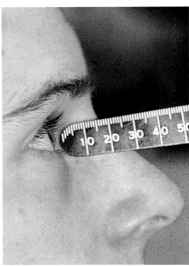

CONGENITAL NYSTAGMUS

Congenital nystagmus may have a pendular or jerky waveform, depending on the direction of gaze. Other characteristic signs are the tendency to have a 'null' point of diminished amplitude, dampening on convergence, absence of oscillopsia, and the reversal of the waveform to optokinetic stimuli.

Congenital nystagmus may be due to a sensory deficit within the visual system, such as ocular albinism, macular aplasia, or stimulus deprivation amblyopia. These patients frequently do not develop nystagmus until two to three months after birth. Other patients show congenital nystagmus with apparently normal eyes and anterior visual pathways. Such patients are sometimes said to have 'motor' nystagmus, and their poorer than normal visual acuity is explained by the difficulty of prolonged foveal fixation and is present soon after birth. Some patients with this type of defect discover ways of reducing the amplitude or frequency of their oscillations, thereby improving their vision. Head shaking, head nodding (spasmus nutans), and holding objects very close to induce convergence are all seen.

Some patients may adopt an abnormal head posture, usually a face turn, to take advantage of a null point. This causes deviation of the eyes to the opposite side and may greatly improve the vision, often by two to three Snellen lines. If the head posture is seen constantly and is cosmetically unsatisfactory, especially when concentrating hard on the object of regard, a suitable next step is to try the therapeutic effect of prisms, with the bases of the prisms located in the direction of the face turn.

If prisms produce an improvement in the head posture, surgery may then effect a permanent improvement. The general principle is to rotate both eyes by an equal amount in the direction of the face turn. Any strabismus present may be corrected at the same time.

Fig. 18.59 Face turn in a patient with congenital nystagmus and abnormal head posture and correction of the condition with prism spectacles.

This girl has a face turn to the left, with ocular deviation to the right to use her null point for viewing objects in the primary position. Prisms with base to the left centralize the eyes and correct the head posture. If their strength is too great for clarity or comfort, surgery is indicated.

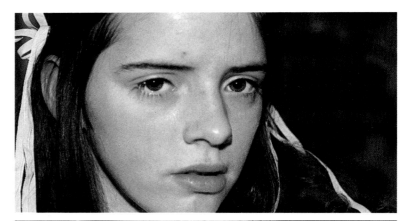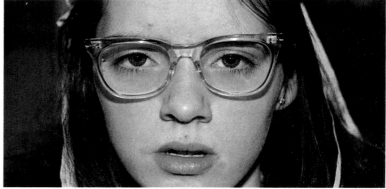

19. Neuro-Ophthalmology

D. J. Spalton

OCULAR MOVEMENT
Introduction
Signals which control ocular movement are initiated in the cerebral hemispheres in a manner analogous to other motor neuronal pathways. They are then transmitted to the gaze centres and ocular motor nuclei in the midbrain and pons, and leave the brain in the third, fourth and sixth cranial nerves. Supranuclear neuronal pathways conduct impulses to the gaze centres; internuclear pathways coordinate the gaze centres with the ocular motor nuclei; and infranuclear pathways lie in the individual ocular motor nerves. A great deal is known about the organisation of horizontal gaze control in the pons, but less is known about vertical gaze mechanisms and still less about the cortical areas involved. Conjugate eye movements (i.e. movements of both eyes as a yoked pair and mediated through supranuclear neuronal pathways) can be divided into saccadic, pursuit or vestibular movements, each of which is generated in a different cerebral area and each has its own velocity and control characteristics.

Supranuclear Gaze Control
Saccadic movements are rapid and relocate fixation of gaze, either by reflex or voluntarily. They are initiated in the contralateral premotor frontal cortex and, once initiated, the movement is irrevocable and ocular position cannot again be modified until the saccade has been completed. A saccadic movement occurs after a latent period of about 200 msec following initiation and has a high velocity of up to 700°/sec. Saccades are tested clinically by commanding the patient to look at a target, or to look right or left.

Pursuit movements are slower and are concerned with keeping ocular fixation locked on the target. They appear to be generated in the ipsilateral occipital cortex but little is known about the supranuclear pathway. Pursuit movements have a latency of about 125 msec from initiation and a maximum velocity of less than 50°/sec. The movement is smooth and is continuously modified according to the speed of the target; if the pursuit movement lags behind the target position, a corrective saccade is inserted to keep up. Pursuit movements are tested by asking the patient to follow a slowly moving target.

Vestibular ocular movements are initiated in the semicircular canals by changes in head posture. They serve to maintain ocular fixation, independent of head and neck posture, and have similar characteristics to pursuit movements, except that they can reach much higher velocities. Thus, vestibular ocular reflexes keep the horizon steady as we walk (the eyes moving in the opposite direction to that of the orbits). In some circumstances the reflex is suppressed and the eyes remain in the same position in the orbit; for example, it would be impossible to read on a train unless one could suppress the vestibular ocular reflex. Vestibular reflexes may be tested either by a 'doll's head' manoeuvre, in which the patient is asked to fixate on a target while the examiner rotates the patient's head, or by caloric stimuli induced by syringing the external auditory meatus with cold or warm water.

Each type of conjugate movement should be examined in both the horizontal and vertical axes. Precise recording of ocular movement by electro-oculographic or infra-red techniques has contributed enormously to the understanding of the physiology of ocular movements but careful examination of ocular motility can supply all the information needed to make a clinical diagnosis. Clinically, horizontal and vertical gaze systems tend to function independently of each other. It is helpful to examine each type of movement in turn, in each axis, to decide whether one is dealing with a problem of either the horizontal or the vertical gaze control, or of both systems. Most diseases disrupt saccadic and pursuit movements initially, with doll's head movements being preserved until relatively later on in the course of events. During examination of ocular control it is important to note whether the patient can hold a steady gaze in the primary or eccentric positions, and also the presence and type of nystagmus, or spontaneous movements, in any position of gaze.

Fig. 19.1 The major inputs to the vertical and horizontal gaze centres are saccadic and pursuit commands from the cerebral hemispheres, and the vestibular ocular reflexes from the vestibular nuclei in the pons. These impulses are then transmitted to the individual ocular motor nuclei in the midbrain and pons. Internuclear pathways coordinate the movements generated in the gaze centres with each other and the third, fourth and sixth nerve nuclei.

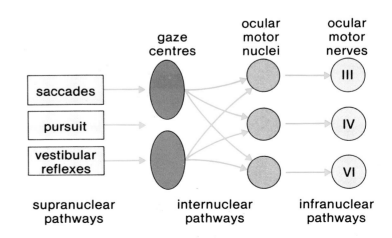

Fig. 19.2 Saccadic movements have been shown biomechanically to consist of impulses in the form of a pulse and step. To change eye position a rapid burst of neuronal signals (the pulse) is fired by the gaze centre and this rapidly moves the eye to the new position. This rapid burst is integrated in the 'pulse-step generator' (a neuronal complex within the gaze centre) to produce an increased tonic discharge (the step) which holds the eye in its new position. Similar responses take place in the agonist of the fellow eye and reciprocal impulses relax the antagonist muscles. These changes are reflected by the EMG recording in an individual nerve. The pulse-step generator exists physiologically in the horizontal gaze centre (otherwise known as the parapontine reticular formation – PPRF) in the pons and various dysfunctions of mismatchings of the pulse to the step signals have been shown to explain some types of nystagmus and eye movement abnormalities.

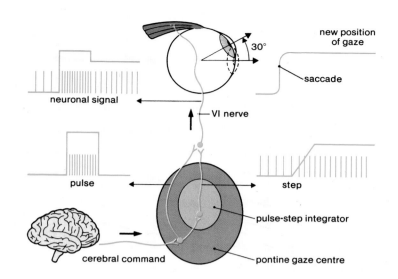

Fig. 19.3 Saccadic and pursuit movements are tested individually, horizontally and vertically, by asking the patient to refixate a stationary target and then to follow it in motion. Vestibular reflexes are tested in a similar manner by the 'doll's head reflex'. Caloric reflexes are produced by stimulating the semicircular canals and vestibular nuclei with warm or cold water and can provide useful information on the integrity of these pathways in the pons. This is especially useful in the neurological assessment of pontine damage in an unconscious patient. In a conscious patient, cold water in the external auditory meatus will generate a nystagmus of both eyes with a fast phase to the opposite side, but in unconscious patients the saccadic phase will be lost and a tonic deviation to the same side will be seen. This indicates an intact pons but results must be interpreted with caution after acute drug overdoses when false negative responses may be seen. Calorics can be adapted to test vertical gaze (and therefore the integrity of the midbrain) by syringing both ears.

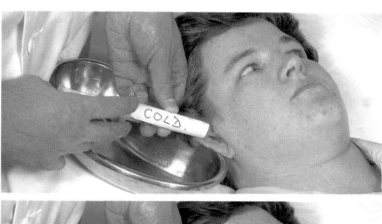

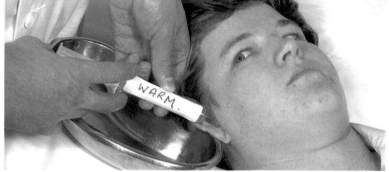

Anatomy of the Ocular Motor Pathways

Fig. 19.4 Saccades are generated in the contralateral hemisphere of the frontal premotor area; thus a saccade to the right is generated in the left frontal lobe, passes through the anterior limb of the internal capsule, and decussates in the midbrain to the horizontal gaze centre in the pons. Pursuit movements appear to be generated in the ipsilateral occipito-parietal area, so that a pursuit movement to the right is controlled by the right hemisphere. Little is known of the neuronal pathway.

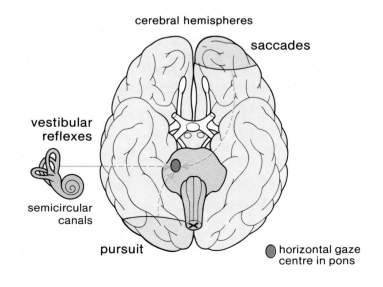

Fig. 19.5 The gaze centres and oculomotor nuclei lie in the midbrain and pons. Vertical gaze is mediated by a nucleus in the posterior commissure, above the superior colliculi; this centre seems to integrate both upward and downward gaze although down gaze is probably generated separately in a nucleus ventral to the aqueduct and inferior to the thalamus (the normal interstitial nucleus of the medial longitudinal fasciculus; 'ri-MLF'). Horizontal gaze is mediated by the horizontal gaze centre (PPRF) at the level of the sixth nerve nucleus in the pons. Thus, defects of vertical gaze tend to be due to lesions of the upper midbrain, whereas defects of horizontal gaze are due to pontine lesions.

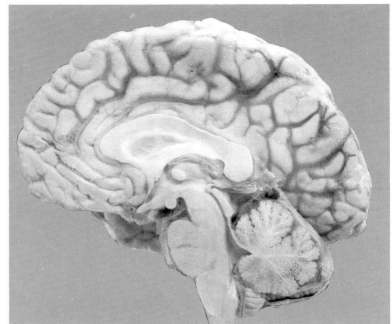

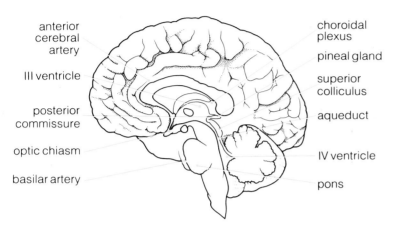

anterior cerebral artery
III ventricle
posterior commissure
optic chiasm
basilar artery

choroidal plexus
pineal gland
superior colliculus
aqueduct
IV ventricle
pons

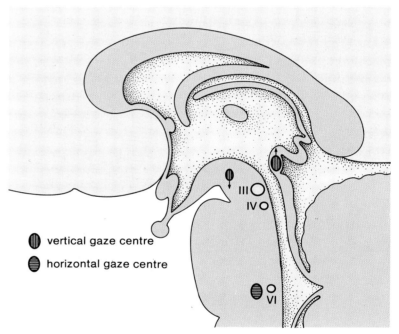

vertical gaze centre

horizontal gaze centre

III
IV
VI

Fig. 19.6 A transverse histological section of the midbrain at the level of the superior colliculus demonstrates the third nerve nucleus inferior to the aqueduct and its efferent fibres. The medial longitudinal fasciculus (MLF), in connecting the third and fourth nuclei and contralateral horizontal gaze centres, is responsible for coordinating horizontal and vertical movements. (Stained to show myelin).

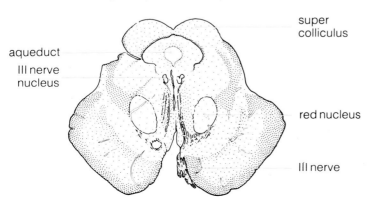

aqueduct
III nerve nucleus

super colliculus

red nucleus

III nerve

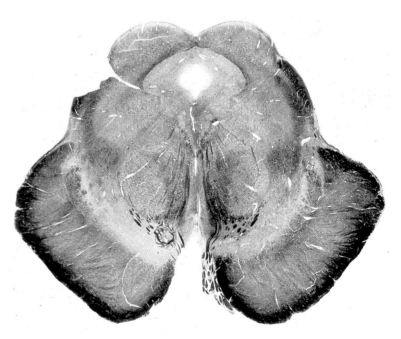

Fig. 19.7 The third nerve nucleus is a complex pool of motor neurones. The parasympathetic nucleus (Edinger-Westphal nucleus) of the pupil lies rostrally and superiorly. The inferior rectus, medial rectus and inferior oblique muscles are all supplied from ipsilateral subnuclei but the superior rectus subnucleus is contralateral. Both levator palpebrae muscles have a single caudal superior nucleus.

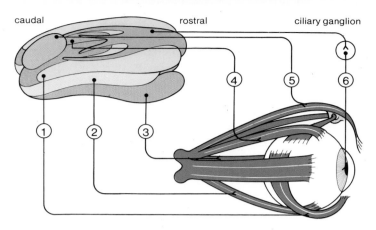

Organisation of Oculomotor Nerve Nucleus

1 inferior oblique muscle	4 superior rectus muscle
2 inferior rectus muscle	5 levator palpebrae muscle
3 medial rectus muscle	6 Edinger-Westphal fibres to pupil

Fig. 19.8 A transverse histological section through the pons at the level of the sixth nerve nuclei demonstrates the medial longitudinal fasciculus (MLF) and the centre for horizontal gaze (PPRF). A command to look left will pass from the left PPRF to the left sixth nucleus and by the MLF to the contralateral third nucleus to stimulate the right medial rectus. Reciprocal inhibitory signals are sent to the left medial rectus and right lateral rectus. (Stained to show myelin).

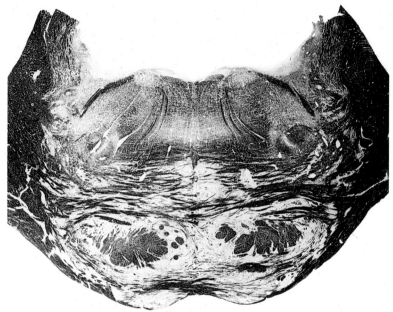

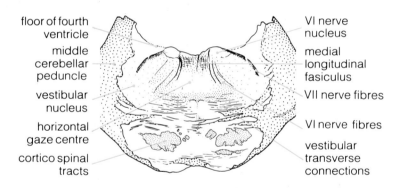

floor of fourth ventricle

middle cerebellar peduncle

vestibular nucleus

horizontal gaze centre

cortico spinal tracts

VI nerve nucleus

medial longitudinal fasiculus

VII nerve fibres

VI nerve fibres

vestibular transverse connections

Fig. 19.9 The third and sixth nerves leave the ventral surface of the brain and pass through the interpeduncular cistern before entering the cavernous sinus. The sixth nerve passes almost vertically upwards and bends forwards under the petroclinoid ligament at the apex of the petrous temporal bone. Here it can be compressed against the bone by raised CSF pressure, or damaged by fractures or disease in the bone.

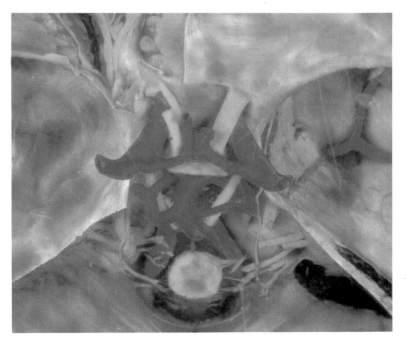

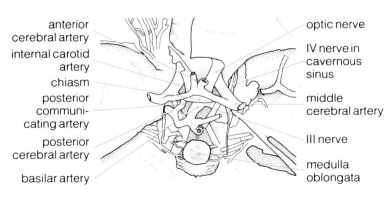

anterior cerebral artery

internal carotid artery

chiasm

posterior communicating artery

posterior cerebral artery

basilar artery

optic nerve

IV nerve in cavernous sinus

middle cerebral artery

III nerve

medulla oblongata

19.5

Fig. 19.10 In this cistern the third nerve passes inferior to the posterior cerebral artery and lateral to the posterior communicating artery. At this position the pupillary fibres lie on the dorsomedial aspect of the nerve; they are readily compressed by a posterior communicating artery aneurysm to produce a third nerve palsy with pupillary dilation. In contrast, vascular disease such as diabetes or hypertension affects the vasa vasorum of the nerve, infarcting central nerve fibres and paralyzing the external ocular muscles but sparing the pupil (cf. Strabismus – Chapter 18).

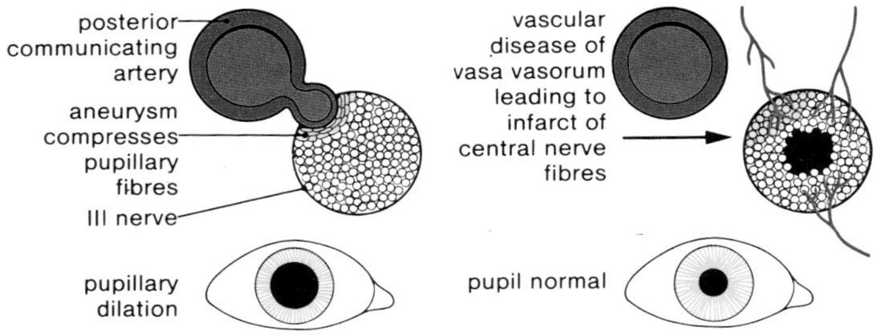

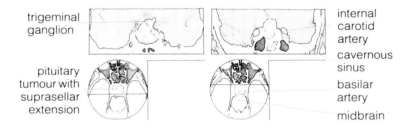

Fig. 19.11 In the cavernous sinus, the third and fourth nerves lie superiorly in the lateral wall; at the anterior end the third nerve divides into superior (superior rectus and lid levator) and inferior branches (inferior and medial rectus, inferior oblique, pupillary and ciliary muscles). At the posterior limit the trigeminal ganglion divides forming the major branches of the fifth nerve; the ophthalmic division then enters the cavernous sinus and passes forwards inferiorly in the lateral wall carrying sensory fibres from the eye and forehead. The internal carotid artery and sixth nerve lie within the sinus.

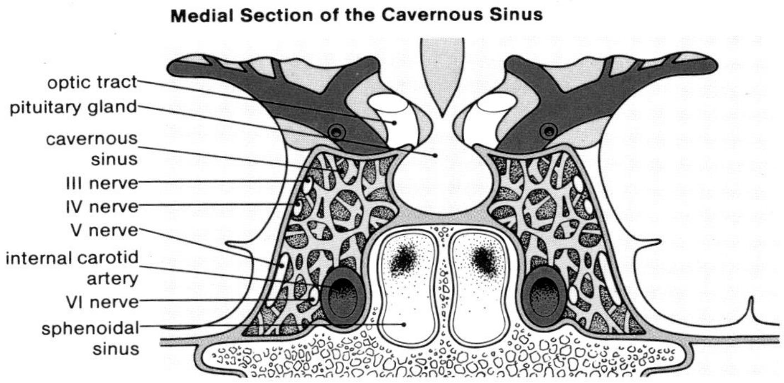

Medial Section of the Cavernous Sinus

Fig. 19.12 High resolution CT scanning with contrast enhancement shows internal details of the cavernous sinus. Lesions in this sinus usually affect the sixth nerve, with variable involvement of the third, fourth and fifth nerves, sympathetic supply, pupil, chiasm or pituitary gland.

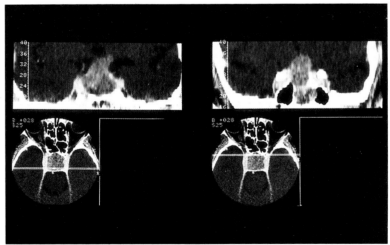

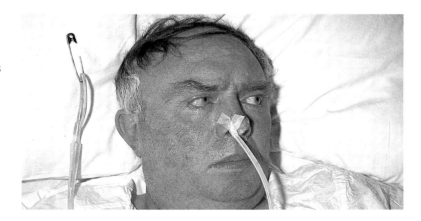

CONJUGATE GAZE PALSIES
Horizontal Supranuclear Palsy

A horizontal gaze palsy results in an inability to make a conjugate ocular movement to one side and may result from a supranuclear or pontine lesion. These can be distinguished from each other by using 'doll's head' or caloric stimuli; the ability to stimulate lateral gaze with these tests depends on the integrity of the pontine pathways and will be preserved in the presence of a supranuclear lesion.

Fig. 19.13 Following an acute cerebrovascular accident involving supranuclear pathways, saccadic gaze is lost in the direction opposite to the side of the lesion and input from the remaining hemisphere deviates the eyes towards the side of the lesion. (Occasionally, irritative lesions, such as cerebral tumours or abscesses, will produce deviation of the eyes to the contralateral side).

Fig. 19.14   On command the patient is unable to make a gaze movement to the target on his right. However, on doll's head rotation to the left, the eyes deviate fully to the right demonstrating intact pontine reflexes and the supranuclear nature of the lesion.

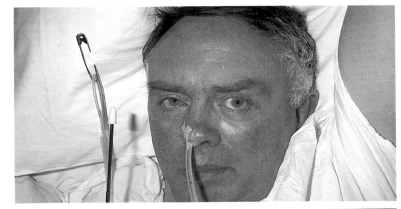

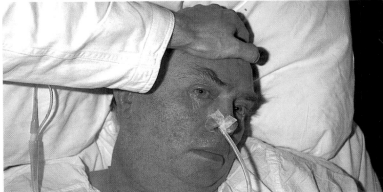

Fig. 19.15   CT scans of the patient seen in Fig. 19.14 show a large infarct in the internal capsule due to the occlusion of middle cerebral artery branches corresponding to lesion 1 in Fig. 19.16. If the patient survives, the acute ocular deviation rapidly recovers. Horizontal gaze becomes full and saccades return to normal. This is probably due to a restoration of control mechanisms by the superior colliculus of the midbrain.

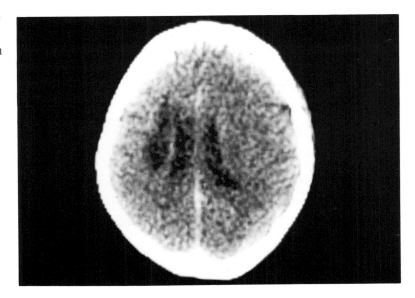

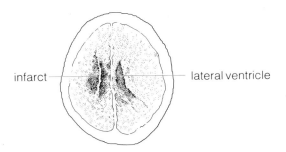

Fig. 19.16   A 'wiring diagram' shows that lesion 1 would result in a right sided supranuclear gaze palsy whereas lesion 2 destroys the pontine gaze centre producing a right sided pontine gaze palsy.

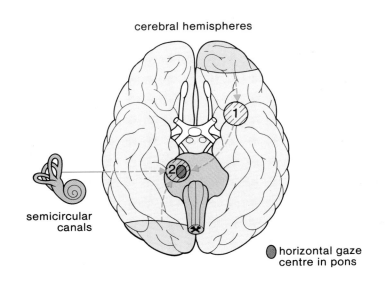

Vertical Gaze Palsy

Vertical gaze palsies are caused by lesions in the area of the upper midbrain and are relatively unusual. They produce a characteristic triad of signs known as Parinaud's syndrome or the dorsal midbrain syndrome; loss of vertical gaze and the pupillary light reflex, with preservation of the near reflex and the bizarre movement known as convergence retraction nystagmus. Vertical gaze is controlled from a centre in the posterior commissure which integrates vertical gaze; there is a downgaze centre caudal to the thalamus but isolated lesions of the area are excessively rare. Most vertical gaze palsies affect both up and down gaze but small or early lesions in the region of the posterior commissure tend to affect upgaze preferentially, especially on saccadic gaze. Lesions may compress the midbrain aqueduct producing hydrocephalus and papilloedema; lateral extension may involve the optic radiations and posterior extension produces ataxia from cerebellar compression. While tumours of the pineal gland are the most common cause of a Parinaud's syndrome, atherosclerosis, embolism, vasculitis or arterio-venous malformations may occasionally be the causal factor.

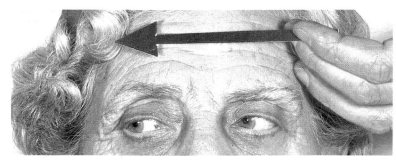

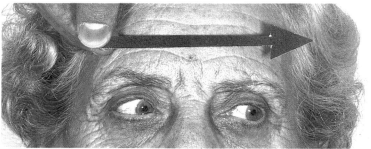

Fig. 19.17   This elderly lady suffered a cerebrovascular accident in the upper midbrain. She retains the ability to make rapid and full horizontal saccades.

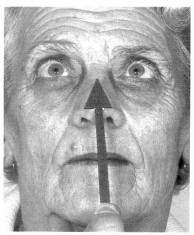
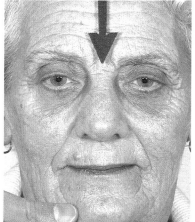

Fig. 19.18   In the same patient, voluntary up and down gaze to saccadic command are lost and compensated for by head movement.

Fig. 19.19   Doll's head rotation shows that vertical movements can be produced and that pontine reflexes are intact.

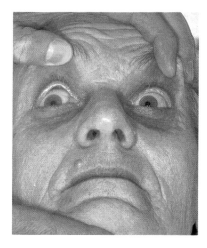

Fig. 19.20 Convergence retraction nystagmus is an interesting ocular movement abnormality sometimes seen with vertical gaze palsies. Bursts of convergence with retraction of both eyes into the orbits, are seen either spontaneously or on attempting an upward saccade. These movements can also be accompanied by accommodative spasm, which accounts for the frequent complaints of blurred vision. Convergence retraction nystagmus is shown particularly well if the patient views a downward rotating optokinetic drum (stimulating upward refixational saccades).

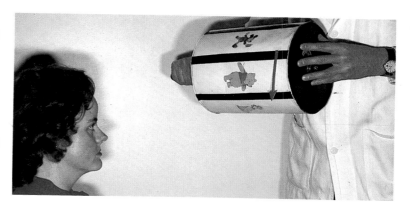

Fig. 19.21 In convergence retraction nystagmus, the lesion is thought to cause disinhibition of the ocular motor nuclei allowing bursts of co-firing of the external ocular muscles. The medial recti muscles are the most powerful of the external ocular muscles and, consequently, the globes converge and retract into the orbits.

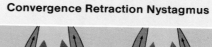

Convergence Retraction Nystagmus

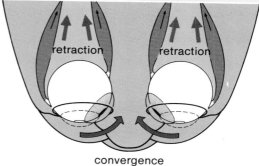

retraction   retraction

convergence

downward rotating drum

Fig. 19.22 Light-near dissociation of the pupils is the third sign of the triad of Parinaud's syndrome. The pupils are normally moderately dilated and show a poor or absent light reaction but preserve the near reaction. It has been suggested that light reflex fibres are more dorsal in the midbrain and are therefore selectively damaged by lesions in this area with comparative sparing of the more ventrally sited near reflex pathways.

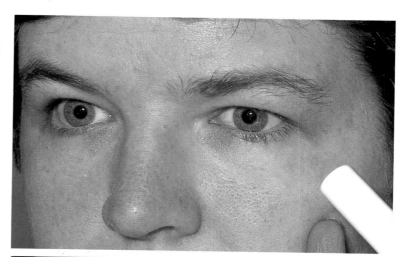

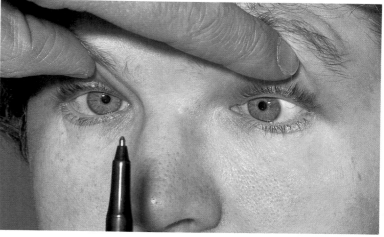

Fig. 19.23 Collier's sign is a bilateral retraction of the upper eyelids sometimes seen with acute upper mid-brain lesions. The upper midbrain is supplied by branches from the posterior cerebral arteries. This elderly man had suffered a cerebrovascular accident of the midbrain region. Horizontal gaze was entirely normal but there was a partial vertical gaze palsy and retraction of both upper eyelids. The patient had dubious long tract signs. The vertical gaze palsy and lid retraction rapidly recovered over 2-3 weeks.

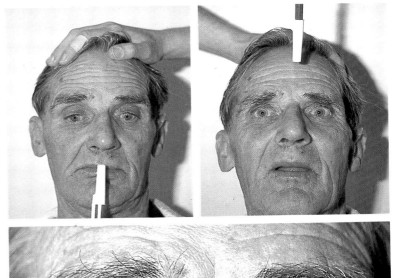

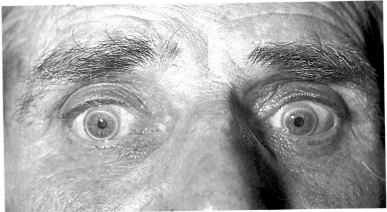

Fig. 19.24 Not unusually, large lesions will damage the third nerve nuclei, as in this boy with a large pineal tumour, producing signs of oculomotor palsy, ptosis or aniscoria as well as signs in the limbs from long tract involvement.

This enhanced CT scan shows an enormous enhancing pinealoma with grossly dilated lateral ventricles from obstruction of the midbrain aqueduct. This patient had a right third nerve palsy, involving the pupil, combined with a vertical gaze palsy and cerebella ataxia.

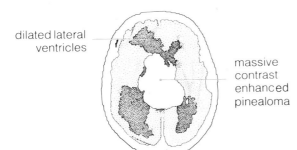

dilated lateral ventricles

massive contrast enhanced pinealoma

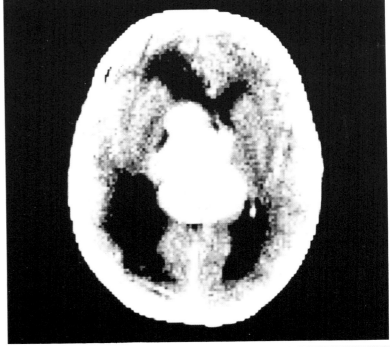

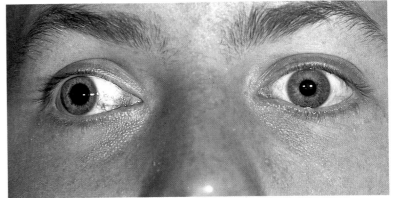

Progressive Supranuclear Palsy
(Steele-Richardson Syndrome)

This is a Parkinsonian-like syndrome in which there is extra pyramidal rigidity (especially of the extensor muscles in the neck and back) pseudo-bulbar palsy, dysarthria and dementia. The importance of the diagnosis lies in the poor prognosis: patients die in a relatively short time from progressive neurological disease whereas Parkinsonian patients will survive for many years with only moderate disability and intact mental function.

An early and diagnostic feature of progressive supranuclear ophthalmoplegia is difficulty in making downgaze saccades with preservation of horizontal saccadic movements and doll's head reflexes. Initial loss of downgaze saccades is followed by complete involvement of vertical, then horizontal gaze. Saccades are lost first, followed by pursuit movement, but doll's head reflexes are preserved until late in the disease. Similar ocular movements can be seen in children with the rare neuronal lipid storage disease (sea blue histiocyte disease).

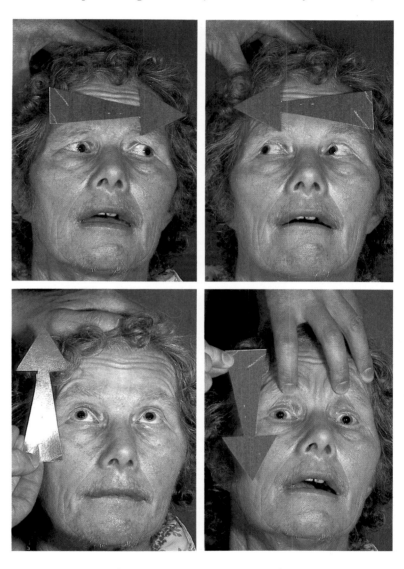

Fig. 19.25 This patient can make an upward saccadic movement, but down gaze saccades are lost. She had extrapyramidal rigidity and an early dementia.

Fig. 19.26 Downgaze is present on doll's head movement showing the supranuclear nature of the lesions. Horizontal movements are intact.

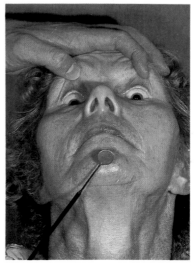

Internuclear Ophthalmoplegia

Lesions in the medial longitudinal fasciculus (MLF) produce poor adduction of the eye on the affected side and abducting nystagmus in the contralateral eye, but although the ocular movements are disconjugate patients rarely, if ever, complain of diplopia. Normal convergence demonstrates the integrity of the medial rectus muscles, providing that the lesion is not too dense, and preservation of convergence does not depend on whether the lesion affects the anterior or posterior part of the MLF. The exact physiology of MLF lesions is complicated and involves defects in pulse-step generation of agonists (Fig. 19.2) and faults in reciprocal inhibition of antagonists; excess tone of the medial rectus of the abducting eye is said to account for the nystagmus on abduction of that eye.

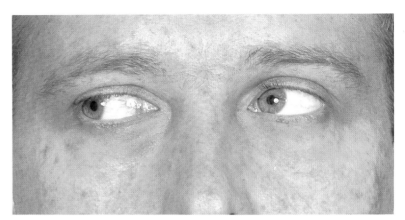

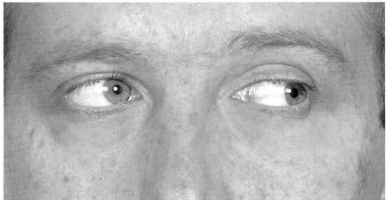

Fig. 19.27 Bilateral internuclear ophthalmoplegia in young people is almost always associated with multiple sclerosis. Vertical nystagmus is usually present on upgaze. Subtle lesions can be demonstrated by getting the patient to make rapid horizontal movements to show the slowness of adduction in each eye.

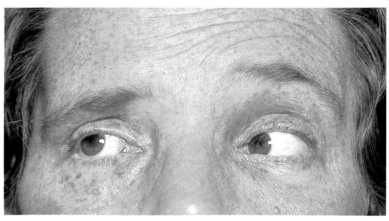

Fig. 19.28 Unilateral internuclear ophthalmoplegia is usually due to a vascular or ischaemic lesion as the basilar artery supplies the pons by lateralizing perforating branches. This hypertensive patient shows a right-sided lower motor neuron seventh nerve palsy, internuclear ophthalmoplegia and partial sixth palsy following a pontine infarct.

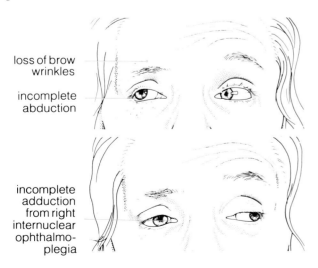

loss of brow wrinkles

incomplete abduction

incomplete adduction from right internuclear ophthalmoplegia

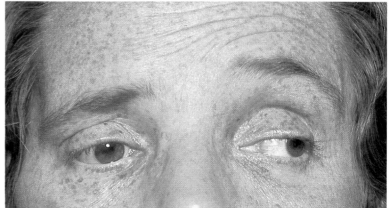

Fig. 19.29 In this recording of a right unilateral internuclear ophthalmoplegia a 30° saccadic movement to the left demonstrates slow adduction of the right eye and abducting nystagmus of the left (small arrows). Return to the primary position shows normal saccadic velocities in each eye but hypermetric overshooting saccades are seen (large arrows) which are then corrected to hold the primary position of gaze. Such overshooting saccades are a common feature of internuclear ophthalmoplegia and can be recognized clinically.

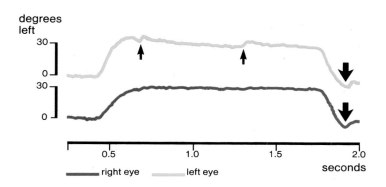

Fig. 19.30 A 'wiring diagram' shows that lesion 1 produces a right unilateral internuclear ophthalmoplegia, whereas lesion 2 causes bilateral internuclear ophthalmoplegia. Note that interneurones from the PPRF pass into the VI nerve neucleus and connect here with the MLF axons rather than passing directly from the PPRF into the MLF.

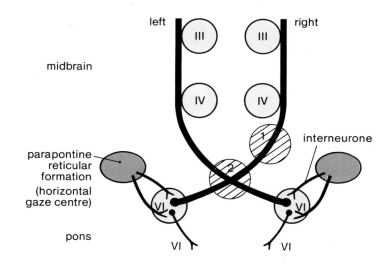

The 'One and a Half' syndrome
(Paralytic Pontine Exotropia)

A more extensive unilateral lesion involving the horizontal gaze centre and MLF will produce a combination of a gaze palsy and internuclear ophthalmoplegia – the '1½ syndrome'. In this situation, the only horizontal movement that the patient can make is abduction of the contralateral eye.

Fig. 19.31 This patient with multiple sclerosis shows a right gaze palsy and right internuclear ophthalmoplegia, with only abduction of the left eye on horizontal gaze remaining. Vertical movements were intact.

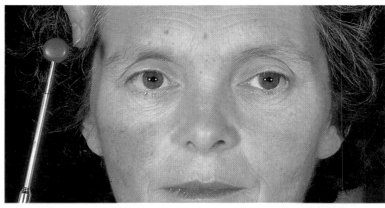

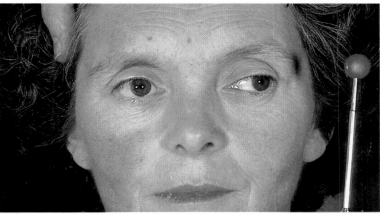

Fig. 19.32 A wiring diagram shows that lesion 3 prevents stimulation of the right PPRF producing a right pontine gaze palsy. Impulses from the cortex to the left PPRF result in stimulation of the left sixth nucleus and abduction of that eye, but stimulation of the right medial rectus through the MLF is blocked. Complete '1½' syndromes are uncommon but the combination of a partial gaze palsy with partial ipsilateral internuclear ophthalmoplegia is not uncommon and is readily observed by getting the patient to attempt rapid horizontal saccadic movements

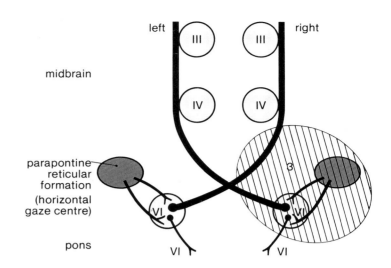

THE PUPIL

The smooth muscle of the pupil is innervated by the sympathetic (dilator pupillae) and parasympathetic systems (constrictor pupillae). Both pupils are normally of the same size but small differences in diameter are seen in about twenty per cent of the normal population and are known as essential aniscoria. Pathological aniscoria is caused by lesions affecting the sympathetic or parasympathetic pathways or by local iris disease. Lesions of the afferent visual system do not produce aniscoria, ie. sectioning one optic nerve does not alter pupillary size in that eye.

Fig. 19.33 Sympathetic impulses are generated in the region of the hypothalamus and transmitted along the spinal cord, synapsing in the lateral grey columns. Pupillary impulses leave the cord in myelinated preganglionic fibres at T1 (some also at C8 and T2) and pass upwards in the sympathetic chain to synapse in the superior cervical ganglion lying at the level of the C1 and C2 vertebrae. Nonmyelinated postganglionic fibres form a plexus on the common carotid artery; vasomotor fibres to the face leave on the external carotid artery at the bifurcation. The internal carotid artery carries sympathetic innervation into the cavernous sinus where the pupillary fibres join the nasociliary branch of the fifth nerve: other sympathetic branches are taken by branches of the ophthalmic artery to the lacrimal glands, Muller's muscles and the orbital vessels.

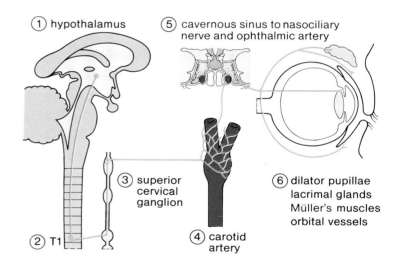

Fig. 19.34 The pupillary light reflexes are mediated through axons from ganglion cells in the retina which pass back in the optic nerve and decussate in the chiasm with the other visual fibres. The pupillary fibres pass through the optic tract and superior brachium to the Edinger-Westphal nucleus of the third nerve; here, they synapse to produce a simultaneous and bilateral response in each third nerve through interneuronal connections. Parasympathetic preganglionic axons run forward in each third nerve and pass into the inferior division at the anterior aspect of the cavernous sinus to the ciliary ganglion where they synapse to supply the constrictor pupillae by the short ciliary nerves. The ratio of light fibres to accommodative fibres in the third nerve is said to be 1:30.

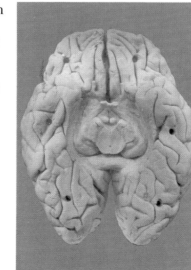
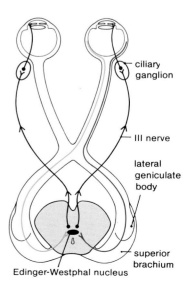

Relative Afferent Pupillary Defect

A relative afferent pupillary defect (RAPD) is an objective sign of an asymmetrical lesion of the afferent visual system (retina, optic nerve, chiasm or tract carrying the pupillary light fibres). An RAPD is seen with major retinal lesions or neurological lesions of the afferent visual pathway. Opacities in the ocular media, such as cataract, do not produce an RAPD but small RAPD's may be seen with a very dense vitreous haemorrhage or dense amblyopia. Thus, the presence of an RAPD in the absence of gross ocular disease indicates a neurological lesion in the afferent visual system and the importance of this physical sign cannot be over emphasised. Corroboration of an RAPD will be found in asymmetrical loss of visual acuity, visual field, colour and brightness sensation and optic disc pallor. Full neurological investigation of such patients is mandatory in order to identify treatable causes of visual failure.

Stimulation of one eye by a bright light produces an equal constricting response in both eyes due to the direct and consensual light reflexes and, if the afferent visual system is normal, transfer of the light to the fellow eye will maintain the same constriction and tone on this pupil. If there is an asymmetrical lesion in the afferent visual pathways on one side (compression, infarct, etc), however, transfer of the light from the good eye to the bad eye will result in 'less' stimulation of the Edinger-Westphal nucleus from that eye and a comparative dilation of both pupils and vice versa. This is seen in practice as an alternating constriction and dilatation of each pupil as the light is swung from eye to eye. A RAPD or optic disc pallor are the only objective clinical signs of disease of the afferent visual system.

Fig. 19.35 A right afferent pupillary defect is seen in this patient with retrobulbar neuritis of the right optic nerve. Stimulation of the left eye produces bilateral pupillary constriction. Transfer of the light to the right eye produces a relative dilation of the pupil in both eyes. If one pupil is damaged or paralysed, an afferent pupillary defect can still be diagnosed by observing whether the size of the response varies in the functioning pupil with alternate stimulation of the two eyes.

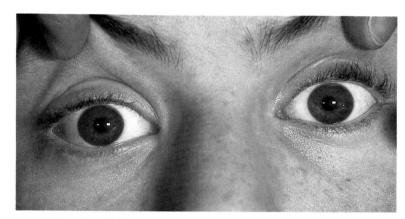

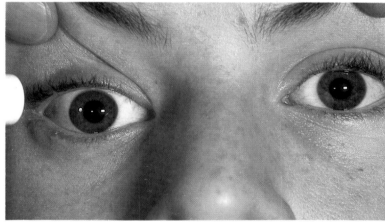

Fig. 19.36 The 'wiring diagram' demonstrates the neurological basis of an RAPD. Stimulation of the normal left eye produces brisk bilateral and equal pupillary constriction by the direct and consensual light reflexes. Rapid transfer to the right eye, where there is an optic nerve lesion, removes some relative input on the Edinger-Westphal nucleus and both pupils dilate. Oscillation of the light from left to right to left to right is seen as tendency for the right pupil to dilate and for the left to constrict.

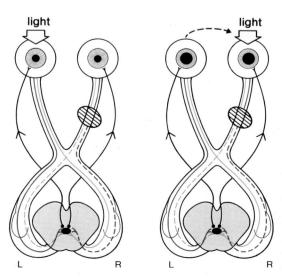

Horner's Syndrome

Horner's syndrome is the result of a lesion in the sympathetic pathway to the eye and may be due to a lesion in the central, pre- or postganglionic neuronal pathways. The features are of miosis and slight ptosis of the upper and lower lid on the affected side; if the branches on the external carotid artery have been affected there is a loss of facial sweating with acute lesions, and facial and conjunctival blood vessels may be dilated.

The diagnosis can be confirmed by instilling G.4% cocaine in both eyes and observing the pupillary

diameters 15 minutes later. The normal pupil dilates and eyelids retract as reuptake of norepinephrine at the synapse is blocked by the cocaine. The diseased eye has no norepinephrine release to be blocked and the pupil size, therefore, does not alter.

Failure to dilate to G hydroxyamphetamine demonstrates a postganglionic lesion; and this is important since preganglionic lesions are often sinister and may accompany lesions such as a Pancroast tumour of the lung.

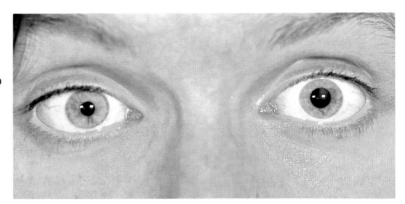

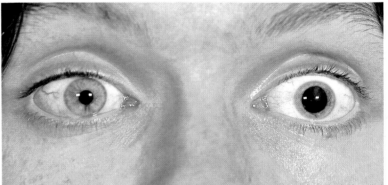

Fig. 19.37 Miosis and ptosis are seen in the affected right eye of a patient with acquired Horner's syndrome. Fifteen minutes after a drop of G.4% cocaine to each eye, the left pupil dilates and the right is unchanged, confirming the diagnosis. Subsequent failure of the right pupil to dilate to G hydroxyamphetamine solution would show that the localization of the lesion was postganglionic. Horner's syndrome does not produce more than about 2mm of ptosis which is due to involvement of Muller's muscle in both the upper and lower lids.

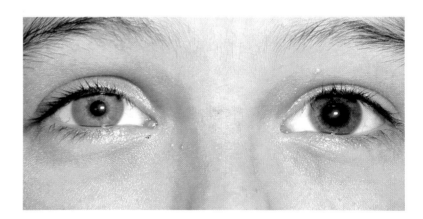

Fig. 19.38 Heterochromia is a feature of congenital Horner's syndrome, the affected iris being lighter in colour.

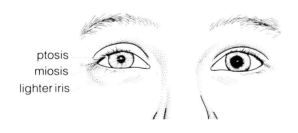

ptosis
miosis
lighter iris

Pupillary Light-Near Dissociation

A poor response of the light reflex with preservation of the near response is a feature of Argyl Robertson pupils, Parinaud's syndrome, Adie's pupils, aberrant third nerve regeneration or uniocular visual loss with intact third nerves.

Argyl Robertson pupils are irregular, miosed and asymmetrical in size with a poor light reflex and brisk near reflex. They are the hallmark of neurosyphilis. However, similar pupils are seen on very rare occasions in diabetics. The lesion is located in the region of the Edinger-Westphal nucleus.

Adie's pupil is due to a lesion of the ciliary ganglion. In the acute stage the pupil is dilated with an absent or poor tonic light reaction, and shows a poor amplitude of

accommodation with a tonic slow pupillary near reflex. With time the pupil becomes miosed and the other eye may be affected. Deep tendon reflexes can be lost. Typical sectorial iris atrophy is seen and is due to sectorial denervation of the iris sphincter following the ciliary ganglion lesion. Slow tonic 'vermicular' or worm-like contractions of the remaining sphincter in response to light or near reflexes are best seen on the slit lamp. The tonicity of the pupillary reflexes is thought to be produced by reinnervation of the iris following the acute lesion by misdirected fibres subserving accommodation in the ciliary ganglion.

Fig. 19.39 Typical sectorial iris palsies seen in two cases of Adie's pupil. Hypersensitivity of the pupil to G⅛%. Pilocarpine substantiates the diagnosis.

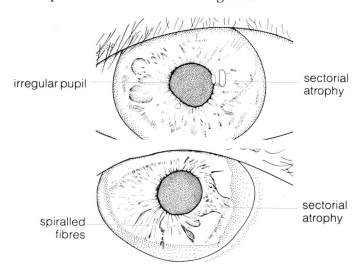

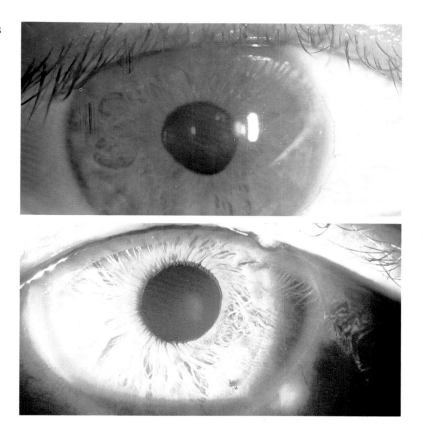

VISUAL FIELD LOSS

Advances in CT scanning have made meticulous charting of visual fields less important as an aid to topographical diagnosis of neurological lesions which affect the visual system. Nevertheless, visual field assessment remains one of the keystones of clinical ophthalmic diagnosis and accurate charting of fields is necessary in the evaluation and follow-up of a wide variety of diseases. Carefully performed confrontation fields provide diagnostic information in the majority of cases but charting by one or other of the standard methods is necessary to identify small defects or provide a permanent record.

Behind the globe, the majority of optic nerve fibres transmit information from the central visual field (60-70% of optic nerve fibres subserve the central 30% of field) and it is therefore in the central field where the subtle and early lesions are usually found. This area of field has a high density of cones and a red target is particularly good for the detection of central field loss. In general, retinal and optic disc field defects are arranged about the horizontal meridian, optic nerve lesions produce a central scotoma and lesions in, or posterior to the chiasm, produce field defects about the vertical meridian.

Fig. 19.40 Lesions at the optic disc will produce arcuate field defects depending on their site. These can be forecast by the identification of the corresponding grooves in the retinal nerve fibre layer or sectorial optic disc pallor with axonal destruction.

Prechiasmal Field Defects

Axons from the retinal ganglion cells converge on the optic disc; they are divided horizontally by the horizontal raphe on the temporal side, but enter radially on the nasal side. The 'maculo-papular bundle', which subserves central vision, runs directly between disc and macula although the horizontal division of nerve fibres is still maintained. Damage to a bundle of axons at the vertical margins of the disc will produce characteristic uniocular 'arcuate' field defects (cf Primary Glaucoma; Chapter 7, and Optic Disc; Chapter 17).

Disease of the retinal ganglion cells preferentially affects the maculo-papular axons and produces central field loss. When this extends from the optic disc to the macula it is known as a centrocaecal scotoma and is seen in toxic or nutritional amblyopias, drug toxicity or inherited optic nerve disease. The results obtained on perimetry may vary according to the target size and colour. A centrocaecal or central scotoma can be produced by manipulation of these so that either field pattern can be obtained and retinal ganglion cell or optic nerve disease cannot be distinguished by perimetry alone.

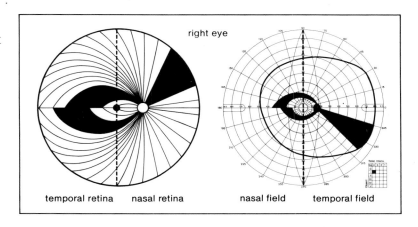

right eye

temporal retina   nasal retina   nasal field   temporal field

Fig. 19.41 This patient with autosomal dominant optic atrophy has a typical centrocaecal pattern of field loss.

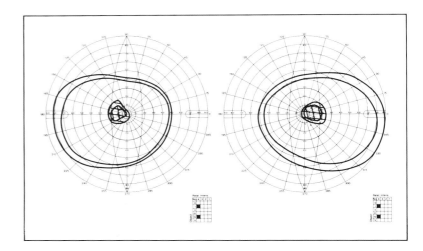

Fig. 19.42 Optic discs of the same patient are myopic but show marked bilateral temporal pallor and loss of the maculo-papular bundles. Acuities were 6/60 right and left with gross colour loss in each eye. Fields remained unchanged over many years.

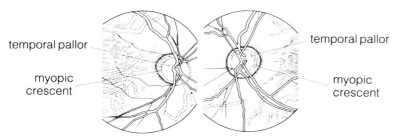

Fig. 19.43 Shortly behind the optic disc, macula fibres come to lie in the centre of the optic nerve and damage to the optic nerve usually produces a central scotoma (cf Optic Disc; Chapter 17). Destruction of nerve fibres in the anterior visual pathway (from the retina to the lateral geniculate body) results in atrophy and loss of retinal nerve fibres about 6 weeks later. This can be seen as

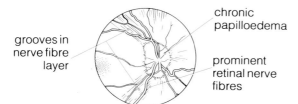

grooves in the nerve fibre layer of a patient with chronic atrophic papilloedema. Nerve fibre defects are most easily observed by using red-free light. Confirmation of optic nerve damage is found in a lowered visual acuity, reduced colour and brightness sensation, a relative pupillary defect and corresponding visual field defects.

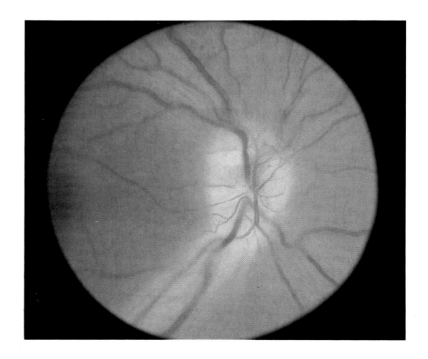

THE CHIASM
Anatomy

Fifty percent of visual fibres from each eye decussate at the chiasm, although albinos have an interesting anomaly with a larger percentage decussation. Field defects produced by chiasmal lesions (most common lesions are pituity adenoma, craniopharyngioma, suprasellar meningioma or aneurysm) will depend on the anatomy of the chiasm and this varies from patient to patient.

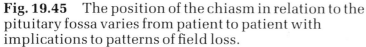

Fig. 19.44   The optic nerves exit from the optic canals at an angle of about 45° to the horizontal and have an intracranial course of about 15mm. The chiasm lies about 10mm above the roof of the pituitary fossa. It follows, therefore, that a pituitary tumour must grow to a considerable extent above the fossa in order to compress the chiasm. For this reason patients with endocrine secreting tumours usually present before they develop field defects while the non-hormone secreting chromophobe adenomas commonly present with visual failure.

Fig. 19.45   The position of the chiasm in relation to the pituitary fossa varies from patient to patient with implications to patterns of field loss.

The chiasm is said to be prefixed if it lies on the tuberculum sellae or diaphragma sella (16% of normals), normally fixed if it lies on the diaphragma projecting backwards onto the dorsum sella (80%) and post-fixed if lying on the dorsum sella, posterior to the fossa (4%). Thus,

a pituitary tumour might compress the posterior chiasm or optic tracts (prefixed chiasm), the anterior chiasm (normally fixed chiasms) or, exceptionally, the optic nerves with posterior fixation. While the anatomy of the chiasm would indicate predictable field defects, surgical inspection of any lesion in this area will show traction and distortion deranging the normal anatomy so that no firm correlation can be made.

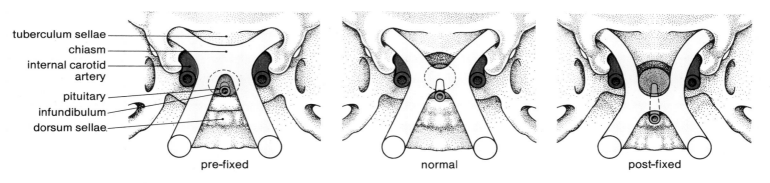

Fig. 19.46   Nasal retinal fibres (temporal field) decussate to the opposite optic tract while temporal retinal fibres (nasal field) remain uncrossed. Inferior nasal fibres (superior temporal fields) decussate anteriorly and superior nasal fibres (inferior temporal fibres) posteriorly. After the superiotemporal field fibres decussate they tend to bend forwards into the fellow optic nerve (von Willebrands's Knee) before passing into the optic tract. The angle between individual optic nerves and the degree of this forward flexion varies accordingly – the narrower angle tends to produce more forward flexion and a wider angle produces less.

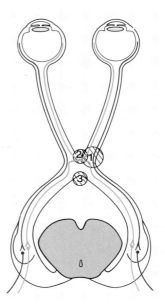

Chiasmal Field Defects

Fig. 19.47 A lesion on the outer lateral aspect of the tuberculum sella, commonly a meningioma, (lesion 1 in Fig. 19.46) may compress not only the optic nerve on the same side but also the inferonasal fibres from the other eye. This produces a 'junctional' field defect – a central scotoma in one eye with superiotemporal loss in the other. Clinically, this implies that a patient with a unilateral central scotoma should have a particularly careful examination of the superiotemporal field in the other eye to exclude intracranial disease.

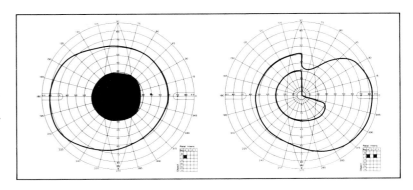

Fig. 19.48 An enhanced CT scan demonstrates a suprasellar meningioma which produced this unusual 'junctional' pattern of field defect. The patient also had a partial sixth palsy and third palsy with aberrant regeneration from invasion of the cavernous sinus. Plain skull x-rays showed hyperostosis of the lesser wing of the sphenoid.

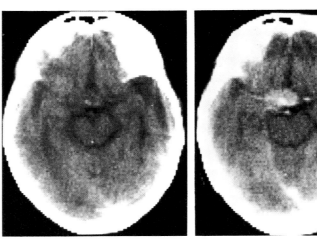

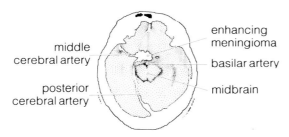

Fig. 19.49 By far the most common cause of chiasmal compression is a large chromophobe pituitary adenoma. This can be easily identified on lateral skull x-ray by an enlargement of the pituitary fossa, a double floor, and undercutting or erosion of the anterior and posterior clinoid processes.

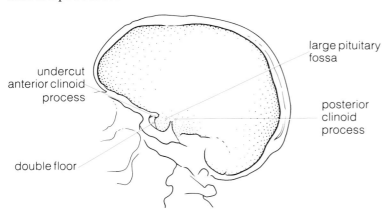

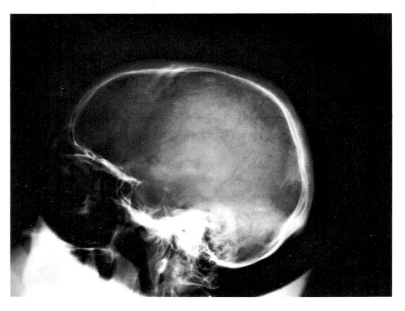

Fig. 19.50 CT scanning is the investigation of choice to confirm the prescence of a pituitary lesion. A contrast enhanced CT scan shows a large cystic chromophobe adenoma expanding the pituitary fossa and extending inferiorly into the sphenoid sinus and superiorly above the sella to compress the chiasm.

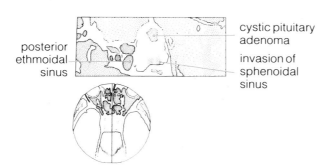

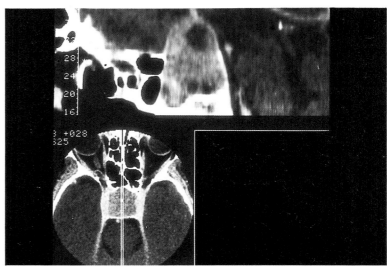

Fig. 19.51 This diagram shows a typical superior bitemporal field defect which would be produced by a lesion at site 2 in Fig. 19.46 (a lesion at site 3 would produce an inferior bitemporal defect). The patient had acuities of 6/18 and 6/24, a left relative afferent pupillary defect (RAPD), poor colour vision in both eyes, but worse in the left, and bilateral optic disc pallor, which was greater in the left eye.

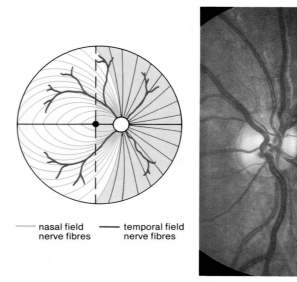

Fig. 19.52 Longstanding chiasmal compression produces characteristic patterns of optic atrophy. Temporal retinal nerve fibres (nasal visual field) arch around the macula and enter the disc vertically, superiorly and inferiorly. Correspondingly, nasal retinal fibres (temporal field) enter the disc horizontally on both sides. Selective optic atrophy from a chiasmal lesion appears initially as a temporal pallor of the disc with retinal grooving from loss of nerve fibres because the macula nerve fibres which are in the temporal field (retina nasal to the fovea) are more dense than those on the nasal side of the disc. The progression of optic disc appearances is therefore initially of temporal pallor followed by horizontal sectorial pallor in a 'bow tie' pattern and eventually total optic atrophy as the tumour completely compresses the optic pathways. The amount of optic atrophy present is a good indication of the visual recovery that the patient can expect following surgical decompression.

— nasal field nerve fibres   — temporal field nerve fibres

Retro-Chiasmal Pathways

All lesions posterior to the chiasm must, by definition, produce a homonymous hemianopic field defect. A complete homonymous hemianopia has no topographical localizing value in the absence of other signs but partial homonymous defects can produce diagnostic information on the localisation of the lesion. It is important to realise that, as macular fibres are represented in both visual cortices, a complete hemianopia always leaves the patient with normal visual acuities.

Optic tract defects are uncommon and usually result from lesions causing chiasmal compression extending posteriorly, or trauma at the time of the surgical removal. These field defects are distinguished by the marked incongruity of the field defect (difference in size and density between the two affected hemifields) in association with an afferent pupillary defect on the same side as the hemianopia from damage to the pupillary fibres in the optic tract, and bilateral optic disc pallor.

Lesions of the lateral geniculate body are excessively rare but produce increasingly complex incongruous homonymous hemianopias.

Fig. 19.53 A right grossly incongruous homonymous hemianopia with a relative afferent pupillary defect in the right eye indicates an optic tract or lateral geniculate body lesion, as seen in this young woman. The posterior cerebral artery contributes to the blood supply of the lateral geniculate body and optic tract and the patient had suffered a recent posterior cerebral artery infarct extending into this region during a severe migrainous attack. The CT scan shows low attenuation and enhancement with contrast in this area.

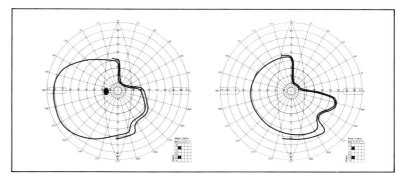

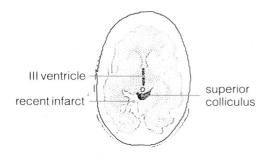

III ventricle —
recent infarct —
superior colliculus

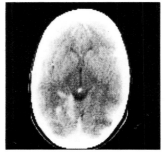

Optic Radiations

After synapsing in the lateral geniculate body, the visual fibres pass posteriorly to the visual cortex on the medial aspect of the occipital lobe; they become better and more tightly organized in their retinotopic projection as they approach the cortex, superior fibres carry inferior fields and vice versa. For this reason, posteriorly placed cortical lesions produce denser and more congruous field defects.

Fig. 19.54 The optic radiation. Inferior fibres loop forwards around the temporal horn of the lateral ventricle (Meyer's loop). The extent of this looping forwards varies and a temporal lobe lesion will only produce a field defect if the loop projects forwards into the lobe.

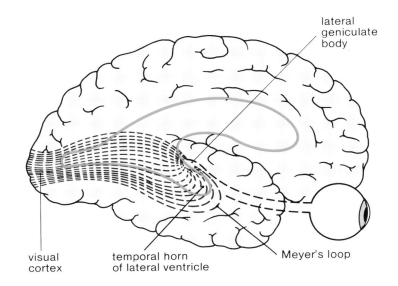

Fig. 19.55 The blood supply of the optic radiations is derived from the middle and posterior cerebral arteries. The anastomosis at the occipital pole between these circulations is thought to account for the phenomenon of macular sparing with occipital lobe lesions. The lateral geniculate body and optic tract are supplied by both posterior and middle cerebral vessels.

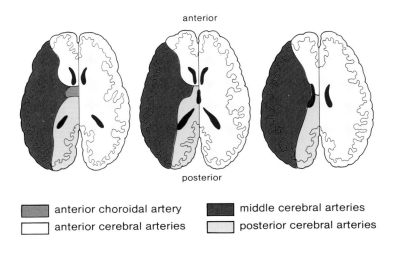

Fig. 19.56 It is unusual for temporal lobe lesions to produce a field defect (Fig. 19.54). They damage the inferior radiation fibres which loop around the temporal horn of the lateral ventricle. This produces an upper quadrantic hemianopia, usually denser in the eye with a nasal defect. Pure temporal lobe field defects must, by definition, have normal pupillary responses as the pupillary fibres have already separated from the visual fibres. However, the temporal lobe and optic tracts lie in close proximity (Fig. 19.34) and share a similar blood supply so that it is not uncommon for temporal lobe lesions to involve the optic tracts. This would be shown by the presence of an afferent pupillary defect in the eye on the side of the lesion.

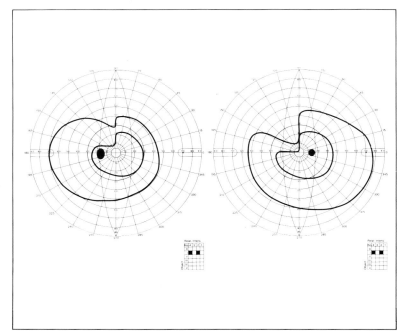

Fig. 19.57 Localized parietal lobe lesions produce an inferior homonymous hemianopia. If the field defect is produced by a space-occupying lesion rather than a vascular infarct, optokinetic nystagmus (OKN) will also be lost and this is a valuable clinical sign in the differential diagnosis of parietal lobe lesions. This is best demonstrated by asking the patient to fixate the stripes on a rotating drum. Under normal circumstances the eyes make a pursuit movement to follow the stripes and a refixational saccade at the end of each traverse to take up fixation on another stripe. The control for both of these normal physiological sequences is generated in the same cerebral hemisphere. Thus, if the patient follows a drum rotating to his right his eyes make a pursuit movement to the right generated by the ipsilateral occipito-parietal lobe, and a refixational saccade to the left generated by the ipsilateral frontal lobe. Thus, rotating the stripes to the patient's right tests the integrity of the right cerebral hemisphere OKN response and vice versa.

Tumours such as this glioma will produce a right homonymous hemianopia with loss of OKN to the right and preservation of the OKN response to the left. If the hemianopic field defect is produced by a vascular infarct the OKN response remains normal to both sides.

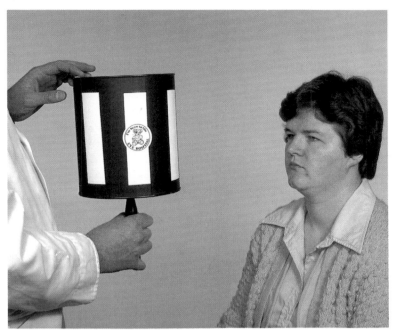

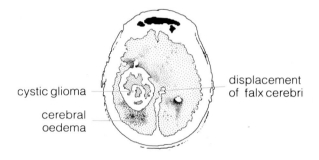

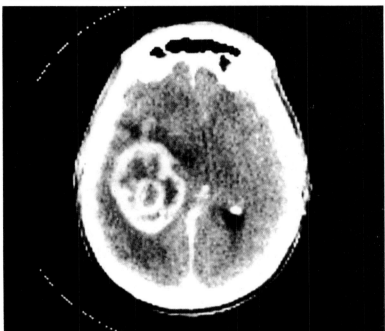

Fig. 19.58 The primary visual cortex (also called the striate cortex due to the line of myelination in area 4) lies above and below the calcarine fissure on the medial surface of the occipital lobe, extending more deeply inferiorly than superiorly. The total length is about 5cm and approximately half of this is concerned with central vision with the macula itself being represented most posteriorly on the superficial surface at the pole of the occipital lobe. The outer temporal 30° of visual field is represented uniocularly in the inner depths of the calcarine fissure.

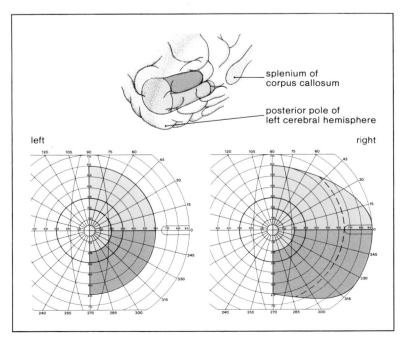

Fig. 19.59 The most common cause of an isolated homonymous hemianopia in the absence of other neurological signs is an occipital lobe infarct from an occlusion in the posterior cerebral artery territory. If macula sparing occurs (preservation of the central 5–10° of visual field from collateral circulation to the occipital pole by the middle cerebral artery) it is diagnostic of an occipital lobe lesion. Sparing of the outer temporal field in the eye on the side of the hemianopia is also a feature of some relatively localized occipital lobe infarcts and is due to unilateral representation of the outer temporal field in the depths of the calcarine fissure (Fig. 19.58).

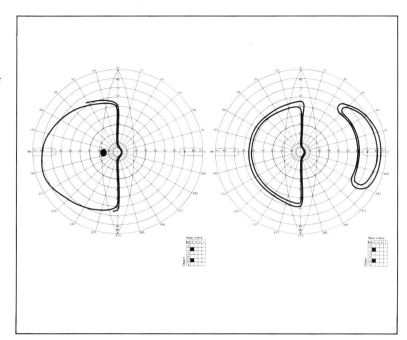

Fig. 19.60 Pre and post contrast enhancement CT scans demonstrate a recent infarct in the right occipital lobe. (Contrast enhancement is due to the hyperaemia surrounding the infarct in the early stages and disappears within a few weeks to leave a non-enhancing low density area).

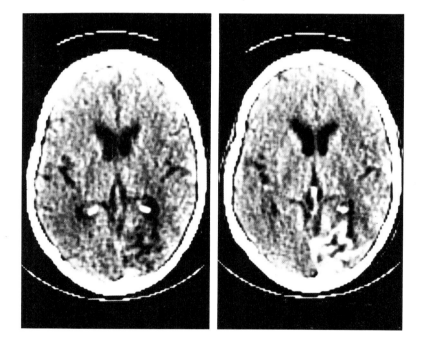

20. The Orbit and Lacrimal System

D. J. Spalton
J. E. Wright

Introduction

The orbit is conical with a volume of approximately 30ml and, in addition to the globe and the optic nerve, contains the external ocular muscles, the ophthalmic artery and its branches, the orbital veins and nerves, and the lacrimal gland. The orbital fat fills the remaining space and acts as a protective cushion: it also contains fibrous septa, which run in planes between the ocular muscles and periosteum and support the orbital contents. Prolapse of the orbital fat with these septa is frequently responsible for the limitations of ocular motility seen following a blowout fracture (cf. Chapter 18 – Strabismus).

The orbit attracts a diverse array of pathology, much of which is uncommon, and it requires an experienced team comprising ophthalmologist, radiologist, neurologist, pathologist and radiotherapist to manage this wide spectrum of disease. Some of the more common conditions are illustrated in this chapter.

ANATOMY

Fig. 20.1   Periosteum covers the orbital bones and is firmly adherent to the anterior rim and to the apex around the optic canal. It is continuous with the dura through the superior orbital fissure and optic canal.

The orbit has a floor and roof, and medial and lateral walls. The lateral wall is formed by the zygomatic bone and greater wing of the sphenoid; the roof by the frontal bone and part of the lesser wing of the sphenoid. The lacrimal fossa lies as a recess in the roof of the frontal bone, just above the junction with the zygoma.

The floor is formed anteriorly by the maxillary process of the zygoma, centrally by the orbital plate of the maxilla, and posteriorly by a small portion of the palatine bone. The infraorbital fissure lies between the greater wing of the sphenoid and the orbital plate of the maxilla and communicates with the pterygopalatine fossa posteriorly. A medial branch, the infraorbital groove, carries the infraorbital nerve (VB) and vessels. The medial wall is formed, from anterior to posterior, by the frontal process of the maxilla, the lacrimal bone (with the lacrimal fossa laying between), the ethmoid and the body of the sphenoid. Radiological enlargement of the bony orbit is a common feature of long-standing (and usually benign) orbital tumours.

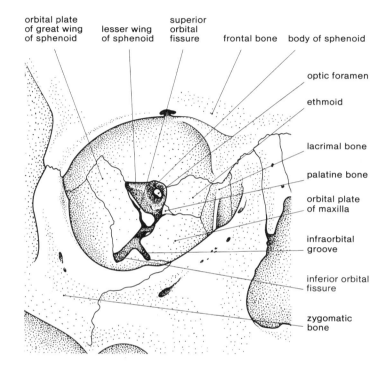

Fig. 20.2   The superior orbital fissure lies between the greater wing of the sphenoid inferiorly, and the lesser wing superiorly. The nerves and blood vessels contained within it can be grouped according to their relationship to the annulus of Zinn: the lacrimal and frontal branches of the fifth nerve, the trochlear nerve and the superior ophthalmic vein are found superiorly and external to the annulus of Zinn; the superior and inferior divisions of the third nerve and the sixth and nasociliary nerves within the annulus. In the body of the sphenoid lies the optic canal. It is lined with dura and transmits only the optic nerve and ophthalmic artery, which lies inferior to the nerve.

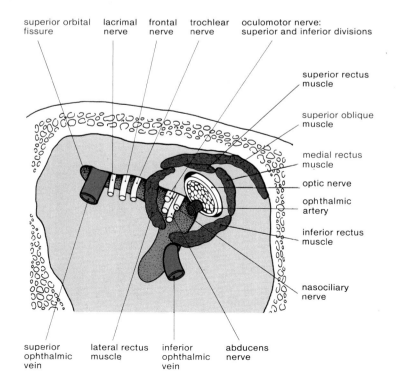

Orbital Blood Supply

Fig. 20.3 The ophthalmic artery arises from the internal carotid artery immediately above the cavernous sinus and enters the orbit through the optic canal inferior to the optic nerve. It then passes laterally and superiorly over the optic nerve to give branches to the lacrimal gland and ocular muscles. The ophthalmic artery continues anteriorly and leaves the muscle cone to anastomose with branches of the external carotid artery in the lids, face and scalp.

The posterior ciliary arteries leave the ophthalmic artery as two branches in the orbital apex, inferior to the nerve, and pass forwards and divide to enter the globe around the disc in 13–20 smaller branches to supply the optic disc and choroid. The central retinal artery also arises from the ophthalmic artery and passes forwards, inferior to the optic nerve, to penetrate the nerve some 10–12mm posterior to the sclera.

The posterior and anterior ethmoidal arteries arise from the ophthalmic artery on the medial side of the orbit and enter the ethmoidal sinuses; the posterior ethmoidal artery lies just anterior to the optic canal and is an important surgical landmark.

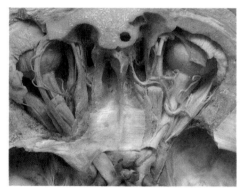
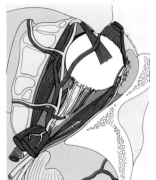

Fig. 20.4 The vortex veins from the choroid drain into the superior and inferior ophthalmic veins which flow into the cavernous sinus posteriorly and pterygopalatine plexus inferiorly. Apsidal veins join the superior and inferior ophthalmic veins in the orbit. Anteriorly, the orbital veins communicate with the frontal vein draining the scalp to form the facial vein, which then drains into the external jugular vein. Orbital veins do not have valves and the free communication between the intra and extracranial venous drainage explains the facility with which infection can spread from the orbit intracranially.

A normal venogram shows dye entering the orbit from the frontal vein through the angular vein to form the superior ophthalmic vein which is in three portions. The first part lies extraconally passing posteriorly to enter the muscle cone superior to the medial rectus, the second part lies intraconally superior to the optic nerve and the third, also intraconal, passes laterally and posteriorly to enter the cavernous sinus through the superior orbital fissure. The inferior ophthalmic vein does not fill routinely. The superior ophthalmic vein lies symmetrically on each side so that distortion, displacement or filling defects from orbital lesions can be compared to the normal side. Lateral views are also sometimes useful.

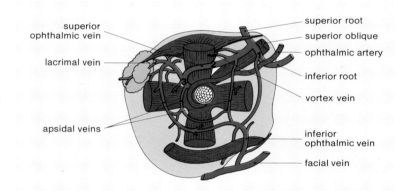
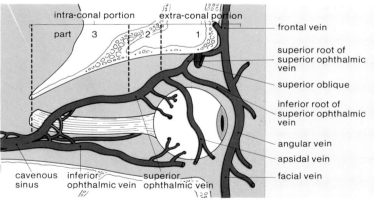
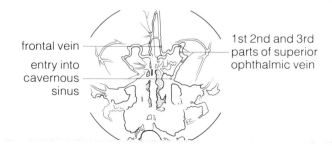
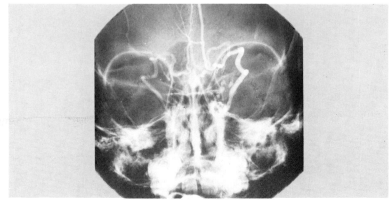

Fig. 20.5 A dissection of the lateral orbit demonstrates the orbital part of the lacrimal gland and its nerve. The lateral rectus muscle and the sixth nerve are retracted to demonstrate the ciliary ganglion and the short ciliary nerves. The ciliary ganglion contains not only the synapses of the parasympathetic fibres to the iris and ciliary body from the third nerve but also the efferent (and non-synapsing) sympathetic fibres to the ocular blood vessels. Afferent sensory fibres from the cornea, iris and ciliary body pass through the ganglion to the nasociliary branch of the ophthalmic nerve.

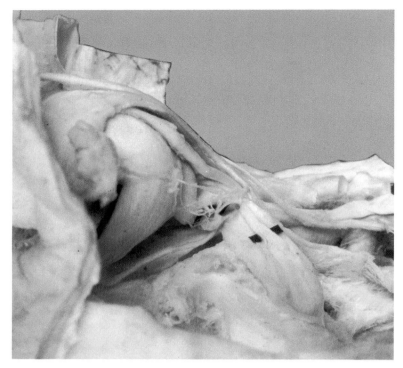

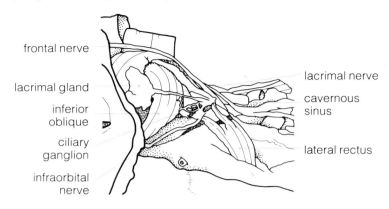

frontal nerve
lacrimal gland
inferior oblique
ciliary ganglion
infraorbital nerve

lacrimal nerve
cavernous sinus
lateral rectus

Fig. 20.6 Anatomical sections enable a clear correlation to be made between the orbital anatomy and the CT scan appearance. Note the close relationship of the frontal lobes to the orbital roof, the anterior and posterior ethmoidal sinuses to the medial orbital wall, and the sphenoidal sinus to the optic canal at the apex.

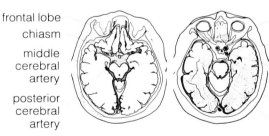

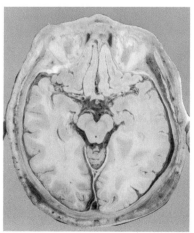

frontal lobe
chiasm
middle cerebral artery
posterior cerebral artery

optic nerve
internal carotid artery
pituitary stalk
cavernous sinus
basilar artery
IV ventricle

Fig. 20.7 The middle cranial fossa and temporal lobes lie posterior to the orbit and are separated from it by the sphenoidal wings. The temporal fossa and muscles lie laterally and the maxillary sinus lies inferomedially.

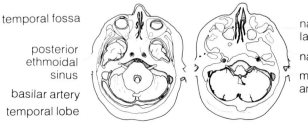

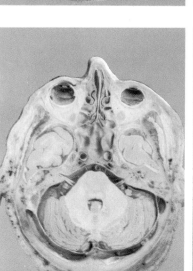

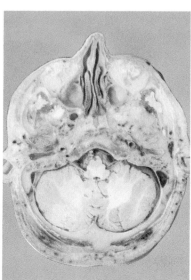

temporal fossa
posterior ethmoidal sinus
basilar artery
temporal lobe

nasal lacrimal duct
nasal cavity
maxillary antrum

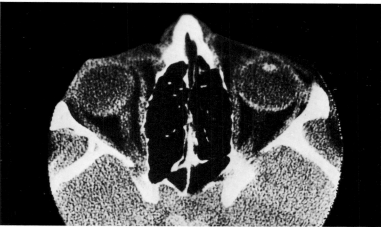

Fig. 20.8 Axial and coronal CT scans demonstrate the neuroradiological anatomy of a normal orbit. Axial scans taken along the line joining the external auditory meatus and inferior orbital rim should cut the globe and lens, optic nerve and optic canal. The superior ophthalmic fissure can be mistaken for the optic canal which lies medially and superiorly, adjacent and medial to the anterior clinoid process. The optic nerve has a sinuous course within the orbit and cannot always be seen on a single tomogram if the section is thin. Similarly, if scans are not interpreted carefully, partial sections of the ocular muscles can resemble a space-occupying mass at the apex.

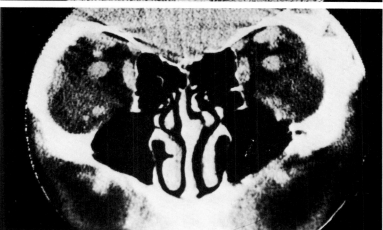

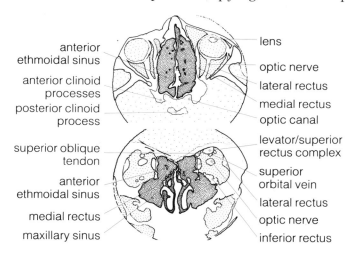

anterior ethmoidal sinus
anterior clinoid processes
posterior clinoid process
superior oblique tendon
anterior ethmoidal sinus
medial rectus
maxillary sinus

lens
optic nerve
lateral rectus
medial rectus
optic canal
levator/superior rectus complex
superior orbital vein
lateral rectus
optic nerve
inferior rectus

EXAMINATION OF THE ORBIT

A careful case history is essential in the diagnosis of orbital problems. Particular attention must be paid to the onset and duration of symptoms and the presence of pain, diplopia or visual failure. The importance of progressive symptoms which indicate an expanding lesion or deteriorating situation cannot be over emphasized. A survey of old photographs of the patient can be extremely useful in dating the onset of long-standing proptosis. Many orbital diseases are related to systemic conditions; a systemic history and examination for disease elsewhere, together with a neuro-ophthalmic examination for associated intracranial disease, is therefore obligatory in the assessment of all patients.

Proptosis must be distinguished from pseudoproptosis due to enlargement of the globe, congenital bony deformity, enophthalmos of the fellow eye, or lid disease. (Occasionally a Horner's syndrome will present as 'proptosis' of the contralateral eye).

Initial examination of a patient with orbital disease should include corrected visual acuities and retinoscopy, colour vision, visual fields and pupillary reflexes, ocular movements and funduscopy with documentation of proptosis and displacement of the globe. Initial investigation of orbital problems usually involves skull radiography and orbital CT scanning; more specialized techniques of ultrasonography, venography and angiography are required in some situations.

Fig. 20.9 The degree of proptosis is measured using an exophthalmometer. The feet of the instrument are placed on each bony lateral orbital margin and the distance between the feet (which is, therefore, the same as the distance between each lateral orbital rim) is recorded to make future comparisons valid. The patient's and observer's eyes are aligned, correcting for parallax (the fellow eye must be occluded if a strabismus is present) and the protrusion of the apex of the cornea in front of the lateral orbital margin is recorded. There is no normal absolute value of proptosis as this distance of the corneal apex varies with individual facial anatomy, but a difference of 2mm or more of proptosis between the two eyes is usually taken as significant.

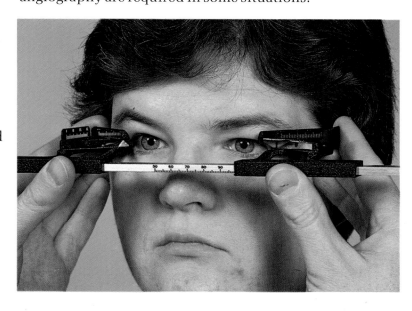

Fig. 20.10 Proptosis may be axial (displacement along the visual axis) or nonaxial (displacement off the visual axis). This can be judged by placing a clear plastic rule horizontally across the bridge of the patient's nose and measuring the horizontal and vertical positions of the visual axis of each eye.

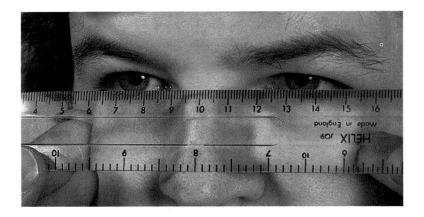

ACUTE PROPTOSIS

Rapid onset of proptosis, accompanied by pain and chemosis of the conjunctiva, is usually caused by orbital cellulitis or inflammatory pseudotumour; retrobulbar haemorrhage or a rapidly infiltrating carcinoma are less common causes. Orbital cellulitis is frequently associated with adjacent sinus infection and requires careful

management to prevent permanent ocular motility problems or the disastrous sequelae of cavernous sinus thrombosis. A sterile obstruction of a paranasal sinus can lead to mucus accumulation with chronic enlargement of the sinus, formation of a 'mucocoele' and encroachment into the orbit to displace the globe.

Fig. 20.11 Acute orbital cellulitis presents with fever and malaise, pain, proptosis, and conjunctival injection and oedema. Patients frequently have a history of sinus infection and occasionally, particularly in elderly patients, an orbital cellulitis may be secondary to a carcinoma infiltrating and obstructing a sinus.

This girl has an acutely swollen and painful upper left

lid with depression of the globe from a cellulitis in the superior orbit, secondary to a frontal sinusitis.

Patients require hospital admission and bacteriological cultures from the nose, pharynx and conjunctiva and blood before starting treatment with the appropriate intravenous antibiotics. If an orbital or subperiosteal abscess develops, this must be drained.

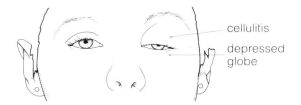

cellulitis
depressed globe

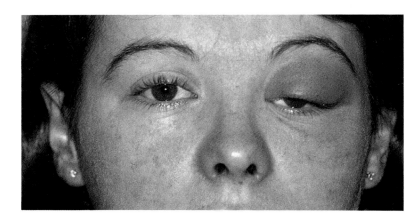

Fig. 20.12 Routine sinus x-rays of the same patient show a fluid level in the frontal sinus and opacity of the ethmoidal and maxillary sinuses. Cavernous sinus thrombosis is now a rare complication of orbital cellulitis but is characterized by meningism, ocular motor palsies and acute inflammatory changes in the cerebrospinal fluid.

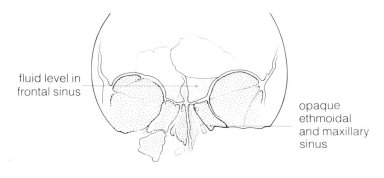

fluid level in frontal sinus

opaque ethmoidal and maxillary sinus

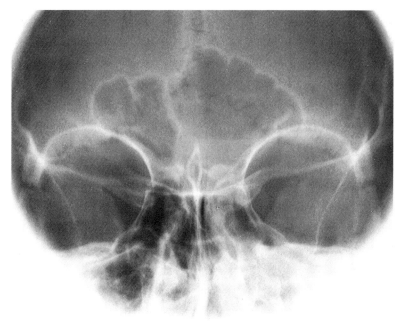

ORBITAL TRAUMA

A blunt injury to the globe can increase intraorbital pressure to produce a 'blowout' fracture into the maxillary or ethmoidal sinuses (cf. Strabismus – Chapter 18).

The optic nerve is easily compressed or traumatized in the tight confines of the orbital apex. This may occur as the direct result of a fracture involving the optic canal or penetrating orbital trauma. It may also result from haematoma formation, usually as a subperiosteal haematoma following fracture or orbital surgery which compresses the optic nerve and produces rapidly progressive visual loss. In this situation, prompt orbital decompression may sometimes prevent loss of sight.

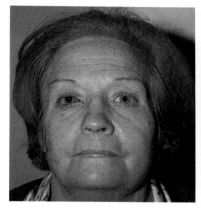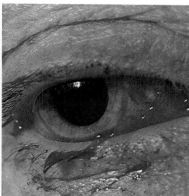

Fig. 20.13 This patient presented with no perception of light in the right eye following a gardening accident in which the right eye was struck by the end of a fine cane support as she bent over. Closer examination shows a conjunctival laceration over the medial aspect of the globe. The tip of the cane displaced the globe laterally and travelled medially along the orbital wall to transect the optic nerve at the orbital apex.

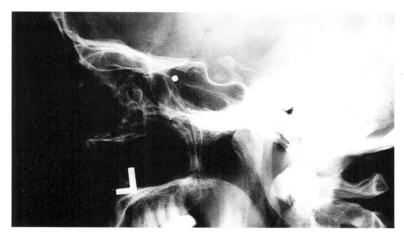

Fig. 20.14 Skull x-rays and CT scans show a shot-gun pellet lodged in the orbital apex following a sporting accident. The patient had an inferior altitudinal field loss in the affected eye which was found to remain unchanged on subsequent follow-up examinations. Surgical removal of the shot pellet is contra-indicated as this would be likely to result in further visual damage.

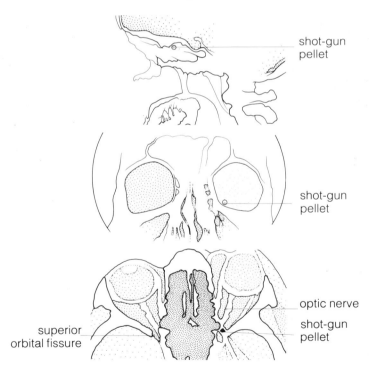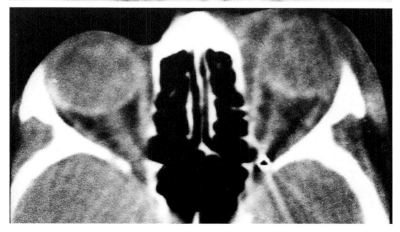

AXIAL PROPTOSIS

Axial proptosis results from a lesion within the external ocular muscle cone caused by a benign or malignant expansion of one of the normal constituents or a metastasis from elsewhere.

Thyroid Eye Disease

The most common cause of axial proptosis is thyroid eye disease which can affect the orbits in a very asymmetrical manner producing apparently uniocular proptosis. Patients may be hypo, eu, or hyperthyroid. T3, T4, thyroid antibodies and a thyrotrophin-releasing hormone test should be performed in all patients, but about fifteen percent of patients have completely normal investigations and in these patients the diagnosis is made on clinical and CT scan findings.

Fig. 20.15 Asymmetrical proptosis in a patient with thyroid eye disease. Lid lag and lid retraction are constant findings whatever the biochemical or immunological status of the patient. This patient shows left-sided proptosis with retraction of the upper and lower lids.

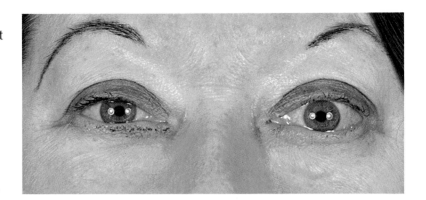

Fig. 20.16 Lateral views demonstrate the markedly asymmetrical proptosis. Patients may have sore eyes from superior limbic keratitis due to disturbance of tear film metabolism, (cf. Chapter 3) or diplopia from infiltration of the external ocular muscles (cf. Chapter 18).

Retraction of the upper and lower eyelids has been attributed to excessive sympathetic stimulation of Müller's muscles. Lateral photographs of the same patient as in Fig. 20.15, shows the left proptosis and lid retraction.

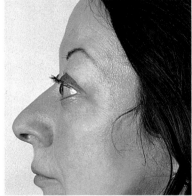
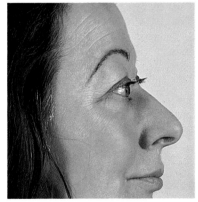

Fig. 20.17 Orbital scans consistently demonstrate enlargement of the external ocular muscles in thyroid eye disease. This is due to an inflammatory cellular infiltrate with oedema which also involves the orbital fat, although usually to a lesser extent. The degree of proptosis can be estimated by comparing the position of the posterior pole of the eye to the lateral orbital margin of the CT scan.

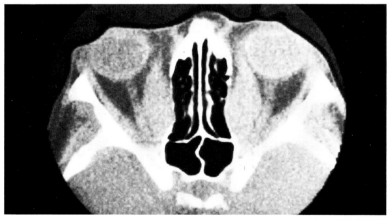

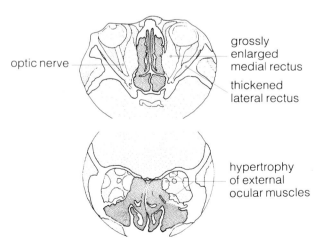

optic nerve

grossly enlarged medial rectus

thickened lateral rectus

hypertrophy of external ocular muscles

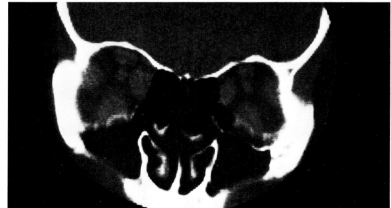

Fig. 20.18 Patients with thyroid eye disease lose vision from either corneal exposure (especially with acute disease) or optic nerve compression. This is due to cramming of the orbital apex by the enlarged muscle bellies and is especially prone to occur in patients who do not have gross proptosis; those with gross proptosis tend to 'decompress' their own orbits. Physical signs of decreasing acuity, colour loss, afferent pupillary defect and field defect suggest optic nerve compression; the optic disc may be swollen, normal or atrophic. Many patients respond to systemic steroids but orbital decompression is indicated if the optic nerve compression is unrelieved.

These CT scans show the pre and postoperative appearances following decompression of the left orbit into the ethmoidal and sphenoidal sinuses, thereby decompressing the orbital apex. Decompression into the maxillary sinus was also performed but cannot be seen on these scans.

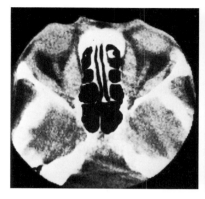
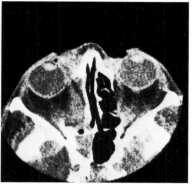

Pre-operative — anterior and posterior ethmoidal sinus, sphenoidal sinus

Post-operative — esotropia, post-operative prolapse of orbital contents into sinuses

Orbital Varices

Congenital orbital venous malformations constitute one of the most common causes of proptosis. Patients usually present with a characteristic history of variable proptosis, the eye protruding with a Valsalva manoeuvre which raises the central venous pressure. Varices are usually unilateral and typically present in young adults; visual loss is uncommon. Accompanying venous malformations are sometimes seen on the eyelids, face or palate.

Fig. 20.19 Variable proptosis of the right eye is demonstrated in this patient on a valsalva manoeuvre. Varices may present with acute painful proptosis if they thrombose or bleed spontaneously.

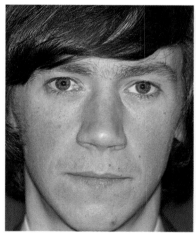
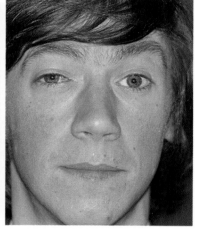

Fig. 20.20 Skull x-rays will usually show an enlarged orbit with phleboliths. A venogram gives the definitive diagnosis and in this case shows a saccular dilatation of the superior ophthalmic vein.

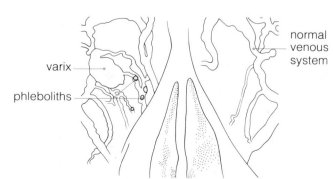

varix

phleboliths

normal venous system

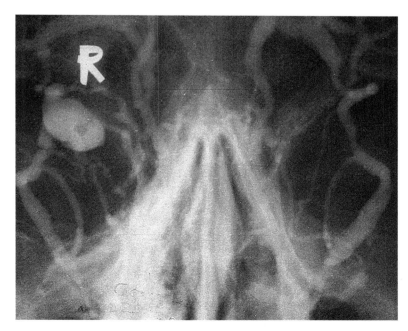

Carotico-Cavernous Fistulas

Arteriovenous fistulas usually result from either trauma to the internal carotid artery in the cavernous sinus in young patients or rupture of an aneurysm in the elderly (this usually produces a high flow rate fistula). They may also occur following a spontaneous rupture of external carotid arterial branches in the dura which produces a communication with the dural veins draining into the cavernous sinus. These dural fistulas occasionally result from excessive straining, such as in childbirth, or from congenital arteriovenous malformations, and tend to have a low flow rate.

The clinical presentation depends on the rapidity of onset, the extent of the vascular shunting, the increase in orbital venous pressure and the consequent orbital or ocular hypoxia. High flow shunts present with bilateral asymmetrical proptosis (which results from communications with the contralateral cavernous sinus), arteriolization of conjunctival vessels, ophthalmoplegia and visual loss from optic nerve ischaemia, or intraocular hypoxia (rubiosis iridis may occasionally be seen). Patients may complain of a bruit. Low flow shunts may present as a glaucomatous eye with arterialized conjunctival vessels (cf. Secondary Glaucoma, Chapter 8).

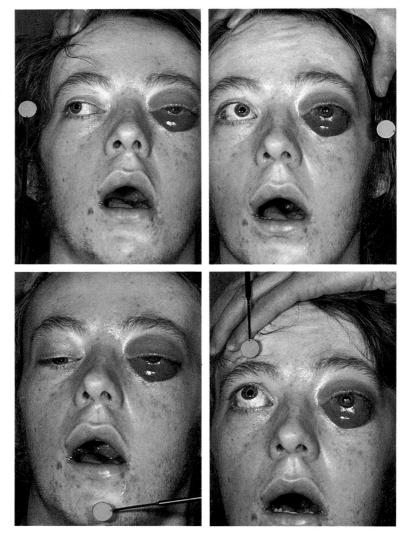

Fig. 20.21 This patient suffered a severe head injury and fracture of the base of the skull in a motor cycle accident. He has asymmetrical proptosis, greater in the left eye, with a total ophthalmoplegia of this eye and a partial ophthalmoplegia of the right. Pulsating exophthalmos was present and an audible bruit could be heard indicating a high flow-rate fistula.

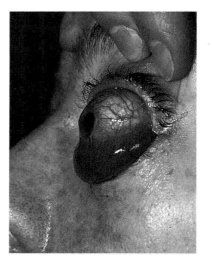

Fig. 20.22 The conjunctiva of the left eye is chemotic and arterialized. The eye was blind, the intraocular pressure was normal but there were signs of ocular hypoxia. The right eye had normal visual acuity.

Fig. 20.23 CT scans show dilatation of the superior ophthalmic vein, a consistent finding in carotico-cavernous fistulae. Carotid angiography demonstrates a massive fistula in the region of the cavernous sinus which was successfully treated by embolisation using a balloon catheter neuroradiological technique. The patient's chemosis, proptosis and ocular movements improved but the vision did not recover.

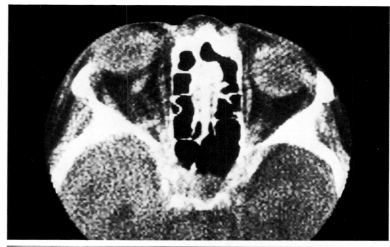

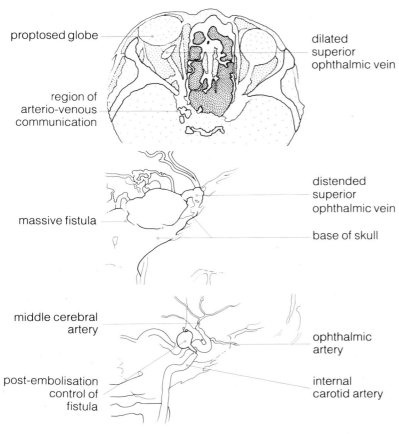

proptosed globe

dilated superior ophthalmic vein

region of arterio-venous communication

massive fistula

distended superior ophthalmic vein

base of skull

middle cerebral artery

ophthalmic artery

post-embolisation control of fistula

internal carotid artery

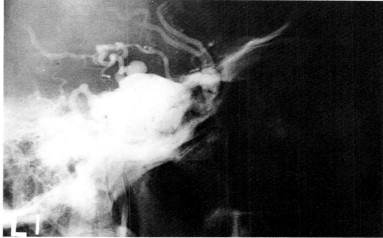

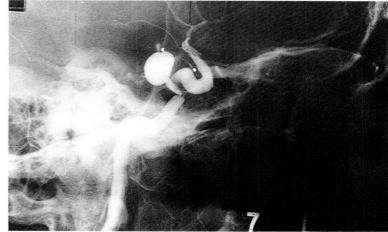

Cavernous Haemangioma

A cavernous haemangioma is the most common orbital tumour and commonly presents as slowly progressive axial proptosis in an adult. The mass is usually sited within the muscle cone, most commonly inferior and lateral to the optic nerve. Patients may have visual symptoms from pressure on the optic nerve, disc or macula.

Fig. 20.24 CT scan shows a typical haemangioma as a discrete circumscribed mass and distinct from the globe and optic nerve. Lesions should enhance uniformly with contrast injection on scanning.

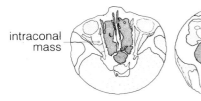

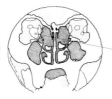

intraconal mass

mass separate and lying inferior and medial to the optic nerve

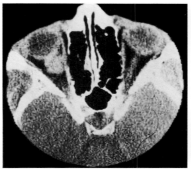

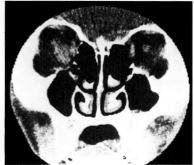

Fig. 20.25   Pathology of the lesion shows large dilated vascular spaces lined by endothelium with thick fibrous walls. The lesion is encapsulated and is readily dissected out of the orbit at lateral orbitotomy.

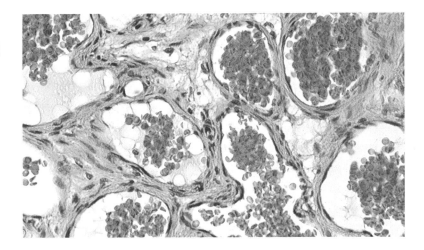

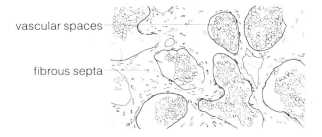

vascular spaces

fibrous septa

Neurofibromatosis

This autosomal dominant condition has an incidence of 1:3000 live births and is inherited with variable penetrance. The disease affects cells derived from the embryological neural crest which form Schwann cells, melanocytes and the adrenal medulla. Patients have a tendency to form neurofibromas and schwannomas of peripheral nerves but also have an increased incidence of meningiomas, gliomas and phaeochromocytomas. The disease has a wide spectrum of involvement but tends to polarise into either peripheral cutaneous or central cranial forms. In the cutaneous form there are multiple

subcutaneous neurofibromas and peripheral nerve tumours and cafe au lait spots, whereas the central form produces intracranial lesions such as optic nerve gliomas, encephalocoeles and meningiomas, with relatively less cutaneous disease. There is considerable overlap, however, between patients and within affected families and there is a wide variation in the spectrum of individual manifestations.

Ocular involvement in neurofibromatosis is common and may affect the lid (cf. Chapter 2) and iris (cf. Chapter 9) as well as the orbit

Fig. 20.26   Neurofibromatosis is associated in some patients with orbital bony malformation, especially the absence of the greater and lesser wings of the sphenoid. In this case the intracranial contents of the middle fossa

(temporal lobe) lie in direct contact with the orbit and produce a characteristic pulsating proptosis from transmission of the cerebral pulse wave.

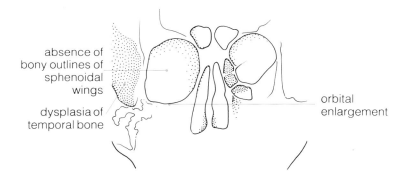

absence of bony outlines of sphenoidal wings

dysplasia of temporal bone

orbital enlargement

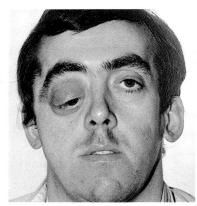

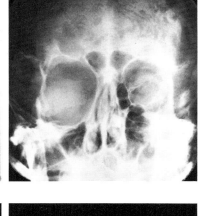

Fig. 20.27   CT scans of the same patient demonstrate an immense bony orbital defect in the sphenoid on the right.

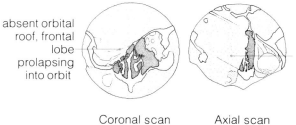

absent orbital roof, frontal lobe prolapsing into orbit

absent posterior orbital wall with temporal lobe prolapsing into orbit and sinuses

Coronal scan   Axial scan

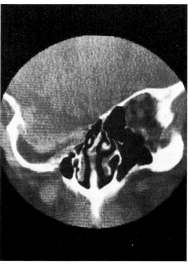

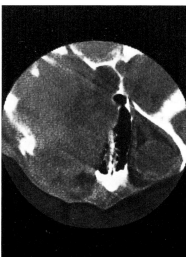

Optic Nerve Gliomas

Optic nerve gliomas are most commonly seen in children or young adults and present with unilateral proptosis and diminished visual acuity (they should not be confused with the rarer malignant glioblastoma seen in middle aged men). About sixty percent of affected children will have cutaneous signs of neurofibromatosis but the tumour is seen independently of this disease. Most optic nerve gliomas behave as benign and indolent hamartomatous lesions originating in the optic nerve which do not appear to spread along the optic nerve to invade the chiasm. However, intracranial invasion is seen occasionally and there is considerable debate as to whether this results from spread from a primary orbital optic nerve tumour or whether it might be part of the original congenital hamartomatous malformation.

All patients with optic nerve gliomas require charting of visual fields, visual evoked responses and CT scanning to detect intracranial involvement and careful follow up with this in mind. Sudden increase in proptosis and visual loss in some patients may result from hydration of mucoid elements in the tumour rather than an aggressive or malignant change. The optic disc may be swollen or atrophic. Indolent tumours are followed by observation. Radical surgical excision of the optic nerve is reserved for progressive enlargement of the tumour with a blind eye in the absence of chiasmal involvement, and extension into the chiasm is usually treated by palliative radiotherapy.

Fig. 20.28 The neuroradiological appearances are characteristic. CT scans show an enlarged orbit with a smooth fusiform enlargement of the optic nerve.

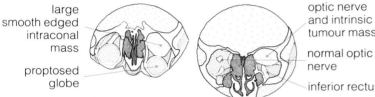

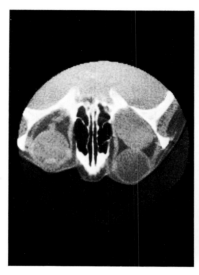
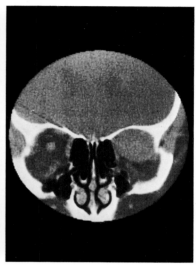

Fig. 20.29 The affected orbit is expanded and the optic foramen may be enlarged, although this usually represents arachnoid hyperplasia of the nerve, and not intracanalicular spread. In patients with neurofibromatosis, associated dysplastic bony changes may be seen in the pituitary fossa or anterior clinoid processes.

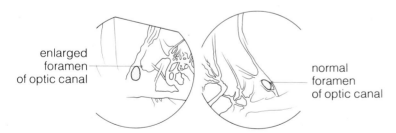

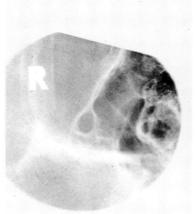
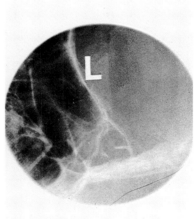

Fig. 20.30 Histology of an optic nerve glioma shows that the optic nerve is replaced by neoplastic astrocytes which have provoked a reactive hyperplasia of the meningeal tissue in the nerve sheath.

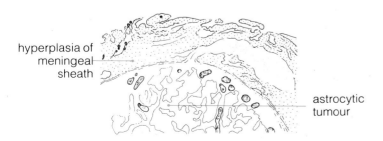

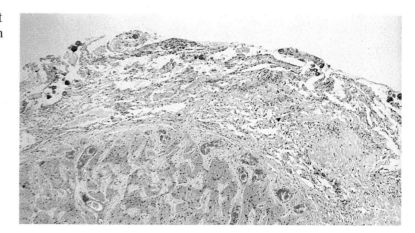

20.13

Meningiomas

Primary optic nerve meningiomas are rare tumours; they arise from the arachnoid within the dura and infiltrate the subarachnoid and subdural space compressing the nerve. Occasionally, the subdural space surrounding the optic nerve may be invaded by the extension of a middle cranial fossa meningioma through the optic canal or superior orbital fissure and this is known as a secondary optic nerve meningioma. The characteristic presentation is of early and slowly progressive visual loss with little proptosis; the optic disc is usually swollen or atrophic. Patients tend to be middle-aged females but optic nerve meningiomas do occur in children and these tend to have a more aggressive and invasive course and require more radical management.

Fig. 20.31 CT scan shows a typical thickened optic nerve sheath from a primary optic nerve meningioma. Calcification can be seen in the sheath and indicates a long-standing tumour. Patients require careful investigation to exclude intracranial spread which is usually seen radiologically as hyperostosis of the optic canal, anterior clinoid processes or superior orbital fissure.

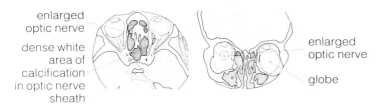
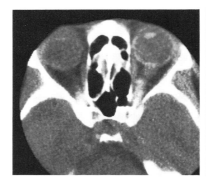
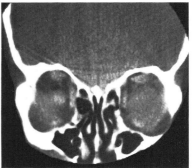

enlarged optic nerve

dense white area of calcification in optic nerve sheath

enlarged optic nerve

globe

Fig. 20.32 The slow strangulation of the optic nerve produces chronic disc oedema followed by optic atrophy. Optico-ciliary collateral vessels (shunting blood from the obstructed central retinal vein to the choroidal circulation) are a common finding. Occasionally, drusen of the disc are also seen in conjunction with optic nerve meningiomas and aggressive meningiomas may even invade the disc.

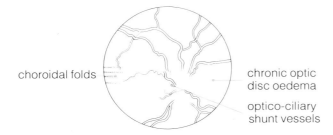
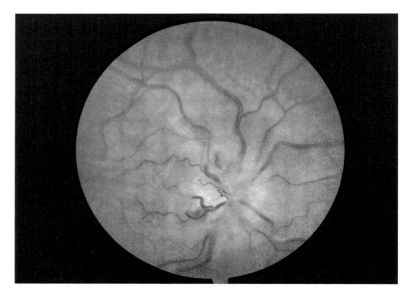

choroidal folds

chronic optic disc oedema

optico-ciliary shunt vessels

Fig. 20.33 Pathology shows an optic nerve meningioma with a syncytial arrangement of cells with oval, vesicular nuclei associated with scattered calcified psammoma bodies. Another example demonstrates meningothelial cells organised in whorls between strands of fibrous tissue. In adults the tumour is slow-growing but locally invasive. Limited surgical exploration or biopsy may risk dissemination of the tumour into the orbital contents and indolent tumours are best either watched or completely excised; both types of treatment have their protagonists.

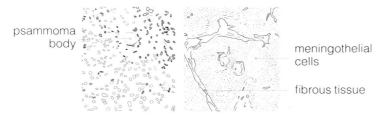
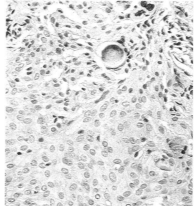
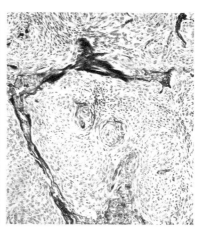

psammoma body

meningothelial cells

fibrous tissue

Fig. 20.34 Sphenoidal ridge meningiomas typically occur in middle-aged females. The meningioma grows *en plaque* producing infiltration and hyperostosis of the bones of the middle cranial fossa and sphenoid. Proptosis is caused by bony encroachment of the orbit and is particularly apparent as hyperostosis of the orbital fissure on routine skull x-rays, or as increased bone density on CT scans.

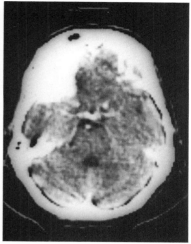

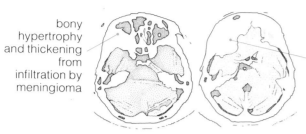

bony hypertrophy and thickening from infiltration by meningioma

bony hypertrophy and thickening from infiltration by meningioma

Fig. 20.35 The meningioma is slow-growing over many years and produces painless proptosis. Swelling of the temporal fossa is a characteristic feature from involvement of the temporal bone. Sphenoidal ridge meningiomas grow *en plaque*, infiltrating bone and

midline structures. The meningiomas cannot usually be completely excised by surgery, indeed, this frequently produces further damage to the nerves in the cavernous sinus or the optic nerve.

sclerosis and narrowing of superior orbital fissure from infiltration of greater and lesser wings of sphenoid by meningioma

displacement of temporal fossa from infiltration of temporal bone

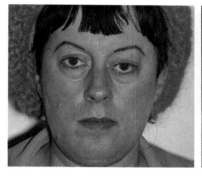

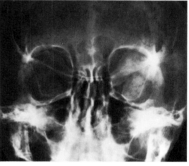

Orbital Pseudotumours

These are defined as non-specific and non-neoplastic inflammatory lesions that occur in the orbit with diverse pathological appearances ranging from that of polymorphous chronic inflammatory lesions to monomorphous lymphocytic masses that may behave as malignant lymphomas. Chronic inflammation associated with known predisposing factors such as endocrine exophthalmos, chronic infection, foreign body reactions

or as a secondary reaction to a vasculitis (such as Wegener's granuloma or polyarteritis nodosa) are not usually included in series of idiopathic pseudotumours. The pathological differentiation between monomorphous lymphocytic lesions, benign lymphoid hyperplasia and malignant lymphoma can be exceptionally difficult; electron-microscopy and immunological cell markers are, therefore, becoming increasingly important in this diagnosis.

Fig. 20.36 Pseudotumours may occur throughout the orbit. Common sites are the lacrimal gland, Tenon's capsule, the intraconal space, external ocular muscles, orbital apex or cavernous sinus. Inflammation in each of these sites produces characteristic symptoms and signs.

In general, pseudotumours commonly present with pain and acute proptosis, chemosis, motility disturbances and deterioration in vision, depending on the precise location of the pseudotumour, but a few present as a chronic painless space occupying lesion.

The orbital apex is a particularly common site for pseudotumours and produces a characteristic syndrome of pain, proptosis and visual loss with third, fourth, fifth and sixth nerve defects, known as the 'orbital apex syndrome'. Lesions found slightly more posteriorly in the cavernous sinus produce the same neurological deficit, but without visual loss.

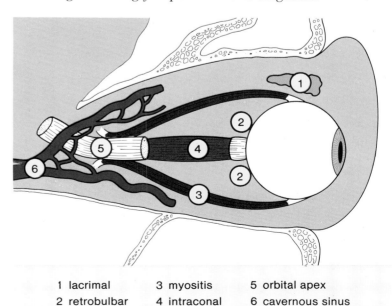

| 1 lacrimal | 3 myositis | 5 orbital apex |
| 2 retrobulbar | 4 intraconal | 6 cavernous sinus |

Fig. 20.37 This middle-aged man presented with painful proptosis and complete ptosis coming on over a few days. There was complete ophthalmoplegia from third, fourth and sixth palsies. The close-up photograph shows the ocular motor paresis with the patient attempting to look right. Note the conjunctival injection and sparing of the pupil with the third nerve palsy which is probably due to a concomitant Horner's syndrome. Visual acuity was reduced by 6/36. Colour sensation was decreased in the left eye; there was a left relative afferent pupillary defect with a relative central scotoma in the visual field. The optic disc appeared normal.

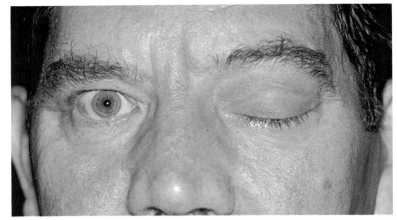

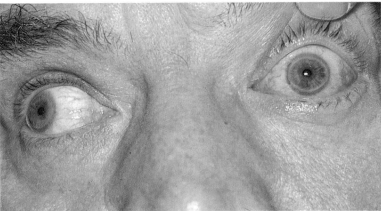

Fig. 20.38 CT scans show an orbital apex mass and thickened horizontal recti. Similar appearances might be seen with malignant lymphomas, metastases, meningiomas or specific granulomas. Patients with a clinical diagnosis of orbital pseudotumour should be biopsied before starting treatment with steroids or radiotherapy.

Orbital apex lesions require urgent medical decompression with steroids to prevent visual loss. Lesions here are relatively inaccessible surgically but failure to make a full clinical recovery is an indication for biopsy to exclude one of the other pathological lesions.

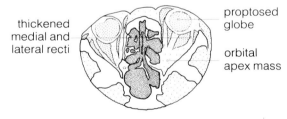

thickened medial and lateral recti

proptosed globe

orbital apex mass

Fig. 20.39. The range of pathological appearances seen with pseudotumours is demonstrated by these three tumours. A picture of reactive lymphoid hyperplasia can be seen on the left. The presence of relatively pale staining germinal centres within the mass of mature lymphocytes is indicative of a non-neoplastic process which would respond satisfactorily to steroid therapy or even resolve spontaneously. The middle picture shows a lymphoid pseudotumour composed of sheets of generally mature lymphocytes and on the right a lymphoma can be seen in which many of the lymphoid cells have thickened nuclear membranes and prominent nucleoli together with some nuclear pleomorphism.

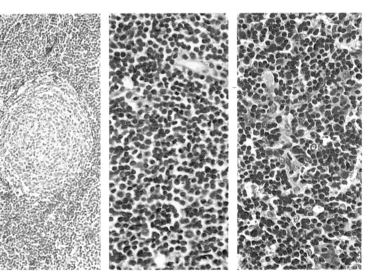

NON-AXIAL PROPTOSIS

Non-axial proptosis is produced by an asymmetrical lesion placed external to the external ocular muscle cone and therefore displacing the globe away from the lesion lying in the orbital tissues or adnexa. Identification of non-axial proptosis is easily performed using a perspex ruler. It localises a lesion and often gives an indication of its likely nature. Careful differential diagnosis of lesions located in the lateral orbit is especially important due to their radically different methods of management.

Fig. 20.40   A dermoid cyst in the superior part of the orbit displaces the right globe inferiorly. The patient was referred as a right 'ptosis' without diplopia.

Dermoid Cyst

Dermoid cysts are common lesions usually presenting in children and young adults. They are formed by epithelial inclusions from malclosure of the embryonic facial clefts and tend to lie in the superior orbit, medially or laterally. They are slow growing and usually painless.

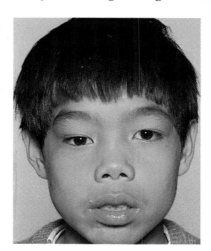

Fig. 20.41   In another patient slow expansion of the cyst produced a bony skull defect with a sharp sclerotic margin readily seen on skull x-ray or CT scan. Dermoid cysts must be evaluated and excised with care as they can

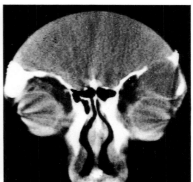

cystic bone defect with well defined walls

dura

dermoid cyst eroding into anterior cranial fossa

globe displaced inferiorly

occasionally penetrate the cranium through to the dura to require a combined neurosurgical excision. Partial excision must be avoided as the remnants produce chronic inflammation with a discharging sinus.

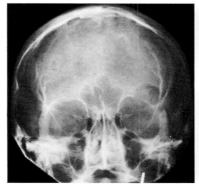

Lacrimal Fossa Lesions

Fig. 20.42   A flow diagram of the differential diagnosis of lacrimal fossa masses based on duration of symptoms and x-ray findings helps to provide a clinical diagnosis. Benign mixed tumours occur in the 20–60 age group and are characterized by a slow, painless, progressively enlarging lacrimal fossa lesion which is usually present for at least a year before presentation. A mass can be palpated and skull x-rays may show diffuse enlargement of the lacrimal fossa without bony invasion. They must be excised en bloc by lateral orbitotomy as biopsy or partial excision leads to local recurrence with invasion of the surrounding structures and a potentially fatal outcome. Carcinomas characteristically have a short progressive history of less than one year and are painful; skull radiography may be normal or show bony invasion or calcification within the tumour. Diagnosis is made by biopsy with the option of radical excision or palliative radiotherapy. Lacrimal gland carcinomas tend to have a very poor prognosis. Other causes of lacrimal fossa masses are viral infection, inflammatory granulomas or pseudotumours.

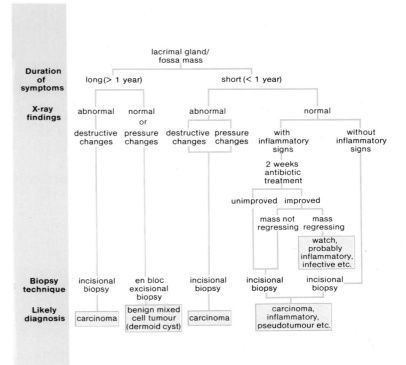

Fig. 20.43 An elderly patient presenting with a painless long-standing mass in the lacrimal fossa shows displacement of the globe downwards and medially, typical of a benign mixed tumour.

A close-up photograph demonstrates the swelling of the tumour more clearly. Skull x-rays showed enlargement of the lacrimal fossa, differentiated from that caused by a dermoid cyst by the absence of a cystic defect with a sharp sclerotic margin.

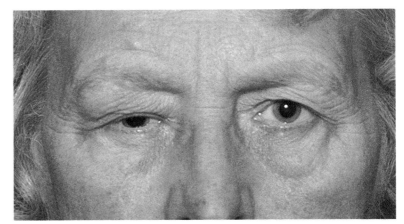

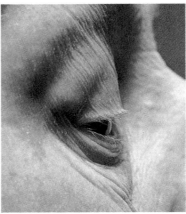

Fig. 20.44 The pathology of a typical benign mixed tumour varies considerably in its appearance within the tumour. Irregular tubule formation is seen with a double layer of epithelium which secretes mucus internally and the myxoid stroma externally. The tumour has a false capsule of compressed normal glandular tissue which is usually invaded by tumour in some areas.

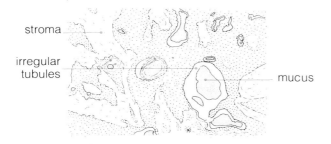

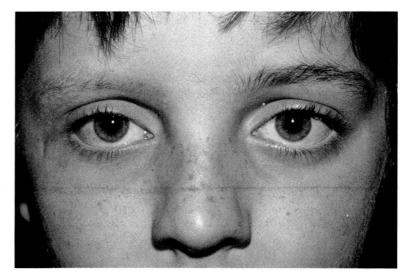

Fig. 20.45 In contrast to a benign mixed tumour, this girl has an adenoid cystic carcinoma which presented with pain in the right lacrimal fossa area and a palpable mass that had been present for a few months. Skull x-rays showed signs of bony destruction and the patient died one year later from intracranial invasion, in spite of radiotherapy.

Fig. 20.46   Pathology of a typical adenoid cystic carcinoma shows irregular islands of poorly differentiated epithelial cells, in a hyaline stroma, which secrete mucin.

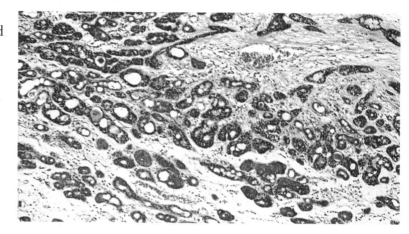

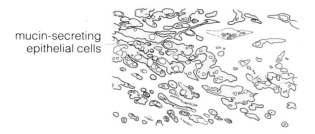
mucin-secreting epithelial cells

Medial Orbital Wall Lesions
The globe is displaced laterally by an external mass in the medial wall of the orbit. The most common lesions are probably mucocoeles and carcinomas of the ethmoidal sinuses in adults, or rhabdomyosarcomas in children.

Fig. 20.47   These two patients have carcinomas of the ethmoidal sinus. Displacement of the globe laterally is demonstrated in the younger man while expansion of the base of the nose is apparent in the older man. Because of the initial non-specific nature of the symptoms (nasal discharge, bleeding etc) patients with paranasal sinus carcinomas tend to present late and consequently have a poor prognosis.

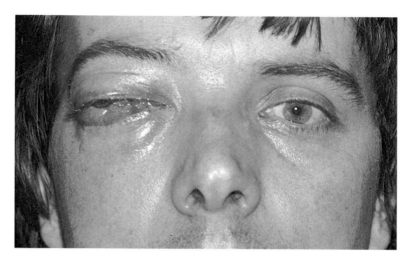

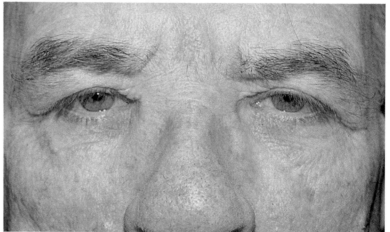

Fig. 20.48   CT scans of another patient show an ethmoidal carcinoma expanding the sinus, destroying the medial orbital wall and invading posteriorly into the middle cranial fossa.

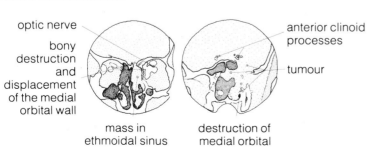
optic nerve
bony destruction and displacement of the medial orbital wall
anterior clinoid processes
tumour
mass in ethmoidal sinus
destruction of medial orbital wall and roof

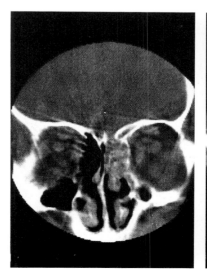
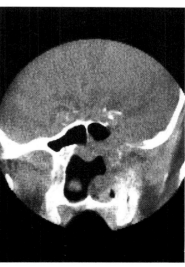

THE LACRIMAL SYSTEM

The basal tear secretion is formed by the accessory lacrimal glands in the conjunctiva with reflex lacrimation coming from the lacrimal gland itself. Tears supply nutrients and oxygen to the cornea; they are responsible for the optical integrity of the corneal surface and are an important barrier to infection, both as a result of their mechanical flushing and their bacteriostatic constituents. The tear film has three physiological layers; an outer oily layer secreted by the meibomian glands to prevent drying, a middle watery layer which carries the oxygen and nutrients which are secreted by the accessory lacrimal glands and an inner layer of mucus secreted by conjunctival goblet cells which acts as a wetting agent, reducing surface tension and spreading the film evenly.

About twenty-five percent of the lacrimal secretion is lost by evaporation and tear secretion declines with age. For these reasons, elderly patients are often asymptomatic in spite of complete obstruction of the nasolacrimal duct. Overflow of tears (epiphora) must be distinguished from oversecretion due to a variety of conjunctival or ocular irritations or to outflow obstruction. Dry eyes are discussed in Chapter 5.

Fig. 20.49   A dissection of the lacrimal system shows the medial palpebral ligament lying across the fundus of the lacrimal sac. The canaliculi lie under this. The nasolacrimal duct passes downwards through the maxilla to enter the inferior meatus of the nose under the turbinate process. Mucosal flaps in the nasolacrimal duct act as valves and prevent air entry into the lacrimal sac.

The puncta lie within the meniscus of the tear film and tears will be drawn into the canaliculi by capillary action. Blinking sweeps the tear film medially and the simultaneous contraction of the palpebral orbicularis oculi fibres inserting into the canaliculi and lacrimal sac ensures that, on blinking, the canaliculi shorten and the sac dilates, sucking tears into the system. It is thought that more tears leave the eye by the lower canaliculus rather than the upper canaliculus but this is not invariable and patients may not be troubled by epiphora so long as the upper canaliculus is patent.

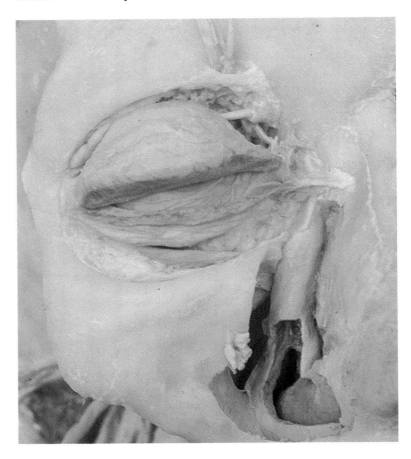

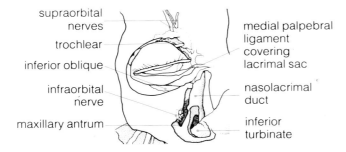

Fig. 20.50   A diagram shows the anatomy in more detail. The upper and lower puncta enter the canaliculus as a short vertical passage which turns medially in the lid margin. The canaliculi have a length of about 8mm. They anastomose to form the common canaliculus which opens by a single orifice into the lateral wall of the lacrimal sac. Palpebral fibres from the orbicularis oculi muscle are inserted into the canaliculus, medial palpebral ligament and fundus of the sac. The nasolacrimal duct has an interosseus length of approximately 12mm and opens into the inferior meatus of the nose.

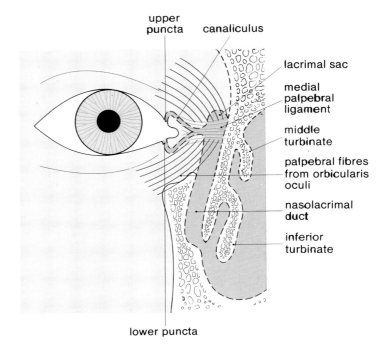

TESTS OF OUTFLOW PATENCY

The patency of the outflow system can be shown by syringing, the Jones' dye tests or dacrocystography (DCG). Whilst syringing is commonly used to diagnose patency it is not performed under normal physiological conditions in that a high pressure is applied to force saline through the system; the Jones' test is conducted under more normal physiological conditions. A DCG demonstrates the anatomy and is particularly useful in planning surgery and in the investigation of canalicular problems or of surgical failures.

Fig. 20.51 The Jones' dye test is a refinement of syringing the nasolacrimal system. It involves instilling one drop of fluorescein into the conjunctival sac. A cotton wool bud, soaked in local anaesthetic, is placed in the inferior meatus and examined for signs of fluorescein every minute for 5 minutes. Positive identification of dye indicates a physiologically patent system. A significant number of normal patients have a negative test at this stage, and if this is the case, excess fluorescein is washed from the conjunctiva and the canaliculi syringed with clear saline. If fluorescein is found to enter the nose this indicates that dye had entered the sac; if clear saline alone is seen then fluorescein has not entered the sac, indicating an obstruction in the puncta or canaliculi. The absence of saline entering the nose indicates a complete obstruction.

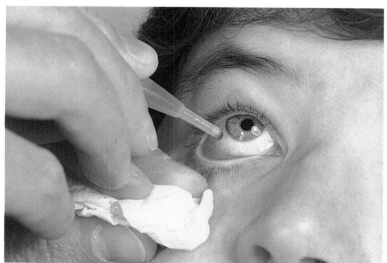

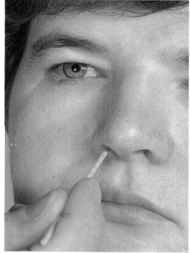
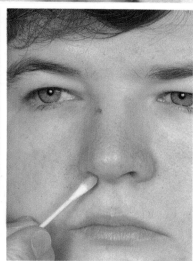

Fig. 20.52 Dacrocystography requires the injection of a radio-opaque dye into the nasolacrimal system. In this patient dye passes normally through the left side but on the right it outlines an obstructed and dilated nasolacrimal sac.

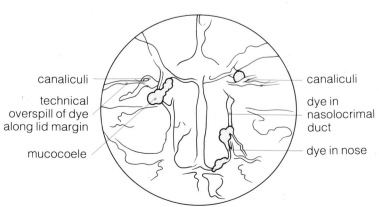

canaliculi — — canaliculi

technical overspill of dye along lid margin — dye in nasolocrimal duct

mucocoele — dye in nose

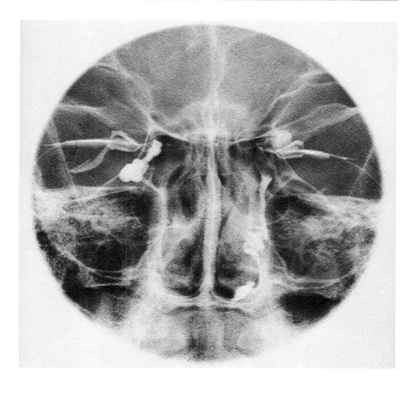

OUTFLOW OBSTRUCTION

Congenital Blockage of the Nasolacrimal Duct

Fig. 20.53   The nasolacrimal duct is formed by a cord of ectoderm which becomes imbedded in mesoderm in the cleft between the maxillary and lateral nasal processes. This cord grows upwards and bifurcates to form the canaliculi which reach the lid margins at the 3rd month of gestation. The central cells of the cord degenerate to leave a lumen and this process extends upwards and downwards to reach the nasal cavity. At birth the process is usually complete, but a membrane may persist at the lower end and fail to perforate leaving the child with a watering eye. If perforation has not occurred spontaneously by a few months of age the duct is cleared by rupturing the membrane with a probe under a general anaesthetic.

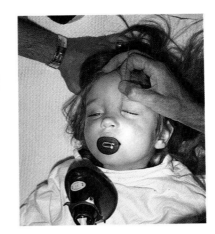

Canaliculitis

Fig. 20.54   Canaliculitis occurs most commonly from Actinomyces infection. The infected canaliculus becomes chronically red, swollen and tender. Pressure over the swelling will sometimes expel pus and 'sulphur granules' from the puncta. Treatment is by incision and curettage of the canaliculus and a course of topical penicillin.

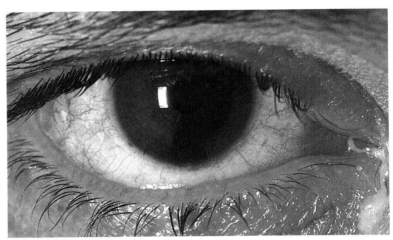

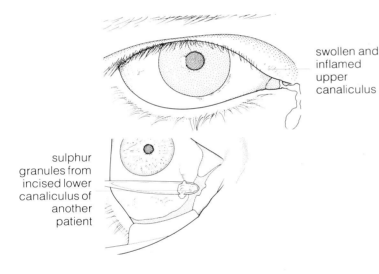

swollen and inflamed upper canaliculus

sulphur granules from incised lower canaliculus of another patient

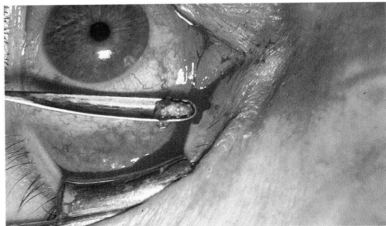

Fig. 20.55   Typical sulphur granules can be seen in the curettings of this patient.

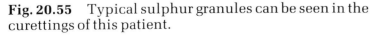

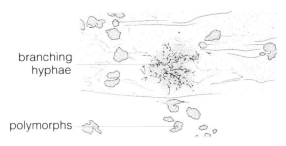

branching hyphae

polymorphs

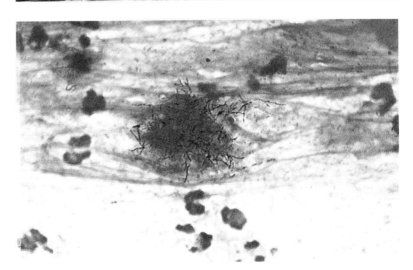

Punctal Stenosis

Fig. 20.56 Punctal stenosis follows conjunctival scarring from such inflammatory causes as trachoma, ocular pemphigoid, herpes simplex, trauma, or topical drugs, such as idoxuridine. Providing the canaliculus is not involved cure lies in dilating and opening the punctum, if necessary, by a '3 snip' operation.

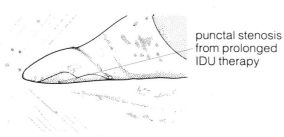

punctal stenosis from prolonged IDU therapy

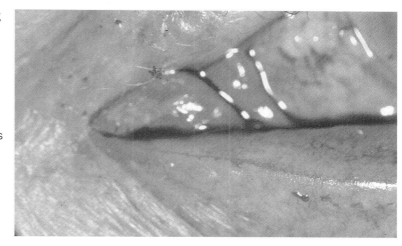

Dacrocystitis

Fig. 20.57 Obstruction of the nasolacrimal duct, usually at the nasal opening, through chronic infection or irritation, may lead to stasis and an acute infection of the lacrimal sac. Patients present with epiphora and an acutely painful, swollen mass over the area of the lacrimal sac; this may form an abscess and require incision, drainage and systemic antibiotics. Dacryocystorhinostomy is necessary to reconstitute lacrimal drainage as soon as the acute inflammation has subsided.

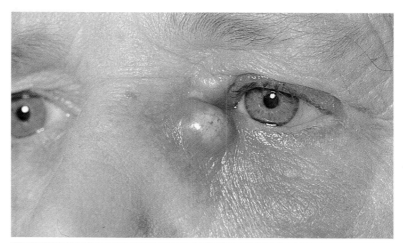

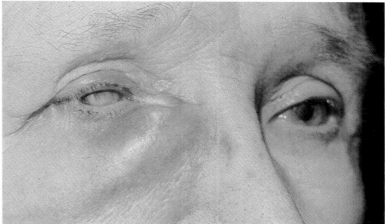

Fig. 20.58 Chronic obstruction of the nasolacrimal duct can lead to a watering eye and a mucocoele of the lacrimal sac. Pressure over the sac causes regurgitation of mucoid material through the puncta (providing the canaliculi are patent).

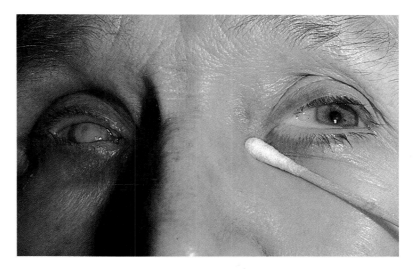

Fig. 20.59 The most common site of outflow obstruction is occlusion of the lower end of the nasolacrimal duct; occlusion requires a dacryocystorhinostomy (DCR) for relief of symptoms. The basis of this procedure lies in removing a large area of the bony medial wall of the lacrimal fossa and lateral wall of the nose in order to anastomose the lacrimal sac to the nasal mucosa thereby bypassing the obstruction at the lower end of the duct. Variations of this operation can be used to relieve canalicular block either in the canaliculi themselves or more commonly at their insertion into the lacrimal sac. Total bypass of the lacrimal outflow system is necessary if the canaliculi are scarred beyond repair and this is achieved by inserting a prosthetic tube (Lester Jones tube) in combination with a DCR procedure.

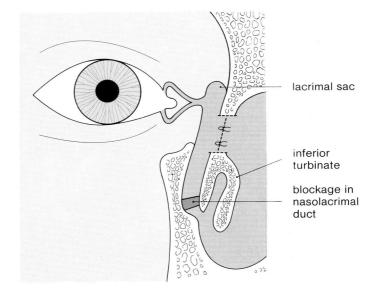

lacrimal sac

inferior turbinate

blockage in nasolacrimal duct

Acknowledgements

We have only been able to assemble this collection of material with the help of friends and colleagues, listed below, who have given freely of their time, advice and clinical material. We would also like to thank our publisher, who initiated the project and had the courage to carry it through, and the staff of Gower Medical Publishing who have committed their time and enthusiasm to ensuring the quality of the book and its completion.

Prof. G. Arden, Department of Electro-Diagnosis, Moorfields Eye Hospital, London, U.K. (Fig. 1.9); **Miss C. Astin,** Contact Lens Dept., Moorfields Eye Hospital, London, U.K. (Fig. 6.60); **Prof. A.C. Bird,** Institute of Ophthalmology, London, U.K. (Fig. 4.54, 14.43 & 14.58); **Mr. R.K. Blach,** Moorfields Eye Hospital, London, U.K. (cover photographs and Fig. 12.15a, 12.30a, 12.55b, 12.56b, 16.34 & 16.35); **Mr. R.J. Buckley,** Moorfields Eye Hospital, London, U.K. (Fig. 3.60, 4.55, 5.7, 5.8, 5.11, 5.12, 5.34, 5.35 & 5.36); Charing Cross Hospital (Department of Anatomy), London, U.K. (Fig. 9.5, 13.1, 13.2, 19.8 & 19.9); **Mr. D.B. Clements,** St. Helen's Hospital, Liverpool, U.K. (Fig. 20.26); **Dr. Gillian Clover,** Institute of Ophthalmology, London, U.K. (Fig. 12.42); **Mr. R.J. Cooling,** Moorfields Eye Hospital, London, U.K. (Fig. 1.27, 12.30b, 12.36b & 12.39); **Prof. S. Darougar,** Institute of Ophthalmology, London, U.K. (Fig. 3.27, 4.6, 4.30, 4.31, 4.32, 4.33, 4.34 & 4.37); **Mr. J. Elston,** Moorfields Eye Hospital, London, U.K. (Fig. 18.9); **Dr. B. Fantl,** Texas, U.S.A. (Fig. 14.48, 14.51b & 14.52b); **Mr. T.J. ffytche,** Moorfields Eye Hospital, London, U.K. (Fig. 6.15, 9.22, 9.23, 9.25, 9.26, 9.30, 10.48, 10.49, 10.59 & 10.60); **Mr. L.G. Fison,** Moorfields Eye Hospital, London, U.K. (Fig. 12.15b, 12.22a, 12.29b & 12.34b); **Dr. J. Fluker,** Charing Cross Hospital, London, U.K. (Fig. 10.16); **Miss S.Ford,** Photographic Dept., Western Ophthalmic Hospital, London, U.K. (Fig. 6.24b); **Prof. A. Garner,** Institute of Ophthalmology, London, U.K. (all pathological material for Chapter 2, 3, 4, 5, 6, 7, 8, 10, & 16 and for Fig. 9.3, 9.19, 9.32, 9.33, 9.34, 9.35, 9.41, 9.46, 9.47, 9.53 & 9.54, 15.2, 15.37, 15.51, 15.58, 15.59, 15.60, 17.21, 17.22, 17.52, 17.55, 17.57, 20.25, 20.30, 20.33, 20.39, 20.44 & 20.46); **Dr. D.G. Green,** Science Vol. 168 June 5 1970, copyright 1970 A.A.A.S. (Fig. 1.8); **Dr. M. Gresty,** National Hospital for Nervous Diseases, London, U.K. (Fig. 19.29); **Dr. I. Grierson,** Institute of Ophthalmology, London,

U.K. (Fig. 7.13, 7.28, 7.33, 8.53, 12.11b & 12.23); **Dr. B. Holden,** School of Optometry, Kensington, New South Wales, Australia (Fig. 1.28 & 1.29); **Mr. B.S. Jay,** Moorfields Eye Hospital, London, U.K. (Fig. 16.59); **Prof. B.R. Jones,** Moorfields Eye Hospital, London, U.K. (Fig. 4.52 & 4.53); **Mr. J.J. Kanski,** King Edward VII Hospital, Windsor, U.K. (Fig. 9.20 & 9.52); **Mr. M. Kerr-Muir,** Moorfields Eye Hospital, London, U.K. (Fig. 1.27 & 6.17a); **Dr. L. Koorneef,** University Eye Hospital, Amsterdam (Fig. 2.5 & 18.54); **Mr. P.K. Leaver,** Moorfields Eye Hospital, London, U.K. (Fig. 12.29a & 12.34a); **Mr W. Lee,** Tennant Institute of Ophthalmology, Glasgow, Scotland; **T.J.K. Leonard,** Charing Cross Hospital, London, U.K. (Fig. 15.52 & 15.53); **Dr. A.C.E. MacCartney,** Charing Cross Hospital, London, U.K. (Fig. 9.1, 9.4, 9.24, 13.9a, 13.10, 13.12, 13.22, 13.27a, 13.29b, 13.30b, 13.31b, 13.32b, 14.27, 17.2 & 17.3); **Mr. P.A. MacFaul,** Middlesex Hospital, London, U.K. (Fig. 3.9, 3.33, 3.34, 3.36, 3.45, 3.50 & 5.1); **Prof. J. Marshall,** Institute of Ophthalmology, London, U.K. (Fig. 6.2, 9.9, 12.1, 12.3, 12.19, 12.26a, 12.41, 12.49, 12.54a, 14.3 & 15.23); **Mr. A.D. McG Steel,** Moorfields Eye Hospital, London, U.K. (Fig. 6.43, 6.50 & 6.53); **Dr. C. McKenzie,** Institute of Tropical Medicine, London, U.K. (Fig. 4.50 & 4.51); **Mr. G. Migdal,** St. Bartholomew's Hospital, London, U.K. (Fig. 10.41, 15.56 & 15.57); **Mr. M. Milliken,** Vice-Principal Optician, Moorfields Eye Hospital, London, U.K. (Fig. 1.22 & 1.23); **Mr. P.A.J. Moriarty,** Royal Victoria Eye and Ear Hospital, Dublin, Eire (Fig. 20.54); **Mr. A. Mushim,** Moorfields Eye Hospital, London, U.K. (Fig. 14.49, 14.50, 14.51a, 14.52a & 16.60); **Dr. G.D. Perkin,** Charing Cross Hospital, London, U.K. (Fig. 19.49, 19.60 & 20.34); **Mr. N.A. Phelps Brown,** Harley Street, London, U.K. (Fig. 6.31b & 6.48); **Mr. M.J.A. Port,** City University, London, U.K. (Fig. 6.7 & 6.59a); **Dr. A.H.S. Rahi,** Moorfields Eye Hospital, London, U.K. (Fig. 5.27, 5.28, 5.29, 5.32 & 5.37); **Miss M. Restori,** Moorfields Eye Hospital, London, U.K. (Fig. 1.56, 1.57, 1.58, 1.59, 9.29, 9.44, 12.5, 12.8b, 12.12, 12.28, 12.38, 12.44 & 12.46); Royal College of Surgeons Department of Anatomy, London, U.K. (Fig. 19.5, 19.34, 20.3, 20.5, 20.6, 20.7 & 20.49); **Mr. M.D. Sanders,** National Hospital for Nervous Diseases, London, U.K. (Fig. 10.43, 10.57, 10.58, 16.58,

19.31, 20.21, 20.22, 20.23 & 20.35); **Mr. J. Sandford-Smith,** Leicester Royal Infirmary, Leicester, U.K. (Fig. 6.22); **Dr. F. Scaravilli,** National Hospital for Nervous Diseases, London, U.K. (Fig. 17.42); **Dr. T. Scott,** Charing Cross Hospital, London, U.K. (Fig. 10.19); **Miss J. Silver,** Principal Optician, Moorfields Eye Hospital, London, U.K. (Fig. 1.13, 1.14, 1.15 & 1.16); **Mr. Mark Smith,** Chelmsford Hospital, Essex, U.K. (Fig. 9.31); **Dr. A. Sommer,** Moorfields Eye Hospital, London, U.K. (Fig. 5.42, 5.44 & 5.45); **Mr. T. Tarrant,** Medical Illustrator, Moorfields Eye Hospital, London, U.K.; **Mr. D.S.I. Taylor,** Great Ormond Street Hospital for Sick Children, London, U.K. (Fig. 9.11, 9.45, 14.55, 17.13, 17.14 & 19.52); **Mr. V. Thaller,** Moorfields Eye Hospital, London, U.K. (Fig. 1.36); **Prof. H.S. Thompson,** University Hospital Iowa, Iowa, U.S.A. (Fig. 19.39); **Dr. M. Viswalingam,** Moorfields Eye Hospital, London, U.K. (Fig. 6.32); **Dr. B. Wigram,** Charing Cross Hospital, London, U.K. (Fig. 10.21 & 10.41); **Dr. E.G. Woodward,** Contact Lens Dept., Moorfields Eye Hospital, London, U.K. (Fig. 6.35b & 6.19b); **Mr. J. Wright,** Moorfields Eye Hospital, London, U.K. (Fig. 18.54); **Mr. P. Wright,** Moorfields Eye Hospital, London, U.K. (Fig. 3.27, 4.42, 6.16, 6.18a, 6.33, 6.41 & 6.44a).

Further Reading

GENERAL

Davson, H.
Physiology of the Eye (4th edn.)
Churchill Livingstone, Edinburgh, U.K.
(1980)

Duane, T.D. (Ed.)
Clinical Ophthalmology
Harper & Row, Philadelphia, U.S.A.
(1982)

Duke-Elder, S.
System of Ophthalmology
Henry Kimpton Publishers, London,
U.K. (1965)

Frisby, J.P.
Seeing: Illusion, Brain and Mind
Oxford University Press, Oxford, U.K.
(1979)

Hogan, M.J., Alvarado, J.A. and
Weddell, J.E.
Histology of the Human Eye. An Atlas &
Textbook.
W.B. Saunders & Co, Philadelphia,
U.S.A. (1971)

Miller, S.J.H. (Ed.)
'Eyes' from 'Operative Surgery:
Fundamental International Techniques'
(3rd edn.)
C. Rob, R. Smith (Gen. Eds.)
Butterworths, London, U.K. (1976)

Moses, R.A. (Ed.)
Adlers Physiology of the Eye: Clinical
Application
Henry Kimpton Publishers, London,
U.K. (1971)

Perkins, E.S. and Hill, D.W. (Eds.)
Scientific Foundation of Ophthalmology
Heinemann Medical Publishing, London,
U.K. (1977)

Peyman, G.A., Saunders, D.R. and
Goldberg, M.F.
Principles and Practice of Ophthalmology
W.B. Saunders Publishers, Philadelphia,
U.S.A. (1981)

Reuben, M. and Woodward, E.G.
Revision of Clinical Optics
Macmillan, London, U.K. (1982)

Spaeth, G.L.S. (Ed.)
Ophthalmic Surgery: Principles and
Practice
W.B. Saunders Publishers, Philadelphia,
U.S.A. (1982)

Wolff, E.
Eugene Wolff's Anatomy of the Eye &
Orbit (7th edn.)
R. Warwick (Ed.)
H.K. Lewis, London, U.K. (1976)

EYELIDS

Beard, C.
Ptosis
C.V. Mosby, St Louis, U.S.A. (1981)

Callahan, M.A. and Callahan, A.
Ophthalmic Plastic and Orbital Surgery
Aesculapius, Birmingham, Alabama,
U.S.A. (1979)

Collin, J.R.O.
A Manual of Systemic Eyelid Surgery
Churchill Livingstone, Edinburgh, U.K.
(1983)

Mustardé, J.C.
Repair and Reconstruction of the Orbital
Region
Churchill Livingstone, Edinburgh, U.K.
(1980)

Reeh, M.J., Beyer, C.K. and
Shannon, G.M.
Practical Ophthalmic Plastic and
Reconstructive Surgery
Lea and Febiger, Philadelphia, U.S.A.
(1976)

Soll, D.B.
Management of Complications in
Ophthalmic Plastic Surgery
Aesculapius, Birmingham, Alabama,
U.S.A. (1976)

ANTERIOR SEGMENT

Grayson, M. (Ed.)
Diseases of the Cornea (2nd edn.)
C.V. Mosby, St Louis, U.S.A. (1979)

Kottow, M.H.
Anterior Segment Fluorescence
Angiography
Williams & Wilkins, Baltimore, U.S.A.
(1978)

Smolin, G. and Thoft, R.A. (Eds.)
The Cornea: Scientific Foundations and
Clinical Practice
Littlebrown & Company, Boston, U.S.A.
(1983)

Waring, G.O., Rodrigues, M.M. and
Laibson, P.R.
Corneal Dystrophies, Parts I and II
Survey of Ophthalmology Vol. 23, Nos. 2
and 3

Watson, P.G. and Hazleman, B.L.
The Sclera and Systemic Disorders
W.B. Saunders Publishers, Philadelphia,
U.S.A. (1976)

Wilson, L.A. (Ed.)
External Diseases of the Eye
Harper & Row, Philadelphia, U.S.A.
(1979)

GLAUCOMA

Grant, W.N. and Chandler, P.A.
Glaucoma (2nd edn.)
Lea & Febiger, Philadelphia, U.S.A.
(1979)

Heilman, K. and Richardson, K.T. (Eds.)
Glaucoma, Conceptions of the Disease,
Pathogenesis, Diagnosis, Therapy
W.B. Saunders Publishers, Philadelphia,
U.S.A. (1978)

Kolker, A.E. and Hetherington, J.
Becker-Schaffer's Diagnosis and Therapy
of the Glaucomas
C.V. Mosby, St. Louis, U.S.A. (1976)

UVEITIS

Friedmann, A.H., Luntz, M.L. and
Henly W.I.
Diagnosis and Management of Uveitis
Williams & Wilkins, Baltimore, U.S.A.
(1982)

Kraus-Mackiw, E. and O'Connor, G.R.
Uveitis: Pathophysiology and Therapy
Grune & Stratton, New York, U.S.A.
(1983)

Rahi, A.H.S. and Garner, A.
Immunopathology of the Eye
Blackwell Scientific Publications,
London, U.K. (1976)

Silverstein, A.M. and O'Connor, G.R.
Immunology and Immunopathology of
the Eye
Masson Publishing, New York, U.S.A.
(1979)

Smith, R.E. and Nozik, R.M.
Uveitis – A Clinical Approach to
Diagnosis and Management
Williams & Wilkins, Baltimore, U.S.A.
(1983)

LENS

Bellows, J.G. MD (Ed.)
Cataract and Abnormalities of the Lens
Grune & Stratton, New York, U.S.A.
(1975)

Elliot, K. and Fitzsimons, D.
The Human Lens in Relation to Cataract
Associated Scientific Publishers, London,
U.K. (1973)

Rosen, E.L.S. (Ed.)
Intraocular Lens Implantation.
C.V. Mosby Co., St Louis, U.S.A. (1983)

RETINA

Bedford, M.A.
A Colour Atlas of Ocular Tumours
Wolfe Medical Publishing, London, U.K.
(1979)

Carr, R.E. and Siegel, I.M.
Visual Electro Diagnostic Testing: A
Practical Guide for the Clinician
Williams & Wilkins, Baltimore, U.S.A.
(1982)

Charles, S.
Vitreous Surgery
C.V. Mosby, St. Louis, U.S.A. (1981)

Chignell, A.H.
Retinal Detachment Surgery
Springer Verlag, Berlin, G.D.R. (1981)

Galloway, N.R.
Ophthalmic Electro-Diagnosis (2nd edn.)
Lloyd-Luke, Medical Books Ltd.,
London, U.K. (1981)

Gass, J.D.M.
Differential Diagnosis of Intra-Ocular
Tumours
C.V. Mosby, St. Louis, U.S.A. (1977)

Gass, J.D.M.
Stereoscopic Atlas of Macular Diseases:
Diagnosis and Treatment.
C.V. Mosby Co., St. Louis, U.S.A. (1977)

Krill, A.E.
Hereditary Retinal and Choroidal
Diseases
Vol. I Evaluation (1972)
Vol. II Clinical Characteristics (1977)
Harper & Row, Hagerstown, Maryland,
U.S.A.

Michels, R.G.
Vitreous Microsurgery
Williams & Wilkins, Baltimore, U.S.A.
(1981)

Shields, J.A.
Diagnosis and Management of
Intraocular Tumours
C.V. Mosby, St. Louis, U.S.A. (1983)

Tolentino, F.I., Schepens, C.L. and
Freeman, H.M.
Vitreoretinal Disorders
W.B. Saunders Publishers, Philadelphia,
U.S.A. (1976)

Wise, G.N., Dollery, C.T. and
Henkind, P.
The Retinal Circulation
Harper & Row, New York, U.S.A. (1971)

Yanuzzi, L.A., Gitter, K.A. and Schatz, H.
The Macula: A Comprehensive Text and
Atlas
Williams & Wilkins, Baltimore, U.S.A.
(1979)

Zinn, K.M. and Marmar, M.F.
The Retinal Pigment Epithelium, Parts I
and II
Harvard University Press, Cambridge,
Massachussetts, U.S.A. (1979)

OCULAR MOTILITY

Burian, H.M. and Von Noorden, G.K.
Binocular Vision and Ocular Motility
(2nd edn.)
C.V. Mosby, St. Louis, U.S.A. (1979)

Helveston, E.M.
Atlas of Strabismus (2nd edn.)
C.V. Mosby, St. Louis, U.S.A. (1977)

Lyle, T.K. and Wybar, K.C.
Practical Orthoptics in the Treatment of
Squints (5th edn.)
H.K. Lewis & Co. Ltd., London, U.K.
(1976)

NEURO-OPHTHALMOLOGY

Glaser, J.S.
Neuro-Ophthalmology
Harper & Row, Philadelphia, U.S.A.
(1978)

Leigh, H.J. and Zee, D.S.
The Neurology of Eye Movements
No. 23 from 'Contemporary Neurology'
series
F.A. Davis & Co., Philadelphia, U.S.A.
(1983)

Moseley, I.F. and Sanders, M.D.
Computerized Tomography in Neuro-
Ophthalmology
Chapman & Hall, London, U.K. (1982)

Rose, F.C. (Ed.)
Medical Ophthalmology
Chapman and Hall, London, U.K. (1976)

Thompson, H.S. (Ed.)
Topics in Neuro-Ophthalmology
Williams & Wilkins, Baltimore, U.S.A.
(1980)

Walsh, F.B. and Hoyt, W.
Clinical Neuro-Ophthalmology, vols. 1-3
(3rd edn.)
Williams & Wilkins, Baltimore, U.S.A.
(1969)

ORBIT

Jones, I.S. and Jakobiec, F.A.
Diseases of the Orbit
Harper & Row, Philadelphia, U.S.A.
(1979)

Krohel, G.B., Stewart, W.B. and
Chavis, R.M.
Orbital Diseases: A Practical Approach
Grune & Stratton, New York, U.S.A.
(1981)

Lloyd, G.A.S.
Radiology of the Orbit
W.B. Saunders, London, U.K. (1975)

LACRIMAL SYSTEM

Veirs, E.R.
Lacrimal Disorders: Diagnosis and
Treatment
C.V. Mosby, St. Louis, U.S.A. (1976)

PATHOLOGY

Apple, D.J. and Rabb, M.F.
Clinico-Pathologic Correlations of Ocular
Disease: A Text and Stereoscopic Atlas,
Chap 6 (2nd edn.)
C.V. Mosby, St. Louis, U.S.A. (1978)

Garner, A. and Klintworth, G.K. (Eds.)
Pathobiology of Ocular Disease: a
Dynamic Approach. Parts A and B
Marcel Decker, New York, U.S.A. (1982)

Greer, C.H.
Ocular Pathology (3rd edn.)
Blackwell Scientific Publishing, London,
U.K. (1979)

Reese, A.B.
Tumours of the Eye (3rd edn.)
Harper & Row, Philadelphia, U.S.A.
(1976)

Yanoff, M. and Fine, B.S.
Ophthalmic Pathology: A Text and Atlas
Harper & Row, Philadelphia, U.S.A.
(1975)

Index

A

A patterns, strabismus 18.10, 18.11, **18.30, 18.31**
AC/A ratio 18.7, **18.19, 18.20**
Accommodation 11.5, 11.6, **11.11, 11.12**
  strabismus 18.6, 18.7, **18.18, 18.20**
Acetylcysteine, vernal disease 5.6, **5.14**
Acne rosacea, blepharitis 4.14, **14.41**
Acropachy, thyroid 18.21, **18.52**
Actinic keratosis 2.10, 2.11, **2.34, 2.35**
  squamous cell carcinoma 2.14, **2.47**
Actinomycosis, canaliculitis 20.22, **20.54, 20.55**
Acute multifocal placoid pigment
  epitheliopathy 10.20, 10.21, **10.47-10.50**
Adenoid cystic carcinoma, lacrimal fossa
  20.18, 20.19, **20.45, 20.46**
Adenoid differentiation, basal cell
  carcinoma 2.13, **2.43**
Adenomas, chromophobe
  chiasmal compression 19.20, **19.49, 19.50**
  visual failure 19.19, 19.20, **19.49, 19.50**
Adenovirus infections 4.2, 4.3, **4.1-4.5,** 6.11, **6.32**
Adie's pupils, light-near dissociation
  19.16, 19.17, **19.39**
Ageing, retinal 13.21, 13.22, **13.44-13.46**
Allergic reactions 5.2-5.11, **5.1-5.20**
Amblyopia
  functional 18.8, **18.23, 18.24**
  haemangioma-induced 2.11
Amiodarone, cornea verticillata 6.11, **6.29**
Ammonia burns 5.12, 5.13, **5.33-5.35**
  corneal plaques 6.7, **6.17**
Amoeboid ulcers, herpetic conjunctivitis
  4.5, **4.12**
Amyloidosis, vitreous 12.5, **12.9**
Angioid streaks, disciform degeneration
  16.13, 16.14, **16.33-16.36**
Angiomas
  capillary, optic disc 17.22, **17.60**
  intracranial 15.16, **15.39**
  choroid haemangioma 9.15, **9.45**
  retinal 15.17, **15.41-15.43**
Angle recession, traumatic 8.14, 8.15, **8.37, 8.38**
Aniridia 7.22, **7.58, 7.59**
Ankylosing spondylitis 10.7, **10.14, 10.15**
Annulus of Zinn, nerve and blood vessel
  relations 20.2, **20.2**
Anterior chamber
  angle 7.5, 7.6, **7.11, 7.12**
  choroidal melanoma 8.7, **8.15**
  cleavage 7.21, 7.22, **7.55-7.59**
  depth measurement 1.12
  epithelialization 8.14, **8.35, 8.36**
Anterior segment
  perforating injuries 9.17, 9.18, **9.51-9.54**
  acute 10.7-10.9, **10.14-10.18**
Anterior uveitis
  associated diseases 10.7
  chronic 10.9, **10.19, 10.20**
  HLA-B27 10.3, **10.4,** 10.7, 10.8
  keratic precipitates 10.4, **10.5-10.7**
  trauma 9.16-9.18, **9.48-9.54**
Anterior vitreous gel, slit lamp
  microscopy 1.10, **1.25**

B

Bacterial infections 4.14-4.16, **4.38-4.47**
Band keratopathy 6.14, **6.41**
BARN syndrome 14.22, **14.58**
Basal cell carcinoma, eyelid 2.12, 2.13, **2.42-2.46**
Basal cell papilloma, eyelid 2.10, **2.32, 2.33**
'Bear tracks' 13.19, **13.40**
Behçet's disease 10.5, 10.12-10.14, **10.29-10.36,** 17.19
Bell's phenomenon 6.6, **6.15**
Benign lymphoid hyperplasia,
  conjunctival 3.13, **3.38, 3.39**
Benign mixed tumour, lacrimal fossa
  20.18, **20.43, 20.44**
Bergmeister's papilla 12.3
Berlin's oedema 14.21, **14.53**
Best's disease 16.22, 16.23, **16.54-16.56**
Bielschowsky head tilt test 18.17, 18.18, **18.45**
Biomicroscopy, slit lamp 1.10, 1.11, **1.24-1.27**
Bitot's spots 5.15, **5.42**
Bjerrum tangent screen, visual fields 1.8, **1.18**
Blepharitis 4.14, 4.15, **4.38-4.43**
  pediculosis 4.18, **4.55**
  ulcerative, vaccinia 4.9
Blepharoconjunctivitis
  herpetic skin lesions 4.4, **4.6, 4.7**
  primary herpetic 4.4, **4.6-4.8**
  staphylococcal 6.12, **6.33,** 6.13, **6.36**
Blepharoplasty, dermatochalasis 2.7
Blindness, vitamin A deficiency 5.15
Bowen's disease 3.11, 3.12, **3.31, 3.32**
Bowman's membrane 6.2
Brain, NMR scan 1.20, **1.60**
  Marcus-Gunn ptosis 2.7
Brown's syndrome 18.12, **18.32, 18.33**
Bruch's membrane
  fragility 16.13, 16.14, **16.33-16.36**
  melanoma breakthrough 9.10, **9.27,** 9.12, **9.31**
  rupture 13.20, **13.41**
Bull's eye macula 16.19, **16.46, 16.47,** 16.20, **16.49**

Second Column continuation

Aphakia 11.19, 11.20, **11.53-11.56**
  pupil block glaucoma 8.5, **8.9,** 8.10
Aponeuroses 2.2, 2.3, **2.1-2.5**
Applanation tonometry 1.13, **1.36**
Apsidal veins 20.3, **20.4**
Aqueous humour
  drug-induced decrease 7.14, **7.35**
  flow 7.3, **7.1,** 7.5, **7.9,** 7.6, **7.13**
  formation 7.2
  outflow increasing drugs 7.14, **7.34**
Arcus juvenilis 6.10, **6.28**
Arcus senilis 6.14, **6.40**
Argyll-Robertson pupils, light-near
  dissociation 19.16
Argyrosis 3.18, **3.53,** 6.7, **6.18**
Asteroid hyalosis 12.5, **12.8**
Atropine hypersensitivity 5.10, **5.26**
Axenfeld's anomaly 6.4, **6.8,** 7.21, **7.55**
Axonal infarction, retinal infarction
  differences 13.12, **13.21**

Buphthalmos (Ox eye) 6.3, **6.5, 6.6,** 7.20,

C

Calcium deposition, corneal 6.7, **6.17,** 6.14, **6.41**
Caloric testing
  vertical gaze 19.3
  vestibular reflexes 19.2, 19.3, **19.3**
Canaliculitis
  actinomycetic 20.22, **20.54, 20.55**
  sulphur granules 20.52, **20.54, 20.55**
Carcinoma
  adenoid cystic 20.18, 20.19, **20.45, 20.46**
  ethmoid sinus 20.19, **20.47, 20.48**
  eyelid 2.12-2.14, **2.42-2.48**
  meibomian glands 2.15, **2.51-2.53**
Carcinoma *in situ*, conjunctiva 3.11, 3.12, **3.31, 3.32**
Carotico-cavernous fistulae, proptosis
  20.10, 20.11, **20.21-20.23**
Cataracts 11.8-11.20, **11.19-11.56**
  capsular (polar) 11.8, 11.9, **11.20, 11.21**
  congenital 11.14, **11.38**
  congenital syphilis 6.12
  coronary 11.13, **11.34, 11.35**
  cortical (cuneiform) 11.8, **11.19,** 11.12-11.14, **11.32-11.37**
  embryonal 11.14, **11.38**
  hypermature 11.18, **11.50**
  nuclear (lamellar) 11.8, **11.19,** 11.14-11.16, **11.34-11.38**
  nuclear sclerotic 11.16, **11.42, 11.43**
  progress and prognosis 11.17-11.19, **11.45-11.51**
  punctate 11.12, 11.13, **11.32-11.35**
  subcapsular (cupiliform) 11.8, **11.19,** 11.9-11.11, **11.22-11.29**
  unilateral congenital 11.19, **11.52**
  visual acuity 1.2
'Cattle trucking' 14.3, **14.6**
Cavernous haemangioma
  proptosis 20.11, 20.12, **20.24, 20.25**
  retinal 15.16, **15.40**
Cavernous sinus
  lesions 19.6, **19.12**
  thrombosis 20.6
Cellophane maculopathy 13.27, **13.57**
Central serous retinopathy 12.12, 13.21, **13.43,** 16.3, 16.4, **16.4-16-7**
Cerebral cortex, visual signalling 1.2
Cervicitis, inclusion conjunctivitis 4.11, **4.30**
Chalazion 2.8, 2.23, 2.24, 4.14, **4.38, 4.39**
Chandler's syndrome 6.16, 8.12, 8.13, **8.33**
  microscopy 6.16, **6.46, 6.47**
Chemical burns 5.12, 5.13, **5.33-5.37**
  cicatricial ectropion 2.4, **2.9**
  eyelid tissue loss 2.16, **2.56**
Chemosis, conjunctival 3.4, **3.8**
  immediate hypersensitivity 5.2, **5.2, 5.3**
'Cherry red spots' 14.2, **14.1,** 14.5, **14.10**
  myoclonus syndrome 16.23, **16.58**
Chiasma 19.19, **19.44-19.46**
  compression, chromophobe adenoma
  19.20, **19.49, 19.50**
  fixation 19.19
  visual field defects 19.20, 19.21, **19.47-19.52**